Continued on back cover

Nutrition and Environmental Health

Volume 2
MINERALS AND
MACRONUTRIENTS

Nutrition and Environmental Health

The Influence of Nutritional Status on Pollutant Toxicity and Carcinogenicity

Volume 2
MINERALS AND MACRONUTRIENTS

Edward J. Calabrese
Environmental Health Program
Division of Public Health
University of Massachusetts

A Wiley-Interscience Publication
JOHN WILEY & SONS
New York   Chichester   Brisbane   Toronto

Library of Congress Cataloging in Publication Data:

Calabrese, Edward J   1946–
  Nutrition and environmental health.

  (Environmental science and technology)
  "A Wiley-Interscience publication."
  Includes indexes.
  CONTENTS: v. 1. The vitamins.—v. 2. Minerals and
macronutrients.
    1. Pollution—Toxicology. 2. Environmentally
induced diseases—Nutritional aspects. 3. Nutrition.
[DNLM: 1. Carcinogens, Environmental. 2. Environmental health. 3. Environmental pollutants—Toxicity.
4. Nutrition. WA671 C141n]

RA566.C28   616.9′8   79-21089
ISBN 0-471-04833-X (v. 1)
ISBN 0-471-08207-4 (v. 2)

Printed in the United States of America

10 9 8 7 6 5 4 3 2 1

To My Wife Mary

Series Preface

Environmental Science and Technology

The Environmental Science and Technology Series of Monographs, Textbooks, and Advances is devoted to the study of the quality of the environment and to the technology of its conservation. Environmental science therefore relates to the chemical, physical, and biological changes in the environment through contamination or modification, to the physical nature and biological behavior of air, water, soil, food, and waste as they are affected by man's agricultural, industrial, and social activities, and to the application of science and technology to the control and improvement of environmental quality.

The deterioration of environmental quality, which began when man first collected into villages and utilized fire, has existed as a serious problem under the ever-increasing impacts of exponentially increasing population and of industrializing society. Environmental contamination of air, water, soil, and food has become a threat to the continued existence of many plant and animal communities of the ecosystem and may ultimately threaten the very survival of the human race.

It seems clear that if we are to preserve for future generations some semblance of the biological order of the world of the past and hope to improve on the deteriorating standards of urban public health, environmental science and technology must quickly come to play a dominant role in designing our social and industrial structure for tomorrow. Scientifically rigorous criteria of environmental quality must be developed. Based in part on these criteria, realistic standards must be established and our technological progress must be tailored to meet them. It is obvious that civilization will continue to require increasing amounts of fuel, transportation, industrial chemicals, fertilizers, pesticides, and countless other products; and that it will continue to produce waste products of all descriptions. What is urgently needed is a total systems approach to modern civilization through which the pooled talents of scientists and engineers, in cooperation with social scientists and the medical profession, can be focused on the development of order and equilibrium in the presently disparate segments of the human environment. Most of the skills and tools that are needed are already in existence. We surely have a right to hope a technology that has created such manifold environmental problems is also capable of solving them. It is our hope that this Series in Environmental Sciences and Technology will not only serve to make this challenge more explicit to the established professionals, but that it also will help to stimulate the student toward the career opportunities in this vital area.

Robert L. Metcalf
Werner Stumm

Preface

This book is the second of a two-volume set concerned with the influence of nutritional status on pollutant toxicity and/or carcinogenicity. While Volume I dealt with the interactions of the vitamins with toxic substances, Volume II details the role of the minerals, protein, fats, carbohydrates, and specific amino acids, as well as fiber and synthetic antioxidants on the adverse effects of pollutants.

This two-volume set comprises the first major synthesis of the general area of nutrition and environmental health. It is intended to be a comprehensive and detailed evaluation of the extent to which nutrients interact with toxic substances in the environment. This volume is organized by nutrient so that each nutrient is given a chapter or a section within a chapter if there is only limited information available on that topic. Within each chapter, the various pollutant interactions with that nutrient are discussed. For example, there are separate chapters on calcium, copper, iron, selenium, and so on. Within each of these chapters there are discussions of how that particular nutrient affects the toxicity of, say, cadmium, fluoride, lead, or nitrosamines, depending on the situation. In general, the pollutants are divided into two categories—inorganic and organic—and then discussed in an alphabetic setting in order to provide a consistent and organized scheme. Furthermore, chapters that have a summary section at the end provide an integrated discussion to a complex series of nutrient-pollutant interactions and an indication of the biomedical significance of the previously discussed findings, as well as a sense of direction for further research. Summary sections were not provided for those sections (i.e., Chapter 6, "Other Minerals" and Chapter 12, "Synthetic Antioxidants") in which the research base is too limited.

This book is not only a comprehensive and critical review of the published literature concerning the role of nutritional status on pollutant toxicity, it is also designed to provide numerous viable and socially relevant research hypotheses for individual investigators to pursue and/or government personnel within research and developmental departments to consider in the formulation of priority allocations.

Governmental regulatory personnel who are concerned with the task of establishing criteria for the development of standards for chemical toxicants should find these volumes of critical interest. In essence, these books provide a vast amount of information on individuals who may be at increased risk to develop adverse effects from pollutant exposures. For whether or not these so-called high-risk groups are specifically protected by standards, they must at least be considered during the standard derivation process.

EDWARD J. CALABRESE

Amherst, Massachusetts
January 1981

Contents

Nutrition and Environmental Health

Volume 2
MINERALS AND
MACRONUTRIENTS

Calcium

A. INORGANIC SUBSTANCES

1. Cadmium

That dietary factors may affect the toxicity of cadmium is well known (Table 1). Considerable research efforts have been directed toward elucidating the influence of various nutrients including ascorbic acid, iron, and zinc on the toxicity of cadmium (Supplee, 1961, 1963; Fox and Fry, 1970; Petering et al., 1971; Maji and Yoshida, 1974; Ragan, 1977; Levander, 1978). An early observation that calcium levels in the diet would modify the toxicity of cadmium was provided by Worker and Mogicovsky (1961), who noted that chickens fed a diet low in calcium and vitamin D exhibited an increased cadmium uptake via the gastrointestinal tract. In the years since this report, there has been a growing concern over the potential interrelationship of calcium and cadmium because (1) cadmium is known to cause demineralization (including decalcification) of bone in both animal models and humans; and (2) cadmium is known to be a cause of hypertension in animal models, while hard water (i.e., water with high levels of calcium) is thought to protect against the development of cardiovascular disease. The following section will show how low levels of dietary

1

Table 1. Relationships between Cadmium and Essential Nutrients

Nutrient	Dietary Intake of Individual Nutrients		
	Normal[a]	Deficiency[b]	Excess[c]
Zinc	+	+	+
Iron	+	+	$+(Fe^{2+})$
Manganese	+	?	?
Copper	+	+	+
Selenium	+	?	+
Calcium	+	+	?
Ascorbic Acid	?	?	+
Vitamin D	?	+	?
Protein	?	+	+

[a]+ Cadmium affects metabolism and/or function of the nutrient, ? No relationship has been established.

[b]+ A deficiency of the nutrient increases the severity of cadmium toxicity.

[c]+ An excess of the nutrient decreases the toxicity of cadmium.

Source: Spivey-Fox, M.R. (1974). Effect of essential minerals on cadmium toxicity. A review. *J. Food Sci.* **39**:322.

calcium enhance the tissue retention and presumably the toxicity of dietary cadmium, as well as how cadmium alters calcium metabolism and how this may be related to the development of osteomalacia.

Influence of Low Levels of Dietary Calcium on Cadmium Retention. Numerous researchers have evaluated the influence of low and normal levels of dietary calcium on the retention of cadmium in a variety of species including the chicken (Worker and Mogicovsky, 1961; Kobayashi et al., 1971; Koo et al., 1978), mice (Suzuki et al., 1969), rats (Itokawa et al., 1973; Pond and Walker, 1975; Washko and Cousins, 1975, 1976; Kello et al., 1979; Hamilton and Smith, 1978), and golden hamsters (Miller et al., 1975), with the predominant research being with the rat model. Although several studies concerning calcium-cadmium interactions preceded the 1970s (Worker and Mogicovsky, 1961; Suzuki et al., 1969; Fleishman et al., 1968), most of the research has been of a very recent nature, getting strong impetus from the reports on cadmium-induced Itai-Itai disease in Japan, which was characterized by osteomalacia with renal tubular damage in women. These women were also found to have diets low in calcium and vitamin D. Thus it was thought that dietary factors (i.e., low levels of calcium and vitamin D) may have enhanced the toxicity of cadmium in the afflicted Japanese women (Emmerson, 1970).

The results of the animal studies have indicated that significantly greater concentrations of cadmium are retained by the tissues of animals reared on diets very low in calcium as compared to animals given normal levels of this mineral. For the most part, the diets low in calcium have been equal to or less than 25% of the rat's recommended allowance (Washko and Cousins, 1975, 1976; Fowler et al., 1975; Omori and Muto, 1977; Larsson and Piscator, 1971; Itokawa et al., 1978). The tissues that retained the most cadmium were the kidney and femur (Table 2), a finding that is in fundamental agreement with previously cited toxicological studies with cadmium. The levels of cadmium employed in the food and drinking water of these animals usually ranged from 20 ppm to 200 ppm, with the exception of the Fowler et al. (1975) study where the levels of cadmium ranged from 0.2 to 200 ppm in drinking water. In fact, even at the 0.2 level in drinking water, the rats reared on the low-calcium diets exhibited higher levels of cadmium retention after 6 weeks of treatment, with the effect becoming greater after 12 weeks. For the most part, individual investigators have utilized one sex during specific experiments and collectively their studies have revealed that both males and females experience enhanced cadmium retention as a result of the low-calcium diets. However, a recently published study by Kello et al. (1979) revealed that female albino rats exhibited enhanced toxicity as compared to males when exposed to cadmium while on low-calcium diets.

Although most studies have considered the influence of diets very low in calcium as compared to those on normal diets, Kello et al. (1979) evaluated the influence of highly variable levels of calcium including an intermediate deficiency (0.3% Ca), normal (0.7%), and at approximately 3.5 times normal on cadmium retention. Their findings revealed that the amount of cadmium retained is inversely related to the level of calcium in the diet. In fact, the group of rats given the supplementary levels of calcium exhibited cadmium values approximately 20% of those of rats on the normal diet while the normally fed rats had approximately 80% of the cadmium values of the intermediate deficient group. Thus, while an intermediate calcium deficiency enhanced the retention of cadmium, consumption of calcium far in excess of normally accepted levels offered exceptional protection from whole-body cadmium retention.

The influence of low-calcium levels in the diet on pregnant rats and their offspring exposed to cadmium (200 ppm in diet) was studied by

Table 2. Cadmium and Calcium Concentration in Femur and Kidney[a]

Group	Diet Calcium	Diet Cadmium	Femur Calcium (mg/g w/w)	Femur Cadmium (μg/g w/w)	Kidney Calcium (μg/g w/w)	Kidney Cadmium (μg/g w/w)
1	Sufficient	–	138.2 ± 3.6^c	0.85 ± 0.09^c	97.0 ± 9.9^c	0.22 ± 0.13^c
2	Deficient	–	$130.7 \pm 4.9^{c,d}$	0.96 ± 0.09^c	109.7 ± 25.7^c	0.21 ± 0.10^c
3	Sufficient	+	124.8 ± 4.3^d	5.52 ± 0.70^d	90.5 ± 6.2^c	47.75 ± 6.85^d
4	Deficient	+	106.8 ± 4.5^c	12.64 ± 1.58^e	104.4 ± 11.8^c	80.12 ± 5.47^e

[a]The same letter superscript in each column denotes no significant difference among groups; different letter superscripts ([c,d,e]) denote significant difference ($P < 0.05$) among groups as based on the one-way analysis of variance. w/w: wet weight.
[b]Values represent mean ± SEM of five rats.

Source: Itokawa, Y.; Nishino, K.; Takashima, M.; Nakata, T.; Kaito, H.; Okamoto, E.; Daijo, K.; and Kawamura, J. (1978). Renal and skeletal lesions in experimental cadmium poisoning of rats. Histology and renal function. *Environ. Res.* **15**:206–211.

Pond and Walker (1975). Previous research had revealed that injections of cadmium into pregnant rats interrupts pregnancy (Chiquoine, 1965; Parizek, 1964) as well as reducing the birth weight of pups (Powers et al., 1973). Pond and Walker (1975) revealed that liver (51.63 vs. 38.35 ppm) and kidney (103.91 vs. 53.08 ppm) cadmium levels were significantly ($p < 0.01$) greater in animals reared on low-calcium diets (0.07%) as compared to controls (0.96% calcium). In addition, the percentage of females producing litters was reduced by 30% in the low calcium-cadmium exposed animals as compared to animals with normal calcium diets and exposed to cadmium. Finally, the pups of the calcium-deficient animals exhibited greater than 2× more cadmium in their tissues, a difference that was significantly different at $p < 0.01$.

In an effort to determine whether the enhanced cadmium deposition and toxicity found in animals reared on low-calcium diets results from increased uptake, differential tissue distribution, or decreased excretion of cadmium, Washko and Cousins (1976) exposed rats that were reared for the previous four weeks on either low or normal levels of calcium to ^{109}Cd either orally or sc. The results of the sc experiment revealed no significant differences in tissue distribution or excretion of ^{109}Cd, with the exception of somewhat higher ^{109}Cd values in the lungs of the low-calcium group. In contrast, Table 3 reveals a markedly greater cadmium retention in rats reared on the low-calcium diet and given cadmium orally. These results support the hypothesis that a calcium deficiency enhanced the gastrointestinal absorption of cadmium. Bredderman and Wasserman (1974) also supported this hypothesis by reporting that the binding affinity of the calcium-binding protein (CaBP) for cadmium was almost as high as that for calcium. Since the CaBP binding activity is increased during a calcium deficiency, it follows that cadmium would replace calcium at the binding sites. According to Washko and Cousins (1976), "this increase in binding capacity would explain the increased ^{109}Cd uptake and the decreased ^{109}Cd content of the feces and colon in the low-calcium rats" (Table 3).

Experiments involving the *in situ* ligated-loop technique with chickens have also suggested that the enhanced retention of cadmium in animals reared on calcium-deficient diets is due to increased gastrointestinal tract absorption. No comprehensive attempt has been made to evaluate the influence of dietary calcium on the excretion of cadmium that is already absorbed into the body. However, whole body ^{115m}Cd retention studies in rats on different calcium diets have suggested a faster excretion rate of cadmium in the calcium-replete diet (Hamilton and Smith, 1978). Thus, although differences in the rate of

Table 3. Effect of Dietary Calcium on the Tissue Distribution and Excretion of Orally Administered ^{109}Cd[a]

	Dietary Group	
Sample	0.6% Calcium	0.1% Calcium
Heart[b]	760 ± 34	1,112 ± 179
Lung[b]	821 ± 59	1,270 ± 81[g]
Liver[b]	9,038 ± 475	16,142 ± 694[g]
Kidney[b]	5,046 ± 458	10,256 ± 753[g]
Spleen[b]	1,949 ± 186	2,026 ± 161
Testis[b]	1,171 ± 254	872 ± 77
Serum[c]	387 ± 4	411 ± 6[f]
Small intestine[b]	2,122 ± 536	5,749 ± 852[g]
Colon[b]	26,830 ± 5,534	7,061 ± 1,386[g]
Feces[d]	2,140,151 ± 101,692	1,567,996 ± 53,319[g]
Urine[e]	5,899 ± 1,539	30,176 ± 4,041[g]

[a] Two groups of 11 rats each were fed either a 0.6 or a 0.1% Ca diet for 4 wk, then each rat was administered an oral dose of 5 μCi of ^{109}CdCl$_2$ 72 hr before sacrifice. Radioactivity is expressed as counts/10 min (mean ± SE).

[b] Radioactivity per gram (wet weight).

[c] Radioactivity per 1 ml.

[d] Radioactivity in total 72-hr collection.

[e] Radioactivity in 3 ml of total 72-hr collection.

[f] Significantly different at $p < 0.05$.

[g] Significantly different at $p < 0.01$.

Source. Washko, P.W. and Cousins, R.J. (1976). Metabolism of ^{109}Cd in rats fed normal and low-calcium diets. *J. Toxicol. Environ. Health* 1:1058.

gastrointestinal absorption of cadmium appears to explain the difference in cadmium retention, it is not possible to eliminate a role of differential excretion rates.

Effect of Cadmium on Calcium Absorption and Excretion. How cadmium affects the development of osteomalacia in animal models as well as humans is of great concern. The adverse effects that cadmium causes to skeletal bones is thought to act via several possible mechanisms including (1) a direct effect of the metal on osseous tissue (Yoshiki et al., 1975), or (2) an indirect effect from disruptions in the calcium-phosphorus balance (Larsson and Piscator, 1971), or both.

A careful examination of the published literature reveals that cadmium may affect (1) enhanced demineralization of bone, (2) increased fecal excretion of calcium, as well as (3) decreased absorption of calcium. The net result of such metabolic effects on calcium metabolism is thought to explain in large part how cadmium induces the occurrence of osteomalacia and bone demineralization in animals and humans. However, as in many cases of scientific inquiry, these generalizable findings are not without critics and some inconsistency.

That cadmium may affect the gastrointestinal absorption and excretion of calcium was suggested by Sugawara (1977) who noted that cadmium-induced osteomalacia is found among those individuals orally exposed to cadmium and not in those exposed to cadmium by inhalation. Several early studies (Ando et al., 1973, 1973a) with rats supported this interpretation since they reported that the amount of calcium in feces and urine of the animals that had been exposed to continuous oral administration of cadmium increased with the duration of the exposure. More recent clinical human studies have confirmed the occurrence of increased urinary calcium excretion in cadmium-exposed workers (Kazantzis, 1979). In addition, Ingersell and Wasserman (1971) have reported that cadmium inhibits calcium transport from the intestinal mucosa to the serosa, thereby providing a possible mechanism to explain the effect of cadmium. These researchers have also demonstrated that the activity of 25-hydroxy vitamin D_3-1α-hydroxylase that synthesizes CaBP is reduced in the cadmium-exposed rats. Comparable findings were reported to occur in chicks (Feldman and Cousins, 1973). Based on these findings, Ando et al. (1977) reasoned that the absorption rate of calcium via the gastrointestinal tract is diminished following exposure to cadmium.

Other recent experiments (Sugawara and Sugawara, 1974, 1974a; Sugawara, 1977; Sugawara et al., 1976; Sakai et al., 1975; Ando et al., 1977; Kobayashi, 1974; Yuhas et al., 1978; Hamilton and Smith, 1977, 1978) have tended to verify the general conclusions of these studies. For example, Ando et al. (1977) reported cadmium-treated (oral) rats excreted considerably more calcium in feces than unexposed controls. In addition, they also reported that most of the labeled calcium given IV was excreted in the feces of cadmium-treated animals. Other investigators demonstrated that 50 ppm of cadmium in the diet caused a rapid reduction in calcium absorption. However, at 10 ppm cadmium it took 270 days before the treatment effected a decrease in calcium absorption (Sugawara and Sugawara, 1974).

As enticing as this proposed mechanism of Ingersell and Wasserman (1971) is, it is not without controversy. Kimura et al. (1974) reported that the hydroxylase activity was not significantly diminished when rats were given smaller amounts of cadmium that more realistically simulate those levels found in cadmium-contaminated diets. In addition, both Feldman and Cousins (1973) and Suda et al. (1974) have reported that when bound to metallothionein, cadmium exhibits no inhibitory influence on the hydroxylation of vitamin D. Furthermore, since cadmium is predominantly bound to metallothionein while in the kidney, the opportunity to effect any significant reduction in 1α-hydroxylase activity is probably limited (Bremmer, 1978).

In addition, Weber and Reid (1969) reported no effect on calcium absorption in mice by cadmium at concentrations of 0, 412, 2060, and 4020 ppm for 3 weeks. More recently, Yuhas et al. (1978) reported that in vivo rat studies revealed no effect of cadmium (1 and 10 ppm) on calcium absorption, but even more surprisingly, at 100 ppm Cd the rats had an enhanced calcium absorption. The reason for the apparent discrepancy between those studies suggesting that cadmium does not affect calcium absorption (Weber and Reid, 1969; Yuhas et al., 1978) and those that do (e.g. Sugawara and Sugawara, 1974) may result from a lack of pair-fed methodology in the Yuhas et al. (1978) and Weber and Reid (1969) study. Since the cadmium-exposed animals in the two dissenting studies consumed much less food than the controls, their absorption efficiency for calcium may have been enhanced. Thus the inhibitory influence of cadmium may have been masked.

It has been reported that cadmium treatment (200 ppm in drinking water) of pregnant rats resulted in increased levels of fetal calcium (Pond and Walker, 1975), while Kelman et al. (1978) have noted no changes in total calcium levels of fetal rats when mothers were exposed to 10 and 25 ppm Cd in drinking water. Although the Cd-exposed fetal tissue did display an increased level of calcium, the mothers exhibited reduced levels of calcium in the kidney (1260 ppm vs. 990 ppm) and liver (117.9 vs. 113.3 ppm). Perhaps this represented a means of adaptation (i.e., enhancing the survival chances of the fetus). Thus the findings of Pond and Walker (1975) may be compatible with the hypothesis that the presence of cadmium reduces the absorption of calcium.

Hard Water and Cadmium-Induced Hypertension.   In light of the earlier studies cited above, Schroeder et al. (1967) evaluated whether an increase in calcium in drinking water (up to 200 ppm),[1] as

---

[1]It should be realized that the addition of the 200 ppm of calcium resulted in a 5.3% increase in calcium exposure. This percentage of the total calcium intake supplied in water to rats was identical to that estimated for humans in 25 hard-water areas (Schroeder, 1966).

may occur from consumption of hard water, influenced the accumulation of cadmium (5 ppm [as well as several other heavy metals] during chronic exposure studies of up to 500 days). The results indicated no significant effect of the calcium on the mean concentrations of cadmium in five organs. However, the occurrence of hypertension was somewhat reduced in male and female rats given the supplemental calcium in the drinking water. Such physiological changes clearly lend support to the epidemiological data suggesting that elements such as calcium in hard water may protect against the development of cardiovascular disease.

Conclusions

Cadmium affects the development of alterations in bony tissue by more than one means. Not only is it thought to directly damage bone tissue but it also reduces the absorption of both calcium and phosphorus, as well as enhancing their excretion. In addition, under conditions of low dietary consumption of calcium, the absorption rate of cadmium is markedly enhanced. Despite these important biomedical findings, data needed to develop precise risk assessments for extrapolation to the human population are quite limited. What is needed are chronic studies in which the dietary levels of calcium range from 10% to 200% of the recommended allowance in rat models as well as Cd exposures that simulate ambient levels. These experiments would not only evaluate the influence of dietary calcium on cadmium body burden but also on cadmium-induced hypertension. It is already known that low levels of calcium in the diet enhance the deposition of cadmium in the kidney and cause constriction of renal vasculature (Fowler et al., 1975). Whether the incidence of hypertension would also be increased is not yet known, but not unexpected.

References

Ando, J.; Matsui, S.; Sayato, Y.; and Tonomura, M. (1973). Hygienic chemical studies on poisonous metal. II. Acute and subacute toxicity of cadmium chloride. *J. Hyg. Chem.* **19**:65–72.

Ando, M.; Sayato, Y.; and Tonomura, M. (1973a). Hygienic chemical studies on poisonous metal. III. Studies on body accumulation of cadmium and relationship between cadmium, calcium and phosphate in excretion by continuous oral administration of cadmium chloride. *J. Hyg. Chem.* **19**:73–81.

Ando, M.; Sayato, Y.; Tonomura, M.; and Osawa, T. (1977). Studies on excretion and uptake of calcium by rats after continuous oral administration of cadmium. *Toxicol. Appl. Pharmacol.* **39**:321–327.

Bredderman, P.J. and Wasserman, R.H. (1974). Chemical composition, affinity for calcium, and some related properties of the vitamin D dependent calcium-binding protein. *Biochem.* **13**:1687.

Bremmer, I. (1978). Cadmium toxicity: nutritional influence and the role of metallothionein. *Wld. Rev. Nutr. Diet* **32**:165–197.

Chiquoine, A.D. (1965). Effect of cadmium chloride on the pregnant albino mouse. *J. Reprod. Fert.* **10**:263–265.

Cousins, R.J. and Feldman, S.L. (1973). Effect of cholecalciferol on cadmium uptake in the chick. *Nutr. Rep. Int.* **8**:363.

Emmerson, B.T. (1970). "Ouch-Ouch" disease: the osteomalacia of cadmium nephropathy. *Ann. Int. Med.* **73**:854–855.

Feldman, S.L. and Cousins, R.J. (1973). Influence of cadmium on the metabolism of 25-hydroxycholecalciferol in chicks. *Nutr. Rept. Intern.* **8**:251.

Fleishman, A.I.; Yacowitz, H.; Hayton, T.; and Bierenbaum, M.L. (1968). Effect of calcium and vitamin D_3 upon the fecal excretion of some metals in mature male rat fed a high fat, cholesterol diet. *J. Nutr.* **95**:19–22.

Fowler, B.A.; Jones, H.S.; Brown, H.W.; and Haseman, J.K. (1975). The morphologic effects of chronic cadmium administration on the renal vasculature of rats given low and normal calcium diets. *Toxicol. Appl. Pharmacol.* **34**:233–252.

Fox, M.R.W. and Fry, B.E., Jr. (1970). Cadmium toxicity decreased by dietary ascorbic acid supplements. *Science* **169**:989.

Hamilton, D.L. and Smith, M.W. (1977). Cadmium inhibits calcium absorption in rat intestine. *J. Physiol.* **265**(1):54.

Hamilton, D.L. and Smith, M.W. (1978). Inhibition of intestinal calcium uptake by cadmium and the effect of a low calcium diet on cadmium retention. *Environ. Res.* **15**:175.

Hennig, A. and Anke, M. (1964). Kadmium-Antimetabolit des Eisens und Zinks. *Arch. Tierernahr.* **14**:55.

Ingersell, R.J. and Wasserman, R.H. (1971). Vitamin D_3-induced calcium-binding protein. *J. Biol. Chem.* **246**:2802–2814.

Itokawa, Y.; Abe, T.; and Tanaka, S. (1973). Bone changes in experimental chronic cadmium poisoning: radiological and biological approaches. *Arch. Environ. Health* **26**:241–244.

Itokawa, Y.; Nishino, K.; Takashima, M.; Nakata, T.; Kaito, H.; Okamoto, E.; Daijo, K.; and Kawamura, J. (1978). Renal and skeletal lesions in experimental cadmium poisoning. Histology and renal function. *Environ. Res.* **15**:206–211.

Kazantzis, G. (1979). Renal tubular dysfunction and abnormalities of calcium metabolism in cadmium workers. *Environ. Health Perspect.* **28**:155–159.

Kello, D.; Dekanic, D.; and Kostial, K. (1979). Influence of sex and dietary calcium on intestinal cadmium absorption in rats. *Arch. Environ. Health* **34**:30–33.

Kelman, B.J.; Walter, B.K.; Jarbue, G.E.; and Sasser, L.B. (1978). Effect of dietary cadmium on calcium metabolism in the rat during late gestation. *Proc. Soc. Exper. Biol. Med.* **158**:614–617.

Kimura, M.; Otaki, N.; Yoshiki, S.; Suzuki, M.; Horiuchi, N.; and Suda, T. (1974). The ısolation of metallothionein and its protective role in cadmium poisoning. *Arch. Biochem. Biophys.* **165**:340.

Kobayashi, J. (1974). Effects of cadmium on calcium metabolism on rats. In: *Trace*

Substances in Environmental Health, p. 263. VII. Edited by D.D. Hemphill. Univ. of Missouri, Columbia, MO.

Kobayashi, J.; Nahahara, H.; and Hasegawa, T. (1971). Accumulation of cadmium in organs of mice fed on cadmium-polluted rice. *Jap. J. Hyg.* **26**:401.

Koo, S.I.; Fullmer, C.S.; and Wasserman, R.H. (1978). Intestinal absorption and retention of ^{109}Cd: effects of cholecalciferol, calcium status and other variables. *J. Nutr.* **108**:1812–1822.

Larsson, S.E. and Piscator, M. (1971). Effect of cadmium on skeletal tissue in normal and calcium-deficient rats. *Israel J. Med. Sci.* **7**:495.

Levander, O.A. (1978). Metabolic interactions between metals and metalloids. *Environ. Health Perspect.* **25**:77–80.

Lorentzon, R. and Larsson, S.E. (1978). Intestinal absorption and tissue retention of cadmium and calcium in normal adult rats and rats given an active metabolite of vitamin D (1,25–dihydroxycholecalciferol). *Clin. Sci. Molec. Med.* **55**:195–198.

Maji, T. and Yoshida, A. (1974). Therapeutic effect of dietary iron and ascorbic acid on cadmium toxicity of rats. *Nutr. Rep. Int.* **10**:139.

Miller, D.W.; Vetter, R.J.; Hullinger, R.L.; and Shaw, S.M. (1975). The uptake and distribution of cadmium-115m in calcium deficient and zinc deficient golden hamsters. *Bull. Environ. Contam. and Toxicol.* **13**(1):40–43.

Muto, Y. and Omori, M. (1977). Nutritional influence on the onset of renal damage due to long-term administration of cadmium in young and adult rats. *J. Nutr. Sci. Vitamin.* **23**:349–360.

Noda, S.; Kubota, K.; Yamada, K.; Yoshizawa, S.; Moriuchi, S.; and Hosoya, N. (1978). The effect of vitamin D_3 and dietary calcium level on the cadmium-induced morphological and biochemical changes in rat intestinal mucosa. *J. Nutr. Sci. Vitamin.* **24**:405–418.

Nordberg, G.F. (editor) for the Task Group on metal interaction (1978). Factors influencing metabolism and toxicity of metals: a consensus report. *Environ. Health Perspect.* **25**:3–41.

Omori, M. and Muto, Y. (1977). Effects of dietary protein, calcium, phosphorus, and fiber on renal accumulation of exogenous cadmium in young rats. *J. Nutr. Sci. Vitamin.* **23**:361–373.

Parizek, J. (1964). Vascular changes at sites of oestrogen biosynthesis produced by parenteral injection of cadmium salts: the destruction of placenta by cadmium salts. *J. Reprod. Fert.* **7**:263–265.

Petering, H.G.; Johnson, M.A.; and Stemmer, K.L. (1971). Studies of zinc metabolism in the rat. I. Dose response effects of cadmium. *Arch. Environ. Health* **23**:93.

Pond, W.G. and Walker, E.F., Jr. (1975). Effect of dietary Ca and Cd level of pregnant rats on reproduction and on dam and progeny tissue mineral concentration. *Proc. Soc. Exper. Biol. Med.* **148**:665–668.

Powers, M.E.; Pond, W.G.; and Walker, E.F., Jr. (1973). Dietary Cd-Ca effects on dam and progeny in rats. *J. Animal Sci.* **37**:369.

Ragan, H.A. (1977). Effects of iron deficiency on the absorption and distribution of lead and cadmium in rats. *J. Lab. Clin. Med.* **90**:700.

Sakai, T.; Miyahara, T.; Sanei, K.; Nomura, N.; and Takayanagi, N. (1975). Hygienic chemical studies on environmental pollution. I. Effect of cadmium ion on chick embryo tibia in tissue culture. *J. Hyg. Chem.* **21**:35–41.

Schroeder, H.A. (1966). Municipal drinking water and cardiovascular death rates. *J. Amer. Med. Assoc.* **195**:81.

Schroeder, H.A.; Nason, A.P.; and Balassa, J.J. (1967). Trace metals in rat tissues as influenced by calcium in water. *J. Nutr.* **93**:331–336.

Spivey-Fox, M.R. (1974). Effect of essential minerals on cadmium toxicity. A review. *J. Food Sci.* **39**:321–324.

Spivey-Fox, M.R. (1978). Nutritional considerations in designing animal models of metal toxicity in man. *Environ. Health Perspect.* **25**:137–140.

Suda, T.; Horiuchi, N.; Ogata, E.; Ezawa, I.; Otaki, N.; and Kimura, M. (1974). Prevention by metallothionein of cadmium induced inhibition of vitamin D activation reaction in kidney. *FEBS Letters* **42**:23.

Sugawara, N. (1977). Inhibitory effect of cadmium on calcium absorption from the rat duodenum. *Arch. Environ. Contamin.* **5**(2):167–175.

Sugawara, C. and Sugawara, N. (1974). Cadmium toxicity for rat intestine, especially on the absorption of calcium and phosphorus. *Jap. J. Hyp.* **28**:511.

Sugawara, N. and Sugawara, C. (1974a). Cadmium accumulation in organs and mortality during a continued oral uptake. *Arch. Toxicol.* **32**:297.

Sugawara, N.; Sugawara, C.; and Miyake, H. (1976). Effects of cadmium on intestinal brush border enzymes and calcium absorption. *Jap. J. Ind. Health* **18**:474–475.

Supplee, W.C. (1961). Production of zinc deficiency in turkey poults by dietary cadmium. *Poultry Sci.* **40**:827.

Supplee, W.C. (1963). Antagonistic relationship between dietary cadmium and zinc. *Science.* **139**:119.

Suzuki, S.; Taguchi, T.; and Yokohashi, G. (1969). Dietary factors influencing upon the retention rate of orally administered [115m]CdCl$_2$ in mice. *Indust. Health* **7**:155–162.

Takashima, M.; Nishino, K.; and Itokawa, Y. (1978). Effect of cadmium administration on growth, excretion, and tissue accumulation of cadmium and histological alterations in calcium sufficient and- deficient rats: an equalized feeding study. *Toxicol. Appl. Pharmacol.* **45**:591–598.

Washko, P.W. and Cousins, R.J. (1975). Effect of low dietary calcium on chronic cadmium toxicity in rats. *Nutr. Repts. Intern.* **11**(2):113–127.

Washko, P.W. and Cousins, R.J. (1976). Metabolism of [109]Cd in rats fed normal and low-calcium diets. *J. Toxicol. Environ. Health* **1**:1055.

Weber, C.W. and Reid, B.L. (1969). Effect of dietary cadmium on mice. *Toxicol. Appl. Pharmacol.* **14**:420–425.

Worker, N.A. and Mogicovsky, B.B. (1961). Effect of vitamin D on the utilization of zinc, cadmium and mercury in the chick. *J. Nutr.* **75**:222–224.

Yoshiki, S.T.; Yanagisawara, T.; Kimura, M.; Otaki, N.; Suzuki, M.; and Suda, T. (1975). Bone and kidney lesions in experimental cadmium intoxication. *Arch. Environ. Health* **30**:559–562.

Yuhas, E.M.; Miya, T.S.; and Schnell, R.C. (1978). Influence of cadmium on calcium absorption from the rat intestine. *Toxicol. Appl. Pharmacol.* **43**:23–31.

A. Inorganic Substances **13**

2. Fluoride

Unlike cadmium and lead, fluoride is not generally considered a serious environmental contaminant. This is especially true in light of the widespread community fluoridation programs to reduce dental caries. In fact, such programs usually result in the addition of fluoride to drinking water so that its levels are approximately 1 mg/L. Nevertheless, there are areas in the United States and other parts of the world, especially India, where naturally occurring levels of fluoride in drinking water considerably exceed the 1 mg/L and to which adverse effects such as skeletal fluorosis have been causally related (Table 4).

In addition, occupational exposure to elevated levels of fluoride has long been known to cause fluorosis in workers and federal regulations have been promulgated to prevent undue exposure (ACGIH, 1976). Thus, even though exposure to elevated levels of fluoride may not cause as much concern as other heavy metals such as cadmium and lead, such exposure may result in a variety of toxicologic responses that may in fact lead to debilitating conditions if exposure is sufficiently high for prolonged periods.

Numerous studies have evaluated the influence of dietary factors on the expression of fluoride-induced toxicity with consideration given to the mineral calcium. That calcium may influence the toxicity of fluoride is not unexpected since fluoride is known to affect the mineralization of bone and soft tissue in a fashion analogous to calcium.

A review of the published data in this area reveals that interest in such calcium-fluoride interactions began in the 1920s and has continued to the present time. Articles have been published on the responses of a variety of animal models including the rat, guinea pig, kitten, sheep, bull, pig, and monkey, as well as humans. This section

Table 4. Adverse Effects Associated with Consumption of Water with Elevated Levels of Fluoride

Adverse Effects	Level of Fluoride in Drinking Water
Dental fluorosis	3–8 mg/L
Bone changes	8–20 mg/L
Crippling fluorosis	>20 mg/L

Source: Public Health Service (PHS) Fluoride. Public Health Service Drinking Water Standards. U.S., HEW, PHS, pp. 41–42, 1962.

will evaluate (1) the influence of differential levels of calcium in the diet on (a) fluoride retention in soft and hard tissue (i.e., its body burden), and (b) fluoride toxicity in different animal species and humans (including the mottling of teeth); and (2) the influence of elevated levels of fluoride on calcium metabolism and requirements.

Dietary Levels of Calcium and Fluoride Body Burden. Several studies have specifically addressed the issue of whether low levels of calcium in the diet enhance the retention or body burden of fluoride (Lawrenz and Mitchell, 1941; Weddle and Muhler, 1954; Wagner and Muhler, 1960; Jowsey and Riggs, 1978; Krylova and Gnoevaya, 1956; Jackson and Train, 1955). In pair-feeding experiments with rats, Lawrenz and Mitchell (1941) revealed that an increase in the calcium content of the diet from 0.23 to 0.75% resulted in a 10–13% reduction in the total carcass retention of fluorine as well as similar reductions in teeth and soft tissue when fluorine was consumed in the diet at variable levels ranging from 9 to 32 ppm. Comparable experiments by Weddle and Muhler (1954) revealed that the presence of 1.0% and 0.1% $CaCl_2$ in the diet diminished the retention of ingested fluorine stored in the carcass by 74 and 47%, respectively, as compared to rats given only 0.01% Ca in the diet. Interestingly, dietary $Ca_2P_2O_7$ (calcium pyrophosphate) did not affect the retention of the fluoride. A similar inverse relationship of dietary calcium with fluoride absorption/retention has been noted by others (Jowsey and Riggs, 1978; Spencer et al., 1975, 1977).

Although these studies indicated that dietary calcium levels affect the body burden of fluoride, they did not provide insight into the mechanism of action. However, Krylova and Gnoevaya (1956) have suggested how calcium may diminish fluoride retention. They noted that the feces fluoride:urine fluoride ratio increased in rats given 0.5 g $CaCO_3$ daily, thereby suggesting that calcium may be inhibiting the gastrointestinal absorption of the fluoride ion. These findings were supported by Wagner and Muhler (1960) who demonstrated a reduction in fluoride retention in weanling rats given 2 mg of calcium orally at 15 to 60 minutes after the oral administration of 2 mg of fluoride.

More recently, normal volunteers, serving as their own controls, were given 30 mg fluoride/day for one week followed by a combination of fluoride and calcium carbonate (i.e., 1.3 g Ca/day). The presence of the combined treatment resulted in a 22% decrease in the serum fluoride levels. However, since excretory samples were not assessed, it is not possible to rule out that the concomitant calcium administration enhanced the net deposition of fluoride in bone (Jowsey and Riggs, 1978).

Based on these studies it is not possible to conclude confidently that various calcium salts reduced the gastrointestinal absorption of fluoride. Carefully designed studies are needed to evaluate the influence of calcium on both the gastrointestinal absorption and the excretory rates of fluoride. Such studies are of particular biomedical importance in light of the suggestion by Havivi (1972) that a low-calcium diet not only increases fluoride absorption but also enhances its retention in rats. Finally, whether dietary levels of calcium affect the retention of fluoride when exposure is between 2–4 mg/day—that is, a normal amount of exposure—is not known since the human studies of Jowsey and Riggs (1978) provided 30 mg/day, a dose 7–15 times the typical human daily exposure to fluoride.

The other research supporting the hypothesis that low levels of dietary calcium enhance fluoride retention was reported by Havivi (1972), Weddle and Muhler (1967), Ericsson (1958), and Jenkins (1967). For example, rats reared on low-calcium diets (1.2 g Ca/kg food) retained 2–3 times more dietary fluoride than similarly exposed rats reared on diets with 14.34 g Ca/kg. These data revealed further that the percent of fluoride absorbed in the low- and high-calcium diet groups was 92.0 and 41.2, respectively, while the percent retained was 14.4 and 4.2, respectively. Consistent with these findings were increased fluoride values in the plasma (28.0 vs. 20.0 μg/g), liver (0.23 vs. 0.10 μg/g), and kidney (0.74 vs. 0.24 μg/g) for rats reared on the low-calcium diets. Such findings imply that low levels of calcium may affect both the absorption and retention of fluoride, a finding not previously demonstrated by other investigators. Similarly, Weddle and Muhler (1967) noted that 21% of fluoride dose was absorbed when it was given together along with a calcium chloride solution as compared with 75% when it was given in distilled water. Likewise, Ericsson (1958) has reported that less fluoride is absorbed from milk (with high levels of calcium) than from water (with considerably less calcium). However, one must be careful not to attribute the entire differential influence of milk on the absorption of fluoride to calcium without systematic assessment of the contribution of the other numerous constituents of milk. Refer to the lead section of this chapter on the influence of milk components on lead absorption for an appreciation of the complexity of such an interaction. Finally, Largent and Heyroth (1949) have reported that most fluoride salts are readily absorbed and that nearly 96% of fluoride from CaF_2 is absorbed, thereby leading Sriranga Reddy and Narasinga Rao (1971) to question whether calcium reduces fluoride absorption via the formation of a salt.

The Influence of Low Levels of Dietary Calcium on Fluoride Toxicity. In light of the studies reported in the previous section, which indicate that low levels of dietary calcium markedly enhance the body burden of elevated levels of dietary fluoride, it may be logically hypothesized that individuals with a diet inadequate in calcium may be at increased risk to adverse effects associated with excessive exposure to fluoride. This hypothesis was supported nearly 50 years ago by a number of researchers including DeEds (1933), who reported that dietary calcium diminishes the toxicity of ingested fluorine as well as by Hauck et al. (1933), who demonstrated that the growth of rats reared on a low-calcium diet was poorer on a diet with 0.15% NaF as compared to rats on a diet with adequate levels of calcium. Other studies supporting the hypothesis that diets inadequate in calcium enhance fluoride toxicity have been reported (Schulz, 1938; Ranganathan, 1941, 1944; Velu, 1933; Majumdar and Ray, 1946). In addition, Pillai et al. (1944) have also noted that the inclusion of sufficient amounts of whole-milk powder and/or bone powder in the diet of rats resulted in a marked protection against fluoride poisoning.

On the whole, these studies have utilized very excessive levels of fluoride, far in excess of any potential human exposure even in the most extreme cases. For example, Ranganathan (1941) exposed rats to 100 mg/kg body weight while the average human exposure may be on the order of 1–5 mg/70kg (or $\sim$ 0.01 mg/1 kg). Of greater relevance to human exposure levels but still quite excessive were more recent studies of Burkhart and Jowsey (1968) in which kittens were given 2.5 mg/kg and Sriranga Reddy and Srikantia (1971) with monkeys that were given 10 mg/kg/day. The degree of calcium deficiency, which varied according to the different studies, generally covered a broad and realistic range from deficient up to adequate.

The specific fluoride-induced adverse health effects that were enhanced in the calcium-deficient animals in these different studies involved (1) reduced survival in rats (Ranganathan, 1941, 1944); (2) development of wide osteoid borders, reduced bone resorption and formation in kittens (Burkhart and Jowsey, 1968); and (3) radiological evidence of fluorosis, elevated levels of serum alkaline phosphatase, and markedly enhanced fluoride body burden in monkeys (Sriranga Reddy and Srikantia, 1971). Unfortunately, there are no data evaluating the influence of moderately deficient calcium diets at levels of fluoride that more closely simulate typical human exposure levels.

Dietary Calcium Levels in Relation to Fluoride-Induced Mottled Enamel. In 1931 Smith et al. provided the first satisfactory explanation for the occurrence of endemic mottled tooth enamel in the United States, which, as is now commonly known, is the consumption of water with elevated levels of fluoride. However, before this relationship was delineated, it was widely hypothesized that the occurrence of the mottled teeth was the result of a dietary deficiency. This notion was supported by the research of Mellanby (1928) who had demonstrated that dental defects frequently result from dietary deficiencies and that nutrition of the tooth is closely associated with its normal development.

Leverton and Smith (1932) reported on a quantitative dietary study of 16 children who exhibited mottled enamel and three children in the same community without mottling. No significant difference in Ca, P, protein, or energy values of the diets of children in the mottled-tooth group were found as compared to the nonmottled group based on either 4 or 7 consecutive-day dietary assessments. Moreover, the nutrient consumption of all the children was considered generally optimal. However, the children with the greatest extent of mottling exhibited a noticeably lower ascorbic acid intake. Although fluoride was the primary cause of the mottled teeth, it was suggested that dietary factors may modify the extent of the fluoride-induced mottling.

There has been some discussion over the years that calcium levels in the diet may influence the occurrence of mottled enamel. In fact, even before it was discovered that excess fluoride exposure was the primary cause of mottled enamel, Pierle (1926) had reported that a diet low in calcium could cause the occurrence of mottled and stained teeth. This finding was supported by Lantz and Smith (1934) who noted that elevated levels of fluoride exposure reduce the capacity of animals to retain the tooth-forming elements such as Ca and P, as inferred by their enhanced excretion of these elements. In fact, it was based on this later report that Smith (1935–36) initiated extensive studies on the influence of variations in Ca and P levels in the diet on the extent of fluoride-induced mottling in rats. The range of experiments was quite broad, involving an assessment of the influence of highly variable levels of Ca and P in the diet; that is, diets were designed to range from very inadequate to amounts that markedly exceeded levels considered adequate for normal growth and development. Fluoride levels ranged upward from the minimum dose known to cause mottling. Regardless of the levels of Ca or P in the diet as well as the extent of fluoride exposure, the levels of Ca or P in the diet did not appear to influence the incidence or severity of fluoride-induced dental fluorosis. Consequently, a suboptimal diet did not enhance the toxicity of fluoride nor did a diet with greater than normal levels offer more protection. However, whenever the Ca or P levels were so inadequate that the mineral deficiency affected normal dental calcification, the fluoride-induced mottling was enhanced. Thus, Smith (1935–36) concluded that "diets faulty in mineral makeup do not render an individual more susceptible to fluoride, but the combination of fluoride damage and that due to inadequate Ca and P intakes may make the teeth doubly inferior and defective in formation and calcification."

In contrast, Greenwood et al. (1946) noted that permanent teeth of puppies fed 5 mg of fluorine/kg of body weight/day as NaF stored excessive fluorides and exhibited dental fluorosis while puppies given the same level of fluoride in bone meal powder and in defluorinated phosphate had sound normal teeth. It was concluded that calcium in the bone meal has a protective action against dental fluorosis. In addition, Hoffman et al. (1942) noted that fluorides given in milk fed to rats resulted in fewer dental changes when compared to the effect of fluorides given through water. In addition to these suggestive animal studies, several investigators had reported other associations of dental mottling with dietary factors (Pandit et al., 1940; Murray and Wilson, 1948; Day, 1940). For instance, Pandit et al. (1940) reported that the deciduous teeth of severely malnourished children were very susceptible to fluoride-induced mottling. Mottled enamel was universal at 1.0 ppm of fluorine or more. In addition, Murray and Wilson (1948) reported the occurrence of mottled enamel in children from low economic levels and inadequate nutritional status. However, mottling was not present in children with good nutritional status living in the same endemic community. Despite this apparent inverse relationship of mottling with nutritional status it was not known whether the enhanced mottling of the enamel resulted from the deficiency of specific dietary components (e.g., calcium) or an overall deficient nutritional status.

A similar epidemiological investigation was undertaken in Italy by Massler and Schour (1952) who reported a markedly enhanced occurrence of dental fluorosis in 12- to 14-year-old children than would have normally been expected to occur at only 1.3 ppm fluoride in drinking water. More specifically, the percentage of children with mottling was 60.0% in the Italian community of Quarto while it was only 25.3% among similarly aged and fluoride-exposed groups in Joliet, Illinois. These authors suggested that the reason for the enhanced occurrence of dental fluorosis in the Italian community was the very poor nutritional status of the population. According to the authors, the calcium intake was quite low because milk was not generally available.

As interesting as these suggestive findings are, they are merely associational inferences. No precise data were presented for the calcium intakes. In addition, there may be important differences relative to susceptibility to tooth mottling between the two groups of 12–14 year olds other than nutritional status. Thus, before any definite conclusions can be drawn, more accurate comparisons between the two study populations would be needed. Despite the striking findings of Massler and Schour (1952), no subsequent human studies concerning the influence of calcium dietary status on fluoride-induced dental mottling have been published. It would seem that this area would be of great public health interest in light of the widespread occurrence of inadequate calcium intake and levels of fluoride in drinking water of approximately 1.3 ppm as they were in Quarto, Italy.

The Influence of Fluoride in Calcium Metabolism. In 1965 Srikantia and Siddiqui demonstrated that patients with fluorosis retain markedly greater amounts of calcium as compared to normal individuals. These findings were subsequently confirmed by Narasinga Rao et al. (1968) who reported that a significant positive calcium balance and low urinary excretion of calcium in three male adults suffering from skeletal fluorosis who were given a standard diet with 800 mg calcium/day for 10 days. Of further interest is that the accumulated excretion of Ca^{45} in urine and feces over the 10-day study was only equal to or less than 4% depending on the specific individual. These values are in marked contrast with the excretory responses (urine and feces) of normal individuals, which were reported by Rinsler et al. (1965) to be 50% or more.

The previously cited studies were primarily of a clinical and not experimental nature. Consequently, Sriranga Reddy and Narasinga Rao (1971) evaluated the hypothesis that fluorosis enhances the retention of calcium in monkeys. In fundamental agreement with previous studies, dietary fluoride (910 mg/kg/day) was found to increase the accretion rate and exchangeable pool size of calcium in monkeys reared on an adequate diet. In addition, monkeys fed a low-calcium diet and exposed to a similar amount of fluoride exhibited an even greater calcium (and Ca^{47}) accretion rate and total calcium retention. Further support for these findings is provided by Cicardo et al. (1955, 1955a) and Dunstone and Payne (1959), as well as by Carlsson (1953) who demonstrated an increased uptake of ^{45}Ca in bones of rats given a low-calcium diet. Finally, positive calcium balances in patients with bone diseases undergoing treatment with fluoride have also been reported by Cohen et al. (1969), Hodge and Smith (1968), and Bernstein et al. (1963).

In contrast to these findings, Neer et al. (1966) noted that fluoride decreased the labile calcium pool size and bone resorption rate. Furthermore, Lengermann and Comar (1963) and Likins et al. (1964) did not find any influence of fluoride on the uptake of ^{45}Ca by bone while Menczel et al. (1963) reported that fluoride reduced the uptake of ^{45}Ca by bones of rats fed a low-calcium diet.

Sriranga Reddy and Narasinga Rao (1971) criticized these nonsupportive studies as not being conducted over a long enough period to evaluate calcium-balance properly. In fact, Spencer et al. (1969) stated that in view of the irregularity in the passage of fecal calcium and the delay in transit time especially in older persons, the influence of sodium fluoride on calcium metabolism is hard to determine in balance experiments of a short duration. This interpretation may explain the nonsupportive studies of Higgins et al. (1965), Lukert et al. (1967), and Spencer et al. (1969) since they were of a short duration. Thus, Higgins et al. (1965) reported that calcium balances were not improved in patients with Paget's disease of the bone given 60 mg fluoride/day for 24–30 days, while Lukert et al. (1967) similarly reported no improvement in calcium balance for patients with osteoporosis receiving 60–120 mg sodium fluoride daily for 3 weeks. However, this criticism is not as valid for the nonsupportive study by Rose (1965) in which patients with osteoporosis were given 120 mg sodium fluoride daily for several months. Yet it should be realized that studies that did indicate a positive calcium balance in humans involved prolonged periods of time including 34 months (Cohen and Gardner, 1964), 12 months (Purves, 1962), and 8 months (Cass et al., 1966).

Summary. The evidence clearly indicates that low levels of calcium in the diet markedly enhance the retention of orally administered fluoride. Although further research is necessary in this area, there is support for the hypothesis of Havivi (1972) that a low-calcium diet enhances not only the gastrointestinal absorption of fluoride but may also be reducing its excretion. Studies with animal models have demonstrated that low levels of dietary calcium result in an increased toxicity of fluoride, most likely because of the enhanced body burden. The uncertain relevance of the animal studies make it difficult to derive reasonably precise human risk assessments. This is because they suffer from the usual problem of excessive fluoride exposure and/or the maintenance of animals on diets very deficient in calcium.

Despite these limitations with much of the data on calcium-fluoride interactions, there have been some comprehensive attempts with animal models (Smith, 1935–36) to evaluate whether fluoride-induced dental mottling may be enhanced by low levels of dietary calcium. While the data of Smith (1935–36) did not support this hypothesis, other animal studies by Greenwood et al. (1946) with dogs and Hoffman et al. (1942) with rats did. In addition, several early epidemiological studies (Massler and Schour, 1952; Murray and Wilson, 1948) have provided at least circumstantial evidence to support this hypothesis. However, the epidemiological as well as toxicological data supporting the view that low levels of calcium in the diet enhance fluoride-induced mottling are not convincing. This is not to say that this view has been discredited. The main problem has been the lack of current research effort, especially from an epidemiological perspective. In light of the fact that hundreds of articles are published every year on some aspect of the fluoridation program, it is odd that the nutrient-fluoride interactions have been totally de-emphasized. In light of the widespread presence of inadequate calcium ingestion in the United States as well as the growing awareness that fluoride consumption has been increasing in fluoridated areas where food processing uses fluoridated water (Spencer et al., 1977), it would appear that epidemiologic investigations of the proposed hypothesis would be of interest. Clearly, further research on this hypothesis is needed in areas of the world where fluorosis is endemic.

Summary of Calcium-Fluoride Interactions

Reference	Animal Model	Comment
1. Elevated Fluoride Exposure Alters the Calcium Levels in Bone, Teeth, and Other Tissue—Animal Studies		
Forbes, 1921	Swine	Reported a reduction in bone ash per cm³ of volume in swine fed rock phosphate containing F.
Tolle and Maynard, 1928	Rats	Found a reduction of 10% in the bone ash of rats after 5 weeks on a ration in which the calcium supplement was supplied by 1.8% rock phosphate.
Chaneles, 1929	Rats	Found an increase in bone ash (5.5%) when NaF was fed in a basal ration of bread and milk, but a 4% decrease in the ash of teeth.

Summary of Calcium-Fluoride Interactions *(Continued)*

Reference	Animal Model	Comment
McClure and Mitchell, 1931	Rats	F at 0.06% of diet decreased the level of calcium retained by 9.8%.
Hauck et al., 1933	Rats	Added 0.15% NaF to diet of young rats with different levels of calcium in diet.
		Bone
		Low-calcium diet—ash content <
		Moderate-calcium diet—ash content <
		High-calcium diet—ash content >
		Teeth
		Low-calcium diet—ash content <
		Moderate-calcium diet—ash content <
		High-calcium diet—ash content <
Schulz, 1938	Rats	Results agreed with Hauck et al., 1933.
Suketa et al., 1977	Rats	Calcium content of kidney markedly increased after fluoride ingestion.

2. Human Balance Studies: Persons with Fluorosis Retain More Calcium

Srikantia and Siddiqui, 1965	Patients with fluorosis retained significantly more calcium than normal subjects did.
Narasinga Rao et al., 1968	Humans with skeletal fluorosis exhibited a high retention of dietary calcium.
Spencer et al., 1969	Ingestion of large quantities of fluoride resulted in reduced absorption of ^{47}Ca; the average decrease in plasma levels was 30%.

Summary of Calcium-Fluoride Interactions *(Continued)*

Reference	Animal Model	Comment

3. Evaluation of the Hypothesis that Low Levels of Calcium Enhance Fluoride-Induced Mottling of Teeth.

Animal Model

Smith (1935–1936)	Rats	Fluorine-induced mottled enamel occurred regardless of calcium supplements; low-calcium diets did not enhance fluorine-induced mottling; only when a calcium deficiency had caused the teeth to be defective did this nutritional status enhance fluorine toxicity.
Hoffman et al., 1942	Rats	Dietary calcium was found to protect against fluoride-induced mottling.
Greenwood et al., 1946	Dog	Calcium levels in the diet were inversely related to the occurrence of dental fluorosis.

Human Studies

Pierle, 1926		A low-calcium diet could enhance mottled and stained teeth.
Day, 1940; Pandit et al., 1940; Murray and Wilson, 1948; Massler and Schour, 1952		Dental mottling was associated with malnourishment, including low-calcium levels.

4. Low Levels of Dietary Calcium Enhance Fluoride Toxicity and/or Calcium Supplementation was Protective

DeEds, 1933		Review of literature; dietary calcium has a protective effect and that calcium-deficient diet enhances the symptoms of fluorosis.
Velu, 1933	Sheep	Dietary calcium protected against fluorine toxicity.
Roholm, 1937	Rats	A diet rich in calcium, phosphorus, and vitamin D was found to reduce fluorine intoxication.

Summary of Calcium-Fluoride Interactions *(Continued)*

Reference	Animal Model	Comment
Ranganathan, 1941, 1944	Rats	Studied relation between calcium intake and the effect of fluorine poisoning in rats; low calcium in diet enhanced fluorine toxicity.
Pillai et al., 1944	Rats	Consumption of milk provided protection against fluoride toxicity.
Majumdar and Ray, 1946	Bulls	Dietary calcium protected against fluoride-induced toxicity.
Wadhwani, 1954	Rats	Calcium and phosphorus in the diet of rats protected the animals against the toxic effects when growth, survival, and the composition and development of bones were considered.
Gabovich and Maistruk, 1963	Guinea pigs	A multivitamin/mineral supplement helped reduce fluoride toxicity.
Burkhart and Jowsey, 1968	Kittens	Elevated levels of calcium in the diet are able to prevent the osteomalacial effects of high levels of fluoride.

5. Evaluation of the Influence of Calcium on the Body Burden of Fluoride

Lawrenz and Mitchell, 1941	Rats	Increasing the calcium level in the diet from 0.23 to 0.73% reduced the total retention of fluorine by 10 to 13% and to a greater extent the deposition of fluorine in teeth and soft tissues; protection was greater in the young.
Weddle and Muhler, 1954	Rats	$CaCl_2$ decreased fluoride storage even at a calcium concentration of 0.1%; calcium pyrophosphate did not alter fluoride storage.

Summary of Calcium-Fluoride Interactions *(Continued)*

Reference	Animal Model	Comment
Jackson and Train, 1955	Rats	Fluoride retention increased in rats placed on a low-calcium diet.
Krylova and Gnoevaya, 1956	Rats	Studied the means by which calcium reduced fluoride retention; they reported that the feces fluoride to urine fluoride ratio increased in rats given 0.5 gm $CaCO_3$. This suggested that calcium and other similarly acting inorganic ions act by inhibiting the absorption of the fluoride ion.
Wagner and Muhler, 1960	Rats	Administration of calcium after fluoride resulted in a decreased retention of fluoride; the degree of fluoride retention was not time dependent.
Sriranga Reddy and Srikantia, 1971	Monkey	The concentration of fluoride in the upper areas of the humerus was greater in animals that had received the low-calcium diet; most animals in the low-calcium group had radiological evidence of fluorosis.
Forsyth et al., 1972	Pigs	Increased levels of calcium in diet decreased fluoride retention.
Havivi, 1972	Rats	Levels of fluoride in soft tissue of the rats kept on low-calcium diets were 2–3 times that of the corresponding tissues of rats kept on high-calcium diets.
Spencer et al., 1975, 1977	Human	In clinical studies of osteoporosis, high-calcium levels did not decrease fluoride absorption.
Jowsey and Riggs, 1978	Human	In clinical studies of osteoporosis, calcium carbonate administration reduced the degree of fluoride absorption.

References

ACGIH (1976). Threshold Limit Values, American Conference of Governmental Industrial Hygienists, Cincinnati, OH.

Anonymous (1974). Skeletal fluorosis and dietary calcium, vitamin C and protein. *Nutr. Rev.* **32**:13–15.

Bernstein, D.S.; Gori, C.; Cohen, P.; Collins, J.J.; and Tamuakopoulos, S. (1963). The use of sodium fluoride in metabolic bone disease. *J. Clin. Invest.* **42**:916.

Burkhart, J.M. and Jowsey, J. (1968). Effect of variation in calcium intake on the skeleton of fluoride-fed kittens. *J. Lab. Clin. Med.* **72**:943–950.

Carlsson, A. (1953). *Acta Pharmacol.* **9**:32 (cited in Sriranga Reddy and Narasinga Rao, 1971).

Cass, R.M.; Croft, J.D.; Perkins, P.; Nye, W.; Waterhouse, C.; and Terry, R. (1966). New bone formation in osteoporosis following treatment with sodium fluoride. *Arch. Intern. Med.* **118**:111.

Chaneles, J. (1929). *Rev. Soc. Argent. de Biol.* v.336 (cited in Hauck et al., 1933).

Cicardo, V.H.; Muraccole, J.C.; and DeLerner, S.J. (1955). *Rev. Soc. Arg. Biol.* (cited in Sriranga Reddy and Narasinga Rao, 1971).

Cicardo, V.H.; Muraccole, J.C.; and DeLerner, S.J. (1955a). *Rev. Assoc. Odontol. Arg.* **43**:307 (cited in Sriranga Reddy and Narasinga Rao, 1971).

Cohen, P. and Gardner, F.H. (1964). Induction of subacute skeletal fluorosis in a case of multiple myeloma. *New Engl. J. Med.* **271**:1129.

Cohen, P.; Nichols, G.L.; and Banks, H.H. (1969). Fluoride treatment of bone rarefaction in multiple myeloma and osteoporosis. *Clin. Orthop.* **64**:221.

Day, C.D.M. (1940). Chronic endemic fluorosis in northern India. *Brit. Dent. J.* **68**:409.

DeEds, F. (1933). Chronic fluorine intoxication. A review. *Med.* **12**:1–60.

Dunstone, J.R. and Payne, E. (1959). Some effects of fluoride on calcium metabolism in the bones of young rats. *Aust. J. Biol. Sci.* **12**:466.

Ericsson, Y. (1958). The state of fluorine in the milk and its absorption and retention when administered in milk. *Acta Odont. Scand.* **16**:51.

Forbes, E.B.; Halverson, J.O.; and Schultz, J.A. et al. (1921). *Ohio Agric. Expt. Sta. Bull.* 347 (cited in Hauck et al., 1933).

Forsyth, D.M.; Pond, W.G.; and Krook, L. (1972). Dietary calcium and fluoride interactions in swine: In utero and neonatal effects. *J. Nutr.* **102**:1639–1646.

Gabovich, R.D. and Maistruk, P.N. (1963). On the therapeutic and prophylactic diet in the fluorine manufacturing industry. *Voprosy Pitaniia* **22**:32–38.

Greenwood, D.A.; Blayney, J.R.; Skinsnes, O.K.; and Hodges, P.C. (1946). Comparative studies of the feeding of fluorides as they occur in purified bone meal powder, defluorinated phosphate and sodium fluoride in dogs. *J. Dent. Res.* **25**:311–335.

Hauck, H.M.; Steenbock, H.; and Parsons, H.T. (1933). The effect of the level of calcium intake on the calcification on bones and teeth during fluorine toxicosis. *Amer. J. Physiol.* **103**:489–493.

Havivi, E. (1972). Effect of calcium and vitamin D on fluoride metabolism in the rat. *Nutr. Metabol.* **14**:257–261.

Higgins, B.A.; Nassim, J.R.; Alexander, R.; and Hilb, A. (1965). Effect of sodium fluoride on calcium, phosphorus, and nitrogen balance in patients with Paget's disease. *Brit. Med. J.* **1**:1159.

Hodge, H.C. and Smith, F.A. (1968). Fluorides and man. *Ann. Rev. Pharm.* **8**:395.

Hoffman, M.M.; Schuck, C.; and Furuta, W.J. (1942). Histologic study on the effects of fluorine administered in dry and moist diets on teeth of young albino rats. *J. Dent. Res.* **21**:157.

Jackson, S.H. and Train, D. (1955). Stabilization of the fluorine concentration of the ash of rats. *Canad. J. Biochem. Physiol.* **33**:93.

Jenkins, G.N. (1967). *Fluoride Wld. Odont. Scand.* **16**:51.

Jolly, S.S.; Singh, B.N.; Mathur, G.C.; and Malhotra, K.C. (1968). Epidemiological, clinical and biochemical study of endemic dental and skeletal fluorosis in Punjab. *Brit. Med. J.* **4**:427.

Jowsey, J. and Riggs, B.L. (1978). Effect of concurrent calcium ingestion on intestinal absorption of fluoride. *Metabolism* **27**:(8):971–974.

Krylova, M.I. and Gnoevaya, V.L. (1956). Fluorine metabolism. *Voprosy Pitaniia* **15**:37.

Lantz, E.M. and Smith, M.C. (1934). The effect of fluorine upon calcium and phosphorus metabolism in albino rats. *J. Physiol.* **109**:645.

Largent, E.J. and Heyroth, F.F. (1949). The absorption and excretion of fluorides. III. Further observations on metabolism of fluorides at high levels of intake. *J. Ind. Hyg. Toxicol.* **31**:134.

Lawrenz, M. and Mitchell, H.H. (1941). The effect of dietary calcium and phosphorus on the assimilation of dietary fluorine. *J. Nutr.* **22**:91–101.

Lengermann, F.W. and Comar, C.L. (1963). Fluoridated water and the skeletal uptake of Sr^{85} and Ca^{45} by young rats. *J. Nutr.* **79**:195.

Leverton, R.M. and Smith, M.C. (1932). The relation of calcium and phosphorus in the diet to the cause of mottled enamel of human teeth. *J. Home Economics* **24**:1091–1097.

Likins, R.G.; Posner, A.S.; and Pakis, G. (1964). Effect of fluoride on crystal texture and radiocalcium uptake of rat bone. *Proc. Soc. Exp. Biol. Med.* **115**:511.

Lukert, B.P.; Meek, J.C.; and Bolinger, R.E. (1967). Acute effect of fluoride on [45]calcium dynamics in osteoporosis. *J. Clin. Endocrinol. Metab.* **27**:828.

McClure, F.J. and Mitchell, H.H. (1931). The effect of fluoride on the calcium metabolism of albino rats and the composition of the bones. *J. Biochem.* **90**:277–326.

Majumdar, B.N. and Ray, S.N. (1946). *Indian J. Vet. Sci. and Animal Husbandry* **18**:107 (cited in Wadhwani, 1952).

Massler, M. and Schour, I. (1952). Relation of endemic dental fluorosis to malnutrition. *J. Amer. Dent. Assoc.* **44**:156–165.

Mellanby, M. (1928). The influence of diet on the structure of the teeth. *Physiol. Rev.* **8**:545–577.

Menczel, J.; Schraer, R.; Pakis, G.; Posner, A.S.; and Likins, R.C. (1963). Effect of low calcium diet on bone crystallinity and skeletal uptake of Ca^{45} in rats. *Proc. Soc. Exp. Biol. Med.* **112**:128.

Murray, M.M. and Wilson, D.C. (1948). Fluorosis and nutrition in Morocco. *Brit. Dent. J.* **84**:97.

Narasinga Rao, B.S.; Siddiqui, A.H.; and Srikantia, S.G. (1968). A study of calcium[45] turnover in skeletal fluorosis. *Metabolism* **17**(4):366–369.

Neer, R.M.; Zipkin, I.; Carbone, P.P.; and Rosenberg, L.E. (1966). Effect of sodium fluoride therapy on calcium metabolism in multiple myeloma. *J. Clin. Endocrin.* **26**:1059.

Pandit, C.G. and Narayana Rao, D. (1940). Endemic fluorosis in South India. Experimental production of chronic fluorine intoxication in monkeys (*Macaca radiata*). *Indian J. Med. Res.* **28**:559.

Pandit, C.G.; Raghavachari, T.N.S.; Subba Rao, D.; and Krishnamurti, V. (1940). Endemic fluorosis in South India. A study of the factors involved in the production of mottled enamel in children and severe bone manifestations in adults. *Indian J. Med. Res.* **28**:533.

Pierle, C.A. (1926). Production of mottling and brown stain. *J. Am. Dent. Assoc.* **13**:999.

Pillai, S.C.; Rajapopalan, R.; and De, N.N. (1944). *Indian Med. Gaz.* **79**:249.

Public Health Service. Public Health Service Drinking Water Standards, pp. 41–42.

Purves, M.J. (1962). Some effects of administering sodium fluoride to patients with Paget's disease. *Lancet* **2**:1188.

Ranganathan, S. (1941). Calcium intake and fluorine poisoning in rats. *Ind. J. Med. Res.* **29**:639–697.

Ranganathan, S. (1944). Studies on experimental fluorine poisoning in rats. *Ind. J. Med. Res.* **32**:233–236.

Rinsler, M.G.; Gwyther, M.; and Field, E.O. (1965). Some aspects of calcium metabolism in malignant disease of bone. *J. Clin. Path.* **18**:69.

Roholm, K. (1937). Fluorine intoxication. In: *Clinical Hygienic Studies.* (Cited in Ranganathan, 1941).

Rose, G.A. (1965). A study of the treatment of osteoporosis with fluoride therapy. *Proc. Roy. Soc. Med.* **58**:436.

Schulz, J.A. (1938). Fluorine toxicosis in the albino rat. *Iowa Agr. Exp. Sta. Res. Bull.* **247**:165–242.

Siddiqui, A.H. (1955). Fluorosis in Nalgonda district, Hyderabad Deccan. *Brit. Med. J.* **2**:1408.

Smith, M.C. (1935–1936). Dietary factors in relation to mottled enamel. *J. Dent. Res.* **15**:281–290.

Smith, M.C.; Lantz, E.M.; and Smith, H.V. (1931). The cause of mottled enamel, a defect of human teeth. Ariz. Exp. Sta. Tech. Bull. No. 32. Also see *J. Dent. Res.* **12**:151, 1932.

Spencer, H.; Lewin, I.; Fowler, J.; and Samachson, J. (1969). Effect of sodium fluoride on calcium absorption and balances in man. *Amer. J. Clin. Nutr.* **22**:381–390.

Spencer, H.; Osis, D.; Kramer, L.; Wiatrowski, E.; and Norris, C. (1975). Effect of calcium and phosphorus on fluoride metabolism in man. *J. Nutr.* **105**:733–740.

Spencer, H.; Wiatrowski, E.; Osis, D. et al. (1977). Studies of the availability of fluoride in man. Presented at the 11th annual conference on Trace Substances in Environ. Health, Univ. of Missouri at Columbia.

Srikantia, S.G. and Siddiqui, A.H. (1965). Metabolic studies in skeletal fluorosis. *Clin. Sci.* **28**:477.

Sriranga Reddy, G. and Srikantia, S.G. (1971). Effect of dietary calcium, vitamin C, and protein in development of experimental skeletal fluorosis. I. Growth, serum chemistry, and changes in composition, and radiological appearance of bones. *Metabolism* **20**:642.

Sriranga Reddy, G. and Narasinga Rao, B.S. (1971). Effect of dietary calcium, vitamin C and protein in development of experimental skeletal fluorosis. II. Calcium turnover with ^{45}Ca; calcium and phosphorus balances. *Metabolism* **20**:651.

Suketa, K.; Mikami, E.; and Hayashi, M. (1977). Changes in calcium and magnesium in the kidney of rats intoxicated with a single large dose of fluoride. *Toxicol. Appl. Pharm.* **39**:313–319.

Tolle, C. and Maynard, L.A. (1928). *Proc. Amer. Soc. of Animal Prod.* **15**:15 (cited in Hauck et al., 1933).

Velu, H. (1933). *Bull. Soc. Path. Exot.* **26**:616 (cited in Wadhwani, 1952).

Wadhwani, T.K. (1952). Mitigation of fluorosis (experimental). *Indian Med. Gaz.* **87**:5–7.

Wadhwani, T.K. (1954). Prevention and mitigation of fluorosis (endemic). II. *J. Indian Inst. Sci.* **36**:64.

Wadhwani, T.K. (1955). Effect of fluorine on the composition of bones: changes in the composition of bones of monkeys (*Macaca radiata*). *Indian J. Med. Res.* **43**:321.

Wagner, M.J. and Muhler, J.C. (1960). The effect of calcium and phosphorus on fluoride absorption. *J. Dent. Res.* **39**(1):49–52.

Weddle, D.A. and Muhler, J.C. (1954). Effects of inorganic salts on F storage. *J. Nutr.* **54**:437.

Weddle, D.A. and Muhler, J.C. (1967). The metabolism of different fluorides in the rat. *J. Dent. Res.* **36**:386.

3. Lead

Introduction. Considerable information has been published about the toxicity of lead in both animal and human systems. Presently there are a variety of health standards including those for ambient and industrial air and drinking water that are designed to prevent undue exposure to lead. That lead toxicity may be affected or modified by a number of biological and environmental factors is now known. For example, lead intoxication may be influenced by seasonal factors, age of the organism, and dietary status, among others (Mahaffey, 1974). With respect to dietary factors, volume 1 has extensively reviewed the influence of the different vitamins on the toxicity of lead. In similar fashion, this volume will demonstrate the influence of numerous nonvitamin nutrients such as certain minerals, protein, fats, carbohydrates, fiber, and other nutrients on the course of lead toxicity in animal models and humans.

Historical Perspectives. That lead intoxication could be modified by calcium or foods with high levels of calcium has long been known. The administration of milk to lead-exposed industrial workers was not uncommon in the early 1900s. In fact, it was strongly recommended by several writers (Feissinger, 1900; McKenna, 1913; Tanquerel des Planches, 1848) and more recently by Hunter (1969) and Krook (1974). According to Stephens and Waldron (1975), the biomedical foundations for such a policy are not well documented but probably originated from the observations "that workers who were poorly fed developed lead poisoning more often than those who were relatively well fed . . . with milk being given to correct deficiencies in the diet."

The recommendation suggesting that milk should be provided to industrial workers exposed to lead has been the source of considerable debate and, of course, much research. The principal problem involved in such an issue is that milk is a very complex substance, being composed in part of calcium, phosphorus, vitamins C and D, protein, fat, citric acid, and lactose, all of which have subsequently been found to affect lead absorption. In fact, as subsequent sections will reveal, milk contains substances that both facilitate and hinder the gastrointestinal absorption of lead with these factors in turn being dependent upon the nutritional status of the subjects being evaluated. Thus it is not too unexpected to find numerous "apparently" conflicting studies with respect to the efficiency of milk as a prophylactic agent in humans exposed to lead. For example, Collier (1952), Dizon et al. (1950), Schweigart (1957), Travers et al. (1956), and Trosi (1950) reported that milk was beneficial in protecting against lead toxicity, while the studies of Boyadzhiev (1960), Lockhart (1963), Schiemann (1960), and Vigliani (1954) did not support that perspective. It naturally follows that similar confusion existed as to whether lead-exposed workers should be given milk as part of an industrial hygiene program (Zielhuis, 1960; Wittgens and Niederstadt, 1954; Sand, 1965; Longley, 1967).

In order to appreciate more fully the influence of milk on lead toxicity, it is necessary to assess the role of its individual components in facilitating the gastrointestinal absorption of lead on the organism. Thus, this section will evaluate the effects of calcium and phosphorus on lead toxicity, while the remaining nutrients will be considered in their respective sections. This type of organization is needed since the specific nutrients are contained in many commonly ingested foods, not only milk. In addition, most studies that have evaluated the interaction of phosphorus and lead have also included calcium and lead within their domain of investigation. Finally, at least from an historical perspective, the role of milk in lead toxicity is an important consideration even though Stephens and Waldron (1975) (along with Kello and Kostial [1973]) concluded that "its overall effect is to promote the absorption of lead from the gastrointestinal tract," that is, that the administration of milk would not be considered an effective prophylactic treatment.

Issues of Critical Importance. In order to get a general perspective on the role of calcium and phosphorus in lead toxicity, several issues should be brought in focus. First, do these minerals affect lead toxicity? If so, then by what mechanism(s)? Do they diminish the lead body burden by decreasing the levels of lead in hard and/or soft tissue? Do calcium and phosphorus differ in their interactions with lead? Do they prevent the absorption of lead via the gastrointestinal tract? Does lead affect the absorption of calcium and/or phosphorus? If deficiencies of both minerals individually enhance lead toxicity, what is the response if both compounds are consumed in less than recommended amounts?

Prevention of Lead Toxicity by Dietary Calcium and Phosphorus. There is a long history demonstrating that both calcium and phosphorus may markedly influence the uptake, retention, and toxicity of dietary lead. Without question the predominance of research has focused on calcium interactions, with phosphorus taking a back seat. Why this is so is not very evident from the literature since research studies have revealed that phosphorus may have a rather profound and frequently equal contribution to that of calcium on lead toxicity. The initial research studies concerning the hypothesis that either element may affect the toxicity of lead were conducted in the late 1930s. On the whole, most of these studies revealed that a high-calcium diet reduced dietary lead retention while low-calcium diets enhanced the retention of dietary lead in a number of animal species, that is, fish, mice, rats, and dogs (Calvery et al., 1938; Grant et al., 1938; Jones, 1938; Tompsett, 1939; Sobel et al., 1940; Lederer and Bing, 1940; Shields and Mitchell, 1941). Of importance in this regard were the findings of Lederer and Bing (1940) who showed that calcium supplementation could reduce the retention of dietary lead in bones and the kidney, but that dietary calcium was unable to affect the retention of lead that had been injected into the abdominal cavity. Such findings have been more recently confirmed in that retention of intraperitoneal ^{203}Pb was not affected by calcium supplementation of the diet (Meredith et al., 1977; Quarterman and Morrison, 1975). Such findings clearly suggest that dietary calcium causes a decreased retention of lead by reducing its absorption via the gastrointestinal tract.

In similar fashion, several studies in the 1930s and 1940s clearly indicated that dietary supplementation with phosphorus resulted in a decreased retention of lead within bones, soft tissue, and carcass as well as a reduction in lead toxicity in animal models (Shelling, 1932; Sobel et al., 1940; Shields and Mitchell, 1941; Sobel and Burger, 1955). However, Lederer and Bing (1940) were not able to confirm the findings that dietary phosphorus levels had any influence on the retention of lead in bone.

Although considerable research interest was generated in the 1930s and 1940s concerning the influence of dietary calcium and phosphorus on lead retention and toxicity, little was published again on the subject until the 1970s, with the obvious exception of a report by Sobel and Burger in 1955. Six and Goyer (1970) speculated that interest had declined in this area of research as a result of the development of chelating agents such as ethylenediaminetetracetic acid (EDTA) used in therapy for Pb poisoning. However, the report of Six and Goyer (1970) initiated a rebirth in this area that has continued through the decade of the 1970s presumably because of the increased recognition of lead as a ubiquitous pollutant and its enhanced toxicity to pregnant women and especially to young children.

The rash of studies in the 1970s has supported the fundamental conclusions of the early research as summarized above. But as expected, they have considerably extended the findings with respect to more accurate dose-response relationships on animal models, more quantifiable risk assessments, and development of epidemiological protocol in attempts to validate the animal studies, as well as research to establish the biochemical basis of the proposed calcium/phosphorus-lead interactions.

In the 1970 study of Six and Goyer, rats were reared on diets with either 0.1 or 0.7% Ca gluconate and exposed to 200 μg Pb/ml of drinking water for 10 weeks. These experimental conditions were selected because previous studies had revealed that this concentration of lead was the maximum dose for a 10-week period that did not cause a significant effect in hematopoiesis or renal size, histology, and function in rats reared on a diet with a 0.9% level of dietary calcium. It should be recognized that 0.1% calcium in the diet represents 20% of the recommended dietary allowance for Ca in the rat. Their findings revealed that rats on diets low in calcium exhibited markedly increased Pb retention in various tissues including blood (Figure 1-1), soft tissue, and bone, increased urinary excretion of Pb and δ-aminolevulinic acid, as well as increasing pathologic changes such as anemia, the frequency and size of intranuclear inclusion bodies in renal tubular cells, kidney size, and aminoaciduria. Subsequent studies have revealed that intermediate deficiencies of calcium of 33% (Quarterman and Morrison, 1975) and 50% (Barltrop and Khoo, 1975, 1976) of normal in the rat likewise result in enhanced lead retention in hard and soft tissue as well as red blood cells. In addition, Quarterman and Morrison (1975) reported that consumption of a diet with only 70% of the recommended level of phosphorus also resulted in a marked retention of lead quite similar to those reported for rats reared on a diet with only 33% of the

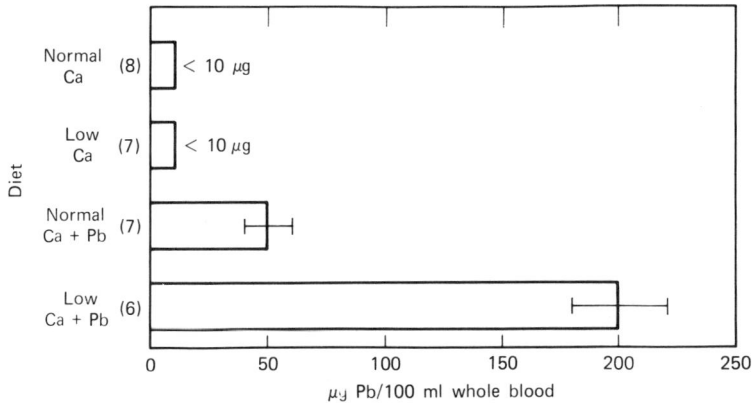

Figure 1-1. Influence of dietary Ca on blood Pb levels. [*Source.* Six, K.M. and Goyer, R.A. (1970). Experimental enhancement of lead toxicity by low dietary calcium. *J. Lab. Clin. Med.* **76**:938.]

recommended calcium levels as previously mentioned. Further studies involving both a calcium (33% of recommended) and phosphorus (70% of recommended) deficiency resulted in an additive effect with respect to lead retention.

While considerable emphasis has been directed toward establishing the influence of lower than required (or recommended) levels of dietary calcium on lead absorption, some researchers have evaluated the influence of supplementary calcium, that is, levels in excess of that recommended in order to see if it offered "extra" protection. Realizing that 0.5% calcium in the diet represents the recommended dietary allowance of calcium for rats, Shields and Mitchell (1941) compared diets with 0.5 and 1.1% calcium with respect to lead retention and found very little difference (p > 0.05) between the groups for total lead in carcass as well as percent of lead intake. In more recent studies, Barltrop and Khoo (1975, 1976) also reported that by increasing the calcium levels in the diet to twice the recommended levels (i.e., 2 × the control values as well) resulted in no difference in Pb retention in blood, kidneys, femur, and liver. However, increasing the calcium values to four times normal and keeping phosphate levels at 0.5% resulted in marked reductions in lead values with respect to whole body without gut (50%), blood (50%), kidneys (30%), femur (60%), and liver (50%) (Table 5).

Interestingly, when recommended levels of phosphate were increased by 100% (to 1.0%), they effected a decrease in lead retention in

Table 5. Effects of Increased Minerals on Lead Absorption (Ratio of Mean Retention Experimental: Control)

Dietary Minerals[a]						
Calcium (%)	Phosphate (%)	Whole Body without Gut	Blood	Kidneys	Femur	Liver
0.7[b]	0.5	1	1	1	1	1
1.4	0.5	1	1	1	1	1
0.7	1.0	1	1	1	1	0.7
1.4	1.0	0.5	1	0.6	0.5	0.6
2.8	0.5	0.5	0.5	0.7	0.4	0.5
0.7	2.0	0.5	0.4	0.3	0.4	0.4
2.8	2.0	0.4	0.4	0.4	0.2	0.5

[a] Added to mineral deficient diet.
[b] Control.

Source: Barltrop, D. and Khoo, H.E. (1976). The influence of dietary minerals and fat on the absorption of lead. *The Science of the Total Environ.* **6**:268.

the liver by 30% while no other tissues were affected. However, when both calcium and phosphate were jointly increased by 100% there resulted marked decreases in lead retention in whole body without gut (50%), kidneys (40%), femur (50%), and liver (40%). Additional supplementation with both calcium and phosphate at four times the recommended levels caused further reductions in lead retention in the kidney (60%) and femur (80%) (Table 5; Barltrop and Khoo, 1976). In addition, Meredith et al. (1977) also reported that calcium supplementation (2× normal) significantly reduced lead retention as determined by short-term radioactivity (Pb^{203}) studies as well as by more chronic exposure experiments by approximately 30% with respect to kidney, liver, and femur lead levels. Finally, a 1978 study by Quarterman et al. also demonstrated that the retention of dietary lead was diminished by 50% when recommended levels of calcium and/or phosphate in the diet were doubled. In partial contrast to Barltrop and Khoo (1975), doubling both calcium and phosphate levels in the same individuals had only a slightly greater reduction in lead levels in blood and in carcass. In addition, research by Hsu et al. (1975) revealed that when dietary calcium was increased from its normal level of 0.7% to 1.1% in weanling pigs, the clinical symptoms of dietary lead toxicity were reduced, thereby implying that high dietary calcium has a protective effect against the adverse effects of dietary lead.

Of further interest with respect to the Quarterman et al. (1978) report was that dietary calcium supplementation did not enhance the release of lead from bones, a position advocated by Aub et al. (1925, 1926, 1935) based on research with lead-intoxicated patients.[2] In fact, Quarterman et al. (1978) suggest "that the efficacy of calcium administration in individuals with lead poisoning may require reexamination." Furthermore, based on their study with rats and previous research with lambs, Quarterman et al. (1978) suggested that lead is lost most quickly from the body when the calcium is given at the normally required quantities. They concluded by stating that "if modifications of dietary calcium and phosphate were to be used to counteract lead poisoning, a distinction may have to be made between prophylactic and curative treatments. To reduce the fraction of ingested lead which is absorbed, dietary calcium and phosphate should be increased to at least twice requirements. If, however, a subject is removed from exposure to lead and it is required to release lead from the body as rapidly as possible, then dietary calcium should be at about requirement level."

[2]From a historical perspective, it was initially thought that lead and calcium had a rather close metabolic relationship. Aub et al. (1926) stated that "it has been shown by chemical studies with animals that an analogy exists in the metabolism of calcium and lead. Various decalcifying agents have been shown to increase lead output. Conversely, the conditions favoring calcium retention also tend to a complete storage of lead in the bones." This statement is based on the observation that no lead could be found in the bones of rachitic rats who were given lead, while rats allowed to recover from rickets exhibited significant lead levels in their bones. It was therefore concluded that situations that permit calcium retention also enhance lead deposition in bones, while the reverse is also true. In the presence of acute symptoms of poisoning, the main objective was to bring about a decrease in the quantity of circulating lead by hastening its storage in harmless deposits in the skeleton. To accomplish this end, a high calcium and phosphorus intake was recommended (Shils, 1948; Shelling, 1932). According to Shelling (1932), the consumption of calcium salts does not guarantee an improved calcification unless the phosphorus level is also closely regulated. In fact, he reports that the "addition of calcium to lead diets which contain an inadequate amount of phosphorus does not lead to improved deposition of either calcium or lead phosphate in the bones but, on the contrary, it inhibits such a process. The deposition of calcium phosphate in the course of normal ossification, or the deposition of other insoluble phosphates such as strontium or lead, can occur only when the phosphorus intake is adequate for their deposition and for the excretion of the excess cations as the insoluble salts in the feces.

"On theoretical grounds alone, it would seem logical that if the aim of therapy in lead poisoning is to deposit or excrete the lead in an insoluble and hence in an innocuous form, i.e. as the phosphate, an abundance of phosphorus or foods containing phosphorus should be supplied."

A potentially important new direction in this area was undertaken by Levander (1979) who investigated the interaction between a calcium and vitamin E deficiency with respect to lead toxicity (Table 6). The experiment revealed that when rats were reared on a diet deficient in vitamin E and with 75% of the daily requirement of calcium, lead toxicity as measured by decreased filterability of red cells in the spleen was markedly enhanced over the respective control groups, thereby suggesting the importance of multiple nutritional factors interacting to enhance lead toxicity. Finally, an enhancement of lead retention by a combined deficiency of minerals and fat has been reported by Barltrop and Khoo (1975) (Figure 1-2).

Dose-Response Relationship of Pb. While it is well established that inadequate levels of dietary calcium enhance the retention of dietary lead, it is necessary to develop a more quantitative dose-response relationship. The first effort to attempt such a quantitative assessment was published by Shields and Mitchell (1941), since all previous work had utilized diets with lead levels greatly in excess of those found in practical human exposure levels. However, the most systematic approach was reported by Mahaffey (1974) who evaluated the influence of varying doses of lead (0, 3, 12, 48, 96, and 200 μg Pb/ml of drinking water) on normal (0.7%) and low-calcium (0.1%) diets for 10 weeks. The levels of Pb in drinking water that resulted in similar degrees of Pb uptake for kidney tissue on normal and low-calcium diets are compared (Table 7). It shows that a 200 μg/ml exposure for a rat on a normal-calcium diet is equivalent to calcium-deficient rats exposed to approximately 12 μg Pb/ml. Table 8 offers a similar comparison for several other parameters of lead effects. These data indicate that lead retention is markedly enhanced at all of the concentrations observed, although the rate was highest at the 96 μg/ml concentration. However, it should be emphasized that although 3 μg/ml "appears" low, it actually represents 3000 μg/L as compared to the EPA drinking-water standard for lead of 50 μg/L. Of particular interest is that even those rats reared on the low-calcium diet with no apparent lead exposure had 3.6 times greater renal Pb levels than the controls. The authors noted that the background levels of dietary lead were less than 1 ppm. This suggests that rats with lead exposure in the diet at $<$ 1.0 ppm are also at risk to greater lead retention if reared on a low-calcium diet.

Human Studies. There have been several case-control epidemiological studies that have attempted to evaluate the influence of dietary calcium levels on the retention of lead in children (Sorrell et al., 1977;

Table 6. Effect of Calcium and Vitamin E Deficiencies on the Filterability of Erythrocytes from Lead-Poisoned and Nonpoisoned Rats[a]

| Dietary Supplement | | Lead in Water (ppm) | Filtration Time (sec) after Incubation for | | | | |
Calcium (%)	Vitamin E (ppm)		0 hr	1 hr	2 hr	4 hr	6 hr
0.5	100	0	13 ± 1[a]	16 ± 1[a]	19 ± 1[a]	26 ± 3[a]	32 ± 3[a]
0.5	100	250	12 ± 0[a]	14 ± 0[a]	18 ± 1[a]	23 ± 2[a]	29 ± 2[a]
0.5	0	0	12 ± 1[a]	17 ± 1[a]	24 ± 3[a]	47 ± 9[a]	> 600[b]
0.5	0	250	13 ± 1[a]	16 ± 1[a]	18 ± 1[a]	29 ± 3[a]	495 ± 62[b]
0.375	100	0	13 ± 1[a]	16 ± 0[a]	19 ± 1[a]	30 ± 1[a]	43 ± 12[a]
0.375	100	250	15 ± 2[a]	18 ± 2[a]	18 ± 1[a]	24 ± 1[a]	35 ± 7[a]
0.375	0	0	12 ± 1[a]	14 ± 1[a]	18 ± 1[a]	34 ± 6[a]	559 ± 42[b]
0.375	0	250	37 ± 20[a]	193 ± 136[a]	222 ± 128[b]	292 ± 111[b]	> 600[b]

[a] Mean values of 4 rats ± SE; means in the same column with different superscript letters differ significantly at the $P <$ 0.05 level (Duncan's multiple range test).

Source: Levander, O. (1979). *Environ. Health Perspect.* **29**:115– 125.

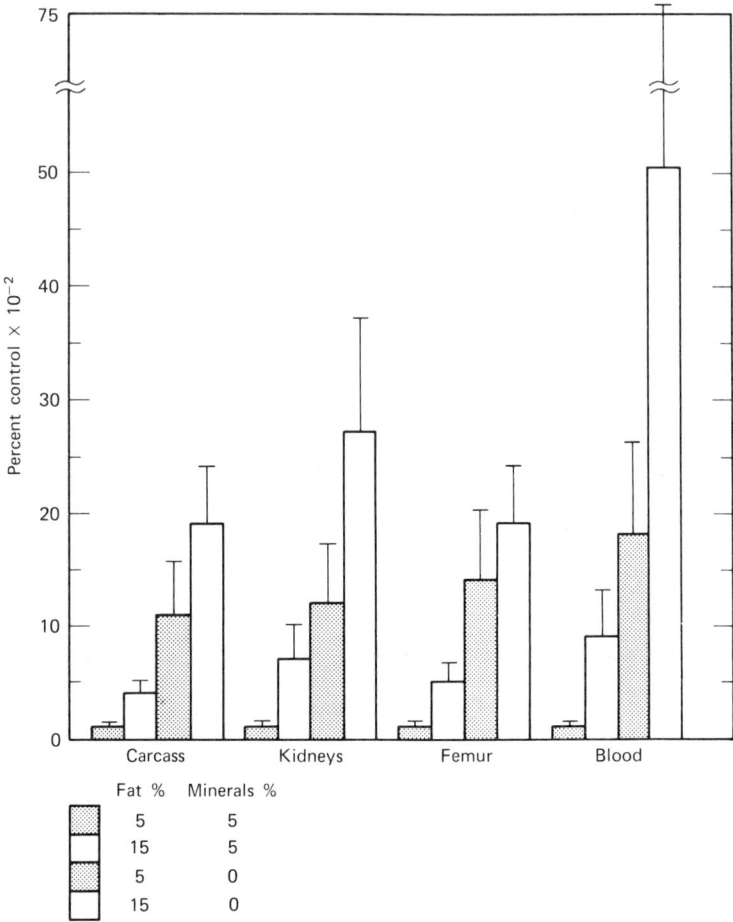

Figure 1-2. Pb uptake in rats fed diets of varying fat and mineral content. Percentage composition of diets calculated from measured addition to a fat and mineral deficient mix. Each value represents a mean + S.D., $n = 6$. [*Source.* Barltrop and Khoo (1976). *Sci. Total Environ.* **6**:268.]

Strehlow and Barltrop, 1978; Johnson and Tenuta, 1979). These epidemiological studies have usually identified young children with variable levels of lead in their red blood cells and then arbitrarily separated them into three groups according to their blood lead levels. At that time an assessment was made of their current intake of a number of nutrients including calcium, which have been associated with lead toxicity. Unfortunately, comprehensive characterization of the child's environment including household lead paint in all areas of access to

Table 7. Renal Pb Content of Animals Fed Normal and Low Ca Diets with Varying Concentrations of Pb

Pb in Drinking Water (μg/ml)	Renal Pb (μg/g wet tissue)[a]	
	Normal Ca Diet	Low Ca Diet
—	1.0 ± 0.1	3.6 ± 0.5
3	1.3 ± 0.1	6.6 ± 1.4
12	1.9 ± 0.1	19.6 ± 2.0
48	5.1 ± 0.4	154 ± 51
96	6.9 ± 0.7	629 ± 170
200	21.3 ± 3.8	942 ± 362
400	20.4 ± 1.9	

[a] Mean $\pm$ 1 SE.
Source: Mahaffey, K.R. (1974). Nutritional factors and susceptibility to lead toxicity. *Environ. Health Perspect.* **7:**107–112. These data were adapted from Mahaffey, K.R. et al., *J. Lab. Clin. Med.* **82:**92–100, 1973.

the child including soil, drinking water, and ambient air have not been compared between the respective groups. Consequently, while these studies have supported previous animal-model investigations, their experimental designs have not been sufficient to yield definitive conclusions.

Finally, in 1943 Kehoe et al. administered to two healthy subjects 1 and 2 mg of soluble lead daily for 40 and 23 months, respectively. Variations in calcium and phosphorus ingestion offered no appreciable effects on the absorption and gross retention of the lead.

Pica and Calcium Deficiency. In 1974 an interesting hypothesis was put forth by Snowdon and Sanderson stating that lead pica behav-

Table 8. The Minimal Concentration of Lead in Drinking Water of Rats Fed a Low Ca Diet that Will Produce Various Signs of Lead Intoxication

	Minimal Toxic Dose (μg/ml)	
	Low Ca Diet	Normal Ca Diet
Inclusions	12	200
Urinary δ-ALA	12	200
Kidney weight	3	200

Source: Mahaffey, K.R. (1974). Nutritional factors and susceptibility to lead toxicity. *Environ. Health Perspect.* **7:**107–112. These data were adapted from Mahaffey, K.R. et al., *J. Lab. Clin. Med.* **82:**92–100, 1973.

ior may be caused in part by a dietary deficiency in calcium. Subsequent testing of this theory revealed that weanling rats reared on a low-calcium diet "voluntarily" ingested solutions of lead acetate significantly more frequently than did a control group on a normal diet and rats reared on an iron-deficient diet. Furthermore, the occurrence of increased consumption of drinking water with elevated lead levels by rats on calcium-deficient diets was in marked contrast to the response of rats reared on normal diets, who found such high levels of lead to be unpalatable.

These findings were subsequently confirmed in monkeys in 1976 by Jacobson and Snowdon. Of importance is that the low-calcium diet was only a marginal deficiency, being 64% of normal. The study revealed that following an initial positive taste response, the normal monkeys rapidly acquired an aversion for the lead solution, while the marginally calcium-deficient monkeys did not develop the aversion for the lead ingestion and continued to ingest the lead at fairly high rates of consumption. However, if the deficient animals were given sufficient calcium to completely overcome their calcium deficiency, then an aversion to the lead solution developed as in the controls. Similar elimination of ingestion of lead solutions by calcium-deficient rats was achieved upon complete restoration of normal calcium levels in the diet, while partial restoration did not eliminate the preferential consumption of the lead solutions (Snowdon, 1976).

Snowdon and Sanderson (1974) have proposed that the voluntary consumption of lead solutions by calcium-deficient rats is an adaptive behavior since the lead may be serving to relieve some of the symptoms of calcium deficiency. They suggested that this relief would offer a reinforcement for continued lead ingestion even after the onset of lead toxicity symptoms. In an attempt to test this hypothesis, Snowdon (1976) reported that calcium-deficient rats, when offered lead solutions to drink, gained significantly more weight than deficient rats not offered the lead solutions.

These data clearly indicate that both rats and monkeys when reared on a calcium-deficient diet voluntarily consume solutions of drinking water with elevated levels of lead. Whether this occurs in children is not known. According to Snowdon (1976) the major limitation of this theory is that children with lead pica have rarely been diagnosed as being deficient in any nutrient other than iron. However, an iron deficiency is more easily recognizable than a calcium deficiency. Thus, if the findings of Snowdon and colleagues applied to humans, a serious situation would exist because of the markedly enhanced retention of lead in individuals with calcium-deficient diets.

Special Sensitivities of the Young. Of particular concern with respect to lead toxicity are the very young because of their potential environmental exposures to lead especially from lead paint, the large number who consume inadequate diets, and the well-known damage that lead may cause to the developing central nervous system. In addition, it is recognized that young animals (i.e., mice and rats) have a more markedly enhanced capacity to absorb heavy metals including lead via the gastrointestinal tract than adults (Shields et al., 1939; Kostial et al., 1973; Forbes and Reina, 1972; Matsusaka, 1972; Kello and Kostial, 1973; Kostial et al., 1975; Jugo, 1975, 1977). Similar trends have also been observed in studies with humans (Alexander et al., 1972, 1974). The magnitude of the differential rate of absorption can be considerable in certain situations. For example, 1-week-old rats exhibited a gastrointestinal tract absorption rate of $^{203}HgCl$ some 40 times greater than adults (Jugo, 1975), while 1-day-old rats displayed a gastrointestinal tract absorption rate for plutonium-239 some 85 times higher than adults (Ballou, 1958). Similar marked increases in animals prior to weaning also occur with other radionuclides such as ^{95}Zr, ^{95}Nb (Shiraishi and Ichikawa, 1972), curium-244, californium-252 (Sullivan, 1973), and radium-226 (Taylor et al., 1962).

Although most of the studies concerning the influence of calcium on dietary lead retention have utilized adult animals, there is some information concerning the influence of calcium on lead uptake in newborn rats (Kostial et al., 1971, 1973). Their data revealed that the retention of lead-203 was about 1.4 times lower in the newborn rats given calcium and phosphate additives than in rats fed an unsupplemented milk regimen. Such findings suggest that newborn rats are at increased risk to lead not only from developmental but also dietary factors. These data should be considered of extreme potential public health significance.

Potential Mechanisms Underlying Calcium/Phosphorus and Lead Interactions. A primary issue is how does consumption of a diet low in calcium enhance the retention of lead (from the diet) as compared to consumption of a diet with normal levels of calcium. It is obvious that a greater retention of lead may be the result of either an enhanced gastrointestinal tract absorption rate[3] or a decreased excretion rate or a combination of both. Until a recent report by Barton et al.

---

[3]Lead is absorbed primarily from the small intestine, with the maximal amount being in the duodenum where bile facilitates the transport of lead across the mucosal epithelial cells of the intestine into the body (Conrad and Barton, 1978).

(1978) (see Goyer [1978] for a related editorial), most researchers seemed to be of the opinion that diets low in calcium facilitated the gastrointestinal absorption of lead. Support for this perspective was given initial impetus by Schroeder (1965) who speculated that the absorption of trace metals by nearly all types of plants and animals is inversely related to the concentration of calcium in the medium from which it is being absorbed. He further suggested the existence of a cellular transport mechanism similar in all organisms that is saturated by calcium ions and regulates the exchange of other cations from the immediate environment. Concurrent investigations by Tidball (1964), which revealed that loosely bound calcium and magnesium in the mucosal membrane control the aqueous permeability of the rat intestinal epithelium, supported the speculations of Schroeder (1965). The interaction of lead with calcium metabolism has been further explored by Mahaffey (1974) who stated that since low dietary levels of calcium enhance the absorption of lead, the existence of an active or passive competition for gastrointestinal absorption is suggested. In this regard, Quarterman et al. (1978) noted that low dietary calcium (as well as low levels of phosphate and vitamin D) stimulate an increase in the concentration of calcium-binding protein (CaBP) in the intestinal mucosa (see Wasserman and Corradino, 1974) and the influence of low dietary calcium levels on lead absorption may be explained, at least in part, if lead is transported by CaBP. Support for such an explanation is provided by Quarterman and Morrison (1975) who reported that the stimulation of lead absorption by vitamin D in rats is inhibited by cycloheximide, a protein-synthesis inhibitor.

In contrast to the assumption that diets low in calcium enhance the gastrointestinal absorption of lead, Barton et al. (1978) have reported that calcium deficiency has little influence on lead absorption by the gastrointestinal tract, but that the predominant influence of low dietary calcium is through reducing lead excretion. While previous studies measured lead retention and inferred absorption, Barton et al. (1978) actually measured absorption via studies with radioactive lead.

These findings of Barton et al. (1978) are striking since they challenge the fundamental thinking of most researchers in this area concerning the manner through which a diet low in calcium enhances the retention of lead. In light of their findings, it is important to ask: Does the extent of reduced lead excretion in rats reared on a calcium-deficient diet explain the exceptional capacity of deficient animals to retain lead? For example, the deficient rats had an increased lead-retention rate of approximately 3% over a 6-week period (Barton et al., 1978). Is this sufficient to explain differences of lead retention in the

Mahaffey et al. (1973) study of over 3–40 times that of the normally fed controls?

The study of Barton et al. (1978) is clearly important in attempting to understand the mechanisms of how dietary calcium affects lead retention. It is imperative that it be replicated and extended in order to more properly assess the influence of gastrointestinal tract absorption and kidney function after lead retention. Particular emphasis should be placed on reevaluating the role of dietary calcium on the production and availability of CaBP in the gastrointestinal tract since it also binds lead, thereby facilitating its absorption, especially in the absence of calcium. This is especially important since Quarterman et al. (1978) had previously theorized that low-calcium diets enhance CaBP, thereby facilitating the absorption of lead while the inverse of this relationship was speculated to occur also; that is, at elevated levels of calcium in the diet, less CaBP would be available (as a result of a biofeedback mechanism), thereby resulting in less lead being absorbed. The Barton et al. (1978) study has seriously challenged this perspective. The resolution of this controversy may answer in large part, how lead may or may not be retained.

Finally, Barton et al. (1978) have mentioned that "there is a diminished excretion of lead associated with calcium deficient diets" citing the following reports (Lederer and Bing, 1940; Grant et al., 1938; Shields and Mitchell, 1941; Willoughby et al., 1972; Six and Goyer, 1970; Quarterman and Morrison, 1975; Quarterman et al., 1978). Careful review of these articles does not reveal support for the Barton et al. (1978) statements. The retention of intraperitoneally administered lead was not significantly affected by dietary calcium (Quarterman and Morrison, 1975; Lederer and Bing (1940), while other studies provided lead exposure orally, thereby making it impossible to differentiate precisely between the effects of absorption and excretion (Six and Goyer, 1970).

Several other metabolic interactions of calcium with lead of biomedical significance occur and should be mentioned in order to achieve a proper perspective.

An interaction of calcium and lead in the kidney takes place, with lead modifying the renal reabsorption of calcium. However, since calcium is primarily reabsorbed in the renal tubule while lead is known to affect the proximal renal tubule (see Goyer and Rhyne, 1973), lead will exhibit less disruption to calcium transport excretion than to phosphorus, glucose, or amino acids. Additionally, Mahaffey (1974) stated that a low-calcium diet enhances the retention of lead in bone to a lesser extent than soft tissue (kidney tissue). This may possibly be explained by an inherently lower total binding capability of bone for lead in animals on the low-calcium diet (Mahaffey, 1974) or by altering the partitioning of lead from the relatively fixed fraction in bone to the diffusable pool in soft tissues (Lin-Fu, 1973). Furthermore, lead and calcium may interact within the parathyroid gland. Hunter (1969) and Aub (1926) have reported that the administration of parathyroid hormone to humans enhances the urinary excretion of Pb as well as Ca. Since parathyroid hormone is thought to influence deposition and reabsorption of the mineral component of bone, mobilization of Pb, as well as Ca, suggests that Pb may be deposited with bone calcium (Sawin, 1969).

There is some evidence to suggest that lead decreases the transfer of calcium and strontium across the duodenal wall of rats and that the decrease is dose dependent (Gruden et al., 1974). Subsequent research by Gruden (1975) revealed that lead causes its effect on calcium absorption by modifying passive (as opposed to active) transport.

Summary and Conclusions. It has been demonstrated that the toxicity of dietary lead is markedly enhanced with diets having less than recommended levels of calcium and phosphorus (Mahaffey et al., 1977; Barltrop and Khoo, 1975, 1976). This has been demonstrated to occur in a variety of species including fish (Jones, 1938), mice (Tompsett and Chalmers, 1939), rats (Barltrop and Khoo, 1975; Grant et al., 1938; Pletscher et al., 1952), pigs (Hsu et al., 1975), dogs (Calvery et al., 1938), lambs (Morrison et al., 1977), and horses (Willoughby et al., 1972). Moreover, increased absorption of lead has also been reported in balance studies, with human infants given diets of normal infant food. Slight reductions in dietary calcium levels enhanced absorption of the lead found in these normal diets (Ziegler et al., 1977).

The extent to which low levels of dietary calcium cause enhanced absorption and toxicity of lead is quite impressive. Rat studies have revealed that a decrease of calcium in the diet to 20% of normal affects a 1600% increase in lead absorption and toxicity indices (Mahaffey, 1974).

A crucial question, then, is what is the incidence of low levels of calcium in the typical American diet? Several nutritional surveys have revealed that calcium is frequently deficient in diets of low-income children. For example, a Texas survey revealed that low-income white children ingested only 73% of the recommended dietary calcium levels, while low-income blacks consumed only 47% of the recommended levels (Stubbs, 1965). Similarly, the 10-state nutritional survey (Ten State Nutrition Survey, 1968–1970) revealed that nearly 30% of children 24–36 months of age from low-income-ratio states consume approximately 50% of the RDA for calcium. In addition, 13.7% were found not to consume even 25% of the RDA. Since low-income children usually have the highest levels of lead exposure, these dietary surveys clearly imply that such children will be at significantly enhanced risk to lead toxicity. The problem of lead-induced toxicity in children is known to be a problem of profound public health significance. The findings reviewed here on the influence of low-calcium levels in the diet seem to dramatically increase the magnitude of its seriousness.

In light of the above data, it appears that the present U.S. EPA-national-drinking-water standard for inorganic lead of 0.05 mg/L (50 ppb) is not justified. This maximum-limit concentration (MLC) was designed to limit lead exposure via water to approximately 25 to 33% of the total lead exposure. However, in the EPA calculation a gastrointestinal absorption rate of 10% for lead was assumed. In light of the enhanced rate of absorption in newborn rats (e.g., up to 60%) and the additional influence of low levels of calcium, it would seem that a considerably lower MLC should have been derived. At the very least, it would seem that EPA should sponsor research to evaluate the influence of dietary levels of calcium and phosphorus on the uptake of lead from drinking water in the range of 1 to 100 ppb. Precise quantitative data in this range are not presently available.

It may be speculated that since low levels of dietary calcium and phosphorus enhance lead retention and since supplementation of those minerals in excess of the RDA by 2-4× offered greater protection than the RDA by about 50% (Quarterman et al., 1978; Barltrop and Khoo, 1975, 1976), that dietary calcium and phosphorus supplementation should be given to young children living in high-risk neighborhoods. As attractive as this proposal may seem, it should be recognized that the data supporting it are primarily with rats, with no such supportive studies conducted with humans. In addition, several potential non-beneficial (i.e., possibly adverse) effects may result from excessive calcium consumption. For example, Kletzien (1940) reported that many salts of calcium greatly diminish the assimilation of iron, while high ratios of calcium to phosphorus produce the same effect (Anderson et al., 1940). Wilgus and Patton (1939) also reported that excess dietary calcium reduces the assimilation of manganese in chicks while Thompson (1936) noted that an excess of calcium will diminish the assimilation of iodine.[4] In addition, the administration of diets high in

---

[4] All these effects of excess calcium should not be considered as adverse because an elevated quantity of dietary calcium in the diet may reduce the toxic effects and elevated levels of iodine (Thompson, 1936) and manganese (Becker and McCollum, 1938).

calcium—low in phosphorus have been found to enhance markedly the removal of lead presumably from bone, resulting in dangerously high levels of lead available to reach sensitive areas in the kidney and nervous tissue (Sobel and Burger, 1955). The burden of proof must certainly fall on those advocating the extra supplementation. It is important to evaluate thoroughly the diverse metabolic interactions of calcium to ensure that the treatment does not cause any new and unsuspected adverse health effects. At the present time such investigations still remain to be conducted.

Finally, it has recently been reported that consumption of a diet low in calcium enhances the occurrence of lead- and zinc-induced chromosomal breaks in mice and monkeys (Deknudt and Gerber, 1979; Deknudt et al., 1977). In light of their findings, Deknudt and Gerber (1979) suggested the need to "ascertain the state of calcium metabolism in persons exposed to heavy metals" and to "recommend a diet rich in calcium for persons with a risk of intoxication by these metals." It should be realized that the monkey study did not include an unexposed low-calcium control group, whereas the mouse study employed an extremely deficient level of calcium (i.e., only about 3% of normal). Consequently, although the findings of these studies are striking, considerably more research must be conducted before adequate human risk assessments may be derived.

References

Alexander, F.W.; Clayton, B.E.; and Delves, H.T. (1974). Mineral and trace metal balances in children receiving normal and synthetic diets. *Quart. J. Med. New Series* **43**:89–111.

Alexander, F.W.; Delves, H.T.; and Clayton, B.E. (1972). The uptake and excretion by children of lead and other contaminants. Proceedings of an International Symposium on Environmental Health Aspects of Lead, Amsterdam, p. 319. Commission of the European Communities, Luxembourg.

Anderson, H. D.; McDonough, K.B.; and Eluehjem, C.A. (1940). Relation of the dietary calcium-phosphorus ratio to iron assimilation. *J. Lab. Clin. Med.* **25**:464–471.

Aub, J.C. (1935). The biochemical behavior of lead in the body. *J. Amer. Med. Assoc.* **104**:87–90.

Aub, J.C.; Fairhall, L.T.; Minot, A.S.; and Reznikoff, P. (1925). Lead Poisoning. Medicine. 4:1.

Aub, J.C.; Fairhall, L.T.; Minot, A.S.; and Reznikoff, P. (1926). Lead Poisoning. Medicine Monographs, Vol. 7. Williams & Wilkins, Baltimore.

Ballou, J.E. (1958). Effects of age and mode of ingestion on absorption of plutonium. *Proc. Soc. Exp. Biol. Med.* **98**:726–727.

Barltrop, D. and Khoo, H.E. (1975). Nutritional determinants of lead absorption. In: *Trace Substances in Environmental Health*, IX, pp. 369–376. Edited by D.D. Hemphill. Univ. Missouri, Columbia.

Barltrop, D. and Khoo, H.E. (1976). The influence of dietary minerals and fat on the absorption of lead. *The Science of Total Environ.* 6:265–273.

Barton, J.C.; Conrad, M.E.; Harrison, L.; and Nuby, S. (1978). Effects of calcium on the absorption and retention of lead. *J. Lab. Clin. Med.* 91(3):366–376.

Becker, J.E. and McCollum, E.V. (1938). Toxicity of $MnCl_2$. $4H_2O$ when fed to rats. *Proc. Soc. Exp. Biol. Med.* 38:740–742.

Boyadzhiev, V. (1960). Vlizanie na kraveto mlyako i maslo vuskhu vuznikraneto i proichaneto na olovonoto otravyane mezhdu akumulatomi rabotnitsi. Nanchni Trud. vissh. med. Inst. Vulko Chervenkov 39:143.

Calvery, H.O.; Laug, E.P.; and Morris, H.J. (1938). The chronic effects on dogs on feeding diets containing lead acetate, lead arsenate, and arsenic trioxide in varying concentrations. *J. Pharmac. Exp. Ther.* 64:364.

Collier, M. (1952). Paralyse de l'accommodation d'origine saturnine: sympathetic oculodigestive. *Revue Oto-Neuro-Ophtal* 24:446.

Conrad, M.E. and Barton, J.C. (1978). Factors affecting the absorption and excretion of lead. *Gastroenterology* 74:735.

Deknudt, Gh.; Coile, A.; and Gerberg, G.B. (1977). Chromosomal abnormalities in lymphocytes from monkeys poisoned with lead. *Mutat. Res.* 45:77–83.

Deknudt, Gh.; and Gerber, G.B. (1979). Chromosomal aberrations in bone marrow cells of mice given a normal or a calcium-deficient diet supplemented with various heavy metals. *Mutat. Res.* 68:163–168.

Dizon, G.D.; Luciano, V.J.; Navarro, J.Y.; Anselmo, J.E.; and Pesigan, D.E. (1950). Lead poisoning among lead workers. *J. Phillipp. Med. Assoc.* 26:417.

Feissinger, M. (1900). Lead poisoning in lapidaries. *Lancet* ii:1466.

Forbes, G.B. and Reina, J.C. (1972). Effect of age on gastrointestinal absorption (Fe, Sr, Pb) in the rat. *J. Nutr.* 102:647–652.

Goyer, R.A. (1978). Calcium and lead interactions: some new insights. *J. Lab. Clin. Med.* 91:363.

Goyer, R.A. and Rhyne, B. (1973). Pathological effects of lead. *Internatl. Rev. Exp. Pathol.* 12:1.

Grant, R.L.; Calvery, H.O.; Laug, G.P.; and Morris, H.J. (1938). The influence of calcium and phosphorus on the storage and toxicity of lead and arsenic. *J. Pharmac. Exp. Ther.* 64:446.

Gruden, N. (1975). Lead and active calcium transfer through the intestinal wall in rats. *Toxicol.* 5:163–166.

Gruden, N.; Stantic, M.; and Buben, M. (1974). Influence of lead on calcium and strontium transfer through the duodenal wall in rats. *Environ. Res.* 8:203–206.

Hsu, F.S.; Krook, L.; Pond, W.G.; and Duncan, J.R. (1975). Interactions of dietary calcium with toxic levels of lead and zinc in pigs. *J. Nutr.* 105:112–118.

Hunter, D. (1969). *The Diseases of Occupations*. 5th edition, p. 279. English Universities Press, London.

Jacobson, J.L. and Snowdon, C.R. (1976). Increased lead ingestion in calcium-deficient monkeys. *Nature* 262:51–52.

Johnson, N.E. and Tenuta, K. (1979). Diets and lead blood levels of children who practice pica. *Environ. Res.* **18**:369–376.

Jones, J.R.E. (1938). The relative toxicity of salts of lead, zinc, and copper to the stickleback (*Gasterosteus aculeatus* L.) and the effect of calcium on the toxicity of lead and zinc salts. *J. Exp. Biol.* **15**:394.

Jugo, S. (1975). Metabolism of lead and mercury in growing organism. Ph.D. dissertation. Medical Faculty of Univ. of Zagreb, Yugoslavia.

Jugo, S. (1977). Metabolism of toxic heavy metals in growing organisms: a review. *Environ. Res.* **13**:36–46.

Kehoe, R.A.; Chola, K.J.; Hubbard, D.M.; Bamback, K.; and McNary, R.C. (1943). Experimental studies on lead absorption and excretion and their relation to the diagnosis and treatment of lead poisoning. *J. Indust. Hyg. Toxicol.* **25**:71.

Kello, D. and Kostial, K. (1973). The effect of milk diet on lead metabolism in rats. *Environ. Res.* **6**:355–360.

Kletzien, S.W. (1940). Iron metabolism I. The role of calcium in iron assimilation. *J. Nutr.* **19**:187–198.

Kostial, K.; Kello, D.; and Harrison, B.H. (1973). Comparative metabolism of lead and calcium in young and adult rats. *Int. Arch. Arbeits Med.* **31**:159–161.

Kostial, K.; Kello, D.; Jugo, S.; and Gruden, N. (1975). The effect of milk diet on toxic trace element absorption in rats. In: "Proceedings of the 18th Intern. Congress on Occupat. Health," Brighton, Eng., Sept. 14–19.

Kostial, K.; Simonovic, I.; and Pisonic, M. (1971). Lead absorption from the intestine in newborn rats. *Nature* **233**:564.

Krook, L. (1974). Calcium protects against lead poisoning. *J. Am. Diet. Assoc.* **64**:397.

Lederer, L.G. and Bing, F.C. (1940). Effect of calcium and phosphorus on retention of lead by growing organisms. *J. Am. Med. Assoc.* **114**:2457.

Levander, O. (1979). Lead toxicity and nutritional deficiencies. *Environ. Hlth. Perspect.* **29**:115–125.

Lin-Fu, J.S. (1973). Vulnerability of children to lead exposure and toxicity—part 2. *New Eng. J. Med.* **289**:1289–1293.

Lockhart, R. (1963). Milk supplementation as a prophylactic in industry. Its use and misuse. *Trans. Assoc. Ind. Med. Offrs.* **13**:65.

Longley, E.O. (1967). Myth about milk. *Factory and Plant* **5**:55.

McKenna, R. (1913). Regulations 6(i) and 31(b). Factory and Workshop Orders. HMSO, London.

Mahaffey, K.R. (1974). Nutritional factors affecting lead toxicity. *Environ. Health Perspect.* **7**:107–112.

Mahaffey, K.R. (1977). Quantities of lead producing health effects in humans: sources and bioavailability. *Environ. Health Perspect.* **19**:285–295.

Mahaffey, K.R.; Goyer, R.; and Haseman, J.K. (1973). Dose-response to lead ingestion in rats fed low dietary calcium. *J. Lab. Clin. Med.* **82**:92–100.

Mahaffey, K.R. et al. (1977). Effect of varying levels of dietary calcium on susceptibility to lead toxicity. Proceedings of the International Conference on Heavy Metals in the Environment. Toronto, Canada.

Mahaffey, K.R. et al. (1979). Differences in dietary intakes of calcium, phosphorus and iron in children having normal and elevated blood lead concentrations. *Amer. J.*

Clin. Nutr. Submitted for publication (Cited in *Environ. Health Perspect.*, Mahaffey, 1977).

Matsusaka, N. (1972). Whole body retention and intestinal absorption of [115m]Cd in young and adult mice. *Med. Biol.* (Japan) **85**:285–289.

Meredith, P.A.; Moore, M.R.; and Goldberg, A. (1977). The effect of calcium on lead absorption in rats. *Biochem. J.* **166**:531–537.

Morrison, J.N.; Quarterman, J.; and Humphries, W.R. (1977). The effect of dietary calcium and phosphate on lead poisoning in lambs. *J. Comp. Path.* **87**:417–429.

NAS (1978). Recommended Dietary Allowance. Ed. 7.

Pletscher, A.; Richterich, R.; Thoelen, H.; Ludin, H.; and Staub, H. (1952). Uber das Verhalten von Amonosaturen und Fermenten bei schwermetall-Vergiftung. 2. Mitteilung an die Wirkung von Calcium and Lavulose bei der experimentellen Bleivergiftung. *Helv. Physiol. Pharmae. Acta* **10**:328.

Quarterman, J. and Morrison, J.N. (1975). The effects of dietary calcium and phosphate on the retention and excretion of lead in rats. *Brit. J. Nutr.* **34**:351–362.

Quarterman, J.; Morrison, J.N.; and Humphries, W.R. (1978). The influence of high dietary calcium and phosphate on lead uptake and release. *Environ. Res.* **17**:60–67.

Rapoport, M. and Rubin, M.I. (1941). Lead poisoning. A clinical and experimental study of the factors influencing the seasonal incidence in children. *Am. J. Dis. Child.* **61**:245.

Sand, T. (1965). Milchgabe an Bleiarbeiter. Eine Literatursichtung. *Zentbl. Arb Med. ArhSchulz* **15**:190.

Sawin, C.T. (1969). *The hormones endocrine physiology*. Little, Brown. London, p. 135.

Schiemann, D. (1960). Prophylaxie. Therapie und Rehabilitation bei Bleiarbeitern. *Z. ges. Hyg.* **6**:20.

Schroeder, H.A. (1965). The biological trace elements, or Peripatetics through the periodic table. *J. Chron. Dis.* **18**:217.

Schweigart, H.A. (1957). Milch bei gewerblichen Vergiftungen inbesondere chronische Bleivergiftung. *Int. J. Prophyl. Med.* **1**:138.

Shelling, D.H. (1932). Effect of dietary calcium and phosphorus on toxicity of lead in the rat: rationale of phosphate therapy. *Proc. Soc. Exp. Biol. Med.* **30**:248.

Shields, J.B. and Mitchell, H.H. (1941). The effect of calcium and phosphorus on the metabolism of lead. *J. Nutr.* **21**:541.

Shields, J.B.; Mitchell, H.H.; and Ruth, W.A. (1939). The metabolism and retention of lead in growing adult rats. *J. Ind. Hyg. Toxicol.* **21**:7–23.

Shils, M.E. (1948). Applying nutrition in industry: diet and resistance to toxic substances. *J. Amer. Diet. Assoc.* **24**:473.

Shiraishi, Y. and Ichikawa, R. (1972). Absorption and retention of [144]Ce and [95]Ar-[95]Nb in newborn, juvenile and adult rats. *Health Phys.* **22**:373–378.

Six, K.M. and Goyer, R.A. (1970). Experimental enhancement of lead toxicity by low dietary calcium. *J. Lab. Clin. Med.* **76**:933–942.

Snowdon, C.T. (1976). A nutritional basis for lead pica. *Physiol. Behavior* **18**:885–893.

Snowdon, C.T. and Sanderson, B.A. (1974). Lead pica produced in rats. *Science* **183**:92–94.

Sobel, A.E. and Burger, M. (1955). The influence of calcium, phosphorus, and vitamin D on the removal of lead from blood and bone. *J. Biol. Chem.* **212**:105–110.

Sobel, A.E.; Yuska, H.; Peters, D.D.; and Kramer, B. (1940). The biological behavior of lead. I. Influence of calcium, phosphorus and vitamin D on lead in blood and bone. *J. Biol. Chem.* **132**:239.

Sorrell, M.; Rosen, J.F.; and Roginsky, M. (1977). Interactions of lead, calcium, vitamin D, and nutrition in lead-burdened children. *Arch. Environ. Health* **32**:160–164.

Stephens, R. and Waldron, H.A. (1975). The influence of milk and related dietary constituents on lead metabolism. *Fd. Cosmet. Toxicol.* **13**:555–563.

Strehlow, C.D. and Barltrop, D. (1978). Nutritional status and lead exposure in a multiracial population. Presented at: 12th Annual Conference on Trace Substances in Environmental Health, University of Missouri, Columbia, June.

Stubbs, A. (1965). Food use and potential nutritional level of 1225 Texas families. Bulletin H-B-1033, Agricultural Experimental Station, Texas A and M University, College Station, TX.

Sullivan, M.F. (1973). Absorption of curium-244 and californium-252 from the gastrointestinal tract of newborn and adult rats. Pacific Northwest Laboratory, Annual Rept. for 1973. BNWL-1850 Pt. 1. UC-48, Richland, WA. pp. 15–77.

Tanquerel des Planches, L. (1848). Lead Diseases: A Treatise with Notes and Additions on the Use of Lead Pipe and its Substitutes. Translated by S.L. Dana, p. 333. Daniel Bixby and Co., Lowell, MA.

Taylor, D.M.; Bligh, P.H.; and Duggan, M.H. (1962). The absorption of calcium, strontium, barium and radium from the gastrointestinal tract of the rat. *Biochem. J.* **83**:25–29.

Ten-State Nutritional Survey, 1968–1970. V. Dietary. U.S. Dept. HEW. Atlanta, GA, 1972.

Thawley, D.G.; Willoughby, R.A.; McSherry, B.J.; MacLeod, G.K.; MacKay, K.H.; and Mitchell, W.R. (1977). Toxic interactions among Pb, Zn, and Cd with varying levels of dietary Ca and vitamin D: hematological system. *Environ. Res.* **14**:463–475.

Thirapatsakun, T. (1970). The influence of dietary calcium and phosphorus on tissue lead distribution in foals. M.S. thesis, University of Guelph, Guelph, Ont., Canada, 1–105.

Thompson, J. (1936). The influence of the intake of calcium on the blood iodine level. *Endocrinol.* **20**:809–815.

Tidball, C.S. (1964). Magnesium and calcium as regulators of intestinal permeability. *Am. J. Physiol.* **206**:243.

Tompsett, S.L. (1939). The influence of certain constituents of the diet upon the absorption of lead from the alimentary tract. *Biochem. J.* **33**:1237–1240.

Tompsett, S.L. and Chalmers, J.N.M. (1939). Studies in lead mobilization. *Br. J. Exp. Path.* **20**:408.

Travers, E.; Rendle-Short, J.; and Harvey, C.C. (1956). The Rotherham lead-poisoning outbreak. *Lancet* **ii**:113.

Trosi, F.M. (1950). Endoarterite obliterante in un fonditone di piombo. *Medna Lav.* **41**:197.

Varanasi, U; and Gmur, D.J. (1978). Influence of water-borne and dietary calcium on uptake and retention by coho Salmon. *(Oncorhynchus kisutch).* *Toxicol. Appl. Pharm.* **46**:65–75.

Vigliani, E.C. (1954). Problemi di alimentazione per i lavoratori esposti all'azione di sostanze tossiche. *Medna Lav.* **45**:423.

Wasserman, R.H. and Corradino, R.A. (1974). Vitamin D, calcium, and protein synthesis. *Vitamin. Horm.* **31**:43–103.

Wilgus, H.S., Jr. and Patton, A.B. (1939). Factors affecting utilization in the chicken. *J. Nutr.* **18**:35–45.

Willoughby, R.A.; Thirapatsakun, T.; and McSherry, B.J. (1972). Influence of rations low in calcium and phosphorus on blood and tissue lead concentrations in the horse. *Amer. J. Vet. Res.* **33**:1165–1173.

Wittgens, H. and Niederstadt, D. (1954). Untersuchung uber der Wert der Vollmilch als angebliches Vorbeugungsmittel gegen gewerbliche Vergiftungen. *Zent. ArbMed. Arb Schutz* **4**:185.

Ziegler, E.E. et al. (1977). Absorption and retention of lead by infants. *Pediatr. Reg.* (in press). (Cited in Mahaffey, 1977).

Zielhuis, R.L. (1960). De Betekenis van de voeding voor het onstaan en het verloop van de industriele lookintoxicatie. *Voeding* **21**:399.

4. Strontium

Considerable concern has emerged with regard to the possible human health hazards resulting from the contamination of the biosphere with strontium 90, which is produced and distributed by atomic explosions. According to Comar et al. (1957), "other fission products have been considered less potentially hazardous because of lower fission yield, shorter half-life or smaller incorporation into biological systems," although there is a serious concern for both radioactive iodine (Dunning, 1956; Comar et al., 1957a) and cesium (Miller and Marinelli, 1956; Anderson et al., 1957). Of particular concern with respect to strontium is that it migrates to calcium in the food chain and is readily absorbed by plants, animals, and humans. Strontium is also known to be transported to and stored in bones as well as being conveyed in milk, thereby reaching the infant. Finally, strontium 90 may be a cause of bone cancer and possibly leukemia. (For an excellent account of the migration of strontium from the atmosphere to soil and finally to humans refer to Comar et al., 1957.)

A variety of dietary factors have been found to affect the body burden of strontium 90. For instance, consumption of milk is known to enhance its gastrointestinal absorption. Likewise, Wasserman et al. (1957) demonstrated that lactose, lysine, and arginine were more efficient at enhancing strontium 90 absorption presumably by markedly enhancing the absorption of calcium. However, of all the dietary factors that are known to affect the body burden of strontium 90, calcium has been studied in the greatest detail.

Although the first references concerning the influence of dietary calcium level on the toxicity of strontium appeared in 1910 by Lehnerdt, very little was published in this area (see Shipley and Park, 1922) until after World War II when considerable above-ground testing of nuclear weapons by the United States occurred. However, these earlier studies did not utilize radioactive strontium.

In 1955, MacDonald et al. hypothesized that calcium might modify the absorption and retention of radiostrontium primarily because of their similarity in metabolic behavior. It was thought that calcium might serve as a "biological carrier" for Sr^{90}. Support for this interpretation was presented by Copp et al. (1947) and Kidman et al. (1952) who noted that a high level of dietary calcium given prior to the administration of the radiostrontium reduced the degree of strontium retention. For example, Kidman et al. (1952) evaluated the influence of diets with low, medium, and high calcium on the retention of a single IV-administered isotope mixture of strontium 89, strontium 90, and yttrium 90 on rabbits of different ages (6 weeks old, 6 and 18 months old). The adult rabbits had been reared on these variable calcium diets since the age of 2–3 months, while the 6-week-old rabbits were the offspring of mothers reared on the variable calcium diets. The data revealed that the extent of strontium retention was inversely proportional to the level of calcium in the diet in all age groupings of the rabbit. The levels of strontium in the urine were markedly elevated in those rabbits given the greater amounts of dietary calcium, thereby providing an explanation of the enhanced retention of strontium in the rabbits reared on the low-calcium diet. Fecal excretion of strontium was less affected by diet, but it was still directly related to the level of calcium in the diet.

The findings that elevated dietary levels of calcium could reduce the retention of strontium were replicated and extended by MacDonald et al. (1955) who employed rats as the animal model in a single-dose oral exposure study. They also noted that the addition of phosphate to the diet enhanced the excretion of the strontium. Despite the findings that strontium retention was inversely proportional to the dietary level of calcium, careful examination of the MacDonald et al. (1955) data reveals that in order to reduce the strontium 90 retention by 50%, it was necessary to raise the calcium level by 2000-fold. In this and other early studies (Kawin, 1956; Catsch, 1957; Wasserman et al., 1956), the calcium carrier and radiostrontium were generally given in a single dose and skeletal retention of radiostrontium determined shortly after. On the whole, these studies did not find any significant influence of calcium on strontium retention. According to Comar et al. (1957) "short term or single dose studies usually indicate that raising the calcium level does not proportionally decrease the strontium burden. . . ." This probably happens because the animal tends to absorb more calcium when the calcium level is raised on a short-term basis.

Longer-term studies as presented by Wasserman et al. (1957) revealed that increased dietary levels of calcium will diminish proportionally the skeletal retention of radioactive strontium in developing rats. When calcium levels ranging from 0.5 to 2.0% in diet were fed for 15 days, this fourfold increase in dietary calcium decreased radiostrontium retention by a factor of 3, while at 45 days a true stoichiometric relationship was reported. Yet even the use of longer-term studies did not immediately end the controversy since Palmer et al. (1958) found that increased levels of dietary calcium did not result in proportional decreases in retained radiostrontium in the mature female rat. However, subsequent studies by Wasserman and Comar (1960) attempted to resolve this apparent conflict by revealing that "(a) in immature rats (as used by Wasserman et al., 1957) elevated dietary calcium levels (within physiological ranges) with or without increased phosphorus levels would almost proportionally reduce the body burden of dietary radiostrontium, (b) in mature rats (as used by Palmer et al., 1958), elevated dietary calcium levels alone would not proportionately reduce the radiostrontium and (c) in mature rats, simultaneous increases in dietary calcium and phosphorus levels would to some degree reduce the ultimate body burden of radiostrontium."

With respect to the influence of dietary calcium on strontium retention in humans, very little research has been published. However, several reports with human subjects do indicate that the intestinal absorption of radiostrontium in humans is inversely related to the dietary intake of calcium (Nordin et al., 1967; Hodgkinson et al., 1967).

The practical implications of these research findings lead one to address the reasonableness of using increased dietary calcium to reduce the amount of strontium in milk for consumption as well as in human tissue. Comar and Wasserman (1956) have already reported on short-term investigations with dairy cows, which revealed that a fourfold increase of dietary calcium resulted in only a 35% decrease of the strontium 90 content of the milk. Based on the research of Wasserman and his colleagues as noted above, it may be reasonably predicted that appropriate supplementation of both calcium and phosphate may diminish to a limited extent the body burden of strontium. Preliminary human studies (Nordin et al., 1967; Hodgkinson et al., 1967; Harrison et al., 1955) actually support this possibility. However, more verification of this point is needed.

The case for supplementation of human diets with additional calcium to reduce the retention of strontium should now be addressed. According to Comar et al. (1957), "it would be much more difficult to justify large increases in dietary calcium for the human population than it would be to justify similar modifications for animal rations." The quantitative data on how much supplementation is necessary to affect precise reductions in strontium retention is not known. Thus, although the concept is of interest, not enough is yet known to make any practical assessment. More importantly, this theoretical discussion should not lead one to conclude that prophylactic and/or therapeutic action is needed as a result of environmental exposure to strontium. Yet, the evidence does suggest that individuals, especially the young who have diets inadequate in calcium, may be at increased risk to retention of greater quantities of strontium than similarly exposed children with a diet adequate in calcium. These findings also lead one to speculate on the influence of other bone-seeking radionuclides such as radium-226, which is commonly found in low levels in most food supplies, especially grains, as well as in the drinking water of certain geographical areas.

References

Alexander, G.V.; Nusbaum, R.E.; and MacDonald, N.S. (1956). The relative retention of strontium and calcium in bone tissue. *J. Biol. Chem.* **218**:911–919.

Anderson, E.C.; Schuch, R.L.; Fisher, W.R.; and Langham, W. (1957). Radioactivity of people and foods. *Science* **125**:1273–1278.

Catsch, A. (1957). Uber den Einfluss isotopischer und nichtisotopischer. Trager auf die Verteifung von Radiostrontium in Organisms der Ratte. *Experientia* **13**:312–313.

Comar, C.L.; Russell, R.S.; and Wasserman, R.H. (1957). Strontium-calcium movement from soil to man. *Science* **126**:485–492.

Comar, C.L.; Trum, B.F.; Kuhn, U.S.G.; Wasserman, R.H.; Noid, M.M.; and Schooley, J.C. (1957a). Thyroid radioactivity after nuclear weapons tests. *Science* **126**:16–18.

Comar, C.L. and Wasserman, R.H. (1956). Progress in nuclear energy series VI, *Biological Sciences* (Pergamon, London). Vol. 1, p. 153.

Comar, C.L.; Wasserman, R.H.; and Nold, M.M. (1956). Strontium-calcium discrimination factors in the rat. *Proc. Soc. Exp. Biol. Med.* **92**:859–863.

Comar, C.L.; Whitney, I.B.; and Lengemann, F.W. (1955). Comparative utilization of dietary-Sr^{90} and calcium by developing rat fetus and growing rat. *Proc. Soc. Exp. Biol. Med.* **88**:232–236.

Copp, D.H.; Axelrod, D.J.; and Hamilton, J.G. (1947). The deposition of radioactive metals in bone as a potential health hazard. *Am. J. Roent. and Radium Therapy.* **58**:10.

Dunning, G.M. (1956). Two ways to estimate thyroid dose from radioiodine in fallout. *Nucleonics* **14**(2):38–41.

Harrison, G.E.; Raymond, W.H.A.; and Tretheway, H.C. (1955). The metabolism of strontium in man. *Clin. Sci.* **14**:681–695.

Hendrix, J.Z.; Alcock, N.W.; and Archibald, R.M. (1963). Competition between calcium, strontium, and magnesium for absorption in the isolated rat intestine. *Clin. Chem.* 9:734–744.

Hodgkinson, A.; Nordin, B.E.C.; Hambleton, J.; and Oxby, C.B. (1967). Radiostrontium absorption in man: suppression by calcium and by sodium alginate. *Canad. Med. Assoc. J.* 97:1139–1143.

Kawin, B. (1956). Biol. Research Annual Rep. Hanford Atomic Products Operation, HW-47,500, pp. 74.

Kidman, B.; Tutt, M.L.; and Vaughan, J.M. (1952). The retention and excretion of radioactive strontium and yttrium (SR[89], Sr[90] and Y[90]) in the healthy rabbit. *J. Path. Bacteriol.* 42:209–227.

Lehnerdt, F. (1910). Zur Frage der Substitution des Calciums im Knochensystem durch Strontium. Beitrage zur Pathologischen Anatomie und zur Allgemeinen Pathologie XLVII, 215 (cited in Shipley and Park, 1922).

MacDonald, N.S.; Spain, P.C.; Ezmirlian, F.; and Rounds, D.E. (1955). The effects of calcium and phosphate in foods on radiostrontium accumulation. *J. Nutr.* 57:555–563.

Miller, C.E. and Marinelli, L.D. (1956). Gamma-ray activity of contemporary man. *Science* 124:122–123.

Nordin, B.E.C.; Smith, D.A.; Shimmins, J.; and Oxby, C. (1967). The effect of dietary calcium on the absorption and retention of radiostrontium. *Clin. Sci.* 32:39–48.

Palmer, R.F.; Thompson, R.G.; and Kornberg, H.A. (1958). Effect of calcium on deposition of strontium-90 and calcium-45 in rats. *Science* 127:1503–1506.

Palmer, R.F.; Thompson, R.C.; and Kornberg, H.A. (1958a). Factors affecting the relative deposition of strontium and calcium in the rat. *Science* 128:1505–1506.

Shipley, P.G. and Park, E.A. (1922). Studies on experimental rickets. XX. The effects of strontium administration on the histological structure of the growing bones. *Johns Hopkins Hospital Bulletin* No. 376:216.

Wasserman, R.H. and Comar, C.L. (1960). Effect of calcium and phosphorus levels on body burdens of ingested radiostrontium. *Proc. Soc. Exp. Biol. Med.* 103:124–129.

Wasserman, R.H.; Comar, C.L.; and Papadopouleu, D. (1957). Dietary calcium levels and retention of radiostrontium in the growing rat. *Science* 126:1180–1182.

Wasserman, R.H.; Schooley, J.C.; and Comar, C.L. (1956). Midyear. Report Oak Ridge Inst. Nuclear Studies Pub. ORINS-16, p. 24.

B. ORGANIC SUBSTANCES

1. Carbon Tetrachloride/Chloroform

An interesting note of historical significance is that dietary levels of calcium are known to affect the occurrence of carbon tetrachloride toxicity (Minot and Cutler, 1928). These authors noted that although very large doses of carbon tetrachloride do not cause acute toxicity in dogs reared on a balanced mixed diet (see Lamson et al., 1923), the same or even much smaller doses caused a highly toxic, even fatal response in dogs on a diet of lean meat without bones (Minot, 1927). Since the fundamental difference between these two diets was thought to be their calcium content, it was hypothesized that low levels of calcium in the diet could markedly enhance the toxicity of carbon tetrachloride.

Minot and Cutler (1928) extended these earlier findings by studying the influence of calcium on the toxicity of carbon tetrachloride, chloroform, and guanidine in dogs. In agreement with the earlier studies, they reported that ingesting large doses of carbon tetrachloride causes acute toxicity in dogs reared on a meat diet noticeably low in calcium. However, with the addition of calcium to such a deficient diet, the extent of the toxicity is markedly diminished. The toxicity characteristics of carbon tetrachloride in the dog include "gastrointestinal irritation, nervous hyperexcitability usually followed by depression, bilirubinemia, a retention of guanidine in the blood and hypoglycemia and severe central necrosis of the liver."[5]

Further investigations revealed that the etiologic agent for much of the toxicity was the retained guanidine. In fact, exposure to guanidine so as to approximate the blood guanidine levels in carbon-tetrachloride-exposed dogs, resulted in comparable toxic symptoms. Furthermore, the administration of calcium was also found to protect against the toxicity of guanidine.

It was speculated by Minot and Cutler (1928) that calcium protects against carbon tetrachloride poisoning by being antagonistic to retained guanidine. It was concluded that "at least three factors contribute to the need for calcium in carbon tetrachloride poisoning: (a) the deficient calcium intake, (b) the need for extra calcium to combat the effects of guanidine, and (c) the reduction of ionized calcium in the blood by combination with retained bile pigments. Practical suggestions for the safe use of carbon tetrachloride would emphasize the importance of a liberal calcium diet and the avoidance of meat which tends to increase guanidine retention."

It must be realized that these investigators utilized levels of carbon tetrachloride that greatly exceed normal occupational exposures as well as diets highly deficient in calcium. Consequently, the recommendations of Minot and Cutler (1928) must be taken in that light. However, because of the paucity of data concerning the influence of dietary factors affecting carbon tetrachloride toxicity in humans, it would seem that a prospective epidemiologic study evaluating the

---

[5]Similar toxicological symptoms appear following exposure to elevated levels of chloroform and when alcohol is given along with carbon tetrachloride.

hypothesis outlined here be initiated. In addition, more realistic evaluations with respect to pollutant exposures and calcium consumption should be undertaken in appropriate animals in chronic toxicity evaluation.

References

Lamson, P.D.; Gardner, G.H.; Gustafson, R.K.; Maire, E.D.; McLean, A.J.; and Wells, H.S. (1923). The pharmacology and toxicology of carbon tetrachloride. *J. Pharmacol. Exper. Therap.* **22**:215.

Minot, A.S. (1927). The relation of calcium to the toxicity of carbon tetrachloride in dogs. *Proc. Soc. Exper. Biol. Med.* **24**:617.

Minot, A.S. and Cutler, J.T. (1928). Guanidine retention and calcium reserve as antagonistic factors in carbon tetrachloride and chloroform poisoning. *J. Clin. Invest.* **6**:369–402.

2.   Microsomal Enzyme Detoxification

Very little research has evaluated the influence of calcium on drug and/or pollutant detoxification or biointoxification via the activity of the hepatic microsomal enzymes. Several major review articles have addressed this issue with respect to minerals including calcium and should be consulted by the reader (Basu and Dickerson, 1974; Campbell and Hayes, 1974). However, the work of Dingell et al. (1966) represents the only original research in this area. They reared weanling rats for 40 days on a calcium-free diet and noted that the activity of hepatic drug-metabolizing enzymes was decreased as compared to pair-fed controls. For example, the livers of the control rats metabolized 13 μmoles of hexobarbital/100 g body weight/unit time as compared to only 7.9 μmoles for the calcium-deficient group. Even though the decreased metabolism of hexobarbital did not occur until 40 days on treatment, sleeping times were increased at 33 days, thereby implying an earlier effect of the calcium deficiency at sites possibly different from the microsomal system. Dingell et al. (1966) speculated that the decreased metabolism of hexobarbital in the calcium-deficient rats may be related to structural modifications in drug-metabolizing enzymes or by a specific inhibition of protein synthesis.

References

Basu, T.K. and Dickerson, J.W.T. (1974). Inter-relationships of nutrition and the metabolism of drugs. *Chem.-Biol. Interactions* **8**:193–206.

Campbell, T.C. and Hayes, J.R. (1974). Role of nutrition in the drug-metabolizing enzyme system. *Pharmacol. Rev.* **26**(3):186.

Dingell, J.V.; Joiner, P.D.; and Horwitz, L. (1966). Impairment of hepatic drug metabolism in calcium deficiency. *Biochem. Pharmacol.* **15**:971–976.

3. Oral Contraceptives

Of potential interest in attempting to understand more fully the inter-relationships of dietary calcium and heavy metals such as cadmium and lead is an assessment of the role of other agents that may affect the gastrointestinal absorption of calcium. Without quantifying the contributions of other dietary or environmental agents on calcium absorption, it would be relatively easy for researchers to overlook potentially confounding variables in the studies. In light of this concern, it is appropriate to comment briefly on the effects of oral contraceptives on the absorption of calcium. Although there is a general lack of information in this area, Caniggia et al. (1970) have reported that an oral contraceptive (i.e., an oral estrogen-progestogen combination) given to 15 postmenopausal women for six months resulted in significantly improved intestinal absorption of calcium. According to Theuer (1972), this enhancing effect of oral contraceptives is consistent with previous observations that estrogen inhibits bone resorption (Anderson et al., 1970; Riggs et al., 1969) and delays the start of osteoporosis (Davis et al., 1966). Since many women in the United States of childbearing age have been reported to consume significantly less than the RDA for calcium, Theuer (1972) concluded that "stimulation of calcium absorption by oral contraceptive agents should be beneficial."

In light of these findings, it would be of interest to evaluate the influence of oral contraceptive usage on the gastrointestinal absorption of heavy metals such as cadmium and lead.

References

Anderson, J.J.B.; Greenfield, J.W.; Posada, J.R.; and Crackel, W.C. (1970). Effect of estrogen on bone mineral turnover in mature female rats as measured by strontium-85. *Proc. Soc. Exp. Biol. Med.* **135**:883–886.

Caniggia, A.; Gennari, C.; Borrello, G.; Bencini, M.; Cesari, L.; Poggi, C.; and Escobar, S. (1970). Intestinal absorption of calcium-47 after treatment with oral estrogen-gestogens in senile osteoporosis. *Brit. Med. J.* **4**:30–32.

Davis, M.E.; Strandjord, N.M.; and Lanzi, L.H. (1966). Estrogens and the aging process. The detection, prevention, and retardation of osteoporosis. *J. Amer. Med. Assoc.* **196**:219–224.

Riggs, B.L.; Jowsey, J.; Kelly, P.J.; Jones, J.D.; and Maher, J. (1969). Effect of sex hormones on bone in primary osteoporosis. *J. Clin. Invest.* **48**:1065–1072.

Theuer, R.C. (1972). Effect of oral contraceptive agents on vitamin and mineral needs: a review. *J. Reprod. Med.* **8**(1):13–19.

4. Pesticides: Chlorinated Hydrocarbons

Decreases in the population size of certain avian species including the peregrine falcon (*Falco peregrinus*) and sparrow hawk (*Accipiter nisus*) since the middle 1940s and early 1950s has been related to chlorinated hydrocarbon insecticide exposure and its capacity to cause eggshell thinning (Ratcliffe, 1967; Potts, 1968; Hickey and Anderson, 1968; Tucker, 1971; Porter and Wiemeyer, 1969; Lehner and Egbert, 1969). That dietary levels of calcium could affect the capacity of chlorinated hydrocarbon insecticides to reduce reproductive success in birds was first suggested by Bitman et al. (1969) who noted that Japanese quail fed a low (0.56%) calcium diet with 100 ppm p,p′ DDT laid eggs with thinner shells and less calcium in their shells than appropriate controls given adequate levels of dietary calcium. These findings were supported in a subsequent report by these same researchers (Cecil et al., 1971). Using the chlorinated hydrocarbon insecticide p,p′ DDT and its metabolite p,p′-DDE, they noted similar though less dramatic effects on egg-shell thinning in Japanese quail given a diet with 2.7% calcium (i.e., a level of calcium sufficient for breeding Coturnix quail) for a 4-month period.

More recently, Robson et al. (1976) reported that low dietary levels of calcium (0.5%) reduced the fertility of eggs, the hatchability of fertile eggs, as well as increased the incidence of cracked eggs in DDT- and/or DDE-treated Japanese quail as compared to their control groups with calcium levels of 3.0% and/or no pesticide. A similar interaction of a low-calcium diet with a different chlorinated hydrocarbon insecticide, dieldrin, was also reported to occur in the Japanese quail (Reading et al., 1976).

In apparent contrast to the above findings, Jefferies (1967) noted that egg production in p,p′-DDT exposed Bengalese finch was not affected by differential levels of calcium in the diet. In addition, Chang and Stokstad (1975) and Scott et al. (1975) also were not able to demonstrate an adverse effect from DDE or DDT on eggshell quality in Japanese quail reared on diets with calcium levels of 2, 3.5, or 3.7%.

Although there is not complete agreement on the matter, there are considerable data that suggest that low levels of dietary calcium (0.5%)

will enhance the toxicity of several chlorinated hydrocarbon insecticides with respect to various parameters of reproductive success for the Japanese quail, such as hatchability of fertile eggs. As usual, the concentration of the pesticides employed markedly exceeded quantities that would normally be encountered in the environment. Whether an enhancement of toxicity would occur at the lower concentrations of insecticide exposure was not tested. Thus the significance of the interaction is not especially striking. Another issue not addressed by the researchers concerns the prevalence of a dietary inadequacy of calcium in birds in their natural habitats. If it could be demonstrated that inadequate dietary calcium intakes are not infrequently encountered, then additional concern could be directed toward more precisely quantifying this potential enhanced-risk condition.

References

Bitman, J.; Cecil, H.C.; Harris, S.J.; and Fries, G.F. (1969). DDT induces a decrease in eggshell calcium. *Nature* **224**:44–46.

Cecil, H.C.; Bitman, J.; and Harris, S.J. (1971). Effects of dietary p,p'-DDT and p,p'-DDE on egg production and egg shell characteristics of Japanese quail receiving an adequate calcium diet. *Poult. Sci.* **50**:657–659.

Chang, E.S. and Stokstad, E.L.R. (1975). Effect of chlorinated hydrocarbons on the shell gland carbonic anhydrase and egg-shell thickness in Japanese quail. *Poult. Sci.* **54**:3–10.

Hickey, J.J. and Anderson, D.W. (1968). Chlorinated hydrocarbons and eggshell changes in raptorial and fish-eating birds. *Science* **162**:271–273.

Jefferies, D.J. (1967). The delay in ovulation produced by p,p' DDT and its possible significance in the field. *Poult. Sci.* **109**:266–272.

Lehner, P.N. and Egbert, A. (1969). Dieldrin and eggshell thickness in ducks. *Nature* **224**:1218.

Porter, R.D. and Wiemeyer, S.N. (1969). Dieldrin and DDT. Effects on sparrow hawk eggshells and reproduction. *Science* **165**:199–200.

Potts, G.R. (1968). Success of eggs of the shag on the Farne Islands, Northumberland, in relation to their content of dieldrin and p,p' DDE. *Nature* **217**:1282–1284.

Ratcliffe, D.A. (1967). Decrease in eggshell weight in certain birds of prey. *Nature* **215**:208–210.

Reading, C.M.; Arscott, G.H.; and Tinsley, I.J. (1976). Effect of dieldrin and calcium on the performance of adult Japanese quail (*Coturnix coturnix japonica*). *Poult. Sci.* **55**:212–219.

Robson, W.A.; Arscott, G.H.; and Tinsley, I.J. (1976). Effect of DDE, DDT, and calcium on the performance of adult Japanese quail (*Coturnix coturnix japonica*). *Poult. Sci.* **55**:2222–2227.

Scott, M.L.; Zimmerman, J.R.; Marinsky, S.; Mullenhoff, P.A.; Rumsey, G.L.; and Rice, R.W. (1975). Effects of PCB's, DDT and mercury compounds upon egg production, hatch ability, and shell quality in chickens and Japanese quail. *Poult. Sci.* **54**:350–368.

Tucker, R.K. (1971). Chlorinated hydrocarbons cause thin eggshells but so may other pollutants. *Utah Sci.* **32**(2):47–49.

C. CALCIUM—POLLUTANT INTERACTIONS—A PERSPECTIVE

It has been shown that dietary calcium affects the toxicity of a variety of substances, especially heavy metals. Without much question, the primary environmental health issues associated with calcium concern how it may affect the retention and toxicity of cadmium and especially lead. It has been amply demonstrated by numerous investigators with a variety of animal models that low levels of dietary calcium markedly enhance the retention of these two heavy metals. Whether this phenomenon occurs in humans is not yet known; however, the animal data are so convincing and the public health significance so great that the burden of proof must fall on those suggesting that humans would respond in a fundamentally different manner than the animal models employed.

Of particular concern with respect to the calcium-lead interaction is that low levels of calcium enhance the retention of lead where it can do the greatest damage; that is, in the soft tissues. In contrast, a deficiency in iron will result in a greater proportion of the retained lead being stored in hard tissue such as bone, causing considerably less immediate damage (Mahaffey, 1974).

The animal studies for the most part have utilized lead exposures that greatly exceed levels normally encountered, while dietary deficient conditions have been fairly realistic with levels of calcium ranging from 20–60% of normal. While the levels of lead exceed normally encountered values, it must be recognized that many children ingest lead in the form of paint chips, which greatly exceed "average" exposure. Thus, these studies should not be deemed "unrealistic." Yet, exposure studies at such elevated levels do not provide EPA decision-makers with an appropriate quantifiable expression of how dietary inadequacies of calcium affect the retention of ambient lead. In establishing health effects criteria for a drinking-water standard for lead, such data are of profound value. Although data are clearly missing at the appropriate ranges of normal lead exposure, all available data imply that low levels of calcium in the diet would most likely enhance lead retention even at low-level exposure. Such theoretical concerns lead one to question the appropriateness of the current lead standard of 50 ppb, which assumes a gastrointestinal tract absorption rate of 10%. Such an assumption is questionable for two groups: (1) the enhanced absorption of heavy metals, including lead in the young of many species and (2) the influence of low levels of calcium enhancing lead retention. It is suggested here that EPA reevaluate the present standard for lead in drinking water since it is obvious that a large number of individuals are at markedly increased risk to retain levels of lead far in excess of what the EPA program purports to prevent. A similar rationale can be adopted for a review of the cadmium-drinking-water standard of 10 ppb as well.

The question naturally arises that if too little calcium enhances the retention of lead then consumption of calcium far in excess of the RDA will probably provide a type of insurance policy against retention of lead, cadmium, strontium, or fluoride. To a certain extent this reasoning has been found to be true. For example, Barltrop and Khoo (1975, 1976) found that consumption of calcium up to 4 times the normal levels caused marked reductions of lead retention, while 2 times normal did not have any effect. In addition, Kello et al. (1979) reported that consumption of calcium 3.5 times normal also markedly reduced cadmium retention in rats.

While there are other studies, as cited in their respective sections, that support the premise that levels of dietary calcium far in excess of the RDA offer a prophylactic potential with regard to lead retention, a strong case can be made against the dietary manipulations of tunnel-visioned individuals looking for a quick fix. For example, numerous researchers have reported that an increase in dietary calcium enhances the magnesium requirement of the rat for survival and normal development (Tufts and Greenberg, 1938; Colby and Frye, 1951; Lengemann, 1959), while Hegsted et al. (1956) reported that a high intake was harmful only when magnesium was fed at a level below the minimum requirements. Similar findings have also been reported to occur in the guinea pig (Morris and O'Dell, 1963; O'Dell et al., 1960), and dog (Bunce et al., 1962). In addition, consumption of large quantities of calcium and phosphorus have been found to cause perosis in chickens by increasing the requirement for manganese (Wilgus and Patton, 1939; Hunter, et al., 1931; Payne, 1932; Wilgus et al., 1937; Caskey and Norris, 1938; Schaible et al., 1938; Wiese et al., 1938). Such findings illustrate the importance of defining more completely the effects that differential levels of dietary calcium may have on other nutrients before recommending the use of dietary calcium supplements far in excess of the RDA in order to prevent undue lead retention. It is clear that further research is needed on the influence of highly variable intakes of dietary calcium on the physiological requirements of other nutrients in human subjects. In light of the widespread and popular usage of excess vitamins and minerals such as calcium, this type of research has important public health implications. In addition, once sufficient information is gained then more rational considerations may be given to utilizing nutrition to modify pollution toxicity.

Considerable evidence was presented concerning the possibility that low levels of calcium in the diet may predispose children exposed to fluoride to develop dental fluorosis. It is surprising that this hypothesis, which has reasonable, although not unequivocal support in animal studies and human epidemiologic investigations, has been almost totally ignored during the past 30 years. Although this may not represent a major human health problem, it does suggest a major aesthetic and social problem, especially if the dental fluorosis was of a serious degree. In light of the millions of Americans who receive community drinking water to which sodium fluoride has been added and the prevalence of inadequate calcium consumption by large segments of the population, it is of importance that further research, especially of an epidemiologic nature, be initiated in this area.

In fact, the results of 10 years of "optimal" fluoridation in Newburgh. New York, indicated "mild" dental fluorosis (mottling) in about 2% of the children who had been born since fluoridation began (Ast et al., 1956). "Mild" dental fluorosis is present when 25 to 50% of the surfaces of two or more teeth are opaque, paper-white. No brown staining from fluoride was noted. However, Dean (1942) found that some brown staining occurs in 1–2% of the children who use a water supply with 1.8 or 1.9 ppm fluoride. The question naturally arises as to why some children were affected and not others. Did these children drink considerably more of the fluoridated water? Did they have a nutritional inadequacy that predisposed them to develop dental fluorosis? At present the answers to these and related questions are not known, yet the idea that nutritional status may affect the occurrence of dental fluorosis is a reasonable hypothesis to evaluate.

References

Ast, D.B.; Smith, D.J.; Wachs, B.; and Cantwell, K.T. (1956). Newburgh-Kingston caries-fluorine study. IV. Combined clinical and roentgenographic dental findings after ten years of fluoride experience. *J. Amer. Dent. Assoc.* **52**:314.

Barltrop, D. and Khoo, H.E. (1975). Nutritional determinants of lead absorption. In: *Trace Substances in Environmental Health*, IX, pp. 369–376. Edited by D.D. Hemphill.

Barltrop, D. and Khoo, H.E. (1976). The influence of dietary minerals and fat on the absorption of lead. *The Sci. of the Total Environ.* **6**:265–273.

Bunce, G.E.; Chiemchaisri, Y.; and Phillips, P.H. (1962). The mineral requirements of the dog. IV. Effect of certain dietary and physiologic factors upon the magnesium deficiency syndrome. *J. Nutr.* **76**:23.

Caskey, C.D. and Norris, L.C. (1938). Further studies on the role of manganese in poultry nutrition. *Poult. Sci.* **17**:433.

Colby, R.W. and Frye, C.M. (1951). Effect of feeding various levels of calcium, potassium, and magnesium to rats. *Am. J. Physiol.* **166**:209.

Dean, H.T. (1942). In: *Fluorine and Dental Health,* pp. 23–32. Edited by F.R. Moulton. Washington, D.C., Assoc. Adv. Amer. Science.

Hegsted, D.M.; Vitale, J.J.; and McGrath, H. (1956). The effect of low temperature and dietary calcium upon magnesium requirement. *J. Nutr.* **58**:175.

Hunter, J.E.; Dutcher, R.A.; and Knandel, H.C. (1931). Further studies on the production of experimental slipped tendons' or hock diseases in chicks. *Poult. Sci.* **10**:392.

Kello, D.; Dekanic, D.; and Kostial, K. (1979). Influence of sex and dietary calcium absorption in rats. *Arch. Environ. Health* **34**:30–33.

Lengemann, F.W. (1959). The metabolism of magnesium and calcium in the rat. *Arch. Biochem. Biophys.* **84**:278.

Mahaffey, K. (1974). Nutritional factors affecting lead toxicity. *Environ. Hlth Perspect.* **7**:107–112.

Morris, E. R. and O'Dell, B.L. (1963). Relationship of excess calcium and phosphorus to magnesium requirement and toxicity in guinea pigs. *J. Nutr.* **81**:175–181.

O'Dell, B.L.; Morris, E.R.; and Regan, W.O. (1960). Magnesium requirement of guinea pigs and rats. Effect of calcium and phosphorus and symptoms of magnesium deficiency. *J. Nutr.* **70**:103.

Payne, L.F.; Hughes, J.S.; and Lienhardt, H.F. (1932). The etiological factors involved in the malformation of bones in young chickens. *Poult. Sci.* **11**:158.

Schaible, P.J.; Bandemer, S.L.; and Davidson, J.A. (1938). The manganese content of feedstuffs and its relation to poultry nutrition. *Mich. St. Col. Agr. Exp. Sta. Tech. Bull.* No. 159.

Tufts, E.V. and Greenberg, D.M,. (1938). The biochemistry of magnesium deficiency. II. The minimum magnesium requirement for growth, gestation, and lactation, and the effect of the dietary calcium level thereon. *J. Biol. Chem.* **122**:715.

Wiese, A.C.; Elvehjem, C.A.; and Hart, E.B. (1938). Studies of the prevention of perosis in the chick. *Poult. Sci.* **18**:33.

Wilgus, H.S., Jr.; Norris, L.C.; and Heuser, G.F. (1937). The effect of various calcium and phosphate salts on the severity of perosis. *Poult. Sci.* **16**:232.

Wilgus, H.S., Jr., and Patton, A.R. (1939). Factors affecting manganese utilization in the chicken. *J. Nutr.* **18**:35–45.

2

Copper

A. INORGANIC SUBSTANCES

1. Cadmium

Introduction. The hypothesis that the nutritional status of copper affects the toxicity of cadmium was first proposed in 1963 by Hill et al. They stated that (1) zinc and copper are interrelated in such a manner that copper can reverse some symptoms of zinc toxicity, and (2) that a zinc-cadmium antagonism is also well known, whereby zinc prevents cadmium toxicity. In light of these observations that zinc is interrelated with copper and cadmium, Hill et al. reasoned that copper and cadmium may also display a comparable interaction.

Interactions of Copper with Iron and Zinc in Preventing Cadmium Toxicity. In testing their hypothesis, Hill et al. (1963) evaluated the influence of the administration of copper and iron to a basal diet on the toxicity of cadmium ranging from 25 to 400 ppm in the diet of chicks. Note that the basal diet contained 25 ppm zinc, 10 ppm iron and 1 ppm copper. Initial studies revealed that in the absence of supplemental copper or iron, 25 ppm Cd administration caused a high incidence of mortality (i.e., 65% vs. 25% in the unexposed controls). At 200 ppm

Cd, 95% of the chicks died within the 17-day observation period. However, supplementation of the basal diet with 40 ppm of copper sulfate markedly reduced cadmium-induced lethality so that no increased mortality incidence occurred up through 100 ppm cadmium relative to the unexposed controls. Supplementation with only 100 ppm iron also reduced cadmium-induced mortality, but not to the extent of the copper. As expected, joint supplementation of both copper (10 ppm) and iron (100 ppm) was highly effective in reducing cadmium intoxication. This level of joint supplementation was quite (but not totally) effective in reducing Cd intoxication up through 200 ppm. Although both copper and iron supplements reduced the occurrence of cadmium-induced mortality, the weight of the chicks was markedly reduced at each increment of cadmium dosage. This finding led Hill et al. to conclude that the depressed weight-gain component of cadmium toxicity was not offset by the supplementation of iron and/or copper.

While it was evident that copper and iron supplementation were quite effective in preventing the toxicity of cadmium, greater supplementation with these elements, such as 50 ppm copper and 100 ppm iron or 10 ppm copper and 200 ppm iron, did not further reduce cadmium-induced mortality. However, a 10 ppm Cu and 500 ppm iron supplementation did further diminish toxicity.

Hill et al. (1963) noted that while both copper and iron were important in preventing cadmium toxicity, additional elements may be needed to prevent other components of cadmium toxicity, especially its effects on growth. Follow-up studies revealed that zinc supplementation prevented cadmium-induced growth depression while having no influence on cadmium-induced mortality. While zinc supplementation was quite specific in preventing cadmium-induced growth depression and copper supplementation was specific for prolonging survival, joint supplementation with both zinc and copper completely prevented cadmium-induced marked atony and elongation of the gizzard.

Hill et al. (1963) finally concluded that their hypothesis that copper dietary status affects the toxicity of cadmium was clearly supported in chicks. With regard to the mechanism by which copper affects cadmium toxicity, they speculated that "cadmium may replace both copper and zinc at active metabolic sites, probably enzymatic, thereby rendering them inactive. In the presence of cadmium, therefore, addition of both copper and zinc to the diet is required to restore the nutritional status of the animal to that of the controls not receiving cadmium. This presumably takes place because the additional copper and zinc displace the interfering cadmium and restores normal metabolism."

Effects of Cadmium on Copper Metabolism.   Following this initial report of Hill et al. (1963), a number of investigators have also supported the occurrence of a copper-cadmium interaction in a variety of species including mice, rats, and sheep (Mills and Dalgarno, 1972, 1972a; Schroeder and Nason, 1974; Bunn and Matrone, 1966; Whanger and Weswig, 1970; Hill and Matrone, 1970). Mills and Dalgarno (1972, 1972a) reported that copper metabolism was markedly affected in pregnant ewes and also in their lambs when they were given cadmium levels ranging from 3.5–12 mg/kg of diet. Copper levels in the liver and whole blood as well as ceruloplasmin levels were significantly reduced by cadmium treatments. However, zinc metabolism was not markedly affected. In contrast, Bremmer and Campbell (1978) found no disruption in the copper metabolism of pregnant ewes given 3 mg Cd/kg of diet. However, they noted that offspring of the cadmium-exposed pregnant ewes had lower birth weights along with signs of skeletal rarefaction and significant reductions in growth, plasma copper levels, and cytochrome-oxidase activities of the liver and duodenal mucosa.

In studies with rats, Campbell and Mills (1974) reported that as low as 1.5 mg Cd/kg of diet decreased plasma ceruloplasmin and kidney copper levels. Increasing the cadmium levels to 18 mg/kg resulted in a progressive reduction in copper levels.

How dietary cadmium may reduce the levels of copper in plasma and tissues has been addressed by several researchers. Van Campen (1966) and Starcher (1969) have proposed that cadmium may inhibit Cu absorption in rats and chicks by reducing the occurrence of copper binding to a low molecular weight protein in the mucosal cytosol. More recent experiments by Davies and Campbell (1977) have shown that cadmium does reduce copper absorption at a molar cadmium:copper ratio as low as 4:1, a ratio that was comparable to the one that produced a copper-deficiency condition in rats (Campbell and Mills, 1974). Davies and Campbell (1977) demonstrated that the binding of ^{64}Cu to the intestinal mucosa was increased even at so low as a 1:1 cadmium:copper ratio. Their data suggested that cadmium may prevent the release of copper from mucosal cells while showing little inhibitory influence on its uptake by the mucosa. While the findings of Davies and Campbell (1977) do not agree with the earlier reports of Van Campen (1966) and Starcher (1969) with respect to the influence of cadmium on the mucosal binding of copper, Bremmer and Campbell (1978) suggest that this apparent discrepancy may be the result of much higher cadmium:copper ratios employed in the earlier investigations.

Proposed Mechanisms of the Copper/Cadmium Antag-onism. An interesting though highly speculative mechanism by which dietary copper may affect the occurrence of cadmium toxicity has recently been proposed. Bremmer and Campbell (1978) have suggested that the well-known disruptions of vitamin D metabolism by cadmium may result from either the "direct inhibition by cadmium of the hydroxylation of vitamin D to the active 1,25-dihy-droxycholecalciferol or indirectly via the creation of a copper deficiency condition." Presumably, the conversion of vitamin D to its active derivative is dependent on mixed-function oxidases whose activity may be decreased both as a result of direct cadmium toxicity (Hadley et al., 1974) and/or by a copper deficiency (Moffitt and Murphy, 1973).

A chemical-physical approach toward developing a conceptual understanding of why copper and cadmium may be antagonistic has been presented by Hill and Matrone (1970). In general, they feel that those substances whose physical and chemical characteristics are alike will be biological antagonists. As for copper, it may occur in either the monovalent or divalent forms. This, of course, means that the monovalent form can accept electrons while the cupric state prefers to donate them. "The $1s$, $2s$, $2p$, $3s$, and $3p$ orbitals are filled with two electrons each. The $3d$ orbitals of the cuprous ion are also filled (Figure 2-1), the arrows in the figure representing electrons and the direction of the arrows the spin state. The cupric ion has one less electron and it happens because of energy considerations that one $3d$ electron is promoted to a $4p$ orbital, leaving a $3d$ orbital as well as the $4s$ orbital without electrons and available for bond formation. The p orbitals tend to be filled in complex formation since the complex then would have the

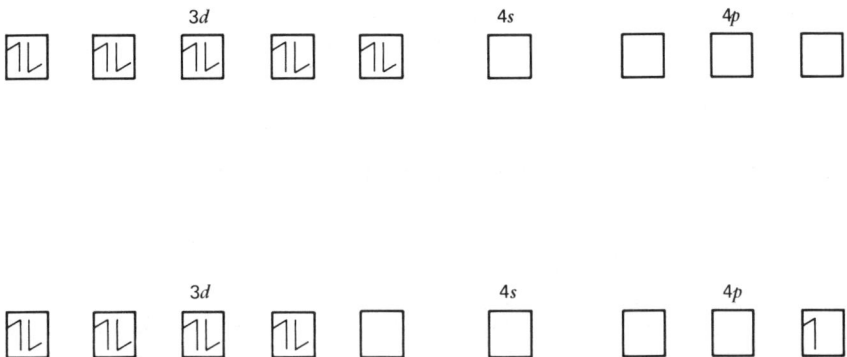

Figure 2-1. Orbital arrangement of cuprous ions (top) and a cupric ion (bottom). [*Source.* Hill and Matrone (1970). *Fed. Proc.* **29**(4):1475.]

structure of the inert, and therefore most stable, krypton. The four empty orbitals indicate that both cuprous and cupric ions should coordinate with four ligands. The structure of the complexes formed in each case, however, will be different. In cuprous complexes the structure is tetrahedral, while the cupric complexes will tend to have a square planar structure. In the former, the four ligands approach the central atom along bisectors of the Cartesian coordinates, while in the square planar complexes the ligands may be thought of as approaching the central atom along the x and y axes."

"The electronic structure of the cuprous and cupric ions is not unique. The Zn^{2+}, Cd^{2+}, and Hg^{2+} ions all have the same electronic structure of the valence shell as the cuprous ion, while the Ag^{2+} ion has the same structure as the cupric ion. . . . All of the ions should be antagonistic to copper."

While the experimental research reviewed above is consistent with the hypothesis of a copper-cadmium antagonism, Hill et al. (1964) have also evaluated the nature of copper interactions with other theoretical antagonists including zinc, silver, and mercury in chicks. In evaluating whether or not one element served as an antagonist of the copper, Hill and Matrone (1970) used the following criterion: that administration of the proposed antagonist may enhance the severity of a copper deficiency. With respect to zinc, Hill et al. (1963) reported that 200 ppm Zn reduced hemoglobin levels in the copper-deficient chicks (i.e., 1 ppm in diet) but not their controls. In addition, 100 ppm Zn caused a marked increase in mortality and a marked decrease in growth in the deficient group but not in the controls. A similar antagonism was found for silver with respect to the cupric ion. Hill et al. (1964) reported that silver reduced growth, elastic control of the aorta, and hemoglobin levels while increasing mortality in copper-deficient chicks.

In contrast to the apparent antagonism of copper with cadmium, silver, and zinc, no antagonism was found for mercury, although it was theoretically predicted to occur as noted above. They found that mercury (400 ppm) did not affect the growth and mortality incidence of chicks reared on a copper-deficient diet. However, mercury reduced the growth of chicks given a copper-supplemented diet (Hill et al., 1964). According to Hill and Matrone (1970), the explanation as to why the predictive antagonism between copper and mercury did not occur may be because the orbitals of mercury (i.e., 6s and 6p) involved were further removed from the nucleus than the 4s and 4p orbitals of the cuprous ion. They further stated that "the wave function of the 6s electrons is less than that of the 4s electrons because of the increased distance from the nucleus, and, therefore, the reactivity of the 6s electrons is much less than that of 4s electrons. The 6s orbitals have been found empirically to be relatively inert. Furthermore, mercury has been found to coordinate with two ligands linearly and form polymeric structures."

References

Anke, M. et al. (1970). The interrelationship between cadmium, zinc, copper and iron in metabolism of hens, ruminants and man. In: *Trace Element Metabolism in Animals,* p. 317. Edited by C.F. Mills. E. and S. Livingstone, Edinburgh.

Bremmer, I. and Campbell, J.K. (1978). Effect of copper and zinc on susceptibility to cadmium intoxication. *Environ. Health Perspect.* **25**:125–128.

Bremmer, I.; Young, B.W.; and Mills, C.F. (1976). Protective effect of zinc supplementation against copper toxicosis in sheep. *Brit. J. Nutr.* **36**:551.

Bunn, C.A. and Matrone, G. (1966). *In vivo* interactions of cadmium, copper, zinc, and iron in the mouse and rat. *J. Nutr.* **90**:395–399.

Campbell, J.K. and Mills, C.F. (1974). Effects of dietary cadmium and zinc on rats maintained on diet low in copper. *Proc. Nutr. Soc.* **33**:15A.

Davies, N.T. and Campbell, J.K. (1977). The effect of cadmium on intestinal copper absorption and binding in the rat. *Life Sciences* **20**:955–960.

Doyle, J.J. and Pfander, W.H. (1975). Interactions of cadmium with copper, iron, zinc, and manganese in ovine tissues. *J. Nutr.* **105**:599–606.

Hadley, W.M.; Miya, T.S.; and Bousquet, W.F. (1974). Cadmium inhibition of hepatic drug metabolism in the rat. *Toxicol. Appl. Pharmacol.* **28**:284.

Hill, C.H. and Matrone, G. (1970). Chemical parameters in the study of *in vivo* and *in vitro* interactions of transition elements. *Fed. Proc.* **29**(4):1474–1481.

Hill, C.H.; Matrone, G.; Payne, W.L.; and Barber, C.W. (1963). *In vivo* interactions of cadmium with copper, zinc, and iron. *J. Nutr.* **80**:227–235.

Hill, C.H.; Starcher, B.; and Matrone, G. (1964). Mercury and silver interrelationships with copper. *J. Nutr.* **83**:107–110.

Mills, C.F. and Dalgarno, A.C. (1972). The influence of dietary cadmium concentration on liver copper in ewes and their lambs. *Proc. Nutr. Soc.* **31**:73A–74A.

Mills, C.F. and Dalgarno, A.C. (1972a). Copper and zinc status of ewes and lambs receiving increased dietary concentrations of cadmium. *Nature* **239**:171–173.

Moffitt, A.E. and Murphy, S.D. (1973). Effect of excess and deficient copper intake on rat liver microsomal enzyme activity. *Biochem. Pharmacol.* *22*:1463.

Schroeder, H.A. and Nason, A.P. (1974). Interactions of trace metals in rat tissues. Cadmium and nickel with zinc, chromium, copper, and manganese. *J. Nutr.* **104**:167–178.

Starcher, B.C. (1969). Studies on the mechanism of copper absorption in the chick. *J. Nutr.* **97**:321.

Van Campen, D.R. (1966). Effects of zinc, cadmium, silver and mercury on the absorption and distribution of copper-64 in rats. *J. Nutr.* **88**:125.

Whanger, P.D. and Weswig, P.N. (1970). Effect of some copper antagonists on induction of ceruloplasmin in the rat. *J. Nutr.* **100**:341–348.

2. Lead

While considerable research has focused on a number of nutrient-lead interactions such as those involving calcium and iron, comparably little research has concerned possible copper-lead interactions. That copper may prevent the toxicity of lead was suggested by earlier studies, which revealed that the administration of copper in salt licks to pregnant ewes was very beneficial in preventing the development of swayback (Dunlop et al., 1939) and that the lead levels in the soil of areas where swayback is common are markedly higher than the soil in the controls' pastures (Innes and Shearer, 1940; Shearer et al., 1940).

The first major effort to evaluate the influence of dietary copper on lead toxicity was published in 1968 by Charka. He reported that dietary copper supplementation reduced the growth inhibitory effects of lead as well as enhancing its urinary excretion. This was followed by a report from Klauder et al. (1972) who exposed weanling male Sprague-Dawley rats to dietary lead (0.5% or 5000 ppm) and copper (0.5 to 2.5 ppm) for an eight-week period. They found that the lead treatment caused a reduction in the growth rate that was inversely related to the levels of copper in the diet. In addition, blood lead values were also inversely related to dietary copper levels; that is, at 0.5 ppm copper the erythrocyte lead value was 231 μg/dl while only 149 and 129 μg/dl at 1.0 and 2.5 ppm Cu, respectively. Finally, they also found that lead caused a reduction of plasma copper and ceruloplasmin levels.

In light of the above findings that (1) increased dietary copper levels prevented signs of lead toxicity, (2) the report of Six and Goyer (1972) that dietary iron could markedly diminish the toxic effects of dietary lead in rats, and (3) numerous reports that indicate that adequate copper ingestion is needed for normal iron utilization (Elveljem and Sherman, 1932; Evans and Abraham, 1973; Klauder and Petering, 1975), Klauder and Petering (1975) evaluated the influence of both dietary copper and iron on dietary lead toxicity. Once again there occurred an inverse relationship between dietary copper levels and the accumulation of lead by erythrocytes (Table 1). However, this only occurred if the dietary levels of iron were adequate. In fact, the protective effects of copper in the presence of adequate iron were not significant as a result of the more pronounced influence of the iron on blood lead levels. They concluded that there is an "additive protective effect by having optimal dietary levels of both copper and iron." Comparable effects of copper and iron on the kidney lead levels were also found (Table 2). Finally, lead-induced decreases in hematocrit and hemoglobin could be partially prevented by both copper and iron dietary supplements.

Table 1. Erythrocyte Lead

Zinc (ppm)	Iron (ppm)	Copper (ppm)	Erythrocyte Lead, μg/100 g wet weight[a]	
			Lead = 0 ppm	Lead = 500 ppm
20	6	0.5	16.0[b]	355[b,g]
20	6	8.5	29.0[c,d]*	412[c,e]
20	40	0.5	16.6[f]	155[g,f]
20	40	8.5	13.0[h,d]*	125[e,h]
140	40	0.5	17.1[i]	158[i]
140	40	8.5	18.6[j]	115[j]

[a]Geometric means given. Matched superscript letters indicate significance at $p < 0.01$; asterisk shows significance at $p < 0.05$.

Source. Klauder and Petering (1975). *Environ. Health Perspect.* **12:**77–80.

Table 2. Kidney Lead

Zinc (ppm)	Iron (ppm)	Copper (ppm)	Lead (ppm)	Kidney lead, μg/g dry weight[a]
20	6	0.5	500	1910[b]
20	6	8.5	500	1490[c]
20	40	0.5	500	126[b]
20	40	8.5	500	111[c]
140	40	0.5	500	112
140	40	8.5	500	90

[a]Geometric means given. Matched superscript letters indicate significance at $p < 0.01$; asterisk shows significance at $p < 0.05$. All control values (no Pb added) were 1–2 μg/g.

Source. Klauder and Petering (1975). *Environ. Health Perspect.* **12:**77–80.

Other research by Klauder and Petering (1975) has suggested that lead acts specifically on copper metabolism, thereby disrupting the normal utilization of iron. The biochemical lesions induced by lead have been characterized as "a reduction of serum iron, elevation of serum iron binding capacity, and an increase in liver iron, all manifestations of system effects related to an interference with copper metabolism."

In marked contrast to the findings of Klauder and his colleagues is the report of Cerklewski and Forbes (1977), which demonstrated that increasing dietary copper (1, 5, and 20 ppm) levels enhanced dietary lead (200 ppm) toxicity in rats. According to both groups of researchers, the conflict may be more apparent than real and may well be explained by differences in experimental protocol that included variations in the time of exposure as well as the dietary regimens employed.

According to Klauder and Petering (1975) the "marked increase in erythrocyte lead when dietary copper and iron are low is an important finding, as this parameter is universally used as the index of lead absorption. When rats are given 500 ppm lead in this deficient diet they actually have an internal exposure which is three times that of rats ingesting the same dose of lead given in a copper- and iron-fortified diet. Since most stock diets are excessive in both copper and iron, it may well be that resistance of rats to lead toxicity is due in large measure to the protective effects of these elements."

References

Cerklewski, F. and Forbes, R.M. (1977). Influence of dietary copper on lead toxicity in the young male rat. *J. Nutr.* **107**:143–146.

Charka, P.A. (1968). The effect of cobalt and copper salts in toxic action of lead on the animal organism. *Voprosy Pitaniia* **27**:29–33.

Dunlop, G.; Innes, J.R.M.; Shearer, G.D.; and Wells, H.E. (1939). "Swayback" studies in North Derbyshire. I. The feeding of copper to pregnant ewes in the control of "swayback." *J. Comp. Pathol. Therap.* **52**(4):259–265.

Elveljem, C.A. and Sherman, W.C. (1932). The action of copper in iron metabolism. *J. Biol. Chem.* **98**:309.

Evans, J.L. and Abraham, P.A. (1973). Anemia, iron storage and ceruloplasmin in copper nutrition in the growing rat. *J. Nutr.* **103**:196.

Innes, J.R.M. and Shearer, G.D. (1940). "Swayback": a demyelinating disease of lambs with affinities to Schilder's encephalitis in man. *J. Comp. Pathol. Therap.* **53**(1):1–39.

Klauder, D.S.; Murthy, L.; and Petering, H.G. (1972). Effect of dietary intake of lead acetate on copper metabolism in male rats. *Trace Substances in Environmental Health* **6**:131–136.

Klauder, D.S. and Petering, H.G. (1975). Protective value of dietary copper and iron against some toxic effects of lead in rats. *Environ. Health Perspect.* **12**:77–80.

Shearer, G.D.; Innes, J.M.; and McDougall, E.I. (1940). Swayback studies in North Derbyshire. *Vet. J.* **96**:309–322.

Six, K.M. and Goyer, R.A. (1972). The influence of iron deficiency on tissue content and toxicity of ingested lead in the rat. *J. Lab. Clin. Med.* **79**:128.

3. Molybdenum-Sulfate

Over forty years ago it was first discovered that naturally occurring molybdenum was the cause of a severe scouring disease of cattle and sheep in certain areas of the United Kingdom (Ferguson et al., 1938). Since this original observation, numerous investigations of molybdenum toxicity have been published. Pitt (1976) has recently summarized the principal pathological and chemical changes caused by molybdenum, and these may include reduced weight gain, anemia, diarrhea, anorexia, alopecia, rough coat, testicular degeneration, and degenerative change of the central nervous system.

Of particular interest was that the symptoms of molybdenum toxicity are very similar to those of a copper deficiency. This suggested that excessive molybdenum may, in fact, be causing toxicity by inducing a copper deficiency. This hypothesis was subsequently supported by Dick and Bull (1945) who experimentally demonstrated that the storage of copper in the livers of sheep and cattle could be markedly reduced by an increase in the molybdenum intake. Furthermore, copper supplementation was found to reduce or prevent molybdenum toxicity in a number of species, including rats (Neilands et al., 1948; Gray and Ellis, 1950; Gray and Daniel, 1954; Halverson et al., 1960; Mills, 1960; Lalich et al., 1965), rabbits (Arrington and Davis, 1953), guinea pigs (Arthur, 1965), cattle (Ferguson et al., 1943; Allcroft, 1952; Cunningham, 1945–1946, 1950; Shirley et al., 1950; Cunningham et al., 1953; Miltimore et al., 1964; Vanderveen and Keener, 1964; Cook et al., 1966; Clawson et al., 1972), and sheep (Goodrich and Tillman, 1966; Hogan et al., 1971; Suttle and Field, 1974).

Dietary sulfate levels or sulfur compounds, in addition to the copper nutritional status, are able to affect molybdenum toxicity. Sulfate prevents molybdenum toxicity in monogastric species while it increases molybdenum toxicity in ruminants. For example, molybdenum toxicity has been reduced by sulfate in the rat (Van Reen, 1959; Miller and Price, 1956; Van Reen and Williams, 1956; Mills et al., 1958; Johnson and Miller, 1961), chick (Davies et al., 1960), and rabbit (Lukashev and Shishkova, 1971). In contrast, sulfate enhanced molybdenum toxicity in sheep (Suttle and Field, 1968; Mills and Fell, 1960; Goodrich and Tillman, 1966) and cattle (Vanderveen and Keener, 1964).

In light of the fact that dietary sulfate may markedly affect the toxicity of molybdenum in both monogastric animals and ruminants in opposite directions, it may be speculated that dietary sulfate levels differentially affect the nature of the molybdenum-copper interaction depending on whether or not the animal is a ruminant.

That sulfate may affect the copper-molybdenum interrelationship was first reported by Dick in 1953 with sheep. He found that the degree of molybdenum toxicity is dependent on the amount of inorganic sulfate in the diet. Inorganic sulfate is needed to allow molybdenum to have a limiting effect on the liver storage of copper. According to Buck and Ewan (1973), the combined effects of copper, molybdenum, and sulfate are considerably less evident in the monogastric animal. They cited the research of Gipp et al. (1967) and Hays and Kline (1969) who did not find any influence of molybdenum and sulfate on the liver storage of pigs fed varying amounts of copper. Other investigators (Dale, 1971; Gray and Daniel, 1964) did report a sulfate-molybdenum-copper interaction in swine and rats, respectively.

In an effort to provide the reader with a clear summary of this complex of mineral interactions, it is advantageous to refer to Buck and Ewan (1973):

In ruminant animals, specifically sheep and cattle, a copper deficiency can be induced by higher than normal dietary levels of molybdenum, but this is not the case with nonruminant animals, such as swine, rats, and poultry. . . . The interactions of copper-molybdenum in ruminants are also dependent upon the presence of adequate dietary inorganic sulfate. The optimum ratio of dietary copper to molybdenum for ruminants is approximately 6:1.

Of what biomedical significance are these findings for humans? According to Pitt (1976), exposure to elevated levels of molybdenum in food in the USSR is associated with a high incidence of gout (see Koval'skii et al., 1961), while Layton and Sutherland (1975) have hypothesized that high-risk areas of multiple sclerosis are associated with a high molybdenum to copper content of soil. In addition to these ecologic findings, molybdenum-induced degenerative changes in the central nervous system of sheep have been reported (Pitt, 1976). Whether these suggestive interrelationships prove to be more than associational remains to be established.

While it has been shown that copper will prevent molybdenum toxicity, it is also important to realize that a low level of molybdenum in the diet enhances the toxicity of copper in ruminants, especially sheep. Buck and Ewan (1973) have indicated this enhancement of copper toxicity in sheep can be a problem in the United States. This is particularly important because copper supplements are permitted as ingredients in feed grains, while molybdenum is not. This extra supplementation may result in a copper:molybdenum ration of 15:1, while a 6:1 ratio is considered optimum.

References

Allcroft, R. (1952). Conditioned copper deficiency in sheep and cattle in Britain. *Vet. Rec.* **64**:17–24.

Arrington, L.R. and Davis, G.K. (1953). Molybdenum toxicity in the rabbit. *J. Nutr.* **51**:295–304.

Arthur, D. (1965). Interrelationships of molybdenum and copper in the diet of the guinea pig. *J. Nutr.* **87**:69–76.

Buck, W.B. and Ewan, R.C. (1973). Toxicology and adverse effects of mineral imbalance. *Clin. Toxicol.* **6**(3):459–485.

Clawson, W.J.; Lesperance, A.L.; Bohman, V.R.; and Layhee, D.C. (1972). Interrelationship of dietary molybdenum and copper on growth and tissue composition of cattle. *J. Anim. Sci.* **34**:516–520.

Compere, R.; Burny, A.R.; Francois, E.; and Vanuytrecht, S. (1965). Copper in the treatment of molybdenosis in the rat: determination of the dose of the antidote. *J. Nutr.* **87**:412–418.

Cook, G.A.; Lesperance, A.L.; Bohman, V.R.; and Jensen, E.H. (1966). Interrelationship of molybdenum and certain factors to the development of the molybdenum toxicity syndrome. *J. Anim. Sci.* **25**:96–101.

Cunningham, H.M.; Brown, J.M.; and Edie, A.E. (1953). Molybdenum poisoning of cattle in the Swan River Valley of Manitoba. *Can. J. Agric. Sci.* **33**:254–260.

Cunningham, I.J. (1945–1946). Copper deficiency in cattle and sheep on peat lands. *N.Z. J. Sci. Technol.* **27A**:381–396.

Cunningham, I.J. (1950). Copper and molybdenum in relation to diseases of cattle and sheep in New Zealand. In: *A Symposium on Copper Metabolism,* pp. 246–273. Edited by W. McElroy and B. Glass. Johns Hopkins Press, Baltimore.

Dale, S.E. (1971). Effect of molybdenum and sulfate on copper metabolism in young growing pigs. M.S. thesis, Iowa State Univ.

Davies, R.E.; Reid, B.L.; Kurnick, A.A.; and Couch, J.R. (1960). The effect of sulfate on molybdenum toxicity in the chick. *J. Nutr.* **70**:193–198.

Dick, A.T. (1953). Influence of inorganic sulphate on the copper-molybdenum interrelationship in sheep. *Nature* **172**:638–639.

Dick, A.T. (1956). Molybdenum in animal nutrition. *Soil Science* **81**:229–236.

Dick, A.T. and Bull, L.B. (1945). Some preliminary observations on the effect of molybdenum on copper metabolism in herbivorous animals. *Austral. Vet. J.* **21**:70–72.

Ferguson, W.S.; Lewis, A.H.; and Watson, S.J. (1938). Action of molybdenum in nutrition of milking cattle. *Nature* **141**:553.

Ferguson, W.S.; Lewis, A.H.; and Watson, S.J. (1943). The teart pastures of Somerset. I. the cause and cure of teartness. *J. Agric. Sci., Camb.* **33**:44–51.

Gipp, W.F.; Pond, W.G.; and Smith, S.E. (1967). Effects of level of dietary copper, molybdenum, sulfate and zinc on body weight gain, hemoglobin, and liver storage of growing pigs. *J. Anim. Sci.* **26**:727.

Goodrich, R.D. and Tillman, A.D. (1966). Copper, sulfate and molybdenum interrelationships in sheep. *J. Nutr.* **90**:76–80.

Gray, L.F. and Daniel, L.J. (1954). Some effects of excess molybdenum on the nutrition of the rat. *J. Nutr.* **53**:43–51.

Gray, L.F. and Daniel, L.J. (1964). Effect of the copper status of the rat on the copper-molybdenum-sulfate interaction. *J. Nutr.* **84**:31.

Gray, L.F. and Ellis, G.H. (1950). Some interrelationships of copper, molybdenum, zinc and lead in the nutrition of the rat. *J. Nutr.* **40**:441–452.

Green, H.H. (1949). Proc. Specialist Conference in Agriculture, Australia, 293. (H.M.S.O., London, 1951).

Halverson, A.W.; Phifer, J.H.; and Monty, K.J. (1960). A mechanism for the copper-molybdenum interrelationship. *J. Nutr.* **71**:95–100.

Hays, V.W. and Kline, R.D. (1969). Copper-molybdenum-sulfate interrelationships in growing pigs. *Feedstuffs* **41**(44):18.

Hogan, K.G.; Money, D.F.L.; White, D.A.; and Walker, R. (1971). Weight responses of young sheep to copper and connective tissue lesions associated with the growing of pastures of high molybdenum content. *N.Z. J. Agric. Res.* **14**:687–701.

Johnson, H.L. and Miller, R.F. (1961). The interrelationships between dietary molybdenum, copper, sulfate, femur alkaline phosphatase activity and growth of the rat. *J. Nutr.* **75**:459–464.

Koval'skii, G.A.; Yarovaya, G.A.; and Shmavonyan, D.M. (1961). Changes in purine metabolism in humans and animals living in biogeochemical areas with high molybdenum concentrations. *Zh. Obshch. Biol.* **22**:179–191. Referat. Zh. Biol. No. 8T404 (1962). Cited from *Biol. Abstr.* **40**:9498 (1962).

Lalich, J.J.; Groupner, K.; and Jolin, J. (1965). The influence of copper and molybdate salts on the production of bony deformities in rats. *Lab. Invest.* **14**:1482–1493.

Layton, W. and Sutherland, J.M. (1975). Geochemistry and multiple sclerosis: a hypothesis. *Med. J. Aust.* **1**:73–77.

Lukashev, A.A. and Shishkova, N.K. (1971). Content of sulfhydryl groups of low-molecular compounds in rabbit tissues in molybdenum poisoning and the effect of sulphate. Trudy Inst. kraev. Patol., Alma-Ata **22**:196–202. Cited from Biol. Abstr. **56**:69,810 (1973).

McElroy, W.D. and Glass, B. (1950). Copper metabolism. A symposium on animal, plant and soil relationships. Johns Hopkins Press, Baltimore.

Marston, H.R. (1952). Cobalt, copper and molybdenum in the nutrition of animals and plants. *Physiol. Rev.* **32**:66.

Miller, R.F. and Price, N.O. (1956). Added dietary inorganic sulfate and its effect upon rats fed molybdenum. *J. Nutr.* **60**:539–547.

Mills, C.F. (1960). Comparative studies of copper, molybdenum and sulphur metabolism in the ruminant and the rat. *Proc. Nutr. Soc.* **19**:162–169.

Mills, C.F. and Fell, B.F. (1960). Demyelination in lambs born of ewes maintained on high intakes of sulphate and molybdate. *Nature,* Lond. **185**:20–22.

Mills, C.F.; Monty, K.J.; Ichihara, A.; and Pearson, P.B. (1958). Metabolic effects of molybdenum toxicity in the rat. *J. Nutr.* **65**:129–142.

Miltimore, J.E.; Mason, J.L.; McArthur, J.M.; and Carson, R.B. (1964). Ruminant mineral nutrition. The effect of copper injections on weight gains and haemoglobin levels of cattle pastured on ground-water soils in the British Columbia interior. *Can. J. Comp. Med.* **28**:108–112.

Nielands, J.B.; Strong, F.M.; and Elvehjem, C.A. (1948) Molybdenum in the nutrition of the rat. *J. Biol. Chem.* **172**:431–439.

Pitt, M.A. (1976). Molybdenum toxicity: interactions between copper, molybdenum and sulfate. *Agents and Actions* **6**(6):758–769.

Shirley, R.L.; Owens, R.D.; and Davies, G.K. (1950). Deposition and alimentary excretion of phosphorus-32 in steers on high molybdenum and copper diets. *J. Anim. Sci.* **9**:552–559.

Stewart, J.; Farmer, V.C.; and Mitchell, R.L. (1946). Molybdenum and copper metabolism of farm animals. *Nature* **157**:442.

Suttle, N.F. and Field, A.C. (1968). Effect of intake of copper, molybdenum and sulphate on copper metabolism in sheep. I. Clinical condition and distribution of copper in blood of the pregnant ewe. *J. Comp. Path.* **78**:351–362.

Suttle, N.F. and Field, A.C. (1974). The effect of dietary molybdenum on hypocupraemic ewes treated by subcutaneous copper. *Vet. Rec.* **95**:165–168.

Vanderveen, J.E. and Keener, H.A. (1964). Effects of molybdenum and sulfate sulfur on metabolism of copper in dairy cattle. *J. Dairy Sci.* **47**:1224–1230.

Van Reen, R. (1959). The specificity of the molybdate-sulfate interrelationship in rats. *J. Nutr.* **68**:243–250.

Van Reen, R. and Williams, M.A. (1956). Studies on the influence of sulfur compounds on molybdenum toxicology in rats. *Arch. Biochem. Biophys.* **63**:1–8.

B. ORGANIC SUBSTANCES

1. Chemical Carcinogens

Does consumption of a diet adequate in all known respects except with a marginally low level of copper affect susceptibility to chemical carcinogenesis? Conversely, will consumption of a diet with excess copper alter sensitivity to environmental carcinogenesis? The first study addressing these issues was published in 1946 by Sharples who demonstrated that increasing the copper levels in the diet of rats given the carcinogen 4-dimethylaminoazobenzene (DAB) resulted in an increase in the induction time (or latent period) for liver tumor formation. Five years later Pedrero and Kozelka (1951) replicated the findings of Sharples (1946), using the more potent carcinogen 3-methyl DAB. Following these two initial reports, several other investigators showed that dietary copper supplementation was effective in preventing adverse effects caused by hepatotoxic and carcinogenic agents (Table 3).

The mechanism by which copper treatment reduces the occurrence of chemically induced tumors is unknown. King et al. (1957) suggested that the protective influence of copper may be due to destroying the azo-dye carcinogen in the diet. However, Fare (1964, 1966) reported that the hepatotoxins are not inactivated by copper salts in vitro during food storage. Further, Brada and Altman (1978) revealed that

Table 3. Effect of Copper on Liver Damage and Carcinogenesis

Toxic Substance	Effect of Copper	Author
4-Dimethylaminoazobenzene	Increased induction time for liver tumor formation	Sharples, 1946 Fare and Woodhouse, 1963
3'-Methyl-4-dimethylamino-azobenzene	Inhibition of tumor formation	Pedrero and Kozelka, 1951 King et al., 1957 Fare and Howell, 1964
Thioacetamide	Minimized damage of liver, restricted it to some portal areas	Fare, 1964
Fluorenylacetamide	Cholangiofibrosis, cholangiocarcinoma, and hepatoma were all absent	Fare, 1966
Dimethylnitrosamine	Protected from ductular cell proliferation and cholangiofibrosis; tumorigenesis not studied	Fare, 1966
	Rats reared on copper-deficient (1 ppm) diet exhibited increased incidence of kidney but not liver tumors, as compared to rats given an excess of copper (800 ppm)	Carlton and Price, 1973
α-Naphthylisothiocyanate	Copper delayed but did not prevent ductular cell proliferation	Fare, 1966
Ethionine	Decreased ductular cell proliferation and cholangiofibrosis; tumorigenesis not studied	Fare, 1966
	Inhibition of tumor formation	Kamamoto et al., 1973

In all cases the copper was administered in salt form in the diet together with the particular toxic substance.

Source. Brada, Z. and Altman, N.H. (1978). The inhibitory effect of copper on ethionine carcinogenesis. In: *Inorganic and Nutritional Aspects of Cancer*, pp. 193–206. Edited by G.N. Schrauzer. Plenum Press, New York.

ethionine and copper acetate form an insoluble complex when combined. In fact, when ethionine is given along with copper acetate in a 1:1 ratio, its rate of absorption is markedly reduced. That copper may interact with carcinogens in the gastrointestinal tract is an important possibility to consider since all the protective findings have occurred when both copper and the carcinogen were present in the diet. However, the one nonsupportive study administered the carcinogen (i.e., 2-aminofluorene) to the skin and not in the diet. In fact, a recent report by Brada and Altman (1978) addressed this issue by feeding both copper and ethionine on alternate weeks over 8 months. They found that the normal protection offered by copper with respect to pathological changes caused by ethionine was markedly diminished, as evidenced by the development of extensive cholangiofibrosis that in certain instances were suggestive of cholangiosarcoma.

Despite the possibility of a copper-carcinogen interaction in the gastrointestinal tract that may affect carcinogenesis, Brada and Altman (1978) have shown that copper also affects the liver metabolism of the carcinogen ethionine; that is, the copper treatment markedly enhanced the hepatic concentration of S-adenosylethionine (S-AE) in rats. These findings are consistent with those of Yamane et al. (1976) who found that the activity of the enzyme-synthetizing S-AE increased in rats given diets with supplemental levels of copper prior to the experiment.

That dietary copper levels may affect the capacity of liver microsomal enzymes to metabolize xenobiotic agents including chemical carcinogens is well established. Table 4 clearly illustrates the influence of dietary copper on the activity of aniline hydroxylase, benzpyrene hydroxylase, hexobarbital oxidase, and on hexobarbital sleeping time. There is a significant reduction in aniline hydroxylase and the concomitant enhancement of benzpyrene hydroxylase activity during copper depletion, along with a diminished *in vivo* metabolism of drugs in copper-deficient rats as indicated by an increase in hexobarbital sleeping times (Moffitt and Murphy, 1973). Once the animals were returned to copper-containing diet for 14 days, all enzyme activities returned to control values.

While considerable research remains to be conducted on the influence of dietary copper on the metabolism of liver microsomal enzymes, enough is known to indicate that at least in certain instances copper may have a profound effect. Thus the hypothesis that copper enhances the detoxication of liver carcinogens such as DAB (Yamane et al., 1969) and ethionine (Brada and Altman, 1978) appears to be a viable one.

Table 4. Effect of Copper Deficiency on Hepatic Microsomal Enzyme Activity

Copper-Deficient Diet	N	In Vitro Activity[a]			Hexobarbital[c] Sleeping Time (min)
		Aniline Hydroxylase	Benzpyrene Hydroxylase	Hexobarbital Oxidase	
0	14	1.70 ± 0.10	3.60 ± 0.15	7.02 ± 0.66	13.0 ± 1.5
21	6	0.80 ± 0.08[b]	4.50 ± 0.27	6.06 ± 0.66	24.1 ± 3.0[b]
42	6	0.66 ± 0.10[b]	4.74 ± 0.27[d]	2.04 ± 0.52[b]	32.3 ± 1.5[b]
42 + Cu (14 days)	4	1.86 ± 0.16	3.90 ± 0.33	7.54 ± 0.38	15.0 ± 2.7

[a]Values represent mean $\pm$ S.E. of N animals per group. Respective enzyme activities are reported as: μmoles p-aminophenol/gm/hr (aniline hydroxylase); pmoles 3-hydroxybenzpyrene/gm/hr (benzpyrene hydroxylase); and μmoles hexobarbital metabolized/gm/hr (hexobarbital oxidase).

[b]Significantly different from pooled control values ($p < 0.01$).

[c]Hexobarbital, 100 mg/kg, intraperitoneally.

[d]Significantly different from pooled control values ($p < 0.05$).

Data calculated from Moffitt, A.E., Jr., and Murphy, S.D.: *Biochem. Pharmacol.* **22:**1463–1476, 1973.

Source. Becking, G.C. (1976). *Medical Clinics of North America* **60**(4):819.

The significance of these findings with regard to human carcinogenesis remains to be established. The data strongly suggest that dietary copper may play an important role in affecting susceptibility to chemical carcinogenesis. Clearly, what is needed are continued studies on the influence of copper on the metabolism of the mixed-function oxidase enzymes as well as additional carcinogenicity studies that more closely simulate patterns of human copper ingestion. In addition, epidemiological research, especially that of an occupational nature, is likely to make valuable contributions to this area.

References

Becking, G.C. (1976). Trace elements and drug metabolism. *Med. Clinics North America* **60**(4):813–830.

Brada, Z. and Altman, N.H. (1978). The inhibitory effect of copper on ethionine carcinogenesis. In: *Inorganic and Nutritional Aspects of Cancer,* pp. 193–206. Edited by G.N. Schrauzer. Plenum Press, N.Y.

Brada, Z.; Altman, N.H.; and Bulba, S. (1974). *Proc. Amer. Soc. Cancer Res.* **15**:145.

Brada, Z.; Altman, N.H.; and Bulba, S. (1975). The effect of cupric acetate on ethionine metabolism. *Cancer Res.* **35**:3172–3180.

Brada, Z. and Bulba, S. (1976). The effect of cupric acetate on L-ethionine metabolism in chronic experiments. *Fed. Proc.* **35**:551.

Carlton, W.W. and Price, P.S. (1973). Dietary copper and the induction of neoplasms in the rat by acetylaminofluorene and dimethylnitrosamine. *Fd. Cosmet. Toxicol.* **11**:827–840.

Clayton, C.C.; King, H.J.; and Spain, J.D. (1953). Effect of dietary copper upon azo dye carcinogenesis and upon some liver components. *Fed. Proc.* **12**:190.

Fare, G. (1964). The protective effects of beef and yeast extract and copper acetate in the diet against rat liver carcinogenesis by 4-dimethylaminoazobenzene. *Brit. J. Cancer* **18**:782–791.

Fare, G. (1966). The effect of cupric oxyacetate on rat liver damage associated with five poisons of unrelated chemical structure. *Brit. J. Cancer* **20**:569–581.

Fare, G. and Howell, J.S. (1964). The effect of dietary copper on rat carcinogenesis by 3-methoxy dyes. 1. Tumors induced at various sites by feeding 3-methoxy-4-aminoazobenzene and its N-methyl derivative. *Cancer Res.* **24**:1279–1283.

Fare, G. and Woodhouse, D.L. (1963). The effect of copper acetate on biochemical changes induced in the rat liver by p-dimethylaminoazobenzene. *Brit. J. Cancer* **17**:512–523.

Goodall, C.M. (1964). Failure of copper to inhibit carcinogenesis by 2-aminofluorene. *Brit. J. Cancer* **18**:777–781.

Howell, J.S. (1958). *Brit. J. Cancer* **12**:594.

Kamamoto, Y.; Makiura, S.; Sugihara, S.; Hiasa, Y.; Arai, M.; and Ito, K. (1973). The inhibitory effect of copper on DL-ethionine carcinogenesis in rats. *Cancer Res.* **33**:1129–1135.

King, H.J.; Spain, J.D.; and Clayton, C.C. (1957) Dietary copper salts and azo dye carcinogenesis. *J. Nutr.* **63**:301–309.

Moffitt, A.E., Jr. and Murphy, S.D. (1973). Effects of excess and deficient copper intake on rat liver microsomal enzyme activity. *Biochem. Pharmacol.* **22**:1463–1476.

Pedrero, E. and Kozelka, F.L. (1951). Effect of copper on hepatic tumors produced by 3′-methyl-4-dimethylaminoazobenzene. *Arch. Path.* **52**:455.

Sharples, G.R. (1946). The effects of copper tumor induction by p-dimethylaminoazobenzene. *Fed. Proc.* **5**:239.

Yamane, Y.; Sakai, K.; and Kojima, S. (1976). *Gann.* **67**:295.

Yamane, Y.; Sakai, K.; Uchiyama, I.; et al. (1969). Effect of basic cupric acetate on the biochemical changes in the liver of the rat fed carcinogenic aminoazo dye. I. Changes in the activities of DAB metabolism by liver homogenate. *Chem. Pharm. Bull.* **17**:2488–2493.

C. COPPER—POLLUTANT INTERACTIONS—A PERSPECTIVE

It has been shown that dietary copper levels may markedly affect the toxicity and/or carcinogenicity of several substances. However, what is most striking about the possible interactions of copper with toxic agents is the general lack of research in this area compared to other essential nutrients such as calcium, iron, selenium, and zinc. The only exception to this generalization has been the widespread recognition of copper toxicity in farm animals and how its toxicity may be modified by the presence of other substances, including sulfate and molybdenum.

Although interest in copper-pollutant interactions has been comparatively modest as compared to the above-mentioned nutrients, there has been very active research since the 1963 study of Hill et al. concerning the capacity of dietary copper to affect cadmium toxicity. In addition, there has been a flurry of activity since the early 1970s concerning copper-lead interactions. While many details remain to be elucidated concerning the interactions of copper with cadmium and lead, it is known that these toxic heavy metals may either reduce the gastrointestinal absorption and/or alter the tissue distribution of copper. Since copper plays a critical role in the functioning of numerous enzymes (e.g., cytochrome C oxidase, tyrosinase, monoamine oxidase, etc.), it is not unexpected that biochemical lesions induced by cadmium and lead may disrupt vital cellular functions, including respiratory metabolism. Whether current ambient exposures of humans to cadmium and lead are sufficient to affect a reduction in copper absorption and/or alterations in copper tissue distribution remains to be evaluated.

While it is too early to derive firm conclusions concerning the interactions of copper with toxic substances, the evidence that is emerging suggests that such interactions are complex. For example, copper nutritional status is known to be affected by several dietary factors including ascorbic acid (Hill and Starcher, 1965; Carlton and Henderson, 1965; Hunt and Carlton, 1965; Van Campen and Gross, 1968), molybdenum and sulfate (Dick, 1956; Gray and Daniel, 1954, 1964), as well as zinc (Van Campen, 1966; Van Campen and Scaife, 1967), and phytate (Davis et al., 1962). In addition, adequate copper intake is necessary for normal iron utilization (Elveljem and Sherman, 1932; Evans and Abraham, 1973).

The magnitude of the interactions of copper with other dietary factors suggests that simple generalizations concerning the nature of copper-pollutant interactions are not likely. In fact, the research by Hill et al. (1963) and Klauder and Petering (1975) has clearly suggested this complexity by showing that copper may interact with iron, zinc, and ascorbic acid in modifying the toxicity of cadmium and/or lead.

In light of what is known about copper-pollutant interactions, where should future research be directed? Several general areas of research may be recommended to yield potentially important interactions between copper and toxic substances:

1. Each agent (plutonium, manganese, benzene, etc.) whose toxicity is affected by dietary iron status should be evaluated with respect to both copper and iron. The findings of Hill et al. (1963) with cadmium and of Klauder and Petering (1975) with lead imply that this would be a fruitful area of research.

2. Of potential public health importance is that adequate levels of copper are necessary for the proper functioning of certain liver microsomal enzymes. Since most foreign compounds are metabolized by the MFO, it is important to further clarify the role of copper in such processes.

3. Since ascorbic acid has been found to decrease the intestinal absorption of copper (Hill and Starcher, 1965; Carlton and Henderson, 1965; Van Campen and Gross, 1968), research should evaluate the possibility that megadoses of ascorbic acid may alter the tissue distribution of copper as well as the activity of the copper-dependent enzymes cytochrome C oxidase and superoxide dismutase.

References

Carlton, W.W. and Henderson, W. (1965). Studies on chickens fed a copper-deficient diet supplemented with ascorbic acid, reserpine and diethylstilbestrol. *J. Nutr.* **85**:67.

Davis, P.N.; Norris, L.C.; and Kratzer, F.H. (1962). Interference of soybean proteins with the utilization of trace minerals. *J. Nutr.* **77**:217.

Dick, A.T. (1956). Molybdenum and copper relationships in animal nutrition. In: *Inorganic Nitrogen Metabolism,* p. 445. Edited by W.D. McElroy and B. Glass. Johns Hopkins Press, Baltimore.

Elveljem, C.A. and Sherman, W.C. (1932). The action of copper in iron metabolism. *J. Biol. Chem.* **98**:309.

Evans, J.L. and Abraham, P.A. (1973). Anemia, iron storage and ceruloplasmin in copper nutrition in the growing rat. *J. Nutr.* **103**:196.

Gray, L.F. and Daniel, L.J. (1954). Some effects of excess molybdenum on the nutrition of the rat. *J. Nutr.* **53**:43.

Gray, L.F. and Daniel, L.J. (1964). Effect of the copper status of the rat on the copper-molybdenum-sulfate interaction. *J. Nutr.* **84**:31.

Hill, C.H.; Matrone, G.; Payne, W.L.; and Barber, C.W. (1963). *In vivo* interactions of cadmium with copper, zinc, and iron. *J. Nutr.* **80**:227–235.

Hill, C.H. and Starcher, B. (1965). Effect of reducing agents on copper deficiency in the chick. *J. Nutr.* **85**:271.

Hunt, C.E. and Carlton, W.W. (1965). Cardiovascular lesions associated with experimental copper deficiency in the rabbit. *J. Nutr.* **87**:385.

Klauder, D.S. and Petering, H.G. (1975). Protective value of dietary copper and iron against some toxic effects of lead in rats. *Environ. Health Perspect.* **12**:77–89.

Van Campen, D.R. (1966). Effects of zinc, cadmium, silver and mercury on the absorption and distribution of copper-64 in rats. *J. Nutr.* **88**:125.

Van Campen, D.R. and Gross, E. (1968). Influence of ascorbic acid on the absorption of copper by rats. *J. Nutr.* **95**:617–622.

Van Campen, D.R. and Scaife, P.U. (1967). Zinc interference with copper absorption in rats. *J. Nutr.* **91**:473.

3

Iron

A. INORGANIC SUBSTANCES

1. Cadmium

That iron nutritional status may affect the expression of cadmium toxicity was first presented by Hill et al. in 1963 in research with chicks. Their discovery was of a serendipitous nature since it was initially hypothesized that copper levels in the diet may reduce cadmium toxicity[1] and that iron was evaluated only because copper requirements can be modified by varying the level of iron in the diet. In the presence of iron, the chick needs less copper. Thus it was originally thought that the addition of iron would enhance the capacity of copper to prevent cadmium-induced toxicity.

Their study revealed that while on the basal diet that contained 10 ppm Fe and 1 ppm Cu, the addition of 25 ppm Cd resulted in a marked increase in mortality. However, supplementation of 100 ppm Fe to the diet markedly reduced the cadmium-induced mortality.

---

[1] These researchers hypothesized that copper may affect cadmium toxicity based on analogy to the interaction of zinc with cadmium, which results in zinc reducing cadmium toxicity. Both of these elements have valence electrons that are isoelectric, with both elements having a coordination number of 4, with tetrahedral configuration (Hill et al., 1963).

With respect to body weight, supplementation with 500 ppm Fe offered even more protection than the 100 ppm Fe level. These data led Hill et al. (1963) to conclude that "there is an iron component of cadmium toxicity."

These findings were verified by Banis et al. (1969) using male and female weanling rats in that supplemental iron at 300 ppm in the diet prevented the adverse effects of cadmium on weight gain and hemoglobin levels. Other investigators have revealed that both oral and intramuscular injections of iron were able to prevent or at least markedly diminish cadmium-induced anemia (Pond and Walker, 1972), decreased hemoglobin and hematocrit values and growth depression in rats (Maji and Yoshida, 1974; Sansi and Pond, 1974), as well as decreased iron levels in the liver of rats (Whanger, 1973; Julshamm et al., 1977) and mice (Bunn and Matrone, 1966).

Table 1 illustrates the expressions of cadmium toxicity prevented in a variety of animal species by the administration of iron. There is such excellent agreement among the responses of these different animal models to cadmium-iron interactions as to confidently conclude that cadmium toxicity can be enhanced by diets low in iron as well as reduced with diets having adequate iron supplements.

Of particular significance among the observations noted above was the finding that low levels of iron in the diet markedly enhanced the

Table 1. Effects of Cadmium Toxicity Prevented by Iron: Findings in Animal Models and Humans

	Chicks	Japanese Quail	Mice	Rats	Pigs	Humans
Intestinal absorption of cadmium	X		X	X		X
Decreased growth			X			
Increased mortality	X					
Decreased weight gain	X			X		
Decreased hemoglobin		X		X	X	
Decreased hematocrit		X		X		
Anemia			X	X		
Increased liver weight				X		
Decreased Fe levels in numerous tissues			X[a]	X		

[a] Kidney only.

absorption and body burden of cadmium in mice (Maji and Yoshida, 1974; Hamilton and Valberg, 1974; Flanagan et al., 1978), and thereby enhanced the expression of cadmium toxicity as compared to controls (see Flanagan et al., 1978). Even at the relatively low cadmium exposure of 1 mg/L of drinking water, mice reared on a low-iron diet exhibited marked reductions in body weight and hematocrit as well as significantly increased the body burden of cadmium including several organs, especially the kidneys (Table 2).

If there is a question as to whether these animal models may provide at least a qualitative prediction for the responses of humans with low-dietary iron intakes, a recent report by Flanagan et al. (1978) provides some insight. They exposed human subjects with markedly different body stores of iron to labeled cadmium (25 μg) that was 50% of the estimated normal daily cadmium intake. Their results revealed that the percentage of labeled cadmium absorbed in volunteers with low-body stores of iron was 8.9%, while only 2.3% in those with normal iron stores.

Since females frequently have lower body-iron stores than males, it would be predicted that as a group they would be at increased risk to cadmium absorption. This prediction was borne out in the Flanagan et

Table 2. Cadmium Content of the Mice and Selected Body Organs

	Cadmium (Mean ± SE) (nmoles)		
	Iron Normal	Iron Deficient	P
Body content[a]	69 ± 4.3	145 ± 7.1	<0.001
Amount absorbed[b]	23 ± 1.6	33 ± 2.3	<0.001
Stomach	0.4 ± 0.03	0.9 ± 0.14	<0.001
Small intestine:			
First 5 cm	3.1 ± 0.46	10.2 ± 0.94	<0.001
Next 10 cm	0.9 ± 0.09	1.3 ± 0.34	>0.1
Remainder	1.3 ± 0.19	1.8 ± 0.19	<0.05
Cecum	1.4 ± 0.16	3.1 ± 0.45	<0.001
Colon	0.5 ± 0.12	0.3 ± 0.11	>0.1
Liver	3.9 ± 0.16	6.7 ± 0.83	<0.001
Kidneys	3.7 ± 0.12	10.2 ± 0.49	<0.001

[a]Determined by whole-body counting before sacrifice.

[b]Determined by counting the carcasses after removal of the gastrointestinal tract.

Source. Flanagan et al., 1978.

al. studies as females exhibited a 3 times greater efficiency of cadmium absorption than males.

Another aspect of the cadmium-iron interrelationship was noted by Spivey-Fox et al. in 1971. They noted that Fe III offered only very little protective action against cadmium toxicity whereas Fe II was particularly effective in preventing the adverse effects of cadmium. It was suggested by these researchers that cadmium may act, in part, by preventing the absorption of Fe III. Furthermore, they predicted that the beneficial effects of ascorbic acid on cadmium toxicity were most likely through the conversion of Fe III to Fe II. Maji and Yoshida (1974) supported this suggestion by demonstrating the strikingly beneficial effects of a joint treatment with 400 ppm Fe and 1% vitamin C in the diet of rats given either 50 or 75 ppm Cd (Table 3).

The studies reviewed here clearly support the hypothesis that low dietary intakes of iron enhance cadmium absorption via the gastrointestinal tract, resulting in an increased body burden of cadmium and an enhancement of its toxicity. Limited human studies have revealed that persons with low body-iron stores absorb dietary cadmium considerably more efficiently than persons with normal body-iron stores. Whether this enhanced capacity to absorb cadmium in persons with low body-iron stores presents a health risk at normal levels of daily cadmium exposure in the diet (70 μg) is not yet known. However, it seems clear that these individuals will have a greater body burden of cadmium. The striking findings of Flanagan et al. (1978) suggest that epidemiological studies should be initiated that are designed to test the hypothesis that those with low body-iron stores actually do have an increased cadmium body burden and if so, whether this enhanced retention of cadmium is related to any adverse health effects such as hypertension. Further research should also be directed toward assessing the influence of iron on the rate of excretion for cadmium that has already been absorbed into the bloodstream from the gastrointestinal and respiratory tracts.

The present findings suggest that menstruating females are at increased risk to developing greater body burdens of cadmium. In addition, it is evident that in any reevaluation of the drinking water standard for cadmium (i.e., 10 ppb), special concern should be directed to quantify the magnitude of the risk from cadmium exposure that people with variable levels of iron in their diets may have. Whether people with low-iron stores absorb cadmium via inhalation more efficiently than normal individuals is unknown but, at least on a conceptual level, not expected. The primary problem seems to involve dietary exposure to cadmium.

Table 3. Effect of Iron and Ascorbic Acid Supplements on Cadmium Accumulation in Tissues

Diet	(1)	(2) 50ppm	(3) 50ppm	(4) 75ppm	(5) 75ppm
Cd	—	50ppm	50ppm	75ppm	75ppm
Fe, Ascorbic Acid	—	—	+	—	+
Male Rats		$\mu g/100g$ body weight			
Liver[a]	ND[e]	31.8 ± 4.6	17.1 ± 2.8	53.3 ± 7.9	31.8 ± 5.5
Kidney[b]	ND	8.43 ± 1.18	5.02 ± 0.82	11.00 ± 1.85	7.69 ± 0.92
Duodenum[c]	ND	6.89 ± 0.76	2.65 ± 1.15	4.47 ± 1.01	3.51 ± 1.37
Female Rats					
Liver[a]	ND	30.9 ± 3.4	17.7 ± 3.5	49.2 ± 14.9	27.1 ± 3.0
Kidney[b]	ND	7.26 ± 0.95	5.42 ± 0.45	10.83 ± 3.17	7.53 ± 1.10
Duodenum[d]	ND	7.20 ± 3.19	4.78 ± 2.19	6.77 ± 2.18	5.18 ± 0.99

[a]$P < 0.01$; (2) vs. (3), (4)   (3) vs. (4), (5)   (4) vs. (5)

[b]$P < 0.01$; (2) vs. (3)   (3) vs. (4), (5)   (4) vs. (5)
 $P < 0.05$; (2) vs. (4)

[c]$P < 0.01$; (2) vs. (3), (4), (5) $P < 0.05$; (3) vs. (4)

[d]$P < 0.01$; (2) vs. (3), (4)   (3) vs. (4), (5) $P < 0.05$; (4) vs. (5)

[e]not detected

Source. Maji and Yoshida, 1974.

Table 4. Dose Effect of Dietary Cadmium Given Before and During Gestation on Fetal Viability and Neonatal Trace-Metal Metabolism

	Number of Pups Born/Stillborn[a]	Live Birth Weight, g ± SE	Metal Concentrations of Whole Pups, μg/g dry wt ± SE			
			Zn	Cu	Fe	Cd
Control	54/0	6.3 ± 0.2	127 ± 3	15.0 ± 0.7	417 ± 15	0.43 ± 0.01
4.3 μg Cd/ml in drinking water	55/0	6.1 ± 0.2	137 ± 3	11.0 ± 0.4[b]	359 ± 14	0.47 ± 0.01
8.6 μg Cd/ml in drinking water	52/0	6.2 ± 0.1	137 ± 3	12.0 ± 0.8[c]	336 ± 9[b]	0.49 ± 0.01
Control	41/0	6.7 ± 0.1	132 ± 4	12.0 ± 0.8	421 ± 19	0.21 ± 0.01
17.2 μg Cd/ml in drinking water	47/1	6.0 ± 0.1[b]	131 ± 2	9.0 ± 0.4[b]	346 ± 14[b]	0.21 ± 0.01
34.4 μg Cd/ml in drinking water	59/1	6.0 ± 0.1[b]	130 ± 2	8.0 ± 0.3[b]	224 ± 8[b]	0.24 ± 0.01

[a]Purina laboratory chow was fed to all adult females. Litters from five pregnant females constituted each group.
[b]Significantly different from controls at $p < 0.01$.
[c]Significanly different from controls at $p < 0.05$.

Source. Petering et al., 1979.

Finally, several recent reports have indicated that both copper and iron metabolism are altered in the fetus and neonate by oral administration of cadmium in drinking water (as low as 4.3 μg Cd/ml) (Martin et al., 1977; Petering, 1974; Petering et al., 1977, 1979). This was reflected in markedly lower copper and iron concentrations in the serum, kidney, and liver of whole pups (Table 4). It must be realized that the present U.S. EPA-drinking-water standard for cadmium is 10 μg/L or .01 μg/ml. Although the exposure to "only" 4.3 μg Cd/ml seems small, it is still far in excess of the current acceptable limit. While further research is needed to evaluate the influence of cadmium on iron metabolism at more realistic exposure levels, it must be realized that even at 4.3 μg Cd/ml the decrease in the iron concentration of the pups was not statistically significant at the .05 level. (Decrease in copper levels was significant at the .01 level, however.) It is interesting to ponder that low body-iron stores enhance cadmium absorption, while cadmium itself reduces body stores of iron. The major question is one of quantification of risks at realistic exposure levels.

References

Banis, R.J.; Pond, W.G.; Walker, E.F., Jr.; and O'Connor, J.R. (1969). Dietary cadmium, iron, and zinc interactions in the growing rat. *Proc. Soc. Exp. Biol. Med.* **130**:802–806.

Bunn, C.R. and Matrone, G. (1966). *In vivo* interactions of cadmium, copper, zinc, and iron in the mouse and rat. *J. Nutr.* **90**:395–399.

Flanagan, P.R.; McLellan, J.S.; Haist, J.; Cherian, G.; Chamberlain, M.J.; and Valberg, L.S. (1978). Increased dietary cadmium absorption in mice and human subjects with iron deficiency. *Gastroenterology.* **74**:841–846.

Freeland, J.H. and Cousins, R.J. (1973). Effect of dietary cadmium binding protein in the chick. *Nutr. Reports Inter.* **8**(5):337–347.

Hamilton, D.L. and Valberg, L.S. (1974). Relationship between cadmium and iron absorption. *Amer. J. Physiol.* **227**(5):1033–1037.

Hill, C.H.; Matrone, G.; Payne, W.L.; and Barber, C.W. (1963). *In vivo* interactions of cadmium with copper, zinc, and iron. *J. Nutr.* **80**:227–235.

Julshamm, K.; Utne, F.; and Braekkan, O.R. (1977). Interactions of cadmium with copper, zinc, and iron in different organs and tissues of the rat. *Acta. Pharmacol. Toxicol.* **41**:515–524.

Maji, T. and Yoshida, A. (1974). Therapeutic effect of dietary iron and ascorbic acid on cadmium toxicity of rats. *Nutr. Reports Inter.* **10**(3):139–149.

Martin, P.G.; Hitchcock, B.B.; and King, J.F. (1977). Interactions of Cd, Zn, Cu, and Fe in the anemic rat. In: *Trace Substances in Environmental Health*, XI, pp. 201–210.

Petering, H.G. (1974). The effect of cadmium and lead on copper and zinc metabolism. In: *Trace Element Metabolism in Animals*, p. 33. Edited by W.G. Hoekstra. Vol. 2. Univ. Park Press, Baltimore.

Petering, H.G.; Choudhury, H.; and Stemmer, K.L. (1979). Some effects of oral ingestion of cadmium on zinc, copper, and iron metabolism. *Environ. Health Perspect.* **28**:97–106.

Petering, H.G.; Murthy, L.; and Cerklewski, F.L. (1977). Role of nutrition in heavy metal toxicity. In: *Biochemical Effects of Environmental Pollutants,* p. 365. Edited by S.D. Lee. Ann Arbor Science, Ann Arbor, MI.

Pond, W.G. and Walker, E.F., Jr. (1972). Cadmium-induced anemia in growing rats: prevention by oral or parenteral iron. *Nutr. Reports Inter.* **5**(6):365–371.

Pond, W.G.; Walker, E.F., Jr.; and Kirtland, D. (1973). Cadmium-induced anemia in growing pigs: protective effect of oral or parenteral iron. *J. Anim. Sci.* **36**(6):1122–1124.

Radi, S.A. and Pond, W.G. (1979). Effect of dietary cadmium on the fate of parenterally administered ^{59}Fe in the weanling pig. *Nutr. Reports. Inter.* **19**:695–701.

Ragan, H.A. (1977). Effects of iron deficiency on the absorption and distribution of lead and cadmium in rats. *J. Lab. Clin. Med.* **90**(4):700–705.

Sansi, K.A.O. and Pond, W.G. (1974). Pathology of dietary cadmium toxicity in growing rats and the protective effect of injected iron. *Nutr. Reports Inter.* **9**(6):407–414.

Spivey-Fox, M.R.; Fry, B.E., Jr.; Harland, B.F.; Schertel, M.E.; and Weeks, C.E. (1971). Effect of ascorbic acid on cadmium toxicity in the young coturnix. *J. Nutr.* **101**:1295–1306.

Whanger, P.D. (1973). Effect of dietary cadmium on intracellular distribution of hepatic iron in rats. *Res. Commun. Chem. Pathol. Pharmacol.* **5**(3):733–740.

2. Lead

Experimental evidence that first indicated that toxicity from oral lead exposure could be modified by dietary levels of iron was reported in 1972 by Mahaffey-Six and Goyer. They became interested in this hypothesis since iron deficiency is commonly found along with childhood lead intoxication, and they wanted to find out which phenomenon came first, the lead poisoning or the poor iron status. It had always been presumed that lead poisoning disrupted iron status by affecting heme biosynthesis; that the level of iron in the diet may enhance lead toxicity was a new concept. In addition, previous research had indicated that iron is related to the toxicity of at least one toxic heavy metal, cadmium (Jacobs et al., 1969).

The experiments of Mahaffey-Six and Goyer (1972) utilized male albino Sprague-Dawley rats (age not given) that were fed purified diets with either 5 or 25 ppm of iron (i.e., ferrous sulfate), and exposed to 200 mg Pb/ml in drinking water for a 10-week period. This level of lead exposure had been previously demonstrated to be the maximum dosage when given for a 10-week period, that did not cause a marked effect in hematopoiesis or size, histology, and function of the kidney in the rat reared on a diet with 198 mg Fe/kg and 0.9% dietary Ca. Their results revealed that the combination of low iron intake and lead exposure acted in a synergistic manner to impair heme synthesis. In addition, rats on the low-iron diet exhibited an increased lead content in the kidneys and bone (Table 5). Another report by Mahaffey (1974), demonstrated differential tissue levels of lead in rats reared on diets deficient in either calcium or iron. These findings revealed that the amount of lead in bone is similar for both types of deficiency, but kidney levels of lead are considerably greater in the calcium-deficient animals (Table 6).

Since these initial reports of Mahaffey, several other investigators have confirmed her striking findings in several strains of rats (Klauder and Petering, 1975; Ragan, 1977; Barton and Conrad, 1977; Conrad and Barton, 1978). Not only does an iron-deficient diet result in the enhanced retention of lead in the liver and kidney (Mahaffey, 1974) but also in many other tissues including the spleen, femur, serum, blood, marrow, muscle, and carcass (Ragan, 1977) (Table 7). Furthermore, Ragan (1977) noted that if tissue levels of lead are considered as a percent of body burden, there is a change in the pattern of lead distribution in the iron-deficient rats. More specifically, femur, marrow, muscle, and spleen contained two or four times more of the body burden than comparable tissue in the normally fed rats.

While these studies were concerned with the influence of low levels of dietary iron on the tissue retention of orally administered lead, Conrad and Barton (1978) evaluated the influence of iron repletion on lead

Table 5. Hematocrit, Urinary δ-Aminolevulinic Acid (δ-ALA), and Renal and Femur Pb Content of Rats Fed Normal and Low-Fe Diets with and without Pb

Dietary Group	N	Hemato-crit[a]	Urinary δ-ALA μg/24 hr[a]	Renal Pb μg/g wet Tissue[a]	Femur Pb μg/g wet Tissue
Normal Fe	9	45.7 ± 0.6	20 ± 5	1.0 ± 0.1	5.6 ± 1.4
Low Fe	8	42.6 ± 1.0	22 ± 5	1.9 ± 0.4	10.6 ± 3.0
Normal Fe and Pb[b]	8	44.2 ± 0.9	180 ± 25	14.5 ± 1.6	75.2 ± 13.1
Low Fe and Pb[b]	8	37.8 ± 0.9	355 ± 50	38.7 ± 4.8	225.2 ± 15.2

[a]Mean ± 1 S.E.

[b]200 μg Pb/ml drinking water.

Source.   Mahaffey, K.R. (1974). Nutritional factors and susceptibility to lead toxicity. *Environ. Health Perspect.* **7**:110.

Table 6. Comparison of Tissue Concentrations of
Lead in Rats Fed Diets Deficient in Calcium
(LCa) and Iron (LFe) and Nutritionally
Adequate Diets (NCa, NFe)

	Pb, g/g	Wet Tissue
Diet	Bone	Kidney
No Pb		
NCa, NFe	2.2 ± 1.0	2.6 ± 1.2
LFe	10.6 ± 3.0	1.9 ± 0.4
LCa	9.7 ± 2.2	4.4 ± 0.6
200 μg Pb/ml H$_2$O		
NCa; NFe	74 ± 12	22 ± 4.3
LFe	225 ± 15	28.7 ± 4.8
LCa	202 ± 202	691 ± 203

Source. Mahaffey, K.R. (1974). Nutritional factors
and susceptibility in lead toxicity, *Environ. Health
Perspect.* **7**:110.

absorption via the gastrointestinal tract with the isolated-duodenal
loop technique. They found that rats reared on an iron-deficient diet
absorbed considerably greater amounts of lead (21.3%) than the control
rats (11.2%). However, rats that were iron-loaded (i.e., rats reared on a
normal diet and loaded with an intramuscular injection of 2 ml of
dextran iron at the initiation of the study) absorbed only 7.7%.

In partial support of these findings of Conrad and Barton (1978) was
a report by Kaplan et al. (1975) that indicated a dose-dependent inhibitory effect of iron at pharmacologic levels on the uptake of lead by
rabbit erythrocytes. At physiologic levels, however, iron did not exhibit
much influence on lead uptake by the erythrocytes. They concluded by
stating that "it is tempting to speculate that diets or therapeutic
agents which elevate serum iron levels could reduce the erythrocyte
uptake of lead level and possibly make lead more readily available to
excretion or binding to other receptors."

Of further interest is that oral exposure of lead did not affect the
mucosal uptake or absorption of iron in adult rats regardless of the
lead concentration employed (Conrad and Barton, 1978) (Table 8). In
fact, lead-exposed rats showed greater iron uptake after weaning (the
22-23 days of life) as compared to controls that fell quickly to adult
values (Dobbins et al., 1978). No adequate explanation was provided as
to how lead enhanced iron absorption immediately after weaning.

Table 7. Retention and Tissue Distribution of ^{210}Pb in Iron-Deficient and Control Rats 48 hr after Gastric Gavage

	% dose/organ					% dose/g ($\times 10^3$)		
	Carcass	Liver	Spleen	Femur	Serum	Blood	Marrow	Muscle
Iron-deficient ($n = 10$)								
$\bar{x}$	26.5	0.63	0.031	0.541	0.296	58.4	5.83	0.90
S.E.M.	6.7	0.17	0.015	0.137	0.221	15.3	1.68	0.32
Control ($n = 10$)								
$\bar{x}$	4.4	0.13	0.003	0.032	0.041	10.5	0.25	0.04
S.E.M.	1.3	0.04	0.001	0.009	0.031	2.4	0.08	0.03
p^a	<0.01	<0.01	NS^b	<0.01	NS	<0.01	<0.01	<0.02

*$\bar{x}$ = mean; S.E.M. = ± standard error of mean.

^{a}Student's t test, two-tail comparisons.

^{b}Not significant.

Source. Ragan, 1977.

Table 8. Lead and Iron Absorption with Various Doses of the Other Metal

Dose[a] (mg)	[203]Pb + carrier Fe[b]	[59]Fe + carrier Pb[b]
1	0.32 ± 0.14	15.32 ± 2.31
0.1	2.83 ± 0.78	17.36 ± 3.16
0.01	11.95 ± 1.98	18.88 ± 2.98
Control	14.35 ± 2.47	17.94 ± 2.57

[a]Quantity of either Pb or Fe added to the test dose of radionuclide.

[b]Percentage of radioisotope in carcass 4 hr after test dose.

Source. Conrad, M.E. and Barton, J.C. (1978). Factors affecting the absorption and excretion of lead in the rat. *Gastroenterology* **74**:735.

However, Dobbins et al. (1978) offered several possible explanations: (1) the lead may have slowed the development of processes within the mucosa of intestinal cells to reduce iron absorption, and (2) lead-induced decreases in the hematocrit and/or hemoglobin levels may have stimulated an adaptive process to maintain high-iron absorption.

Several investigators have proposed possible mechanisms by which iron deficiency may enhance lead uptake and toxicity. Mahaffey (1974) hypothesized that increased lead absorption from the gastrointestinal tract may be the mechanism by which diets deficient in iron enhance tissue retention of oral lead exposure (Figure 3-1). This hypothesis is supported by observations that diets low in iron enhance the gastrointestinal absorption of a variety of metals including manganese (Diez-Edward et al., 1968; Pollack et al., 1965), cobalt (Pollack et al., 1965; Valberg et al., 1969), and zinc (Pollack et al., 1965). This perspective was strongly supported by the isolation of heat-stable intestinal mucosal protein that binds both iron and lead *in vitro* and *in vivo*. Moreover, this protein was found to bind iron more avidly than lead. It was hypothesized that the presence of this protein "may explain why iron diminishes lead absorption but that iron absorption is not significantly altered by either the addition of lead to test doses of radioiron or in lead laden animals" (Barton and Conrad, 1978). More recent findings by Flanagan et al. (1979) suggest a more complex association involving two simultaneous processes: the first being a diffusion-type mechanism while the second is carrier mediated, displaying saturation kinetics.

Human Studies.   Although there is strong support from research with animal models that dietary iron status affects the retention of

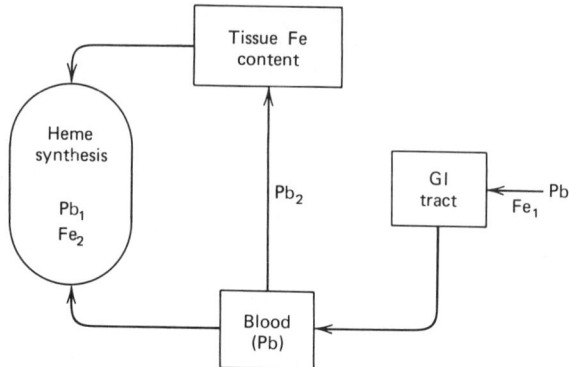

Figure 3-1. Interaction of lead and iron metabolism. Fe = increased Pb absorption in Fe deficiency; Pb_1 = inhibition of heme synthesis by Pb; Fe_2 = addition of Fe to reticulocytes *in vitro* reduces Pb_1 effect; Pb_2 = mild hemolytic anemia in Pb poisoning increases serum Fe and tissue Fe. [*Source.* Mahaffey, 1974.]

lead, there are very limited human data available on this subject (Strehlow and Barltrop, 1978; Angle et al., 1975; Mooty et al., 1975). Epidemiological studies using the case-control methodology have been utilized by Mooty et al. (1975) who compared the dietary status of children (aged 2–4 years) whose blood-lead levels markedly differed; that is, the mean blood-lead levels of the controls and cases were 20.4 and 56.9 $\mu g/dl$, respectively. With respect to ethnicity, the control group was made up of 12 Puerto Rican, 8 Black, and 5 Caucasian children, while the case group was composed of 4 Puerto Rican, 17 Black, and no Caucasian children. Dietary status was determined by interviews with the mothers of the children. In addition, data on demographic and social characteristics such as employment, education of parents, and maternal history of pica were obtained. With respect to mean iron intake no statistically significant differences were noted between the groups. However, it was reported that the cases consumed 59.1% of the RDA while the controls averaged 68.3% of the RDA. In addition, 62% of cases and 56% of controls had values 2/3 of the RDA for iron.

The authors concluded that the differential level of lead body burden could not be explained by differences in dietary iron intake. Thus the hypothesis that individuals with elevated levels of lead retention may have their condition, in part, because of poor iron nutrition was not supported. However, it should be realized this study was very limited in its perspective and that the strength of its conclusions are quite modest. For example, no effort was made to determine the difference in environmental lead exposure between the two groups. In addition, the presence of different proportions of racial subgroups between the cases and controls creates even further difficulties in properly assessing the actual contribution of dietary, genetic and cultural factors in differential lead retention.

In an experimental approach to assess a possible relationship between iron deficiency and blood-lead levels among iron-deficient children without anemia (i.e., serum Fe below 80 μg/dl and Hb > 10.5 g%), Angle et al. (1975) evaluated (1) the influence of increased blood-lead levels on the response to iron treatment and (2) the influence of iron supplementation on blood-lead levels. The results indicated that the presence of a moderate elevation of blood-lead levels (i.e., 20–40 μg/dl) did not increase the severity of iron deficiency as compared to individuals with blood-lead levels below 20 μg/dl. Other findings indicated that iron supplementation (i.e., 200 mg $FeSO_4$ daily for 4 months) did not diminish the seasonal increase of blood-lead levels as compared to control children not given such supplementation. In fact, in six of the seven pairs of children studied, the iron-supplemented ones exhibited a greater increase in blood-lead levels, thereby suggesting that oral iron was enhancing the retention and/or absorption of lead.

Not only do the findings of Angle et al. (1975) not support the hypothesis that low-dietary levels of iron enhance the retention of lead, but their data in fact suggest the opposite. Why there should be lack of agreement between the animal-model studies and the clinical report of Angle et al. (1975) needs to be resolved. In fact, based on the data of Angle et al. (1975), Levander (1979) concluded that "additional investigation is needed before any large scale iron supplementation trials are begun in an attempt to minimize the incidence of lead poisoning in children." However, it should be noted that Angle et al. (1975) did not comment on the possible differential environmental exposures to lead of their participants. For example, no mention was made of determining lead levels in their respective drinking water, house paint, soil, and so on. Clearly, this is an important factor that requires monitoring in order to ensure comparability of the experimental groups. It is not adequate to assume similar environmental exposure to lead. In addition, the groups may have differed in other dietary factors such as calcium, which could affect lead retention. Thus, although the data of Angle et al. (1975) are of great concern, the strength of their conclusions must be placed in perspective in light of the obvious limitations of their experimental design.

Other research with human subjects has also addressed the issue of the role of iron status in the development of a lead body burden in secondary-lead smelter workers (Lilis et al., 1978). These researchers did not find any correlation between total iron-binding capacity and serum iron levels with blood-lead levels in exposed and nonexposed individuals and concluded that the lead body burdens were not related to an iron deficiency. As in the case of Angle et al. (1975), the legitimacy of such a conclusion is weakened by the lack of quantitative exposure data within the lead-exposed group, lack of dietary history especially with respect to the mineral calcium, as well as other potentially confounding variables (see Zielhuis et al., 1978). In addition, while Lilis et al. (1978) cited the research of Mahaffey-Six and Goyer (1972) as supporting the rationale of their study, it should be pointed out that research with animal models such as those of Mahaffey-Six and Goyer (1972) involved exclusively gastrointestinal exposure to lead while the primary, though not exclusive, route of exposure to their worker population was respiratory. Finally, the hypothesis has been supported by the work of Delves et al. (1973), who found a negative correlation between blood-lead level and serum-iron levels in children thought to be lead poisoned and by Wibowo et al. (1976) who also found a negative correlation between blood-lead and serum-iron levels in healthy nonexposed young males.

This represents an important area in environmental health because of the prevalence of lead intoxication, especially among the very young and also because of the widespread consumption of diets inadequate in iron. In fact, iron deficiency is well recognized as one of the most common nutritional inadequacies in children, especially in those from lower socioeconomic backgrounds (Lin-Fu, 1973).

Further research is needed to establish what possible role iron deficiency and supplementation may have with respect to the development of lead intoxication. Development of appropriate models other than the rat should also be encouraged. Epidemiologic investigations must recognize the limitations of presently reviewed studies and incorporate a rigorous attempt to determine the extent of potential environmental-lead exposure between cases and controls as well as other confounding variables in order to make valuable new contributions to this area.

Finally, it has been proposed that iron deficiency plays a role in human lead pica (Watson et al., 1958), but Snowdon (1977) found no support of this hypothesis in studies with rats reared on iron-deficient diets.

References

Angle, C.R. and McIntire, M.S. (1974). More on the relevance of the concentration of lead in plasma versus that in blood. *J. Pediat.* **85**:286–287.

Angle, C.R. and McIntire, M.S. (1975). Blood lead level of iron deficient children—increase following iron supplementation. *Pediat. Res.* **9**:257.

Angle, C.R.; Stelmak, K.L.; and McIntire, M.S. (1975). Lead and iron deficiency. *Trace Substances in Environmental Health* IX, pp. 377–386.

Barton, J.C. and Conrad, M.E. (1977). Effects of an intestinal metal binding protein upon lead and iron absorption. *Blood* **50**(5), Suppl. I., p. 89.

Conrad, M.E. and Barton, J.C. (1978). Factors affecting the absorption and excretion of lead in the rat. *Gastroenterology* **74**:731–740.

Delves, H.; Bicknell, J.; and Clayton, B. (1973). The excessive ingestion of lead and other metals by children. In: *Environmental Health Aspects of Lead*, CEC, Luxembourg, p. 345.

Diez-Edward, M.; Weintraub, L.R.; and Crosby, W.H. (1968). Interrelationship of iron and manganese metabolism. *Proc. Soc. Exp. Biol. Med.* **129**:448.

Dobbins, A.; Johnson, D.R.; and Nathan, P. (1978). Effect of exposure to lead on maturation of intestinal iron absorption of rats. *J. Toxicol. Environ. Health,* **4**:541–550.

Flanagan, P.R.; Hamilton, D.L.; Haist, F.; and Valberg, L.S. (1979). Interrelationships between iron and lead absorption in iron deficient mice. *Gastroenterology* **77**:1074–1081.

Jacobs, R.M.; Fox, M.R.S.; and Aldridge, M.H. (1969). Changes in plasma proteins associated with the anemia produced by dietary cadmium in Japanese quail. *J. Nutr.* **99**:119–128.

Kaplan, M.L.; Jones, A.G.; Davies, M.A.; and Kopito, L. (1975). Inhibitory effect of iron in the uptake of lead by erythrocytes. *Life Sciences* **16**:1545–1554.

Klauder, D.S. and Petering, H.G. (1975). Protective value of dietary copper and iron against some toxic effects of lead in rats. *Environ. Health Perspect.* **12**:77–80.

Kochen, J. and Greener, Y. (1975). Interaction of ferritin with lead and cadmium. *Pediat. Res.* **9**:323 (Abst.).

Lamola, A.A. and Yamane, T. (1974). Zinc protoporphyrin in the erythrocytes of patients with lead intoxication and iron deficiency anemia. *Science* **186**:936.

Levander, O.A. (1979). Lead toxicity and nutritional deficiencies. *Environ. Health Perspect.* **29**:115–125.

Lilis, R.; Eisinger, J.; Blumberg, W.; Fishbein, A.; and Selikoff, I.J. (1978). Hemoglobin, serum iron, and zinc protoporphyrin in lead-exposed workers. *Environ. Health Perspect.* **25**:97–102.

Lin-Fu, J.S. (1973). Vulnerability of children in lead exposure and toxicity. *N.E. J. Med.* **289**(24):1289–1293.

Mahaffey, K.R. (1974). Nutritional factors and susceptibility to lead toxicity. *Environ. Health Perspect.* **7**:107–112.

Mahaffey, K.R. (1977). Quantities of lead producing health effects in humans: sources and bioavailability. *Environ. Health Perspect.* **19**:285–295.

Mahaffey-Six, K. and Goyer, R.A. (1972). The influence of iron deficiency on tissue content and toxicity of ingested lead in the rats. *J. Lab. Clin. Med.* **79**:128–136.

Mooty, J.; Ferrand, C.F., Jr.; and Harris, P. (1975). Relationship of diet to lead poisoning in children. *Pediat.* **55**(5):636–639.

Pollack, S.; George, J.N.; Reba, R.C.; Kaufman, R.M.; and Crosby, W.H. (1965). The absorption of nonferrous metals in iron deficiency. *J. Clin. Invest.* **44**:1470.

Ragan, H.A. (1977). Effects of iron deficiency on the absorption and distribution of lead and cadmium in rats. *J. Lab. Clin. Med.* **90**:700–706.

Robertson, I.K. and Worwood, M. (1978). Lead and iron absorption from rat small intestine: the effect of dietary Fe deficiency. *Brit. J. Nutr.* **40**:253–260.

Snowdon, C.T. (1977). A nutrition basis for lead pica. *Phys. Behavior* **18**:885.

Strehlow, C.D. and Barltrop, D. (1978). Nutritional status and lead exposure in a multiracial population. Presented at 12th Annual Conference on Trace Substances in Environmental Health, Univ. Missouri at Columbia.

Szold, P.D. (1974). Plumbism and iron deficiency. *N.E. J. Med.* **290**:520.

Valberg, L.S.; Ludwig, J.; and Olatunbosun, D. (1969). Alteration in cobalt absorption in patients with disorders of iron metabolism. *Gastroenterology* **56**:241.

Watson, R.J.; Decker, E.; and Lichtman, H.C. (1958). Hematologic studies of children with lead poisoning. *Pediat.* **21**:40.

Wibowo, A.A.E. et al. (1976). Interaction between lead and iron metabolism, a probable cause of female susceptibility to inorganic lead. Paper presented at 2nd International Workshop on Permissible Limits for Occupational Exposure to Lead, Amsterdam.

Zielhuis, R.L.; del Castilho, P.; Herber, R.F.M.; and Wibowo, A.A.E. (1978). Levels of lead and other metals in human blood: suggestive relationships, determining factors. *Environ. Health Perspect.* **25**:103–109.

3. Manganese

The toxic effects of direct manganese exposure are usually found only in occupational settings. In reported cases of manganese toxicity, miners have been exposed to manganese dusts for various lengths of time from about a year to greater than a decade (EHRC, 1975). The frequency of industrial manganism is reportedly quite low. It is often characterized by a self-limited psychiatric disorder, at the end of which neurological symptoms appear. These symptoms may persist even after the excess manganese becomes cleared from the tissues (Mena et al., 1969).

Several studies have indicated that animals reared on diets deficient in iron tended to absorb and/or retain significantly more manganese than control groups given diets with sufficient iron. The iron-deficient rats tend to incorporate the excess manganese into the porphyrin part of the hemoglobin molecule of the red blood cell (Borg and Cotzias, 1958; Pollack et al., 1965; Diez-Ewald et al., 1968; Chandra and Tandon, 1973; Mena et al., 1969; Thomson et al., 1971).

The only experimental animal model utilized has been the adult male rat, although the sex was not stated by several investigators (Thomson et al., 1971; Pollack et al., 1965). The iron-deficiency condition has been induced by either (1) feeding the animal on a diet low or deficient in iron for several weeks (Pollack et al., 1965; Chandra and Tandon, 1973) or for up to several months (Thomson et al., 1971), or (2) by bleeding the animal [3.5 ml over 3 days (Pollack et al., 1965) or 20 ml over 8 days (Diez-Ewald et al., 1968)]. Exposure to the manganese was either by per OS feeding (Pollack et al., 1965; Chandra and Tandon, 1973) or by injection during isolated intestinal loop studies (Diez-Ewald et al., 1968; Thomson et al., 1971). Despite these methodological differences among the various studies, their collective findings indicated that the iron-deficient rats had enhanced absorption and/or retention of manganese. However, there was disagreement on the influence of iron-loading on the gastrointestinal absorption of manganese, with Diez-Ewald et al. (1968) reporting an inverse relationship (i.e., the iron-loading reduced manganese absorption), while Thomson et al. (1971) did not find any difference.

The extent to which the presence of an iron deficiency enhances the absorption of manganese relative to normally fed controls ranged from 2.2% (Pollack et al., 1965) to 11.9% (Diez-Ewald et al., 1968). The biological significance of these findings was further explored by Chandra and Tandon (1973) who reported that a dietary-induced iron deficiency in rats exposed to manganese resulted in an increased retention of manganese in the liver, kidney, and testis (Table 9), with histopathological changes being more evident in the liver and kidneys of the iron-deficient rats.

Investigations with human subjects have also suggested that iron dietary status affects the absorption of manganese (Thomson et al., 1971; Mena et al., 1969). For example, in a study involving 36 human subjects of various nutritional status, anemic individuals absorbed manganese at a 150% greater rate than "normal" individuals: 3.0% versus 7.5% (Table 10) (Mena et al., 1969). The authors suggested that if an individual became anemic while being exposed to high levels of manganese, the person's tissue concentrations of this metal would quickly become excessive. Consequently, it was concluded that workers with iron deficiencies would be at high risk with respect to manganese toxicity (Mena et al., 1969).

Although the animal model and human studies clearly support the hypothesis that poor iron status enhances the gastrointestinal absorption of manganese as well as its retention, several studies (Mahoney and Small, 1968; Diez-Ewald et al., 1968) have revealed that the rate of

Table 9. Correlation of Morphological Alterations with the Manganese Concentration in Liver, Kidney, and Testis of Rats Fed with Manganese Chloride (10 mg/kg) for 15 Days

Group	Liver		Kidney		Testis	
	Histological Grading	Manganese[c] Concentration	Histological Grading	Manganese[c] Concentration	Histological Grading	Manganese[c] Concentration
I (normal rats)	0	1.98 ± 0.08 (6)	0	0.98 ± 0.03 (6)	0	0.47 ± 0.03 (6)
II (MnCl$_2$-fed rats)	+	2.45 ± 0.12 (6)[a]	0	1.61 ± 0.11 (6)[a]	0	0.54 ± 0.06 (6)
III (iron deficient, MnCl$_2$-fed rats)	++	3.12 ± 0.08 (6)[b]	+	2.17 ± 0.11 (6)[b]	0	0.88 ± 0.07 (6)[b]

[a]Significantly differed from Group I ($P < 0.02$).
[b]Significantly differed from Group II ($P < 0.001$).
[c]Amount of Mn expressed as mean ± S.E. in µg/g fresh tissue. Figure in parenthesis indicates number of animals used.

Source. Chandra, S.V. and Tandon, S.K. (1973). Enhanced manganese toxicity in iron-deficient rats. *Environ. Physiol. Biochem.* **3:**231.

Table 10. Results of Intestinal Absorption Studies of Orally Administered ^{59}Fe and ^{51}Mn, Retention of ^{54}Mn, and Concentration of ^{55}Mn in the Erythrocytes

Subjects	Number of Subjects	% Intestinal Absorption				Total body turnover of ^{54}Mn		Natural ^{53}Mn	
		^{59}Fe	P	^{51}Mn	P	T½ (days)	P	(µg./l. of erythros)	P
Normal individuals	11	11 ± 10		3.0 ± 0.5		37 ± 7		20 ± 6	
Anemic patients	13	64 ± 22	>0.001	7.5 ± 2.0	>0.001	23 ± 3	>0.01	130 ± 40	>0.001
Manganism victims	6	32 ± 8	>0.01	4.0 ± 1.0	>0.2	34 ± 5	>0.4	25 ± 2	>0.4
Healthy miners	6	19 ± 17	>0.2	3.0 ± 0.1	>0.5	15 ± 2	>0.001	55 ± 3	>0.001

Source. Mena, I.; Horivchi, K.; Burke, K.; and Cotzias, G.C. (1969). Chronic manganese poisoning: individual susceptibility and absorption of iron. *Neurology* **19**:1003.

manganese excretion is enhanced in iron-deficient animals while it is reduced in those given an iron load. According to Diez-Ewald et al. (1968), "the body appears to compensate for the changes in manganese absorption by increased manganese excretion in the iron-deficient state and decreased manganese excretion in the iron-loaded state." However, based on the research of Chandra and Tandon (1973), this compensation was not sufficient to reduce the level of manganese retention at least with respect to the liver and kidneys, where the manganese levels were 2.5 and 2 times greater in the iron-deficient rats.

Although the major occasions for exposure to excessive manganese is via occupation, the potential of manganese becoming a community health problem has recently emerged with the adoption of the catalytic converter. In order to permit the catalyst to operate as it was designed, lead must be removed from gasoline. However, in order to keep the gasoline at the proper octane levels without lead, it has been necessary to replace the lead with manganese (EHRC, 1975). Consequently, the release of considerable quantities of manganese into the environment as a result of the combustion of unleaded fuels is now a reality. In fact, in 1978, Joselow et al. presented evidence that young children in urban areas of New Jersey showed direct correlations between blood-lead levels and blood-manganese levels. These authors suggested that the elevated levels of manganese in the blood of these children were best explained by the manganese emitted from automobiles burning unleaded fuels. Since manganese is homeostatically regulated, one would not expect to find a buildup of manganese as found by Joselow et al. (1978) unless there was the concomitant presence of an inadequate iron-nutritional status. Unfortunately, these researchers did not evaluate the iron status of their participants. Further research to confirm the interesting findings of Joselow et al. (1977) should evaluate the influence of dietary iron intake on manganese retention.

Note: The use of the manganese fuel additive, MMT, in catalytic converter equipped automobiles was banned by the EPA on October 1, 1979 because it adversely affects hydrocarbon emissions.

References

Borg, D.C. and Cotzias, G.C. (1958). Incorporation of manganese into erythrocytes as evidence for a manganese porphyrin in man. *Nature* **182:**1677.

Chandra, S.V. and Tandon, S.K. (1973). Enhanced manganese toxicity in iron-deficient rats. *Environ. Physiol. Biochem.* **3:**230–235.

Diez-Ewald, M.; Weintraub, L.R.; and Crosby, W.H. (1968). Interrelationship of iron and manganese metabolism. *Proc. Soc. Exp. Biol. Med.* **129**:448–451.

Environmental Health Resource Center (EHRC) (1975). Health effects and recommended ambient air standard for manganese. Illinois Institute for Environmental Quality, 309 W. Washington St., Chicago, IL.

Joselow, M.M.; Tobias, E.; Koehler, R.; Coleman, S.; Bogden, J.; and Gause, D. (1978). Manganese pollution in the city environment and the relationship to traffic density. *Amer. J. Pub. Health* **68**(6):557–560.

Mahoney, J.P. and Small, W.J. (1968). Studies on manganese. III. The biological half-life of radiomanganese in man and factors which affect this half-life. *J. Clin. Invest.* **47**:643.

Mena, I.; Horivchi, K.; Burke, K.; and Cotzias, G.C. (1969). Chronic manganese poisoning: individual susceptibility and absorption of iron. *Neurology* **19**:1000.

Pollack, S.; George, J.N.; Reba, R.C.; Kaufman, R.M.; and Crosby, W.H. (1965). The absorption of nonferrous metals in iron deficiency. *J. Clin. Invest.* **44**(9):1470–1743.

Thomson, A.B.R.; Olatunbosun, D.; and Valberg, L.S. (1971). Interrelation of intestinal transport system for manganese and iron. *J. Lab. Clin. Med.* **78**(4):642–655.

4. Plutonium

An interesting recent study by Ragan (1975) concerned the influence of a dietary iron deficiency on the gastrointestinal absorption and body burden of plutonium. According to Ragan (1975), the widespread prevalence of iron-deficiency anemia along with the increased development of nuclear power reactors makes it important to evaluate conditions (i.e., dietary factors) that enhance the incorporation of radionuclides such as plutonium in the body.

Several earlier reports have demonstrated that plutonium has a high binding constant to transferrin, ferritin, and hemosiderin (Stover et al., 1968; Stevens et al., 1968; Boocock et al., 1970). Consequently, based on these observations, Ragan (1975) speculated that plutonium absorption may be inversely associated with dietary iron status.

To test this hypothesis, Ragan (1975) exposed iron-deficient adolescent mice to orally administered plutonium. He reported that the total body burden of plutonium after 24- and 96-hours exposure was about 4 times greater in the iron-deficient mice as compared to controls (Figure 3-2). Furthermore, he also noted a quicker translocation of plutonium from soft tissues to bone in the deficient group after 96 hours of exposure.

The increased body burden of plutonium in the iron-deficient mice was thought to be due to an enhanced absorption. Unfortunately, urinary excretion data were not collected. However, it would appear that these relatively large differences in body burdens did not result from

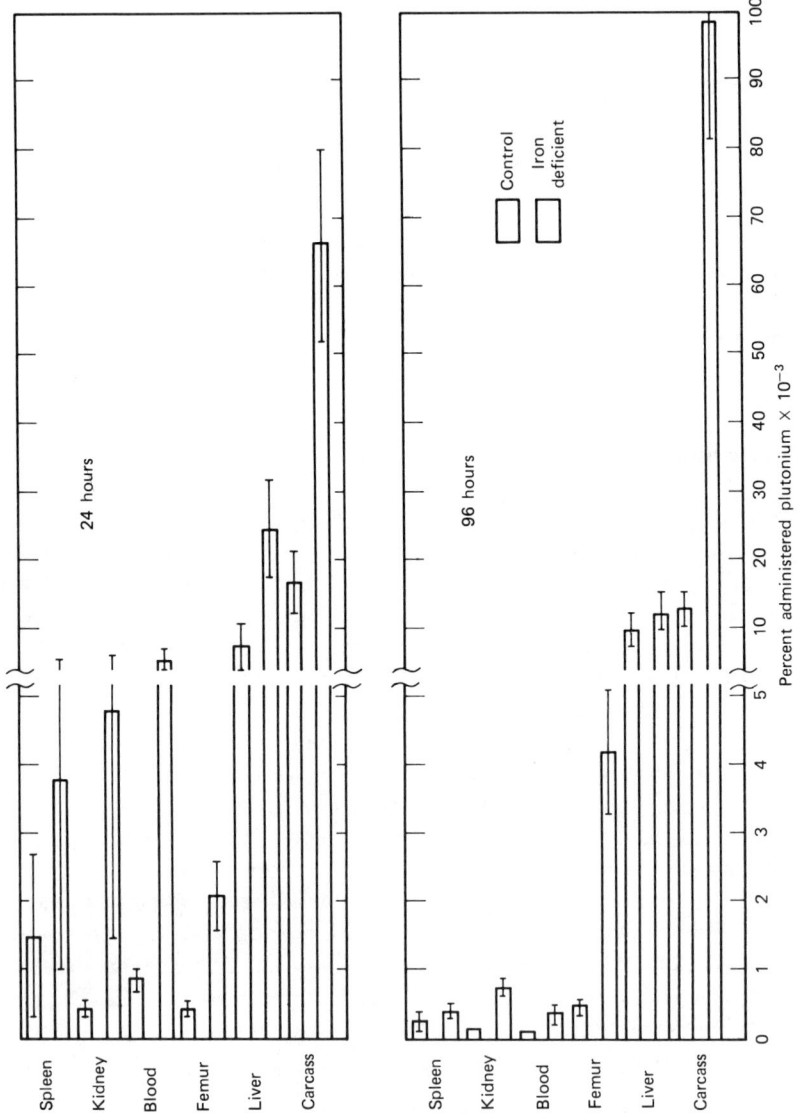

Figure 3-2. Percentage of ^{239}Pu citrate administered to iron-deficient and control mice by gastric gavage found in various tissues 24 and 96 hours later (mean ± SEM). [*Source.* Ragan, H.A. (1975). Enhanced plutonium absorption in iron-deficient mice. *Proc. Soc. Exp. Biol. Med.* **150**:36.]

decreased plutonium excretion in iron-deficient mice. This is supported by findings from a subsequent experiment in which iron-deficient mice, given plutonium by intraperitoneal injection, exhibited a greater urinary excretion rate (3x) of plutonium than the similarly exposed iron-replete group. According to Ragan (1975), it is reasonable to assume similar excretion differences occurred following the oral exposure to plutonium, in which case absorption may actually have been greater than that indicated from total body-burden analyses. However, these statements by Ragan (1975), while reasonable, lack experimental confirmation.

The results by Ragan (1975) have important public health implications in our nuclear age. Whether these experiments with mice provide a good indication of how iron-deficient humans would respond is unknown. It is imperative that studies be initiated not only to replicate and extend Ragan's study in mice but also in other species. Of interest would be whether consumption of a low-iron diet would enhance the susceptibility to plutonium-induced cancer.

References

Boocock, G.; Danpure, C.J.; Popplewell, D.S.; and Taylor, D.M. (1970). The subcellular distribution of plutonium in rat liver. *Radiol. Res.* **42**:381–396.

Ragan, H.A. (1975). Enhanced plutonium absorption in iron-deficient mice. *Proc. Soc. Exp. Biol. Med.* **150**:36.

Ragan, H.A. (1977). Body iron stores and plutonium metabolism. In: *Biological Implications of Metals in the Environment.* Edited by H. Drucker and R. Wildung. Conf. No. 750929. National Technical Information Service, Virginia.

Stevens, W.; Bruenger, F.W.; and Stover, B.J. (1968). *In vivo* studies on the interactions of PuIV with blood constituents. *Radiol. Res.* **33**:490.

Stover, B.J.; Bruenger, F.W.; and Stevens, W. (1968). The reaction of PuIV with the iron transport system in human blood serum. *Radiol. Res.* **33**:381–394.

B. ORGANIC SUBSTANCES

1. Benzene

In light of the widespread controversy concerning the hypothesis that benzene is a chemical carcinogen on the blood-forming organs, it is especially important to consider dietary factors that may alter the severity of benzene-induced metabolic changes. Evidence has been reported that ascorbic acid, protein, methionine, and pyridoxine may alleviate the occurrence of adverse effects from benzene exposure

(Friedman et al., 1977). Knowledge of this kind is of interest since it may help to identify groups of individuals who may be at enhanced risk to benzene intoxication and carcinogenicity. Quite recently the first indication that iron-deficient red blood cells may be at increased risk to benzene-induced inhibition of protein synthesis has been reported by Friedman et al. (1979). They demonstrated that iron-deficient rabbit reticulocytes incubated with 0.1 M benzene exhibited only approximately 1/3 the heme-synthesis activity of red blood cells of unexposed control animals with normal levels of iron. An iron deficiency alone or benzene exposure alone resulted in approximately 1/2 and 3/4 the heme synthesis of the control, respectively, thereby indicating the enhanced susceptibility of the iron-deficient red blood cell to benzene toxicity. Similar enhanced susceptibility of the iron-deficient, benzene-exposed reticulocytes with respect to reticulocyte protein synthesis was also shown.

According to the authors, the benzene level (0.1 M) (880 mg/dl) employed in this study would be fatal in normal situations. However, because benzene is highly lipid soluble, this exposure may be reachable in the bone marrow (Friedman et al., 1977). Based on these findings, Friedman et al. (1979) concluded that iron-deficient people might have an enhanced susceptibility to develop a benzene-induced anemia. Clearly, these findings are of great interest and suggest that epidemiological investigations should not overlook the influence of dietary factors, including the nutritional status of iron in the development of any risk assessment for benzene exposure.

References

Friedman, M.L.; Cohen, H.S.; Ibrahim, N.G.; and Gruenspecht, N. (1979). Ethanol, lead, and benzene inhibition of rabbit reticulocytes heme and protein synthesis increased *in vitro* toxicity in iron-deficient cells. *Environ. Res.* **18**:291–299.

Friedman, M.L.; Wildman, J.M.; Rosman, J.; Eisen, J.; and Greenblatt, D.R. (1977). Benzene inhibition of *in vitro* rabbit reticulocyte haem synthesis at δ-aminolevulinic acid synthetase. Reversal of benzene toxicity by pyridoxine. *Brit. J. Haematol.* **35**:49–60.

2. Dimethylhydrazine

While much research has been directed toward elucidating the influence of iron-deficiency anemia on the retention of a variety of heavy metals, especially cadmium and lead, little attention has focused on any interaction of iron with chemical carcinogens. However, the presence of iron deficiency has been associated with either metastases or with premalignant lesions. For instance, iron-deficiency-induced defects in immune competency have been hypothesized as being involved either in the development of neoplasia or in metastases (Vitale et al., 1978).

Since iron deficiency has been related with changes associated with the development of neoplasms, Vitale et al. (1978) decided to evaluate whether a dietary-induced iron deficiency may predispose rats to the carcinogenic effects of dimethylhydrazine (10 mg/kg/twice weekly starting at four weeks of age). They reported that all iron-deficient rats treated with dimethylhydrazine developed "what appeared to be neoplastic changes" in the liver after four months. In contrast, control animals given the carcinogen or reared on the iron-deficiency diet alone did not develop any neoplastic lesions during the period of observation.

In light of these interesting findings and the prevalence of iron-deficiency anemia within society, further research concerning the role of dietary iron as an agent in the expression of chemical carcinogenesis should be aggressively pursued.

References

Vitale, J.J.; Broitman, S.A.; Vavrousek-Jakuba, E.; Rodday, P.W.; and Gottlieb, L.S. (1978). The effects of iron deficiency and the quality and quantity of fat on chemically induced cancer. In: *Inorganic and Nutritional Aspects of Cancer*, pp. 229–242. Edited by G.N. Schrauzer. Plenum Press, New York.

3. Microsomal Enzyme Activity

That iron deficiency may affect the metabolism of xenobiotics was first demonstrated by Catz et al. (1970) who reported that chronic iron deficiency[2] caused a statistically significant increase in hexobarbital side-chain oxidation, aminopyrene N-demethylation, and microsomal cytochrome b_5 concentration, but no significant modification in either sleeping times or in the levels of cytochrome P-450. In addition, they reported no significant changes in the mixed-function oxidase metabolism of aniline, 3,4 benzopyrene, and p-nitrobenzoic acid, or in the conjugations of the o-p-aminophenols.

In contrast, Becking (1972) reported that aniline metabolism in rats

---

[2]The hemoglobin and hematocrit values in whole blood were reduced from 35 to 50% that of the controls.

is enhanced both *in vitro* and *in vivo* as soon as 18 days following feeding a deficient diet or when hemoglobin levels were diminished to about 65% of the controls. Aminopyrine N-demethylation was likewise enhanced in rats reared on the iron-deficient diet, but only when the deficiency was further advanced. Although pentobarbital metabolism *in vivo* and *in vitro* was not altered, the deficient animals displayed longer sleeping times than the controls. In addition, p-nitrobenzoic acid reduction was not changed. In agreement with Catz et al. (1970), Becking (1972) noted that cytochrome-reductase activities were enhanced following the development of an advanced iron deficiency. They observed that in an iron deficiency the activity of the mixed-function oxidase enzymes are either increased or left unaltered.

No adverse effects on drug metabolism occurred after feeding a diet with 1.5 times the normal iron content for 35 days. Becking (1972) stated that since this study was not carried out for a prolonged time period, it is not possible to conclude "that 1.5 times the normal intake of iron is harmless to the young adult rats" used in his study. Because a statistically significant reduction in growth rate occurred in the iron-supplemented rats as compared to the controls, he cautioned against possible dangers with the consumption of high levels of iron.

Other studies by Wills (1969, 1972) have provided some insight into the mechanism by which iron affects the activity of mixed-function oxidase enzymes. He noted that excess iron enhances the rate of lipid peroxidation, an activity that is closely associated with diminished rates of oxidative demethylation of aminopyrine and p-chloro-N-methyl aniline. The iron-induced lipid peroxidation was speculated to result in a disruption of the endoplasmic reticulum membrane, which itself affected a reduction in mixed-function oxidase hydroxylation and demethylation. Thus, hypothetically, the presence of a dietary iron deficiency causes a stabilizing of endoplasmic reticulum membranes and thereby enhances mixed-function oxidase enzyme activities and subsequent protection from peroxidative attack.

References

Becking, G.C. (1972). Influence of dietary iron levels on hepatic drug metabolism *in vivo* and *in vitro* in the rat. *Biochem. Pharmacol.* 21:1585–1593.

Campbell, T.C. and Hayes, J.R. (1974). Roles of nutrition in the drug-metabolizing enzyme system. *Pharmacol. Reviews* 26(3):171–197.

Catz, C.S.; Juchau, M.R.; and Yaffe, S.J. (1970). Effects of iron, riboflavin and iodide deficiencies on hepatic drug-metabolizing enzyme systems. *J. Pharmacol. Exp. Therap.* 174:197–205.

Wills, E.D. (1969). Lipid peroxide formation in microsomes. III. Relationship of hydroxylation to lipid peroxide formation. *Biochem. J.* **113**:333.

Wills, E.D. (1972). Effects of iron overload on lipid peroxide formation and oxidative demethylation by the liver endoplasmic reticulum. *Biochem. Pharmacol.* **21**:239–247.

C. OTHER: EXCESS IRON EXPOSURE

Hemochromatosis. While the principal problem associated with dietary iron is that of a nutritional inadequacy, medical problems can be caused by an excessive intake and subsequent accumulation of iron, which is termed secondary hemochromatosis and is characterized by pathologic changes in liver structure or function. Secondary hemochromatosis is common in African Bantu adults because of a dietary iron intake that frequently is in excess of 100 mg/day, a quantity nearly seven times greater than the daily requirement of iron (Bothwell and Finch, 1962). The majority of this excess intake of iron comes from the iron utensils used in cooking and in the preparation of alcoholic beverages (e.g., Kaffir beer). In addition, there has been a high incidence of hemochromatosis in persons with alcoholic cirrhosis, presumably because wines made in Europe or the United States contain from 5 to 22 mg of iron per liter. Furthermore, extensive deposition of iron pigment in numerous organs has been found in persons with Kaschin-Beck disease living in Asia, especially in Manchuria, where water and food have a high iron content [0.3 to 10 mg per liter (Hiyeda, 1939)]. Although pathologic changes associated with hemochromatosis are not present, this disease is recognized by recurrent attacks of polyarthritis in adolescence with symmetric joint deformities and shortness of stature.

It thus appears that ingestion of iron far in excess of the normal daily requirements for a prolonged period can result in serious pathological disorders to the liver (i.e., secondary hemochromatosis). Whether an excess of ingestion of iron on the order of only 2–5 times the RDA for long periods would cause any adverse health effects remains to be assessed. However, in light of the highly efficient regulation of iron absorption in periods of either deficiency or apparent repletion, this would not appear to be a serious concern (Underwood, 1971). Whether consumption of iron in quantities that exceed the RDA would reduce the retention and/or toxic effect of cadmium or lead is also unknown. If it is true that these metals interfere with the absorption of iron via competition for binding sites in the intestinal mucosa (Underwood, 1971), it would seem logical that the presence of excess iron in the gastrointestinal tract may serve to reduce the opportunity of these toxic heavy metals to reach binding sites and to be absorbed. Such speculation needs to be evaluated experimentally.

References

Bothwell, T.H. and Finch, C.A. (1962). *Iron Metabolism*. Little, Brown. Boston.

Caroli, J. and Andre, J. (1964). Surcharge ferrique dans les cirrhosis (a l'exclusion de l'hemochromatose idiopathique). In: *Iron Metabolism*, p. 326. Edited by F. Gross. Springer-Verlag, Berlin.

Hiyeda, K. (1939). The cause of Kaschin-Beck's disease. *Jap. J. Med. Sci.* 4:91.

MacDonald, R.A. (1964). *Hemochromatosis and Hemosiderosis*. Charles C. Thomas, Springfield, IL.

Underwood, E.J. (1971). *Trace Elements in Human and Animal Nutrition*. Academic Press, N.Y.

Carcinogenicity.   While the study of Vitale et al. (1978) evaluated the influence of iron deficiency on the incidence of dimethylhydrazine carcinogenicity, other researchers have been concerned with the role of excessive iron overload in carcinogenesis. For instance, numerous studies have noted a very high incidence of primary carcinoma of the liver (11.5 to 42.9%) in groups with hemochromatosis (Warren and Drake, 1951; Berk and Lieber, 1941; Finch and Finch, 1955; Willis, 1941; Stewart, 1931), while the incidence of this cancer in nonpigmentary cirrhosis is considerably lower (Berk and Lieber, 1941). Although the etiology of primary carcinoma of the liver in hemochromatosis is not yet elucidated, the presence of excessive iron in the liver is thought to be somehow related.

That excess iron may affect the toxicity and/or carcinogenicity of environmental agents has been demonstrated by several studies. For example, the animal carcinogen acetamide was found to cause the development of small, tumorlike nodules only along with hepatic siderosis. However, the acetamide was shown to be relatively innocuous even when given for long periods of time, provided there was an absence of an excess of liver iron (Timme, 1972). Other research implicating a role of excess iron in affecting pollutant toxicity was noted by Goldberg and Smith (1960) who reported that the combination of excess iron and ethionine causes an increase in the severity and speed of ethionine-induced cirrhotic changes in the liver of rats.

In contrast, Dunn (1967) found that iron-dextran injections in rats did not enhance the development of ethionine-induced tumors. Similarly, Timme (1974) was unable to demonstrate that prior iron overload influenced the carcinogenic effects of p-dimethylaminoazobenzene in rats.

With respect to human studies, several reports have indicated that iron does not seem to contribute to the frequency of primary liver carcinoma in the indigenous black races of South Africa (Becker and Chatgidakis, 1961; Higginson and Steiner, 1961; Steiner, 1960). However, it has been reported that Bantu siderosis may be related to hepatic fibrosis as well as a portal-type cirrhosis (Higginson et al., 1957). The issue therefore of whether industrial exposure to excessive iron dust that results in the development of siderosis enhances the carcinogenic and/or toxic effects of certain industrial substances in humans remains to be further evaluated, since animal-model studies provide inconsistent findings while human studies are also not yet adequate to fully answer this question.

References

Becker, B.J.P. and Chatgidakis, C.B. (1961). Primary carcinoma of the liver in Johannesburg. *Acta Un. Int. Cancer* **17**:650–653.

Berk, J.E. and Lieber, M.L. (1941). Primary carcinoma of liver in hemochromatosis. *Amer. J. Med. Sci.* **202**:708–714.

Dunn, W.L. (1967). Iron-loading fibrosis and hepatic carcinogenesis. *Arch. Path.* **83**:258–266.

Finch, S.C. and Finch, C.A. (1955). Idiopathic hemochromatosis, an iron storage disease. *Medicine* (Baltimore). **34**:381–430.

Goldberg, L. and Smith, J.P. (1960). Iron overloading and hepatic vulnerability. *Amer. J. Path.* **36**:125–150.

Higginson, J.; Grobbelaar, B.G.; and Walker, A.R.P. (1957). Hepatic fibrosis and cirrhosis in man in relation to malnutrition. *Amer. J. Path.* **33**:29–54.

Higginson, J. and Steiner, P. (1961). Cirrhosis and primary liver cancer in the non-white population of Johannesburg, South Africa. *Acta Un. Int. Cancer* **17**:654–666.

Steiner, P. (1960). Cancer of the liver and cirrhosis in Trans-Saharan Africa and the United States of America. *Cancer* **13**:1085–1166.

Stewart, M.J. (1931). Precancerous lesions of alimentary tract (Croonian lecture). *Lancet.* **2**:565.

Timme, A.H. (1972). The action of acetamide on the iron-laden rat liver. *S. African Med. J.* **46**:871–876.

Timme, A.H. (1974). Aspects of experimental hepatocarcinogenesis. Part III. Iron overload and hepatocarcinogenesis. *S. African Med. J.* **48**:1293–1294.

Vitale, J.J.; Broitman, S.A.; Vavrousek-Jakuba, E.; Rodday, P.W.; and Gottlieb, L.S. (1978). The effects of iron deficiency and the quality of fat in chemically induced cancer. In: *Inorganic and Nutritional Aspects of Cancer*, pp. 229–242. Edited by G.N. Schrauzer. Plenum Press, N.Y.

Warren, S. and Drake, W.L. (1951). Primary carcinoma of the liver in hemochromatosis. *Amer. J. Path.* **27**:573–592.

Willis, R.A. (1941). Hemochromatosis, with special reference to supervening carcinoma of liver. *Med. J. Aust.* **2**:666–669.

D. IRON—POLLUTANT INTERACTIONS—A PERSPECTIVE

It has been shown that low levels of dietary iron markedly enhance the toxicity and/or body burden of several heavy metals including cadmium, lead, manganese, and plutonium, and the carcinogenic expression of dimethylhydrazine, while modifying the capacity of the mixed-function oxidase enzymes of the liver to metabolize a number of xenobiotic drugs and hydrocarbon pollutants. The greatest amount of research in this area has been with cadmium and lead. In both instances, it has been found that a low dietary intake of iron for as short as a several-week period markedly enhances the tissue retention of these two toxic heavy metals, provided exposure is via the oral route. The present studies suggest that this knowledge has direct implications concerning exposure via food and drinking water. Studies employing airborne lead or cadmium on animals with variable consumption of iron have not been performed. Whether individuals with poor dietary status for iron would be at increased risk to airborne lead is not known, but would not be expected except through the ultimate passage of the airborne lead from the respiratory tract to the alimentary canal.

Consequently, the decision of the EPA not to consider the potential increased sensitivities of those with nutritional inadequacies (including iron) in establishing the ambient lead standard is not considered inappropriate (*Federal Register*, December 14, 1977). Although the present ambient air standard for lead probably did not need to consider those with nutritional inadequacies in the standard setting process, the data do suggest that the current drinking-water standards for lead and cadmium may be grossly inadequate to protect those with iron- (as well as calcium) deficient diets. It must be emphasized that the prevalence of inadequate iron consumption in the United States is striking, especially among the poor. Table 11 indicates the cumulative percentages of children aged 2–3 from low-income states not consuming one-quarter, half, and three-quarters of the recommended dietary intake of iron. Incredible as it seems, only 2% of this group received their RDA level of iron while 24.1% consumed only about one-fourth of the RDA. Development of a more precise quantification of the influence

Table 11. Cumulative Percentage of Distribution of Calcium and Iron Ingestion for Children 2 to 3 Years of Age from Low-Income Ratio States[a]

Calcium		Iron	
Ingestion (mg/day)	Percentage of Children	Ingestion (mg/day)	Percentage of Children
200	13.7	3.9	24.1
400	28.9	7.9	67.3
600	50.1	11.9	90.9
800[b]	65.9	15.0[b]	98.0

[a]Data derived from the Ten State Nutrition Survey, 1968–1970 (Ten State Nutrition Survey, 1972).

[b]Recommended dietary allowances for children 2 to 3 years old, 1968 (NAS, 1968).

Source. Mahaffey (May, 1974).

of this dietary condition over a wide range of lead exposures should be a high priority for EPA. In addition, the influence of multiple nutrient inadequacies such as calcium and iron in affecting heavy metal retention and toxicity is also of importance (see Levander, 1978). Finally, the mechanisms by which diets low in iron enhance the retention of heavy metals such as cadmium and lead need to be evaluated. To date this has been generally overlooked and it appears that important contributions to our understanding of iron-cadmium (lead) interactions could be made in this area.

The public health significance of enhanced plutonium and manganese retention resulting from low dietary intakes of iron remains to be evaluated. While exposure to plutonium will hopefully approach zero, exposure to manganese did rise with the implementation of the catalytic converter and the use of manganese fuel additives. While it is true that manganese is an essential trace element that is homeostatically regulated, this regulatory process apparently becomes disrupted under conditions of an iron deficiency. Prolonged exposure of individuals with inadequate levels of dietary iron to elevated levels of manganese has been reported to result in excessively heavy burdens of manganese with resulting toxic symptoms. If the EPA did not recently ban the use of MMT, it would have been quite proper to strongly recommend the EPA to sponsor research to evaluate the hypothesis that children with diets poor in iron living in areas heavily traveled with catalytic-converter-equipped automobiles may have an increased body burden of manganese.

In light of the increased susceptibility of individuals with low levels of iron in the diet to developing greater body burdens of cadmium and lead, would it not be wise to consume more than the RDA just for "extra" protection? At this point, sufficient data are not available on which to make that assessment. For even if extra iron did reduce cadmium or lead body burdens even more than consumption of a normal dietary intake of iron, it would still leave the nagging question about what else the excess iron would affect. According to Spivey-Fox (1979), "the use of nutrient supplements in excess of requirement must be approached with . . . caution. Numerous antagonisms and interactions between essential minerals themselves and between essential minerals and other nutrients continue to be recognized. Virtually nothing is known about dietary imbalances that may have an adverse effect on the function of the newly recognized essential elements, such as silicon, arsenic, and nickel. Some of our recent data illustrate the type of interaction problem that might arise with a nutrient supplement. Supplements of zinc and ascorbic acid have been shown to be very beneficial individually in counteracting the toxicity of cadmium. A combined supplement of these would seem to be useful; however, we have recently found that the combination is much more antagonistic to copper than either alone." This quote by Spivey-Fox (1979) expresses a legitimate caution that counsels against the substitution of a cure that may be worse than the disease.

References

Federal Register (1977). Environmental Protection Agency Proposed National Ambient Air Quality Standard for Lead. December 14, 1977.

Levander, O.A. (1978). Metabolic interactions between metals and metalloids. *Environ. Health Perspect.* **25**:77–80.

Mahaffey, K.R. (1974). Nutritional factors and susceptibility in lead toxicity. *Environ. Health Perspect.* **7**:107–111.

Spivey-Fox, M.R. (1979). Nutritional influences on metal toxicity—cadmium as a model toxic element. *Environ. Health Perspect.* **29**:95.

4

Selenium

A. INORGANIC SUBSTANCES

1. Arsenic

During the 1930s researchers at the South Dakota Agricultural Experiment Station reported that the cause of the "alkali disease" common to certain sections of the Great Plains was the consumption of plants with elevated levels of selenium (Moxon and Rhian, 1943). In further studies the combined toxicities of selenium with a variety of heavy metals were evaluated. Quite unexpectedly, it was found that the presence of arsenic (in the form of sodium arsenite) at 5 ppm in drinking water was able to provide full protection against dietary selenium-induced (11 ppm) liver damage in male and female rats (Moxon, 1938; Moxon and DuBois, 1939).

These findings were of some potential practical significance since many animals suffered from selenium intoxication as a result of consuming plants grown in areas where the soil had very high levels of this element. Consequently, a search for substances that would offset selenium toxicity was of great importance to those managing cattle, sheep, and horses. As a result of this initial report that arsenic could prevent selenium intoxication in rats, there evolved a series of new questions.

What forms of arsenic could prevent selenium toxicity? Are all forms of selenium equally affected? Does arsenic prevent selenium toxicity in all economically important farm animals? By what mechanism could arsenic reduce selenium toxicity?

Effect of Different Arsenicals. In the subsequent years of research, it was found that a number of arsenic compounds were effective in preventing selenium toxicity. DuBois et al. (1940) reported that both sodium arsenite and sodium arsenate were able to reduce the toxicity of several types of selenium compounds including seleniferous wheat as well as sodium selenite and selenocystine. In contrast, several arsenic sulfides (AsS_2, AsS_3) were ineffective as prophylactic agents.

While several inorganic forms of arsenic are capable of preventing the toxic effects of selenium, the toxicity of these inorganic arsenicals precluded their general usage on farms and ranches in seleniferous areas. However, organic arsenicals as therapeutic agents had long been used in the treatment of diseases such as syphilis and as growth stimulants for some farm animals and were known to be of lower toxicity than inorganic forms (Hendrick et al., 1953). As a result of the reduced toxicity of organic arsenicals compared to the inorganics, Hendrick et al. (1953) speculated that use of organic arsenicals may be a practical prophylactic treatment against selenium intoxication. Subsequent reports did in fact reveal that the use of several organic arsenicals [neoarsphenamine (Moxon et al., 1947), arsenilic acid, and 3-nitro, 4-hydroxyphenylarsonic acid (Hendrick et al., 1953; Wahlstrom and Olson, 1959; Wahlstrom et al., 1955)] were also effective in reducing selenium toxicity.

Effects on Various Species. While initial findings of an arsenic-selenium interaction were demonstrated by Moxon (1938) with experiments using rats, later researchers extended considerably the types of similarly affected animal species. Among the animals in which arsenic treatment reduced selenium toxicity were poultry (Moxon, 1941; Moxon and Wilson, 1944; Carlson et al., 1962; Thaper et al., 1969), ewes (Muth et al., 1971); pigs (Wahlstrom et al., 1955, 1956; Wahlstrom and Olson, 1959); cattle (Olson, 1960), dogs (Rhian and Moxon, 1943), and of course numerous experiments with rats (Moxon et al., 1945; Olson et al., 1963; Petersen et al., 1950; Moxon et al., 1947; Obermeyer et al., 1971).

Mechanism of Action. Since a number of arsenic compounds were capable of preventing selenium intoxication, what mechanisms of detoxification were involved? The earliest hypothesis was that arsenic forms a complex with selenium in the gastrointestinal tract, thereby diminishing the absorption of selenium (Anonymous, 1940). If this were accurate, then subcutaneous arsenic treatment would be expected to be ineffective in preventing selenium toxicity. Conversely, oral administration of arsenic would not be expected to reduce the toxicity of selenium given subcutaneously. However, Moxon et al. (1945) discredited the theory of an arsenic-selenium complex in the gastrointestinal tract by showing that detoxification was not dependent on the route of administration of either substance.

It was not until the 1960s that a coherent picture began to emerge concerning the mechanism by which arsenic diminished the toxicity of selenium. Ganther and Baumann (1962) reported that arsenic treatment prevented the production of volatile selenium compounds while both reducing the retention of selenium in the liver and increasing its level in the gastrointestinal tract. These findings of Ganther and Baumann (1962) were in fundamental agreement with the earlier research of Palmer and Bonhorst (1957) which revealed that arsenic treatment reduced the transport of selenium to the liver and with that of Kamstra and Bonhorst (1953), that arsenic administration reduced the exhalation of volatile selenium compounds. While an arsenic-induced reduction of selenium in the liver was consistent with a decrease in hepatotoxicity, the arsenic-induced reduction in selenium volatilization[1] did not appear consistent with the concept that arsenic offsets selenium toxicity. This seemed especially confusing since the elimination of selenium compounds via exhalation was long considered an important means of detoxification. For example, Schultz and Lewis (1940) reported that when adult rats were injected with 2.5 to 3.5 mg of selenium/kg as selenite, they exhaled 17 to 52% of the selenium within 8 hours.

In attempting to further resolve the question of how arsenic reduces selenium toxicity, Levander and Baumann (1966) demonstrated a dose-dependent relationship in which as the size of arsenic administration increased the level of selenium in the liver was diminished, while the levels of selenium in the gastrointestinal tract were increased (Table 1). Subsequent experimentation by Levander and Baumann (1966a) revealed that administration of inorganic arsenicals especially

[1]Selenium compounds may be excreted via exhalation in the following manner. Selenite is reduced to selenide, which is then methylated by methyl transferase enzymes to the volatile product, dimethyl selenide. Arsenite is thought to inhibit the synthesis of the dimethyl selenide via its inhibitory action on the methyl transferase enzymes (Levander, 1977; Ganther and Hsieh, 1974).

Table 1. Distribution of Selenium in Rats Given Various Doses of Arsenic[a]

| Dose of Arsenite (mg As/kg) | Proportion of the Dose of Selenium (%) | |
	In Liver	In Gastrointestinal Contents plus Feces
0.0	24.9 ± 2.5	8.7 ± 0.3
1.0	17.8 ± 2.0	11.2 ± 1.4
2.0	13.9 ± 1.4	25.4 ± 6.2
3.0	8.0 ± 0.9	22.4 ± 2.1
5.0	8.6 ± 1.0	25.8 ± 0.5

[a] All animals received 2 mg Se/kg as sodium selenite 10 min after injection with saline or sodium arsenite; length of experiment was 10 hr.

Source. Levander, O.A. and Baumann, C.A. (1966). Selenium metabolism. V. Studies on the distribution of selenium in rats given arsenic. *Toxicol. Appl. Pharmacol.* **9:**98–105.

sodium arsenite followed in effectiveness by sodium arsenate considerably enhanced the biliary excretion of selenium in rats (Table 2). Organic arsenicals were generally less effective. Of further interest was that selenite enhanced the biliary excretion of arsenite while also reducing its concentration in the liver.

According to Levander (1977), "the most appealing explanation [for the mechanism by which arsenic detoxifies selenium] is that selenium and arsenic react in the liver to form a detoxification conjugate which

Table 2. Effect of Arsenic on the Biliary Excretion of Selenium[a]

| | Proportion of the Dose of Selenium, % | |
	Saline only	Selenite
Bile	4.0 ± 0.4	40.8 ± 7.2
Liver	51.3 ± 3.0	20.9 ± 3.0
Gastrointestinal contents	1.7 ± 0.3	1.5 ± 0.3
Bile volume (ml)	3.0 ± 0.2	3.8 ± 0.5

[a] All animals received 0.5 mg Se/kg as sodium selenite 10 min before injection with either saline or 1 mg As/kg as sodium arsenite.

Source. Levander, O.A. and Baumann, C.A. (1966a). Selenium metabolism. VI. Effect of arsenic on the excretion of selenium in the bile. *Toxicol. Appl. Pharmacol.* **9:**98–105.

is excreted into the bile. Such an explanation would be consistent with the fact that arsenic and selenium increase the biliary excretion of the other. How or whether this mechanism is related to the inhibitory effect of arsenite on the methyl transferase responsible for the formation of dimethyl selenide is unknown. However, if the methyl transferase were blocked, excessive levels of hydrogen selenide might be generated in the liver, which then could react with any arsenite present in a manner akin to the reaction between arsenite and thiols. Such a selenoarsenite might then be the detoxification conjugate . . . that is excreted into the bile."

Based on the numerous studies previously cited that indicated that arsenic administration could diminish tissue levels of selenium, it has been hypothesized that arsenic treatment may be used to precipitate a selenium deficiency in animals reared on diets low in selenium. Despite the apparent logic of this hypothesis, a number of studies (Scott et al., 1967; Halverson and Palmer, 1975; Whanger et al., 1976) have been unable to support this suggestion regardless of the type of arsenic employed or the clinical end point measured (i.e., gizzard myopathy in turkey poults, liver necrosis in rats, white muscle disease in lambs). Finally, while the previous discussions have dealt exclusively with how arsenic detoxifies selenium, several reports have indicated that arsenic may actually enhance the toxicity of methylated selenium compounds (Obermeyer et al., 1971; McConnell and Portman, 1952).

Practical Applications and Future Considerations. In his excellent review of this topic, Levander (1977) stated that there were three general areas where the knowledge of arsenic-selenium interactions may have some possible significance:

1. Industrial hygiene—either arsenic or selenium could be used as an antidote for acute poisoning by the other. However, the probability of acute poisoning in the industrial environment by these substances is quite unlikely. The real question is whether diets chronically low or high in either element affect the body burden and toxicity of the other compound. Since arsenic is considered a carcinogen by OSHA, and EPA considers both arsenic and selenium as potential carcinogens, it would appear that such organizations would not advocate the use of dietary supplements of either element to prevent the toxicity of the other. However, because evidence for the carcinogenicity of both arsenic (Frost, 1978) and selenium is not particularly impressive, especially that of selenium (Lafond and Calabrese, 1979), it would seem that further animal experimenta-

tion and human epidemiological studies should be conducted with the intention of evaluating their mutually antagonistic properties and their potential application to industrial hygiene practice.

2. The reports that arsenic enhances the toxicity of methylated selenium compounds are of concern from an ecological as well as human-health-effects perspective. It is obvious that greater research efforts need to be directed into this area.

3. From the agricultural perspective, it had been hoped that arsenicals, especially the organic types, might be of use in preventing selenium toxicity in farm animals. However, Olson, in a personal communication to Levander (1977), reported that this had not proved feasible. However, this statement was not supported.

4. The recent hypothesis of Ganther (1978) that arsenic in tuna fish may contribute to a reduction in the toxicity of fish with elevated levels of mercury should be investigated.

References

Anonymous (1940). Progress in the selenium problem. *JAMA* **114**:1083.

Carlson, C.W.; Gross, P.L.; and Olson, O.E. (1962). Selenium content of chick tissues as affected by arsenic. *Poult. Sci.* **41**:1987–1989.

DuBois, K.P.; Moxon, A.L.; and Olson, O.E. (1940). Further studies on the effectiveness of arsenic in preventing selenium poisoning. *J. Nutr.* **19**:477–482.

El-Begearmi, M.M.; Ganther, H.E.; and Sunde, M.L. (1975). More evidence for a selenium-arsenic interaction in modifying mercury toxicity. *Poult. Sci.* **54**:1746.

Frost, D.V. (1960). Arsenic and selenium in relation to the food additive law of 1958. *Nutr. Rev.* **18**:129–132.

Frost, D.V. (1965). Selenium and poultry: an exercise in nutrition toxicology which involves arsenic. *World's Poult. Sci. J.* **21**:139–156.

Frost, D.V. (1978). The arsenic problems. In: *Inorganic and Nutritional Aspects of Cancer,* pp. 259–279. Edited by G.N. Schrauzer. Plenum Press, N.Y.

Ganther, H.E. (1978). Modification of methyl mercury toxicity and metabolism by selenium and vitamin E: possible mechanisms. *Environ. Health. Perspect.* **25**:71–76.

Ganther, H.E. and Baumann, C.A. (1962). Selenium metabolism. I. Effects of diet, arsenic and cadmium. *J. Nutr.* **77**:210–216.

Ganther, H.E. and Hsieh, H.S. (1974). Mechanisms for the conversion of selenite to selenides in mammalian tissues. In: *Trace Element Metabolism in Animals,* p. 339. Edited by W.G. Hoekstra, J.W. Suttie, H.E. Ganther, and W. Mertz. Univ. Park Press, Baltimore.

Halverson, A.W. and Palmer, I.S. (1975). The effect of substances which protect against selenium toxicity in selenium utlization by rats. *Proc. South Dakota Acad. Sci.* **54**:148–156.

Hendrick, C.; Klug, H.L.; and Olson, O.E. (1953). Effect of 3-nitro, 4-hydroxyphenyl arsonic acid and arsanilic acid on selenium poisoning in the rat. *J. Nutr.* **51**:131–137.

Holmberg, R.E. and Ferm, V.H. (1969). Interrelationships of selenium, cadmium, and arsenic in mammalian teratogenesis. *Arch. Environ. Health* **18**:873–877.

Howell, G.O. and Hill, C.H. (1978). Biological interaction of selenium with other trace elements in chicks. *Environ. Health Perspect.* **25**:147–150.

Kamstra, L.D. and Bonhorst, C.W. (1953). Effect of arsenic on the expiration of volatile selenium compounds by rats. *Proc. South Dakota Acad. Sci.* **32**:72.

Klug, H.L.; Lampson, G.P.; and Moxon, A.L. (1950). The distribution of selenium and arsenic in the body tissues of rats fed selenium, arsenic, or selenium plus arsenic. *Proc. South Dakota Acad. Sci.* **29**:57.

Klug, H.L.; Moxon, A.L.; Petersen, D.F.; and Potter, V.R. (1950). The *in vivo* inhibition of succinic dehydrogenase by selenium and release by arsenic. *Arch. Biochem. Biophys.* **28**:253–259.

Krista, L.M.; Carlson, C.W.; and Olson, O.E. (1961). Effect of arsenic on selenium deposition in chicken eggs. *Poult. Sci.* **40**:1365–1367.

Lafond, M. and Calabrese, E.J. (1979). Is the selenium drinking water standard justified? *Med. Hypoth.* **5**(8):877–899.

Levander, O.A. (1965). Studies on the distribution of selenium in rats given arsenic. Ph.D. dissertation, Univ. of Wisconsin, Madison.

Levander, O.A. (1977). Metabolic interrelationships between arsenic and selenium. *Environ. Health Perspect.* **19**:159–164.

Levander, O.A. and Argrett, L.C. (1969). Effect of arsenic, mercury, thallium, and lead on selenium metabolism in rats. *Toxicol. Appl. Pharmacol.* **14**:308.

Levander, O.A. and Baumann, C.A. (1965). The influence of arsenic on the biliary excretion of selenium. *Federat. Proc.* **24**:373.

Levander, O.A. and Baumann, C.A. (1966). Selenium metabolism. V. Studies on the distribution of selenium in rats given arsenic. *Toxicol. Appl. Pharmacol.* **9**:98–105.

Levander, O.A. and Baumann, C.A. (1966a). Selenium metabolism. VI. Effect of arsenic on the excretion of selenium in the bile. *Toxicol. Appl. Pharmacol.* **9**:106–115.

McConnell, K.P. and Carpenter, D.M. (1971). Interrelationship between selenium and specific trace elements. *Proc. Soc. Exp. Biol. Med.* **137**:996–1001.

McConnell, K.P. and Portman, J.W. (1952). Toxicity of dimethyl selenide in rat and mouse. *Proc. Soc. Exp. Biol. Med.* **79**:230.

McDowell, L.R.; Froseth, J.A.; and Piper, R.C. (1978). Influence of arsenic, sulfur, cadmium, tellurium, silver and selenium on the selenium-vitamin E deficiency in the pig. *Nutr. Rept. Intern.* **17**:19–35.

Moxon, A.L. (1938). The effect of arsenic on the toxicity of seleniferous grains. *Science* **88**:81.

Moxon, A.L. (1941). Some factors influencing the toxicity of selenium. III. The toxicity of arsenic and its influence upon the toxicity of selenium in chicks. Ph.D. dissertation, Univ. of Wisconsin.

Moxon, A.L. (1941a). The influence of arsenic on selenium poisoning in hogs. *Proc. South Dakota Acad. of Sci.* **21**:34–36.

Moxon, A.L. and DuBois, K.P. (1939). The influence of arsenic and certain other elements on the toxicity of seleniferous grains. *J. Nutr.* **18**:447–457.

Moxon, A.L.; Jensen, C.W.; and Paynter, C.R. (1947). The influence of germanium, gallium, antimony and some organic arsenicals on the toxicity of selenium. *Proc. South Dakota Acad. Sci.* **26**:21–26.

Moxon, A.L.; Paynter, C.R.; and Halverson, A.W. (1945). Effect of route of administration on detoxification of selenium by arsenic. *J. Pharm. Exp. Therap.* **84**:115–119.

Moxon, A.L. and Rhian, M. (1943). Selenium poisoning. *Physiol. Rev.* **23**:305.

Moxon, A.L.; Rhian, M.A.; Anderson, H.D.; and Olson, O.E. (1944). Growth of steers on seleniferous range. *J. Anim. Sci.* **3**:299.

Moxon, A.L. and Wilson, W.O. (1944). Selenium-arsenic antagonism in poultry. *Poult. Sci.* **23**:149–151.

Muth, O.H.; Whanger, P.D.; Weswig, P.H.; and Oldfield, J.E. (1971). Occurrence of myopathy in lambs of ewes fed added arsenic in a selenium-deficient ration. *Amer. J. Vet. Res.* **32**:1621–1623.

Obermeyer, B.D.; Palmer, I.S.; Olson, O.E.; and Halverson, A.W. (1971). Toxicity of trimethyl selenonium chloride in the rat with and without arsenite. *Toxicol. Appl. Pharmacol.* **20**:135–146.

Olson, O.E. (1960). Selenium and the organic arsenicals. *Feed Age* **10**:49.

Olson, O.E.; Schulte, B.M.; Whitehead, E.I.; and Halverson, A.W. (1963). Effect of arsenic on selenium metabolism in rats. *J. Agricult. Food Chem.* **11**:531–534.

Palmer, I.V. and Bonhorst, C.W. (1957). Modification of selenite metabolism by arsenite. *J. Agricult. Food Chem.* **5**:928–930.

Petersen, D.F.; Klug, H.L.; Harshfield, R.D.; and Moxon, A.L. (1950). *Proc. South Dakota Acad. Sci.* **29**:123.

Rhian, M. and Moxon, A.L. (1943). Chronic selenium poisoning in dogs and its prevention by arsenic. *J. Pharm. Exper. Therap.* **78**:249–264.

Rossner, P.; Bencko, V.; and Havrankora, H. (1977). Effect of the combined action of selenium and arsenic on suspension culture of mice fibroblasts. *Environ. Health Perspect.* **19**:235–237.

Schultz, J. and Lewis, H.B. (1940). The excretion of volatile selenium compounds after the administration of sodium selenite to white rats. *J. Biol. Chem.* **133**:199.

Scott, M.L.; Olson, G.; Krook, L.; and Brown, W.R. (1967). Selenium-responsive myopathies of myocardium and of smooth muscle in the young poult. *J. Nutr.* **91**:573.

Thaper, N.T.; Guenthner, E.; Carlson, C.W.; and Olson, O.E. (1969). Dietary selenium and arsenic additions to diets for chickens over a life cycle. *Poult. Sci.* **48**:1988.

Wahlstrom, R.C.; Kamstra, L.D.; and Olson, O.E. (1955). The effect of arsanilic acid and 3-nitro-4-hydroxyphenyl arsonic acid on selenium poisoning in the pig. *J. Anim. Sci.* **14**:105–110.

Wahlstrom, R.C.; Kamstra, L.D.; and Olson, O.E. (1956). The effect of organic arsenicals, chlortetracycline and linseed oil meal on selenium poisoning in swine. *J. Anim. Sci.* **15**:794.

Wahlstrom, R.C. and Olson, O.E. (1959). The relation of prenatal and pre-weanling treatment to the effect of arsanilic acid on selenium poisoning in weanling pigs. *J. Anim. Sci.* **18**:578–582.

Whanger, P.D.; Weswig, P.H.; Schmitz, J.A.; and Oldfield, J.E. (1976). Effects of selenium, cadmium, mercury, tellurium, arsenic, silver and cobalt on white muscle disease in lambs and effect of dietary forms of arsenic on its accumulation in tissues. *Nutr. Rept. Intern.* **14**:63–72.

2. Cadmium

In 1957, Parizek first reported that the acute toxicity of cadmium to the testis of rats could be prevented by the administration of zinc. While this initial striking finding was soon confirmed by a number of investigators (Kar et al., 1960; Gunn et al., 1961; Mason et al., 1964), a search for other substances that would protect against cadmium toxicity also ensued. Reports concerning possible interactions of cadmium with other elements revealed that sodium, calcium, or copper (Parizek, 1957) could not offset cadmium-induced toxicity. However, several reports emerged that clearly suggested that selenium was able to prevent cadmium toxicity and, in fact, that it was even more efficient in this regard than zinc (Kar et al., 1960; Mason et al., 1964). The findings that selenium prevents the toxicity of cadmium along with an infrequently cited but similarly supportive study by Tobias et al. (1946) initiated considerable interest in further elucidating the extent, nature, and potential public health significance of selenium-cadmium interrelationships.

In research with both mouse and rat models, it was shown that selenium was remarkably efficient in not only reducing but also in preventing the occurrence of cadmium-induced testicular damage (Gunn et al., 1968, 1968a; Mason et al., 1964; Kar et al., 1960). However, it was a curious phenomenon that the selenium treatment *did not* reduce the level of cadmium reaching the testis but actually dramatically increased it. In fact, the selenium treatment resulted in a striking 150 to 250% increase (p<0.005) in the uptake of cadmium by the testis as compared to controls given only cadmium, thereby implying the formation of a selenium-cadmium complex. Comparison with other agents (e.g., cysteine and zinc) that also protect the testis from cadmium-induced damage revealed that neither reduced the level of cadmium in the testis, while cysteine also increased it by 38% (Figure 4-1) (Gunn et al., 1968). Among five agents (i.e., which were found to protect against cadmium-induced testicular damage) selenium was clearly the most effective, by completely preventing testicular lesions in a dosage ratio of 2:1 (Gunn et al., 1968a).

Not only does selenium administration prevent cadmium-induced testicular damage, but Gunn et al. (1968) have also revealed that it prevents cadmium-induced lethality in mice (20 weeks old), in agreement with the earlier findings of Tobias et al. (1946). In addition, Parizek et al. (1968) reported that selenium administration prevented cadmium-induced renal toxicity and placental damage in pregnant rats and lethality to their fetuses when both compounds were given on the 21st day of gestation. In similar fashion as with the testicular

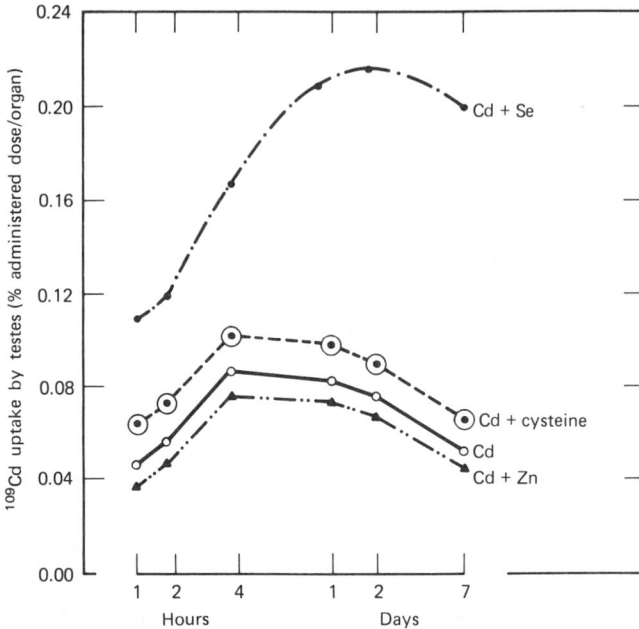

Figure 4-1. The effect of zinc acetate (0.3 mmole/kg), cysteine (6.0 mmole/kg) and selenium dioxide (0.024 mmole/kg) on the uptake of ^{109}Cd in cadmium chloride (0.012 mmole/kg) by testes of CD-1 male mice. [*Source.* Gunn, S.A., et al. (1968). Mechanisms of zinc, cysteine, and selenium protection against cadmium-induced vascular injury of mouse testis. *J. Reprod. Fert.* **15**:67.]

studies, it was found that the selenium exposure enhanced the presence of cadmium in affected tissues (e.g., placenta) while paradoxically decreasing toxicity.

Analyses of cadmium levels of other tissues in the rats protected by selenium treatment revealed that the blood-cadmium levels were also markedly increased and that the cadmium was tightly bound to the macromolecular fraction of blood plasma (Parizek et al., 1968a). Based on these findings, Parizek et al. (1968) suggested that selenium treatment may in fact result in an alteration of the binding of cadmium and thereby reduce (or at least change) the toxicity of cadmium.

While concomitant treatment with selenium and cadmium was found to cause a marked increase in the cadmium levels of several tissues including the testis (3×), blood (22×), and plasma (32×), Chen et al. (1975) found that the selenium administration reduced cadmium

Table 3. Cd Concentrations in Rat Tissues[a]

	ng Cd/ml or g Fresh Tissue				
Treatment	Blood	Plasma[b]	Liver	Kidney	Testis
Control	138	148	7675	1430	114
Se-pretreated	3025	4830	4012	1260	299

[a]The amounts of Cd were calculated according to the specific activity of ^{109}Cd in the injection solution.

[b]The plasma contained 59% and 88% of the blood Cd in the control and Se-pretreated rats, respectively, as calculated by assuming that the whole blood contained 46% of its volume as erythrocytes.

Source. Chen, R.W. et al. (1975). Selenium-induced redistribution of cadmium binding to tissue proteins—a possible mechanism of protection against cadmium toxicity. *Bioinorg. Chem.* **4:**127.

levels in the liver by 48% and in the kidney by 12% (Table 3). In agreement with and in extension of the studies of Parizek et al. (1968), Chen et al. (1974, 1975) and Whanger (1979) reported that selenium was able to alter the tissue distribution and protein-binding capacity of cadmium in the testis, kidney, and liver (Table 4).

It is important to note that most of the studies concerned with elucidating the selenium-cadmium interaction have exposed animal models via injection. According to Whanger (1979), "the environ-

Table 4. Subcellular Cd Distribution in Rat Tissues

		ng Cd/g Tissue		
Subcellular	Treatment	Liver	Kidney	Testis
Crude nuclear	Cd	1130	210	54
	Cd + Se	1522	352	76
Mitochondrial	Cd	1259	228	2
	Cd + Se	431	144	7
Microsomal	Cd	966	123	3
	Cd + Se	403	111	21
Soluble	Cd	4431	795	48
	Cd + Se	1690	583	190

Source. Chen, R.W. et al. (1975). Selenium-induced redistribution of cadmium binding to tissue proteins—a possible mechanism of protection against cadmium toxicity. *Bioinorg. Chem.* **4:**127.

mental significance of these injection experiments, however, is questionable, since oral dosing with selenium and cadmium or inclusion in the diet do not cause a diversion of cadmium binding in tissue. Since animals (and man) are exposed to heavy metals in the environment either through the oral or pulmonary route, selenium must counteract metals such as environmental cadmium by other mechanisms besides diverting their binding in tissue protein."

While it is apparent that selenium alters the intracellular tissue distribution of cadmium as well as its protein-binding capacity, thereby modifying its toxicity, other investigators have also attempted to further elucidate the manner in which selenium may affect cadmium toxicity. Stowe (1976) reported that selenium enhances the biliary excretion of cadmium, possibly contributing to reduced toxic effects. He stated that "the elevated levels of cadmium present in the bile following selenium pretreatment . . . are consistent with elevated blood cadmium levels and a reduced amount of cadmium bound in the liver [as seen by Chen et al., 1975]." Other researchers have found that selenium treatment does not influence the effects of cadmium on tissue iron levels (Whanger, 1979), while selenium (as selenite) does seem to require a GSH-dependent transformation probably to glutathion selenotrisulfide before being able to affect binding with cadmium (Gasiewicz and Smith, 1976, 1978).

Conclusions.   Selenium administration has been shown to be able to reduce and prevent, depending on the dosages employed, the toxicity of cadmium in a variety of tissues (Table 5). Of particular interest and importance are those findings that have shown that cadmium-induced testicular damage (Gunn et al., 1968; Ganther et al., 1972) and hypertension (Perry et al., 1974) have been preventable by selenium supplementation. Not only does selenium supplementation reduce cad-

Table 5.   Toxic Effects of Cadmium Prevented by Selenium Administration

Lethality in adult and fetal mice	Gunn et al., 1968
Testicular damage	Gunn et al., 1968
	Mason et al., 1964
Hypertension	Perry et al., 1974
Altered pancreas function	Merali and Singhal, 1975
Liver enzyme changes	Merali and Singhal, 1975
Respiratory disease	Reddy et al., 1978
Renal damage	Parizek et al., 1968
Teratogenic effects in hamsters	Holmberg and Ferm, 1969

mium toxicity, its deficiency in the diet markedly enhances cadmium toxicity (Reddy et al., 1978).

The mechanisms by which selenium administration reduce cadmium toxicity are not precisely known. Considerable evidence does exist, however, that suggests that selenium alters both the tissue distribution and protein-binding capacity of cadmium. Conceivably these changes in cadmium metabolism could be wholly or partly responsible for its altered toxicity in the presence of selenium.

It is difficult to assess the public health significance of the findings presented here for several reasons. The doses of cadmium employed have been much larger than normal human exposure, while the routes of exposure have often been via injection. Such factors only increase the difficulty of assessing human risk. This may be especially important since there are differences in the binding of cadmium according to the route of exposure (Whanger, 1979). There is also a general lack of chronic exposure studies. Information from such studies could add immeasurably to the current state of knowledge in this area. In addition, the impressive findings of Perry et al. (1974) that cadmium induces hypertension in animal models have not been effectively replicated by other investigators, even using hypertension-prone rats and in a chronic experimental exposure (see Whanger, 1979).

Finally, since elevated levels of selenium exposure definitely pose a toxicologic hazard, it would seem that the emphasis in research should be directed from the use of very elevated levels of selenium exposure to diets containing adequate and marginally deficient amounts of selenium. Such studies could probably be conducted with industrial populations exposed to cadmium.

References

Chen, R.W.; Wagner, P.A.; Hoekstra, W.G.; and Ganther, H.E. (1974). Affinity labeling studies with [109]cadmium in cadmium-induced testicular injury in rats. *J. Reprod. Fertil.* **38**:293.

Chen, R.W.; Whanger, P.D.; and Weswig, P.H. (1975). Selenium-induced redistribution of cadmium binding to tissue proteins—a possible mechanism of protection against cadmium toxicity. *Bioinorg. Chem.* **4**:125–133.

Ganther, H.E. and Baumann, C.A. (1962). Selenium metabolism. Effects of diet, arsenic, and cadmium. *J. Nutr.* **77**:210–216.

Ganther, H.E.; Wagner, P.A.; Sunde, M.L.; and Hoekstra, W.G. (1972). Protective effects of selenium against heavy metal toxicities. In: *Trace Substances in Environmental Health*, pp. 247–252. Edited by D.D. Hemphill, Univ. of Missouri, Columbia.

Gasiewicz, T.A. and Smith, J.C. (1976). Interactions of cadmium and selenium in rat plasma *in vitro*. *Biochem. Biophys. Acta* **428**:113.

Gasiewicz, T.A. and Smith, J.C. (1978). Interaction between cadmium and selenium in rat plasma. *Environ. Health Perspect.* **25**:133–136.

Gunn, S.A. and Gould, T.C. (1967). Specificity of response in relation to cadmium, zinc, and selenium. In: *Selenium in Biomedicine.* Edited by O.H. Muth. The Avi Publishing Co., Westport, CT.

Gunn, S.A.; Gould, T.C.; and Anderson, W.A.D. (1961). Zinc protection against cadmium injury to rat testis. *Arch. Path.* **71**:274.

Gunn, S.A.; Gould, T.C.; and Anderson, W.A.D. (1968). Mechanisms of zinc, cysteine, and selenium protection against cadmium-induced vascular injury of mouse testis. *J. Reprod. Fert.* **15**:65–70.

Gunn, S.A.; Gould, T.C.; and Anderson, W.A.D. (1968a). Specificity in protection against lethality and testicular toxicity from cadmium. *Proc. Soc. Exp. Biol. Med.* **128**:591–595.

Hill, C.W. (1975). Interrelationships of selenium with other trace elements. *Fed. Proc.* **34**:2096–2100.

Holmberg, R.E. and Ferm, V.H. (1969). Interrelationships of selenium, cadmium, and arsenic in mammalian teratogenesis. *Arch. Environ. Health* **18**:873–877.

Kar, A.B.; Das, R.P.; and Mukerji, F.N.I. (1960). Prevention of cadmium induced changes in the gonads of rats by zinc and selenium—a study in antagonism between metals in the biological system. *Proc. Natl. Instit. Sci. India* B. 26, Suppl., 40.

Magos, L. and Webb, M. (1976). Differences in distribution and excretion of selenium and cadmium or mercury after their simultaneous administration subcutaneously in equimolar doses. *Arch. Toxicol.* **36**:63.

Mason, K.E. and Young, J.O. (1967). Effectiveness of selenium and zinc in protecting against cadmium-induced injury of the rat testis. In: *Selenium in Biomedicine.* Edited by O.H. Muth. The Avi Publishing Co., Westport, CT.

Mason, K.E.; Young, J.O.; and Brown, J.E. (1964). Effectiveness of selenium and zinc in protecting against cadmium-induced injury of the rat testis. *Anat. Record* **148**:309.

Merali, Z. and Singhal, R.L. (1975). Protective effect of selenium on certain hepatotoxic and pancreotoxic manifestations of subacute cadmium administration. *J. Pharmacol. Exp. Therap.* **195**:58–66.

Parizek, J. (1957). The destructive effect of cadmium on testicular tissue and its prevention by zinc. *J. Endocrinol.* **15**:56.

Parizek, J. (1976). Interrelationships among trace elements. In: *Effects and Dose-Response Relationships of Toxic Metals,* pp. 498–510. Edited by G.F. Nordberg. Elsevier Scientific Publishing Co., Amsterdam.

Parizek, J.; Benes, I.; Kalouskova, J.; Ostadalova, I.; Lener, J.; Babicky, A.; and Benes, J. (1968a). Metabolic interrelations of certain trace elements in the organism: cadmium, zinc, selenium and mercury. *Cslka Fysiol.* cited in Parizek et al., 1968.

Parizek, J.; Ostadalova, I.; Benes, I.; and Babicky, A. (1968). Pregnancy and trace elements: the protective effect of compounds of an essential trace element—selenium—against the peculiar toxic effects of cadmium during pregnancy. *J. Reprod. Fert.* **16**:507–509.

Parizek, J.; Ostadalova, I.; Benes, I.; Babicky, A.; and Benes, J. (1967). The protective effect of trace amounts of selenite in the intoxication with compounds of cadmium and bivalent mercury. *Cslka Fysiol.* **16**:41.

Perry, H.M., Jr.; Perry, E.F.; and Erlanger, M.W. (1974). Reversal of cadmium-induced hypertension by selenium or hard water. In: *Trace Substances in Environmental Health,* pp. 51–57. Edited by D.D. Hemphill. Univ. of Missouri, Columbia.

Reddy, K.A.; Omaye, S.T.; Hasegawa, G.K.; and Cross, C.E. (1978). Enhanced lung toxicity of intratracheally instilled cadmium chloride in selenium-deficient rats. *Toxicol. Appl. Pharmacol.* 43:249–257.

Stowe, H.D. (1976). Biliary excretion of cadmium by rats: effects of zinc, cadmium, and selenium pretreatments. *J. Toxicol. Environ. Health* 2:45–53.

Tobias, J.M.; Lushbaugh, C.C.; Patt, H.M.; Postel, S.; Swift, M.N.; and Gerard, R.W. (1946). The pathology and therapy with 2,3-dimercaptoproponal (BAL) on experimental Cd poisoning. *J. Pharmacol. Exp. Therap.* Suppl. 87:102–118.

Whanger, P.D. (1976). Selenium versus metal toxicity in animals. In: *Proceedings, Symposium Selenium-Tellurium in the Environment,* p. 234. Industrial Health Foundation, Pittsburgh, PA.

Whanger, P.D. (1979). Cadmium effects in rats on tissue iron, selenium, and blood pressure; blood and hair cadmium in some Oregon residents. *Environ. Health Perspect.* 28:115–121.

3. Fluoride

It is certainly well known that consumption of drinking water with levels of fluoride at approximately 1 mg/L markedly reduces the occurrence of decayed, missing, and filled teeth in children as compared to those receiving water with lower levels of fluoride. Epidemiological investigations, however, have suggested that the elevated levels of selenium in drinking water may reduce the effectiveness of fluoride in preventing dental caries (Tank and Storvick, 1960). However, later studies with animal models revealed that the proposed adverse effects of selenium on the cavity-fighting functions of fluoride did not seem to be caused by a decreased uptake of fluoride (Hadjimarkos, 1967) since selenium did not affect the retention of fluoride in bone, nor does selenium (3 ppm) appear to enhance the toxicity of 50-ppm fluoride (Hadjimarkos, 1969).

In light of these findings, it must be tentatively concluded that experimental evidence derived from research with animal models does not support the hypothesis that dietary selenium in food or drinking water affects the retention of fluoride or its toxicity.

References

Hadjimarkos, D.M. (1967). Selenium-fluoride interaction in relation to dental caries. *Arch. Environ. Health* 14:881.

Hadjimarkos, D.M. (1969). Selenium toxicity: effect of fluoride. *Experientia* 25:485.

Tank, G. and Storvick, C.A. (1960). Effect of naturally-occurring selenium and vanadium on dental caries. *J. Dent. Res.* 39:473.

4. Lead

Several investigators have suggested that dietary selenium may be expected to affect the toxicity of lead since both substances are known to display a high affinity for sulfur-containing proteins. Other heavy metals such as cadmium and mercury, like lead, also exhibit a strong binding attraction for sulfur-containing compounds and selenium is known to diminish their toxicity. With this type of rationale to support their endeavors, several research teams independently set out to evaluate the hypothesis that selenium may reduce lead toxicity (Cerklewski and Forbes, 1976; Stone and Soares, 1976; Rastogi et al., 1976).

The findings of these investigations indicated that dietary selenium affects the tissue retention of lead as well as modifying several of its effects on biochemical processes. For instance, all three studies indicated that selenium supplementation (1 to 10 ppm) markedly enhanced the retention of lead in several tissues including the blood and kidney in rats and quail. However, Cerklewski and Forbes (1976) reported that the 0.5-ppm selenium treatment resulted in a diminished retention of lead in the blood, liver, kidney, and tibia of rats. Selenium supplementation also reduced the extent to which lead diminished the activity of ALAD in blood, liver, and kidney tissue in rats (Rastogi et al., 1976), while being unable to prevent lead-induced decreases in ALAD activity of red blood cells in quail (Stone and Soares, 1976).

In partial contrast to the findings of Rastogi et al. (1976), Cerklewski and Forbes (1976) reported that selenium supplementation (up to 1 ppm) resulted in a reduction of the inhibitory effect of lead on ALAD activity in liver tissue only and not in the kidney and blood. Subsequent research by Levander et al. (1977) and Sifri and Hoekstra (1978) have also revealed a limited but definite interaction between dietary selenium (approximately 0.5 ppm) and lead, especially with respect to preventing lead-induced changes in red-cell function and lipid peroxidation.

The general conclusions of these findings are that selenium supplementation in rats of up to at least 0.5 ppm may result in a slight reduction in the retention and toxicity of elevated exposures to lead (200 to 250 ppm in drinking water) (Levander et al., 1977; Cerklewski and Forbes, 1976; Sifri and Hoekstra, 1978). Studies involving more elevated levels of selenium supplementation in which from 1 ppm to 10 ppm are employed in the diet become less practical with respect to human dietary implications because evidence does exist that selenium becomes toxic at levels as low as 1.25 ppm (Witting and

Horwitt, 1964). In fact, Levander et al. (1977) reported that selenium supplements as low as 0.5 ppm to vitamin E-supplemented lead-poisoned rats resulted in quantifiable adverse health effects (i.e., slight increase in spleen size and decrease in hematocrit). These findings led Levander et al. (1977) to conclude that "although excess levels of selenium do have some protective effects against lead poisoning in vitamin E-deficient rats, the levels of selenium that are needed to demonstrate an effect are toxic in themselves."

While the conclusion of Levander et al. (1977) is in concert with the reported findings of published studies, it would seem that further research should continue to evaluate the influence of dietary selenium on lead intoxication. However, the emphasis should be toward assessing how diets marginally deficient, adequate, or with slightly greater than adequate amounts of selenium affect lead toxicity resulting from chronic low-level exposure.

References

Cerklewski, F.L. and Forbes, R.M. (1976). Influence of dietary selenium on lead toxicity in the rat. *J. Nutr.* **106**:778–783.

Levander, O.A. and Argrett, L.C. (1969). Effects of arsenic, mercury, thallium, and lead on selenium metabolism in rats. *Toxicol. Appl. Pharmacol.* **14**:308–314.

Levander, O.A.; Morris, V.C.; and Ferretti, R.J. (1977). Comparative effects of selenium and vitamin E in lead-poisoned rats. *J. Nutr.* **107**:378–382.

Rastogi, S.C.; Clausen, J.; and Srivastava, K.C. (1976). Selenium and lead: mutual detoxifying effects. *Toxicol.* **6**:377–388.

Sifri, M. and Hoekstra, W.G. (1978). Effect of lead on lipid peroxidation in rats deficient or adequate in selenium and vitamin E. *Fed. Proc.* **37**:757.

Stone, C.L. and Soares, J.H., Jr. (1976). The effect of dietary selenium level on lead toxicity in the Japanese quail. *Poult. Sci.* **55**:341–349.

Witting, L.A. and Horwitt, M.K. (1964). Effects of dietary selenium, methionine, fat level and tocopherol on rat growth. *J. Nutr.* **84**:351–360.

5. Mercury

Among the numerous interactions that selenium is known to have with toxic substances in the environment, none has been researched and discussed as much as the one with mercury. Not including review articles on the subject, approximately 50 original research articles have evaluated this interaction. The reasons for such interest are certainly conjectural, but are probably related to a combination of events including (1) the initially encouraging findings that selenium supplementation markedly reduces mercury intoxication, (2) the widespread scientific and public attention provided to several tragic incidences of human intoxication by mercury, and (3) the recognition that methylmercury was present in appreciable quantities in both tuna and swordfish.

That selenium supplementation could prevent mercury intoxication was first reported by Parizek and Ostadalova in 1967. In previous reports, Parizek had revealed that selenium was highly effective in reducing the toxicity of cadmium (see cadmium section of this chapter), and he wanted to see if this detoxifying capacity of selenium was more generalizable. The report of Parizek and Ostadalova (1967) revealed that sodium selenite prevented mercuric chloride-induced acute toxicity and pathological changes in the kidneys and intestines. This finding was subsequently confirmed and extended by numerous researchers.

Since the magnitude of these investigations is considerable, an attempt will be made to present several generalizations concerning the thrust of the research designs employed. On the whole, these investigations have evaluated both inorganic and organic mercury interactions with selenium, with the usual forms being mercuric chloride and methylmercury, respectively. Occasionally, a researcher may employ a different type of organic mercury such as the phenyl form, but this is clearly the exception. The levels of mercury employed in the experimental studies in all cases grossly exceed the usual levels of human exposure. While the average daily human intake of mercury (most of it being the methyl form) is approximately 3 μg/day, the usual level of methylmercury used in the diet or drinking water of these studies has been between 20–40 ppm, while for inorganic mercury the levels used most commonly are between 50–400 ppm. With respect to selenium, it is a rare exception to find a form other than sodium selenite.

The levels of selenium used are highly variable, depending on the purpose of the investigations. For instance, the range of selenium used goes from a dietary deficiency to levels that would normally be grossly intoxicating by themselves (i.e., up to 28 ppm). However, a common range is between 3–8 ppm, since researchers realize that prolonged exposure to these levels will be toxic to many laboratory species. However, since the levels of mercury are so high, a large amount of selenium is thought to be needed for detoxification. Also, the studies using large amounts of selenium are also of a short-term nature, thus precluding the occurrence of selenium toxicity. The more prolonged studies have, as expected, used levels of selenium below 1.0 ppm.

While there are several studies of human subjects and the relationship of selenium and mercury in their respective tissues, nearly all information concerning the selenium-mercury interaction is derived from animal models. In general, the use of rats has predominated with the Wistar and Sprague-Dawley strains being used most often. The next most frequent model has been the Japanese quail (usually unsexed), primarily because it grows very quickly and is ideal for generational studies. Other models considered have been chicks (especially for embryological damage), mice, pigs, cats, and chubs (the final three with just one study each).

These investigations have usually been of short duration (i.e., less than several weeks). However, there are a number of exceptions to this generalization, especially the multigenerational studies of Ganther and his associates at the University of Wisconsin using the Japanese quail as their model. With this summary information as a start, we may proceed to consider the nature of the selenium-mercury interaction and its public health implications.

From a theoretical perspective it is not unexpected that selenium and mercury should interact in the environment as well as within the body. Beijer and Jernelov (1978) have noted that heavy metals such as mercury, which are relatively large along with possessing a high degree of polarizability and several readily excited outer electrons, frequently form covalent bonds with the so-called soft-base elements; that is, elements of large size with accessible low-lying empty orbitals such as selenium (and sulfur).

With such physiochemical complementarity, it follows that in all investigated species of mammals, birds, and fish, mercury is accompanied by selenium and not by other substances analyzed, including Cd, As, Zn, and Sb. In fact, it has been suggested that increases in mercury and selenium concentrations occur in a $1:1$ molecular ratio (Beijer and Jernelov, 1978; Koeman et al., 1975).

Recognition of the fact that mercury is "accompanied by" selenium led Ganther et al. (1972) to evaluate the toxicity to Japanese quail of tuna with high levels of methylmercury (20 ppm) and selenium (0.49 ppm) as compared with the toxicity of a corn-soya diet to which a similar amount of methylmercury had been added. The most striking finding of their study was that consumption of the tuna diet did reduce the toxicity of methylmercury in those quail. Quail given the tuna diet exhibited 7% mortality after 4–6 weeks, while those on the corn-soya diet had a 54% mortality rate for the same time period (Table 6). Furthermore, these findings were replicated in a second-generational study.

While these findings suggest that the high selenium content may have been the primary factor responsible for offsetting the mercury

Table 6. Delayed Onset of Mortality in Japanese Quail Fed 20 ppm Hg in Tuna Diet Compared to Corn-Soya Diet

		Cumulative Mortality (%)[a]			
		Generation 1		Generation 2	
Week	Period (days)	Tuna	Corn-soya	Tuna	Corn-soya
5	29–35	0	4 (1)	0	0
6	36–42	7 (2)	54 (13)	0	12 (3)
7	43–49	41 (9)	77 (6)	4 (1)	54 (10)
8	50–56	63 (6)	92 (4)	29 (6)	83 (7)
9	57–63	81 (5)	100 (2)	50 (2)	83 (0)
10	64–70	96 (4)	100	79 (7)	87 (1)

[a] Figure in parentheses is number of deaths per group during period, out of approximately 25 in each group retained at 4 weeks. Hg (20 ppm) was present in diets in the form of methylmercury continuously from day 1.

Source. Ganther, H.E. and Sunde, M.C. (1974). Effect of tuna fish and selenium on the toxicity of methylmercury: a progress report. *J. Food Sci.* **39**:2.

toxicity, there may have been other nutritional differences as yet undefined that were of even more significance. In addressing this issue, Ganther and his associates reported that the addition of 0.5 ppm sodium selenite to purified diets enhanced the growth and delayed the occurrence of mortality in rats provided with up to 25 ppm of methylmercury in drinking water (Ganther et al., 1972, 1973). These researchers also demonstrated that the addition of selenite to the corn-soya diets of the Japanese quail also provided a type of protection similar to the tuna diet (Table 7) (El-Begearmi et al., 1973, 1974; Ganther and Sunde, 1974).

Numerous reports have confirmed the findings of Ganther and his associates as well as the earlier reports of Parizek, using both methylmercury or mercuric chloride (Stillings et al., 1972, 1974; Potter and Matrone, 1974; Iwata et al., 1973; Stoewsand et al., 1974; Ohi et al., 1976; Kling and Soares, 1978, 1978a). Table 8 lists examples of the types of mercury-induced toxicity that have been reported to be prevented by concomitant treatment with selenium. It is quite obvious that selenium treatment is capable of reducing the toxicity of a wide range of adverse effects induced by mercury. Of particular interest were the findings that selenium treatment was able to reduce the well-known symptoms of renal (Groth et al., 1972; Parizek and Ostadalova, 1967) and neurotoxicity (Ohi et al., 1976; Kasuya, 1976), as

Table 7. Decreased Toxicity of Methylmercury in Corn-Soya Diets Supplemented with Sodium Selenite

Added to C-S Diet[a]			Percentage of Quail Surviving					
			4–8 weeks[b]		4–12 weeks[b]		4–16 weeks[b]	
Hg (ppm)	Se (ppm)	0–4 week	M	F	M	F	M	F
0	0	95	100	100	100	100	100	100
0	6	100	100	100	100	91	100	91
20	0	55	0	3	0	0	0	0
20	0.35	95	36	35	7	12	0	6
20	0.70	100	67	60	17	40	8	30
20	1.50	100	88	100	41	50	6	25
20	3.00	95	83	85	28	77	11	46
20	6.00	98	100	90	67	50	25	15

[a]Basal diet contains about 0.15 ppm Se.

[b]Based on number present in group at 4 weeks.

Source. Ganther, H.E. and Sunde, M.C. (1974). Effect of tuna fish and selenium on the toxicity of methylmercury: a progress report. *J. Food Sci.* **39**:2.

Table 8. Some Examples of Mercury Toxicity Prevented by Selenium

Lethality
Lack of weight gain and growth
Lesions in kidney and intestine
Enzyme inhibition (GSH peroxidase)
Neurological disorders
In vitro nerve changes
Proteinuria
Mercury accumulation in fetus

well as transplacental passage and fetal toxicity (Ganther and Sunde, 1974).

Since it is generally without dispute that the presence of selenium either in the diet, drinking water, or via injection reduces the toxicity of both inorganic and organic mercury, the next question is how does it accomplish this end? Does selenium diminish the gastrointestinal absorption of mercury; does it enhance its excretion, or its sequestration in relatively harmless locations, or does selenium alter the pattern of tissue distribution, thereby affecting toxicity?

At the present time there is no evidence to suggest that selenium reduces the absorption of methylmercury (Skerfving, 1978). However, there is evidence that selenium treatment results in enhanced concentrations of mercury in rats, presumably via a decreased rate of elimination in urine and feces (Eybl et al., 1969; Moffitt and Clary, 1974; Parizek, 1978). Comparable changes also occurred in rats with methylmercury (Stillings et al., 1972, 1974). Yet a selenium enhancement of mercury retention cannot explain the protective nature of selenium.

Other research has been more promising in attempting to explain how selenium modifies mercury toxicity. It is now well established that selenium administration results in pronounced changes in the tissue distribution of mercury in rats. When mercuric chloride is given in single injections, selenite, selenate, and selenomethionine treatment resulted in a rather large reduction of kidney mercury levels, while mercury levels of several other organs such as the liver and muscle increased (Magos and Webb, 1978; Parizek et al., 1971). In Table 9, Chen et al. (1974) clearly illustrated the dramatic changes in mercury tissue distribution as influenced by selenium administration. Not only are the mercury levels dependent on the presence of selenium, but also upon the selenium dosage as seen for blood, liver, kidney, and spleen in Figure 4-2 (Moffitt and Clary, 1974). In contrast to these findings were several reports that indicated that repeated administration of selenium and mercuric mercury in rats and mice actually increased the levels of mercury in the kidney (Skerfving, 1978; Wada et al.,

Table 9. Hg Concentrations in Rat Tissues

| Treatment | ng Hg/ml or g Fresh Tissue | | | | |
	Blood	Plasma[a]	Liver	Kidney	Testis
Control	780	314	1549	12824	58
Se-Pretreated	2297	2527	1623	1196	111

[a]The plasma contained 22% and 61% of the blood Hg in the control and Se-pretreated rats, respectively, as calculated by assuming that the whole blood contained 46% of its volume as erythrocytes.

Source. Chen, R.W. et al. (1974). Diversion of mercury binding in rat tissues by selenium; a possible mechanism of protection. *Pharmacol. Res. Commun.* **6:**573.

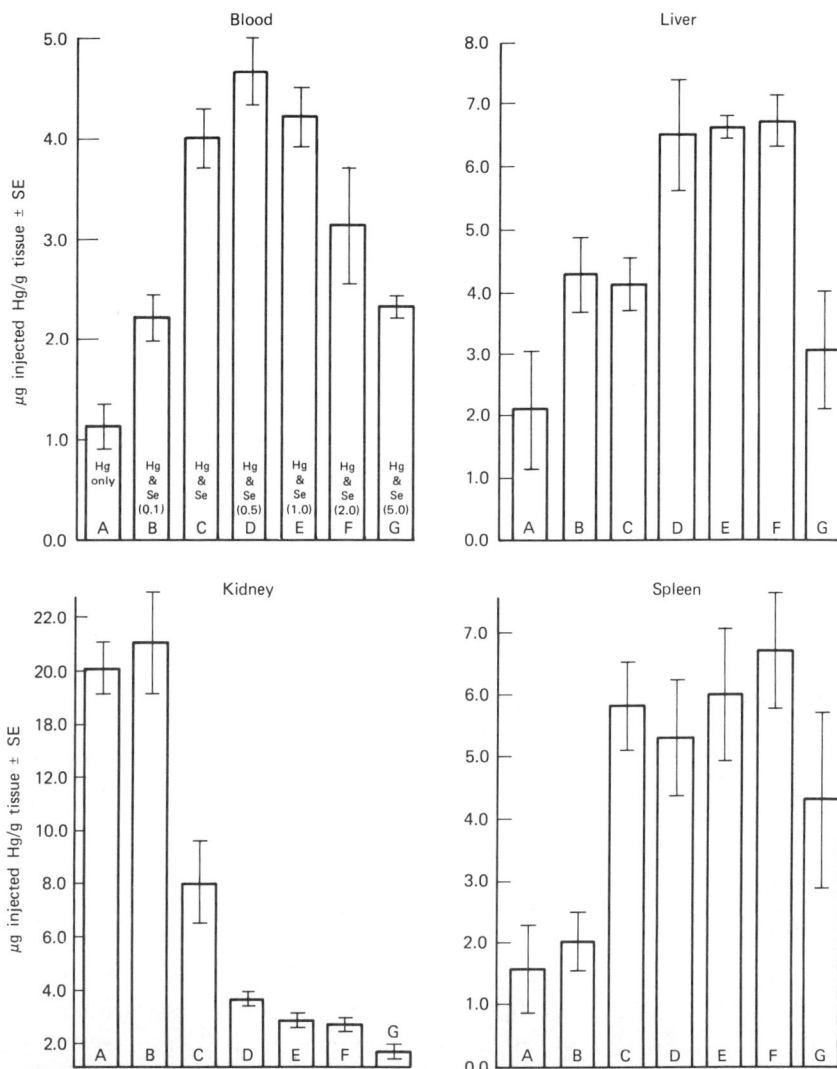

Figure 4-2. Effect of variation in selenite dosage on the binding of ^{203}Hg to blood, liver, kidney, and spleen 24 hours after dosing. ^{203}HgCl$_2$ was administered i.p. at a dose of 1 mg/kg. Simultaneously, sodium selenite was administered i.p. at the doses given in the figure (0.1, 0.4, 0.5, 1.0, 2.0, and 5.0 mg/kg). Each value represents the mean ± S.E. of 5-6 animals per group. [*Source.* Moffitt, A.E., Jr., and Clary, J.J. (1974). Selenite-induced binding of inorganic mercury in blood and other tissues in the rat. *Res. Comm. Chem. Pathol. Pharmacol.* **7**(3):593–603.]

1976). Furthermore, Skerfving (1978) has succinctly summarized ten relevant studies and reported that the "total mercury levels in tissues in animals repeatedly exposed to methylmercury were not greatly affected by selenium administration; in no study did the effect exceed a factor of 2" (Table 10).

Even though the findings of Skerfving (1978) did not reveal any "major effects attributable to selenium on tissue mercury levels," Stoewsand et al. (1974) revealed that selenium-treated quail are less susceptible to mercury-induced mortality, thereby implying that methylmercury is less toxic in selenium-treated quail. They concluded by saying that high methylmercury levels do not necessarily reveal that birds will exhibit evidence of methylmercury toxicosis. If differences in absorption, excretion, and tissue distribution cannot account for the protection that selenium provides against mercury intoxication, perhaps selenium-induced changes in the subcellular constituents can. Chen et al. (1974) demonstrated that selenite treatment altered the subcellular distribution arrangement of mercuric mercury in rats. In Table 11, it is shown that the crude nuclear, mitochondrial, and microsomal fraction levels are increased while the soluble fraction content is decreased for the liver. In contrast, all subcellular fractions are decreased in the kidney, while the reverse is true for the testis. In addition, the selenium treatment diverted much of the mercury in the soluble fraction from small molecular proteins (i.e., probably metallothionein) to larger ones. In marked contrast to these findings with inorganic mercury, selenium pretreatment did not markedly alter the subcellular distribution of methylmercury nor its distribution among various molecular weight proteins of the soluble fraction in tissues other than the kidney (Chen et al., 1975).

Despite this apparent lack of understanding of how selenium reduces methylmercury toxicity, a new hypothesis has been proposed by Ganther (1978). He states that methylmercury neurotoxicity results from free radicals formed in part by the breakdown of methylmercury. These free radicals may "be taken up by membranes in target tissues such as the brain in close proximity to lipids. It would then initiate a chain reaction peroxidation of various lipid constituents . . . the onset of neuropathologic changes would be preceded by a lag phase during which the various systems defending against lipid peroxidation would be overcome, followed by a rapid and progressive degeneration of the tissue." Presumably both vitamin E and selenium would be part of the "various systems" defending against the lipid peroxidation. Ganther (1978) states that selenium, in its role as a component of glutathione

Table 10. Effect of Selenium on Tissue-Total Mercury (Hg) Levels and of Methylmercury on Tissue-Total Selenium (Se) Levels

Species	Exposure Time (days)	Hg (mg/kg food)[a]	Se (mg/kg food)[a,b]	Mercury Accumulation[c] Brain	Liver	Kidney	Muscle	Selenium Accumulation[d] Brain	Liver	Kidney	Muscle
Japanese quail	28	20	0.7 T[e]	1.0	0.9	1.1	0.9	—	—	—	—
	35	20	5	1.1	1.2	1.5	—	—	—	—	—
	23	20	8	1.6	1.0	—	1.0	—	—	—	—
Chicks	25	20	8	1.0	0.7	—	0.6	—	—	—	—
Rats	8	10 mg/ kg-day[f]	0.5 mg/ kg-day[f]	1.7[g]	1.0[g]	1.0[g,i]	—	—	—	—	—
	28	25	3	—	1.8	—	—	10	1.0	2.0	1.2
	21	10–40	5	—	1.0–1.7	0.6–1.0	—	—	—	—	—
	14	25	0.6	0.7	1.1	0.5	0.8	—	—	—	—
	70	20	1.0 T	1.5	1.1	1.5	—	2.3	4.8	3.7	—
	70	20	1.0	1.4	1.2	1.4	—	4.2	4.0	4.2	—
Pigs[h]	42–49	7 mg/kg (single dose)	5[i]	<1	<1	<1	<1	—	<1	<1	<1

[a] If not indicated otherwise.
[b] T denotes that Se was given as tuna; in other studies it was given as selenite.
[c] Level in group given Hg and Se/level in group given Hg only.
[d] Level in group given Se and Hg/level in group given Se only.
[e] Level in control group ("low Se") 0.4 mg Se/kg. In most other cases, Se levels in "control group" were not given.
[f] Subcutaneous administration.
[g] Methylmercury levels.
[h] Scanty information.
[i] Se levels in "controls" 0.03–0.05 mg/kg.

Source. Skerfving, S. (1978). Interaction between selenium and methylmercury. *Environ. Health Perspect.* **25**:57–65.

Table 11. Subcellular Hg Distribution in Rat Tissues

Subcellular Fraction	Treatment	ng Hg/g Fresh Tissue[a]		
		Liver	Kidney	Testis
Crude nuclear	Hg	399 (26)	2515 (20)	18 (31)
	Se + Hg	496 (31)	278 (23)	21 (19)
Mitochondrial	Hg	261 (17)	1900 (15)	5 (9)
	Se + Hg	319 (20)	175 (15)	8 (7)
Microsomal	Hg	203 (13)	1261 (10)	3 (5)
	Se + Hg	320 (20)	243 (20)	11 (10)
Soluble	Hg	665 (43)	7314 (57)	32 (55)
	Se + Hg	402 (25)	474 (40)	68 (61)

[a] Numbers in parentheses indicate percentage distribution.

Source. Chen, R.W. et al. (1974). Diversion of mercury binding in rat tissues by selenium; a possible mechanism of protection. *Pharmacol. Res. Commun.* **6:**571–579.

peroxidase, would retard the breakdown of methylmercury by decomposing peroxides.

Conclusions. It has been unequivocally demonstrated that sodium selenite administration either by injection or within the diet markedly diminishes the toxicity of both inorganic and organic mercury in a variety of species, especially the rat and Japanese quail. The mechanism by which selenium acts to reduce mercury toxicity is not precisely known, although it is clear that there are differences between the interaction of selenium and the different forms of mercury. While considerably more research is necessary to elucidate the mechanism of the selenium-mercury interaction, it appears that selenium may be able to affect toxicity by altering tissue-distribution patterns as well as changing the subcellular distribution of mercury. However, whether these selenium-induced changes in mercury tissue levels and subcellular distribution are causally related to the reductions in mercury toxicity has not been demonstrated.

Most of the studies concerning the use of selenium to prevent mercury toxicity have been of a short-term nature with the notable exception being those of Ganther et al., and have used relatively high doses of selenium. These two components of most research studies reduce the ability of investigators to confidently predict their relevance for human populations; for while selenium is an essential nutrient, it is also a highly toxic agent at elevated doses. In fact, while the animal studies reported herein used selenite at levels between 0.1 to 8.0 mg/kg, the average daily human intake is approximately 200 μg/day, or only about 0.1 mg/kg. Since the recommended maximum daily intake of selenium is 500 μg (or about .25 mg/kg), one can see that the doses used in many of the animal studies cannot be considered of practical significance in human terms. Thus while Moffitt and Clary (1974) talk about the possibility of a "therapeutic usage of selenium compounds in mercury toxicity," it is quite clear that long-term supplementation at doses beyond 500 μg/day cannot be recommended as a prophylactic measure. Certainly there is no evidence to suggest that at 3 μg of daily mercury exposure there is any demonstrable adverse human health effect for which selenium supplementation may be needed or useful. However, the question of therapeutic usage of selenium compounds in case of mercury intoxication is certainly a legitimate area of further research. However, since selenium does not enhance the excretion of mercury, investigators may not be totally satisfied with it.

It is interesting to note that Ganther and Sunde (1974) feel "that those who must attempt to define the safe level of mercury for the human population [should] consider the effect of selenium. It would not be valid, for example, to estimate the minimum toxic level of mercury intake from fish on the basis of a human population poisoned from eating mercury-treated seed. Essentially no selenium would accompany the mercury ingested in treated seed, whereas selenium faithfully accompanies mercury in tuna."

While there is a compelling logic to the conclusions of Ganther and Sunde (1974), their perspective may not be transferable to the problems of setting standards for exposure to mercury in drinking water and in the industrial environment. However, limited human studies (Kosta et al., 1975; Rossi et al., 1976) have shown that persons industrially exposed to inorganic mercury tended to retain considerably more selenium in the kidney, brain, pituitary, and thyroid glands than nonexposed comparison groups, thereby implying that occupational exposure to mercury enhances the retention of selenium, which in turn may diminish the toxicity of mercury. Certainly, research concerning the role of dietary selenium on the retention and toxicity of mercury to humans from various environmental sources remains to be conducted.

Addendum. A recent report by Nobunaga et al. (1979) revealed that MeHg-induced teratogenic effects in mice may be either enhanced or reduced by selenite depending on their respective doses. Since these findings do not support the large body of evidence indicating that selenium uniformly reduces MeHg toxicity, a concerted effort should be made to resolve this issue.

References

Alexander, J. and Norseth, T. (1979). The effect of selenium on the biliary excretion and organ distribution of mercury in the rat after exposure to methyl mercuric chloride. *Acta Pharmacol. Toxicol.* **44**:168–176.

Ansari, M.S. and Britton, W.M. (1974). Effect of dietary selenium and mercury and [203]Hg metabolism in chicks. *Poult. Sci.* **53**:1134–1137.

Beijer, K. and Jernelov, A. (1978). Ecological aspects of mercury-selenium interactions in the marine environment. *Environ. Health Perspect.* **25**:43–45.

Berlin, M. (1978). Interaction between selenium and inorganic mercury. *Environ. Health Perspect.* **25**:67–69.

Burk, R.F.; Jordan, H.E., Jr.; and Kiker, K.W. (1977). Some effects of selenium status on inorganic mercury metabolism in the rat. *Toxicol. Appl. Pharmacol.* **40**(1):71–82.

Chen, R.W.; Lacy, V.L.; and Whanger, P.D. (1975). Effect of selenium on methylmercury binding to subcellular and soluble proteins in rat tissues. *Res. Com. Chem. Pathol. Pharmacol.* **12**:297–308.

Chen, R.W.; Whanger, P.D.; and Fang, S.C. (1974). Diversion of mercury binding in rat tissues by selenium: a possible mechanism of protection. *Pharmacol. Res. Commun.* **6**:571–579.

Chmielnicka, J. and Brzeznicka, E.A. (1978). The influence of selenium on the level of mercury and metallothionein in rat kidneys in prolonged exposure to different mercury compounds. *Bull. Environ. Contam. Toxicol.* **19**:183–190.

Chmielnicka, J.; Hajdukiewicz, Z.; Komstra-Szumska, E.; and Lukaszek, S. (1978). Whole-body retention of mercury and selenium and histopathological and morphological studies of kidneys and liver of rats exposed repeatedly to mercuric chloride and sodium selenite. *Arch. Toxicol.* **40**:189–199.

El-Begearmi, M.; Ganther, H.E.; and Sunde, M.L. (1974). Effect of some sulfur amino acids, selenium and arsenic on mercury toxicity using Japanese quail. *Poult. Sci.* **53**:1921.

El-Begearmi, M.; Ganther, H.E.; and Sunde, M.L. (1975). More evidence for a selenium, arsenic interaction in modifying mercury toxicity. *Poult. Sci.* **54**:1756.

El-Begearmi, M.; Goudie, C.; Ganther, H.E.; and Sunde, M.L. (1973). Attempts to quantitate the protective effect of selenium against mercury toxicity using Japanese quail. *Fed. Proc.* **32**:886.

Eybl, V.; Syora, J.; and Mertl, F. (1969). Einfluss von natrium-selenite, natrium-tellurit und natriumsulfit auf retention und verteilung von Queksilber bei Mäusen. *Arch. Toxikol.* **25**:296–305.

Ganther, H.E. (1978). Modification of methylmercury toxicity and metabolism by selenium and vitamin E: possible mechanism. *Environ. Health Perspect.* **25**:71–76.

Ganther, H.E.; Goudie, C.; Sunde, M.L.; Kopecky, M.; Wagner, P.; Oh, S-H.; and Hoekstra, W.G. (1972). Evidence that selenium in tuna decreases mercury toxicity. *Fed. Proc.* **31**:725 (Abstract).

Ganther, H.E.; Goudie, C.; Sunde, M.L.; Kopecky, M.J.; Wagner, P.; Oh, S-H.; and Hoekstra, W.G. (1972a). Selenium: relation to decreased toxicity of methylmercury added to diets containing tuna. *Science* **174**:1122–1124.

Ganther, H.E. and Sunde, M.L. (1974). Effect of tuna fish and selenium on the toxicity of methylmercury: a progress report. *J. Food Sci.* **39**:1–5.

Ganther, H.E.; Wagner, P.A.; Sunde, M.L.; and Hoekstra, W.G. (1973). Protective effects of selenium against heavy metal toxicities. In: *Trace Substances in Environmental Health*, pp. 247–252. Edited by D.D. Hemphill. Univ. of Missouri, Columbia.

Groth, D.H.; Stettler, L.; and MacKay, G. (1976). Interactions of mercury, cadmium, selenium, tellurium, arsenic, and beryllium. In: *Effects and Dose-Response Relationships of Toxic Metals*, pp. 527–543. Edited by G.F. Nordberg. Elsevier Scientific Publishing Co., Amsterdam.

Groth, D.H.; Vignati, L.; Lowry, L.; MacKay, G.; and Stokinger, H.E. (1972). Mutual antagonistic and synergistic effects of inorganic selenium and mercury salts in chronic experiments. In: *Trace Substances in Environmental Health*, pp. 187–189. Edited by D.D. Hemphill. University of Missouri, Columbia.

Gunn, S.A.; Gould, T.C.; and Anderson, W.A.D. (1968). Specificity in protection against lethality and testicular toxicity from cadmium. *Proc. Soc. Exp. Biol. Med.* **128**:591–595.

Iwata, H.; Okamoto, H.; and Ohsawa, Y. (1973). Effect of selenium on methylmercury poisoning. *Res. Commun. Chem. Pathol. Pharmacol.* **5**:673–680.

Kasuya, M. (1976). Effect of selenium on the toxicity of methylmercury on nervous tissue in culture. *Toxicol. Appl. Pharm.* **35**:11–20.

Kim, J.H.; Birks, E.; and Heisinger, J.F. (1977). Protective action of selenium against mercury in northern creek chubs. *Bull. Environ. Contam. Toxicol.* **17**(2):132–136.

Kling, L.J. and Soares, J.H., Jr. (1978). Mercury metabolism in Japanese quail. I. The effect of dietary mercury and selenium on their tissue distribution. *Poult. Sci.* **57**:1279–1285.

Kling, L.J. and Soares, J.H., Jr. (1978a). Mercury metabolism in Japanese quail. II. The effects of dietary mercury and selenium on blood and liver glutathione peroxidase activity and selenium concentration. *Poult. Sci.* **57**:1286–1287.

Koeman, J.H.; van de Ven, W.S.M.; de Goeij, J.J.M.; Tjioe, P.S.; and van Haaften, J.L. (1975). Mercury and selenium in marine mammals and birds. *Science Total Environ.* **3**:279.

Komsta-Szumska, E.; Chnielnicka, J.; and Piotrowski, J.K. (1976). The influence of selenium on binding of inorganic mercury by metallothionein in the kidney and liver of the rat. *Biochem. Pharmacol.* **25**:2539–2540.

Kosta, L.; Byrne, A.R.; and Zellenko, V. (1975). Correlation between selenium and mercury in man following exposure to inorganic mercury. *Nature* **254**:238–239.

Levander, O.A. and Argrett, L.C. (1969). Effects of arsenic, mercury, thallium, and lead on selenium metabolism in rats. *Toxicol. Appl. Pharmacol.* **14**:308–314.

Magos, L. (1978). Mercury: an environmental and dietary hazard. *J. Human Nutr.* **32**:179–186.

Magos, L. and Webb, M. (1978). Theoretical and practical considerations on the problem of metal-metal interactions. *Environ. Health Perspect.* **25**:151–154.

Moffitt, A.E., Jr. and Clary, J.J. (1974). Selenite-induced binding of inorganic mercury in blood and other tissues in the rat. *Res. Comm. Chem. Pathol. Pharmacol.* **7**(3):593–603.

Nobunaga, T.; Satoh, H.; and Suzuki, T. (1979). Effects of sodium selenite on methylmercury embryotoxicity and teratogenicity in mice. *Toxicol. Appl. Pharm.* **47**:79–88.

Nutr. Rev. (1973). Mercury toxicity reduced by selenium. *Nutrition Reviews* **31**:25–27.

Ohi, G.; Nishigaki, S.; Seki, H.; Tamura, Y.; Maki, T.; Konno, H.; Ochiai, S.; Yamada, H.; Shimamura, Y.; Mizoguchi, I.; and Yagyu, H. (1976). Efficacy of selenium in tuna and selenite in modifying methylmercury intoxication. *Environ. Res.* **12**:49–58.

Ohi, G.; Nishigaki, S.; Seki, H.; Tamura, Y.; Maki, T.; Maeda, H.; Ochiai, S.; Yamada, H.; Shimamura, Y.; and Yagyu, H. (1975). Interaction of dietary methylmercury and selenium on accumulation and retention of these substances in rat organs. *Toxicol. Appl. Pharmacol.* **32**:527–533.

Parizek, J. (1978). Interactions between selenium compounds and those of mercury or cadmium. *Environ. Health Perspect.* **25**:53–55.

Parizek, J. and Ostadalova, I. (1967). The protective effect of small amount of selenite in sublimate intoxication. *Experientia* **23**:142–143.

Parizek, J.; Ostadalova, I.; Kalouskova, J.; Babicky, A.; Pavlik, L.; and Bibr, B. (1971). Effect of mercuric compounds on the maternal transmission of selenium in the pregnant and lactating rat. *J. Reprod. Fert.* **25**:157–170.

Piotrowski, J.K.; Bem, E.M.; and Werner, A. (1977). Cadmium and mercury binding to metallothionein as influenced by selenium. *Biochem. Pharmacol.* **26**:2191–2192.

Potter, S.D. and Matrone, G. (1974). Effect of selenite on the toxicity of dietary methylmercury and mercuric chloride in the rat. *J. Nutr.* **104**:638–647.

Potter, S.D. and Matrone, G. (1977). A tissue culture model for mercury-selenium interactions. *Toxicol. Appl. Pharm.* **40**:201–215.

Prohoska, J.R. and Ganther, H.E. (1977). Interactions between selenium and methylmercury in rat brain. *Chem.-Biol. Interact.* **16**:155–167.

Rossi, L.C.; Santaroni, G.; and Clementa, G.F. (1976). Mercury and selenium distribution in a defined area and in its population. *Arch. Environ. Health* **31**:160–165.

Sell, J.L. and Horani, F.G. (1976). Influence of selenium on toxicity and metabolism of methylmercury in chicks and quail. *Nutr. Rept. Intern.* **14**(4):439–447.

Shiramizu, M.; Yamaguchi, S.; and Kaku, S. (1976). Health effect of long-term diet of mercury contaminated tuna. Part II. Accumulation and retention of mercury and selenium in organs and clinical symptoms. *Jap. J. Ind. Health* **18**:123–135.

Skerfving, S. (1978). Interaction between selenium and methylmercury. *Environ. Health Perspect.* **25**:57–65.

Stillings, B.R.; Lagally, H.; Bauersfeld, P.; and Soares, J. (1974). Effect of cystine, selenium, and fish protein on the toxicity and metabolism of methylmercury in rats. *Toxicol. Appl. Pharmacol.* **30**:243–254.

Stillings, B.R.; Lagally, H.; Soares, J.; and Miller, D. (1972). Effects of cystine and selenium on the toxicological effects of methylmercury in rats. In: Proceedings of the IX Internat. Congress of Nutrition, p. 206. Summaria, Mexico City.

Stoewsand, G.S.; Anderson, J.L.; Gutemann, W.H.; and Lisk, D.J. (1977). Form of dietary selenium on mercury and selenium tissue retention and egg production in Japanese quail. *Nutr. Rept. Intern.* **15**:81–87.

Stoewsand, G.S.; Bache, C.A.; and Lisk, D.J. (1974). Dietary selenium protection of methylmercury intoxication of Japanese quail. *Bull. Environ. Contam. Toxicol.* **11**(2):152–156.

Sukra, Y.; Sastrohadinoto, S.; Budiarso, I.T.; and Bird, H.R. (1976). Effect of selenium and mercury on gross morphology and histopathology of chick embryos. *Poult. Sci.* 55:2424–2433.

Sukra, Y.; Sastrohadinoto, S.; and Haeruman, H., Jr. (1976a). Effect of selenium and mercury on survival of chick embryos. *Poult. Sci.* 55:1423–1428.

Sunde, M.L.; Goudie, C.; and Ganther, H. (1972). Methylmercury effects in Japanese quail fed tuna. *Fed. Proc.* 31:725 (Abstract).

Wada, O.; Yamaguchi, N.; Ono, T.; Nagahashi, M.; and Morimuri, T. (1976). Inhibitory effect of mercury on kidney glutathione peroxidase and its prevention by selenium. *Environ. Res.* 12:75–80.

Welsh, S.O. and Soares, H.H., Jr. (1976). The protective effect of vitamin E and selenium against methylmercury toxicity in the Japanese quail. *Nutr. Rept. Internat.* 13:43–51.

Yamane, Y.; Fukino, H.; Aida, Y.; and Imagawa, M. (1977). Effects of selenium on metabolism of mercury compounds. *Yakugaku Zasshi* 97(6):667–670.

6. Ozone

Ozone is a powerful environmental oxidant that causes irritation to the lining of the respiratory tract as well as a range of systemic effects such as chromosomal damage to circulatory lymphocytes and changes in the structure of red blood cell membranes. Considerable research effort has attempted to evaluate how the influence of vitamin E and other antioxidants can modify ozone toxicity (see Volume 1, Chapter 5, "Vitamin E"). However, while considerable theoretical support could be rationalized for the possibility of a selenium-deficient diet enhancing the toxicity of oxidants such as ozone, very little has been published on this topic. In a study evaluating the potentially protective effects of 18 antioxidants against ozone toxicity in mice, Pagnotto and Epstein (1969) tested the capacity of a sodium selenite pretreatment (0.01 mg on 4 occasions) to prevent ozone-induced (8.8–10.3 ppm for 4 hours) mortality. Their findings revealed a slight (4%) but insignificant (p > .05) decrease in mortality.

While this finding was not especially encouraging, it certainly was limited in scope so as to insufficiently evaluate the influence of selenium on ozone toxicity.

Another study concerning the influence of selenium on ozone toxicity was recently reported by Chow (1977) who evaluated the effect of dietary selenium and vitamin E on the biochemical response of lung tissue in ozone-exposed (0.7–1.2 ppm for 2–4 days) male rats. His findings revealed that the ozone-exposed rats reared on either a selenium- or vitamin E-deficient diet exhibited greater biochemical changes (e.g., GSH, GSHpx, GSH reductase) than animals given normal or supplemented diets. The presence of both a selenium- and vitamin E-deficient diet was found to be additive with respect to susceptibility to oxidant stress.

Future studies should be designed to evaluate the influence of a wide range of dietary intakes of selenium and vitamin E on the toxicity of ozone in both lung tissue and red blood cells in appropriate animal models. This is certainly an area that may provide knowledge not only of a practical nature but also one that adds to our understanding of how cells deal effectively with oxidant stress.

References

Chow, C.K. (1977). Effect of dietary selenium and vitamin E on the biochemical responses in the lungs of ozone-exposed rats. *Fed. Proc.* **36**:1094 (Abstract no. 4347).

Pagnotto, L.D. and Epstein, S.S. (1969). Protection by antioxidants against ozone toxicity in mice. *Experientia* **25**:703.

7. Radiation

Because selenium may function as an antioxidant, it is not unexpected that investigators would be interested in evaluating the capacity of selenium to reduce toxicity resulting from exposure to radiation. In fact, selenium compounds (i.e., selenomethionine and selenocystine) have been shown to diminish damage from free radicals generated by ionizing radiation *in vitro* (Shimazu and Tappel, 1964, 1969). In addition, several studies have revealed that pretreatment with injected selenium compounds has prolonged the life spans of irradiated animal models (Breccia et al., 1969; Hollo and Zlatarov, 1960). More recently, Badiello et al. (1975) similarly reported that pretreatment by injection of selenourea reduces the adverse effects of ionizing radiation in rats as measured by changes in protein content, protein pattern, and plasma enzyme activity. In contrast to these positive findings, Hurt et al. (1970, 1971) were not able to find an important protective effect of dietary selenomethionine (0.5 ppm) on the toxicity of chronic whole-body irradiation as compared to controls reared on a diet with very low selenium levels. No significant differences occurred between treatment groups in hematocrit, erythrocyte, or leucocyte levels or in the length of survival. According to the authors, their study is probably more valid than other *in vivo* supportive studies with respect to whether selenium may offer a protective effect against irradiation exposure, since this study was a "more natural approach of regulating selenium" because it used diet instead of the injections of other studies.

While the findings discussed here are ambivalent to the potentially protective action of selenium compounds on radiation toxicity, there are sufficient data that indicate that some type of interaction may be occurring, at least when the selenium compounds were injected. Studies concerning the role of dietary selenium on radiation-induced toxicity should be conducted, especially in light of the essentially negative findings of Hurt et al. (1970, 1971). Additionally, the possibility that selenium may reduce radiation-induced cancer may be worth evaluating.

References

Badiello, R.; Gattavecchia, E.; Mattii, M.; and Tamba, M. (1975). Further observations on *in vivo* radioprotection of rats by selenourea. *Biochemie Biophysik.* **29**(9–10): 647–648.

Breccia, A.R.; Dadiello, A.; Trenta, A.; and Mattii, M. (1969). On the chemical radioprotection by organic selenium compounds *in vivo*. *Radiat. Res.* **38**:483–492.

Hollo, M.A. and Zlatarov, S. (1960). Prevention of deaths by means of selenium salts administered after roentgen irradiation. *Borgy Venerol. Szemle* **36**:204.

Hurt, H.D.; Allaway, W.H.; and Cary, E.E. (1970). The effects of dietary selenium on the survival of rats exposed to whole body irradiation. *Fed. Proc.* **29**:499.

Hurt, H.D.; Cary, E.E.; Allaway, W.H.; and Visek, W.J. (1971). Effect of dietary selenium on the survival of rats exposed to chronic whole body irradiation. *J. Nutr.* **101**:363–366.

Shimazu, F.; Kumta, V.S.; and Tappel, A.L. (1964). Radiation damage to methionine and its derivatives. *Radiat. Res.* **23**:276–277.

Shimazu, F. and Tappel, A.L. (1964). Selenoamino acids as radioprotectors *in vitro*. *Radiat. Res.* **23**:210–217.

Shimazu, F. and Tappel, A.L. (1969). Seleno-amino acids: decrease of radiation damage to amino acids and proteins. *Science* **143**:369.

8. Silver

Within the past decade it has become known that selenium may interact with a wide range of potentially toxic substances of importance to the public health. Those elements whose toxicity has been alleviated by interactions with selenium include mercury, cadmium, and lead. Another potentially toxic substance that also interacts with selenium, but about which considerably less is known, is silver.

Despite its apparent obscurity in toxicological literature relative to heavy metals such as cadmium, lead, and mercury, it is well known that the addition of silver to either rations or drinking water of weanling rats (Diplock et al., 1967; Bunyan et al., 1968; Grasso et al., 1969; Shaver and Mason, 1951; Wagner et al., 1975), chicks (Bunyan et al., 1968; Peterson and Jensen, 1975, 1975a), turkey poults (Jensen et al., 1974), and swine (Van Vleet, 1976) may induce characteristics of a selenium-vitamin E deficiency such as hepatic lesions in rats and swine, exudative diathesis in chicks, and gizzard and cardiac myopathy in turkeys. As expected, supplementation of the diet with either selenium or vitamin E partially or completely prevented the adverse effects induced by the silver.

However, not only does selenium offset the toxic effects of silver, but silver prevents the toxicity of selenium as well (Jensen, 1974, 1975). This is not unique for silver, since other highly toxic elements including mercuric chloride, cupric sulfate, and cadmium sulfate may also reduce the toxicity of selenium (Hill, 1974). Thus it is known that selenium and silver interact in such a manner as to diminish the toxicity of each other in animal systems.

The manner in which these biochemical antagonisms occur has been evaluated by various research groups. Jensen (1975) has reported that high levels of silver may reduce the absorption and/or alter the metabolism of selenium in chicks. He speculated that "selenium may form a relatively insoluble compound with silver either in the intestinal tract or in the tissues, which would reduce the availability of silver ions for interacting with other trace elements and for interfering with normal enzymic reactions in the tissues." This hypothesis is supported by observations of diminished storage of selenium in many organs (i.e., liver, kidney, pancreas, intestinal tract, heart and breast muscle, and blood) of chicks fed silver. In addition to possibly preventing the uptake of selenium, silver is thought to alter the chemical form of selenium from selenite to the more insoluble selenide, thereby altering the toxicity of selenium. However, no experimental evidence has been presented to substantiate this statement.

While such effects of silver administration may assist in preventing the toxicity of elevated levels of dietary selenium, high levels of silver markedly reduce the activities of selenium-dependent enzymes such as glutathione peroxidase in both the red blood cells and kidney and may contribute to the occurrence of silver-induced toxicity symptoms (Wagner et al., 1975). Selenium supplementation was able to prevent the occurrence of growth depression in rats given 76 and 751 ppm silver in drinking water. Interestingly, the selenium supplementation increased the accumulation of silver in the liver and kidney, leading the authors to suggest that selenium was probably not reducing silver toxicity by preventing its uptake and retention.

Despite the obvious fact that the biochemical mechanisms involved in the selenium-silver antagonism are not well understood, Wagner et al. (1975) attempted to develop a conceptual model that would provide a working scheme for assessing further their interaction. They stated that "a diversion of silver by selenium from critical targets to nontoxic binding sites and of selenium by silver to biologically inactive forms within the cell could explain the increased tissue concentration of silver, the concomitant modification of the silver toxicity, and the induction of selenium-deficiency defects."

References

Bunyan, J.; Diplock, A.T.; Cawthorne, M.A.; and Green, J. (1968). Vitamin E and stress. 8. Nutritional effects of dietary stress with silver in vitamin E deficient chicks and rats. *Brit. J. Nutr.* **22**:165–182.

Diplock, A.T.; Green, J.; Bunyan, J.; McHale, D.; and Muthy, I.R. (1967). Vitamin E and stress. 3. The metabolism of D-α-tocopherol in the rat under dietary stress with silver. *Brit. J. Nutr.* **21**:115–125.

Grasso, P.; Abraham, R.; Hendy, R.; Diplock, A.T.; Goldberg, L.; and Green, J. (1969). The role of dietary silver in the production of liver necrosis in vitamin E-deficient rats. *Exp. Mol. Pathol.* **11**:186–199.

Hill, C.H. (1974). Reversal of selenium toxicity in chicks by mercury, copper, and cadmium. *J. Nutr.* **104**:593–598.

Jensen, L.S. (1974). Interactions of silver and copper and selenium in chicks. *Fed. Proc.* **33**:694.

Jensen, L.S. (1975). Modification of a selenium toxicity in chicks by dietary silver and copper. *J. Nutr.* **105**:769–775.

Jensen, L.S.; Peterson, R.P.; and Falen, L. (1974). Inducement of enlarged heart and muscular dystrophy in turkey poults with dietary silver. *Poult. Sci.* **53**:57–64.

NAS (1977). *Drinking Water and Health.* National Academy of Sciences, Washington, D.C., pp. 289–292.

Peterson, R.P. and Jensen, L.S. (1975). Induced exudative diathesis in chicks by dietary silver. *Poult. Sci.* **54**:795–798.

Peterson, R.P. and Jensen, L.S. (1975a). Interrelationship of dietary silver with copper in the chick. *Poult. Sci.* **54**:771–775.

Shaver, S.L. and Mason, K.E. (1951). Impaired tolerance to silver in vitamin E deficient rats. *Anat. Rec.* **109**:382–388.

Tabershaw, I.R.; Utidjian, M.; and Kawahara, B. (1977). Chemical hazards. In: *Occupational Diseases.* Edited by M.M. Key, H.F. Henschel, J. Butler, R. Ligo, and I.R. Tabershaw. NIOSH. Washington, D.C.

Van Vleet, J.F. (1976). Induction of lesions of selenium-vitamin E deficiency in pigs fed silver. *Am. J. Vet. Res.* **37**:1415–1420.

Wagner, P.A.; Hoekstra, W.G.; and Ganther, H.E. (1975). Alleviation of silver toxicity by selenite in the rat in relation to tissue glutathione peroxidase. *Proc. Soc. Experim. Biol. Med.* **148**:1106–1110.

B. ORGANIC SUBSTANCES

1. Aflatoxin

Consumption of diets with either an excess or a deficiency of selenium is known to result in liver damage to animal models (Harr, 1967; Schwartz and Foltz, 1957). Because of this capacity of dietary extremes of selenium to adversely affect liver function, Newberne and Conner (1974) became interested in the possibility that dietary selenium in either minimal and/or excess levels may influence the occurrence of liver lesions resulting from exposure to hepatotoxins. In order to evaluate this possibility, these researchers studied the effects of highly variable levels of dietary selenium (minimal [0.03 ppm], adequate [0.10 ppm], excessive [1.00 ppm], and very excessive [5.00 ppm]) on the hepatotoxicity of aflatoxin B_1 to rats. Additional reasons for selecting aflatoxin B_1 as the hepatotoxic agent for study were that its adverse effects can be modified by several dietary factors and that in certain situations aflatoxin B_1 may occur in diets that may be either deficient or excessive in selenium. Unfortunately, this latter point was not elaborated on.

Their study revealed that the two highest concentrations of selenium (1.0 and 5.0 ppm) caused significantly reduced growth as indicated by body-weight gain 2 weeks after treatment. However, the administration of 1.0 ppm selenium markedly reduced the incidence of aflatoxin B_1-induced mortality relative to all other experimental groups. The groups with minimal (0.03 ppm) and very excessive (5.0 ppm) levels of selenium appeared to enhance the toxicity of aflatoxin B_1 relative to those adequately (0.10 ppm) fed. In addition, both groups with excessive levels of dietary selenium appeared to enhance the occurrence of aflatoxin B_1-induced renal lesions that were not evident in the other experimental groups.

At this point the data are too limited to make any generalizations beyond the obvious statement that dietary selenium levels may affect the occurrence of aflatoxin B_1-induced liver and renal damage as well as mortality incidence. While it appears that diets either deficient in or with excessive levels of selenium enhance toxicity, the precise relationships are too unclear. Further study designed to elucidate this interaction is warranted.

Finally, Lalor et al. (1978) have recently reported that both aflatoxin B₁ and sodium selenite modify duodenal serotonin metabolism either singly or together. These findings are certainly worthy of further investigation since changes in serotonin levels have been associated with intestinal neoplasia (Brown, 1977; Thompson, 1977); and while selenium may protect against intestinal cancer (Schrauzer et al., 1977; Shamberger et al., 1973), aflatoxin B₁ may be a cause of such cancer (Ward et al., 1975).

References

Aleksandrowicz, J.; Dobrowolski, J.; Lisiewicz, J.; Smyk, B.; and Skotnicki, A. (1975). The effect of selenium on the growth of carcinogenic fungi and cytotoxic action of aflatoxin B₁ in cell cultures of lymphocytes and on the embryonal development of *Xenopus laevis. Pol. Arch. Med. Wewn.* **53**:209.

Brown, H. (1977). Serotonin-producing tumors. In: *Serotonin in Health and Disease*, p. 353. Edited by W.B. Essman. Vol. IV. *Clinical Correlations*. Spectrum Publications, N.Y.

Harr, J.R. (1967). Selenium toxicity in rats. I. Growth and longevity. In: *Selenium in Biomedicine*. Edited by O.H. Muth. Avi Publishing Co., Westport, CT.

Lalor, J.H.; Kimbrough, T.D.; and Llewellyn, G.C. (1978). Induction of duodenal serotonin production by dietary sodium selenite and aflatoxin B₁. *Fd. Cosmet. Toxicol.* **16**:611–613.

Newberne, P.M. and Conner, M.W. (1974). Effect of selenium in acute response to aflatoxin B₁. In: *Trace Substances in Environmental Health*, VIII, pp. 323–328. Edited by D.D. Hemphill. University of Missouri at Columbia.

Schrauzer, G.N.; White, D.A.; and Schneider, C.J. (1977). Cancer mortality correlation studies. III. Statistical associations with dietary selenium intakes. *Bioinorg. Chem.* **7**:23.

Schwartz, K. and Foltz, C.M. (1957). Selenium as an integral part of factor 3 against dietary necrotic liver degeneration. *J. Amer. Chem. Soc.* **79**:3292.

Shamberger, R.J.; Rukovena, E.; Longfield, A.K.; Tytko, S.A.; Deodhar, S.; and Willis, C.E. (1973). Antioxidants and cancer. I. Selenium in the food of normals and cancer patients. *J. Natl. Cancer Inst.* **50**:863.

Thompson, J.H. (1977). Serotonin (5-hydroxytryptamine) and the alimentary system. In: *Serotonin in Health and Disease*. Vol. IV. *Clinical Correlates*, p. 201. Edited by W.B. Essman. Spectrum Publications, N.Y.

Ward, J.M.; Sontag, J.M.; Weisburger, E.K.; and Brown, C.A. (1975). Effect of lifetime exposure to aflatoxin B₁ in rats. *J. Natl. Cancer Inst.* **55**:107.

2. Benzene

A highly controversial debate within recent years has been the hypothesis that occupational exposure to benzene results in an increased leukemogenic risk. The major reason for the intense debate is of course the widespread usage of benzene in industry and the economic cost of instituting engineering controls to ensure decreased exposures. While there is still much uncertainty as to whether benzene is a carcinogen in humans, there is certainly no question that prolonged exposure to benzene may result in toxic changes to the hematopoietic system including bone-marrow aplasia, leucocytosis, and granulocytopenia.

That selenium supplementation may affect the toxic effects of benzene on blood elements was first proposed by Aleksandrowicz et al. (1977). They noted that Sarnari et al. (1969) reported fewer adverse effects of benzene on the morphotic elements of blood, as well as the leucocytic and the megakaryocytic system via the action of phytohemagglutinin (PHA).[2] This was followed by a report from Aleksandrowicz et al. (1975) that selenium, which has immune-stimulating properties, enhanced the capacity of PHA to increase blastic transformation of lymphocytes and a report by Astaldi et al. (1974) who proposed that immunologically activated lymphocytes may become precursors of marrow cells.

In light of the theoretical capacity of selenium to enhance the transformation of immunologically activated lymphocytes to become precursors of bone marrow and the capacity of benzene to adversely affect bone marrow by inhibiting cell division and differentiation processes, Aleksandrowicz et al. (1977) evaluated the effect of selenium on benzene-induced changes in the hematopoietic system of rats.

These researchers found that selenium (5 μg/kg) given for 10 consecutive days prior to benzene exposure (1200 mg/m^3—6 hrs daily for 12 weeks) prevented the occurrence of lymphocytopenia and retarded the occurrence of thrombocytopenia as compared to groups similarly exposed to benzene but given either 0.0 or 1.0 μg selenium/kg.

Subsequent studies have also shown that selenium supplementation prevents some of the toxic effects of chronic benzene exposure. For instance, Moszczynski and Starek (1978) also reported that selenium prevented both lymphocytopenia and destruction of lysosomes in peripheral-blood lymphocytes, while Moszczynski et al. (1978) reported that selenium supplementation (1.0 μg/kg) prevented several enzymatic changes (i.e., acid phosphatase and alkaline phosphatase in peripheral-blood neutrophils) caused by chronic (5 months) exposure to benzene (1200 mg/m^3).

---

[2]PHA—is a mucoprotein from the red kidney bean that stimulates the transformation of small lymphocytes of human peripheral blood-tissue culture into large, morphologically primitive blastlike cells capable of undergoing mitosis.

These findings are of extreme interest since they may help to provide a greater understanding of differential susceptibility to benzene within the human population. Clearly these findings need to be extended, especially with respect to evaluating whether selenium supplementation may prevent benzene-induced cancer. Moszczynski et al. (1978), while recognizing the need for continued research in this area, clearly implied that future research may result in the prophylactic use of selenium supplements in persons occupationally exposed to benzene and its homologues.

References

Aleksandrowicz, J.; Dobrowolski, J.; Lisiewicz, J.; Smyk, B.; and Skotnicki, A. (1975). Influence of selenium on the growth of carcinogenic fungi and cytotoxic action of aflatoxin B_1 in cell structure of lymphocytes, and on the embryonal development of *Xenopus Laevis. Pol. Arch. Med. Wewn.* **53**:209.

Aleksandrowicz, J.; Starek, A.; and Moszczynski, P. (1977). The effect of selenium on peripheral blood picture in rats chronically exposed to benzene. *Work Med.* **28**(6):453–459.

Astaldi, G.; Karanovic, D.; Vettori, P.P.; Karanovic, J.; and Piletic, O. (1974). Phytohemagglutinin (PHA) stimulation of peripheral-blood lymphocytes and stem-cell. *Bioll. Ist. Sieroter. Milanese* **53**:599 (Cited in Aleksandrowicz et al, 1977).

Moszczynski, P. and Starek, A. (1978). Activity of lysosomal betaglucuronidase in leukocytes of rats exposed to benzene and sodium selenate. *Folia Haematol.* **105**:230–238.

Moszczynski, P.; Starek, A.; Czarnobilski, Z.; and Aleksandrowicz, J. (1978). Activity of acid and alkaline phosphatase in neutrophils of rats exposed to benzene and treated with selenium. *Folia Haematol.* **105**(4):489–496.

Sarnari, V.; Bianchi, A.; Cupini, G.; and Rapone, P. (1969). Phytohemagglutinin and hemopoietic system. *Polizlinico* **76**:58.

3. Carbon Tetrachloride

Carbon tetrachloride (CCl_4) is a well-known hepatotoxic agent in both animal models and humans. Similarly, a chronic dietary deficiency of selenium is known to contribute to the development of hepatic necrosis in a variety of species including the mouse, rat, rabbit, and pig (Schwarz and Mertz, 1959). In addition, selenium often displays a sparing influence on the effects of a vitamin E deficiency, a deficiency that also enhances CCl_4-induced hepatotoxic effects (Hove et al., 1949). In light of these findings, Muth (1960) hypothesized that a dietary deficiency or inadequacy of selenium would be likely to result in an enhancement of the hepatotoxic and possibly other adverse effects of CCl_4.

Since this hypothesis was first proposed in 1960, six studies have been published that have addressed this issue. In all cases the results of these studies have tended to support the concept that a selenium deficiency enhances CCl_4 toxicity. These studies have demonstrated that supplements of selenium either in the diet or by injection reduced the occurrence of acute toxic effects of CCl_4 as measured by mortality in rats (Seward et al., 1966; Gallagher, 1961, 1962) and ewes (Muth, 1960), as well as hepatotoxic effects in the same animal models (Fodor and Kemeny, 1965; Muth, 1960). In addition, Seward et al. (1966) found that selenium supplementation also reduced the occurrence of CCl_4-induced tooth discoloration in rats. Joint supplementation of both selenium and vitamin E was found to be more effective than either antioxidant alone in reducing toxicity and tooth discoloration.

Recent studies by Hafeman and Hoekstra (1977, 1977a) have provided some insight into how selenium prevents some of the toxic effects of CCl_4. They showed that selenium as well as vitamin E and methionine were able to prevent CCl_4-induced lipid peroxidation (as measured by the evolution of ethane). In fact, vitamin E, selenium, and methionine diminished ethane evolution from CCl_4-treated rats by 82%, 74%, and 60%, respectively. Presumably the methionine and selenium protect against CCl_4-induced toxicity by maintaining intracellular levels of glutathione and the activity of glutathione peroxidase.

In contrast to the findings of Seward et al. (1966), Hafeman and Hoekstra (1977) found no additive effect when both selenium and vitamin E were given together, either with or without methionine. However, in the absence of vitamin E, selenium provided a partial sparing effect. It is also important to note that much of the beneficial effects of *supplemental* vitamin E in preventing CCl_4-induced toxicity is diminished in the presence of optimal levels of either vitamin E and/or selenium. According to Hafeman and Hoekstra (1977), "difference in prior vitamin E or selenium nutritional status may explain existing disagreements in the literature regarding the effectiveness of vitamin E administration against CCl_4 toxicity" (McLean, 1967; Green et al., 1969; Cawthorne et al., 1970).

References

Cawthorne, M.A.; Bunyan, J.; Sennitt, M.V.; and Green, J. (1970). Vitamin E and hepatotoxic agents. 3. Vitamin E, synthetic antioxidants and carbon tetrachloride toxicity in the rat. *Brit. J. Nutr.* **24**:357–384.

Fodor, G. and Kemeny, G.L. (1965). On the hepato-protective effect of selenium in carbon tetrachloride poisoning in albino rats. *Experientia* **21**:666–667.

Gallagher, C.H. (1961). Protection by antioxidants against lethal doses of carbon tetrachloride. *Nature* **192**:881–882.

Gallagher, C.H. (1962). The effect of antioxidants on poisoning by carbon tetrachloride. *Austral. J. Exp. Biol.* **40**:241–254.

Green, J.; Bunyan, J.; Cawthorne, M.A.; and Diplock, A.T. (1969). Vitamin E and hepatotoxic agents. I. Carbon tetrachloride and lipid peroxidation in the rat. *Brit. J. Nutr.* **23**:297–307.

Hafeman, D.G. and Hoekstra, W.G. (1977). Protection against carbon tetrachloride-induced lipid peroxidation in the rat by dietary vitamin E, selenium, and methionine as measured by ethane evolution. *J. Nutr.* **107**:656–665.

Hafeman, D.G. and Hoekstra, W.G. (1977a). Lipid peroxidation *in vivo* during vitamin E and selenium deficiency in the rat as monitored by ethane evolution. *J. Nutr.* **107**:666–672.

Hove, E.L.; Copeland, D.H.; and Salmon, W.D. (1949). A fatal vitamin E deficiency disease in rats caused by massive lung hemorrhage and liver necrosis. *J. Nutr.* **39**:397–412.

McLean, A.E.M. (1967). The effect of diet and vitamin E on liver injury due to carbon tetrachloride. *Brit. J. Exp. Pathol.* **48**:632–636.

Muth, O.H. (1960). Carbon tetrachloride poisoning of ewes on a low-selenium ration. *Amer. J. Vet. Res.* **21**:86–87.

Schwarz, K. and Mertz, W. (1959). Terminal phase of dietary liver necrosis in the rat (hepatogenic hypoglycemia). *Metabolism* **8**:79–87.

Seward, C.R.; Vaughan, G.; and Hove, E.L. (1966). Effect of selenium on incisor depigmentation and carbon tetrachloride poisoning in vitamin E-deficient rats. *Proc. Soc. Exp. Biol. Med.* **121**:850.

4.   Dimethylhydrazine and Related Carcinogens

The role of selenium in health and disease is a highly controversial subject. Selenium is certainly universally recognized as a highly toxic agent at elevated levels of exposure, while more recently it has also become accepted as an essential nutrient. Similarly, selenium has been suspected of being a carcinogen in animal models, while within the past 10 to 15 years evidence has emerged that suggests that selenium may actually protect against the occurrence of cancer in both animal models and humans (Frost, 1972; Shamberger, 1969, 1970). The intention of this section is to assess the role of selenium in the enhancement or prevention of chemically induced cancer.

That selenium may affect the occurrence of chemical carcinogenesis was first reported by Clayton and Baumann in 1949, who reported that dietary sodium selenite (5 ppm) resulted in a 50% reduction in the incidence of dimethylaminoazobenzene- (DAB) induced hepatic lesions in rats. However, other experiments did not reveal a consistent influence of selenium when given either with or before the carcinogenic azo dye. Despite this interesting although ambivalent start, it was not until 1966 that the next report in the literature appeared concerning the influence of selenium on chemically induced cancer.

Since 1966 there has been a continuing interest in the notion that selenium may be a chemopreventive agent with respect to cancer. This hypothesis has received support from a variety of research studies, including those with bacterial systems (i.e., mutagenicity testing), animal-carcinogenicity studies with a variety of well-known chemical carcinogens, and human epidemiological investigations.

In 1966, two reports were published that indicated that sodium selenite either in the diet (100 ppm) or dermally applied (0.0005%) markedly reduced the occurrence of DMBA- and BAP-induced papillomas in ICR Swiss mice (Shamberger and Rudolph, 1966; Shamberger, 1966). Subsequent research by Shamberger (1970) and Harr et al. (1972, 1973, 1973a) supported these earlier reports by finding that sodium selenite reduced the carcinogenicity of BAP, DMBA, 3-methylcholanthrene, and N-2 fluorenyl-acetamide in rats. In fact, Shamberger et al. (1973) reported that sodium selenite reduced the incidence of DMBA-induced chromosomal breaks in human leucocyte cultures by 42%.

More recently Jacobs and her colleagues (1977, 1977a, 1977b, 1978) have clearly shown that selenium diminished dimethylhydrazine- (DMH) induced colon cancer incidence, reduced the occurrence of carcinogen-induced mutagenesis in the Ames test, and prevented carcinogen-induced sister-chromatid exchanges in human lymphocytes. More specifically, Jacobs (1977) reported that 1,2-dimethyl-hydrazine- (DMH) induced colon cancer incidence in rats was diminished from 87% to 40% and the total number of colon tumors reduced by a factor of 3 with a 4 ppm selenium supplementation to the drinking water. In similar fashion, the selenium treatment reduced the total number of methylazoxymethanol- (MAM) induced tumors by twofold.

Several theoretical mechanisms by which selenium may reduce the incidence of DMH- and MAM-induced colon cancer have been proposed by Jacobs (1977). For instance, DMH requires bioactivation through azomethane and azoxymethane (AOM) before formation of MAM, the ultimate carcinogen. Since disulfiram and related compounds have been reported to prevent the oxidation of azomethane to AOM and the hydroxylation of AOM to MAM (Fiala et al., 1976; Fiala, 1977), Jacobs (1977) suggested that selenium may also act to prevent the formation of MAM by inhibiting the metabolism of DMH at either or both of these sites. However, no experimental evidence was presented to support this possibility. Jacobs (1977) also evaluated the influence of selenium on the mutagenicity of 2-acetylaminofluorine (AAF), N-OH-AAF, and N-OH-aminofluorine (N-OH-AF) because (1) the DMH-to-MAM-activation scheme closely paralleled that of AAF through N-OH-AAF to N-OH-AF, and (2) neither DMH nor MAM were mutagenic in the *Salmonella typhimurium* TA 1538 strain while AAF was mutagenic in this strain.

These findings revealed that the mutagenic frequency of the three substances was decreased in the presence of selenium. Additions of 4 and 20 mM selenium to 4.5 mM AAF diminished the activity to about 80 and 65%, respectively, of the nonselenium AAF-exposed control. Further increases in selenium concentration to 40 mM did not further reduce the mutagenicity. A similar pattern of selenium-induced reductions in mutagenicity was found for N-OH-AF. However, a progressive dose-dependent reduction of NA-OH-AAF induced mutagenicity was observed (Figure 4-3).

Finally, in assays with human lymphocytes in culture it was determined that selenium was able to reduce the frequency of sister-chromatid exchanges (SCE) induced by methylmethane sulfonate by approximately 75–80% (p < 0.01). Such findings are consistent with the chemopreventive characteristics of selenium as demonstrated in both animal carcinogenicity studies as well as the mutagenicity experiments.

The findings presented here clearly indicate that selenium either topically applied or within the diet is capable of preventing the carcinogenicity of a number of well-known chemical carcinogenic agents in mice and rats. These chemopreventive findings have also been extended recently by Jacobs (1977), by showing that selenium prevents chemically induced mutations in human and bacterial chromosomes. In addition, a chemoprotective function of selenium against cancer has been inferred from ecologic-epidemiological studies so that there has been an increased incidence of colon, rectal, breast, and other cancers in humans in areas of the United States where selenium is generally quite low (Shamberger and Willis, 1971; Jansson et al., 1975, 1976). Similar ecologic studies have also shown that such selenium-cancer relationships are apparent in other countries. For example, selenium-deficient regions such as Denmark, the southern part of Sweden, New Zealand, and South Australia have high colo-rectal and breast-cancer rates, while selenium-adequate countries (i.e., Japan) have low rates of these cancers (Jansson et al., 1976). Finally, Von Evler et al. (1956) reported a regression of rat ascites sarcomata by feeding selenite with

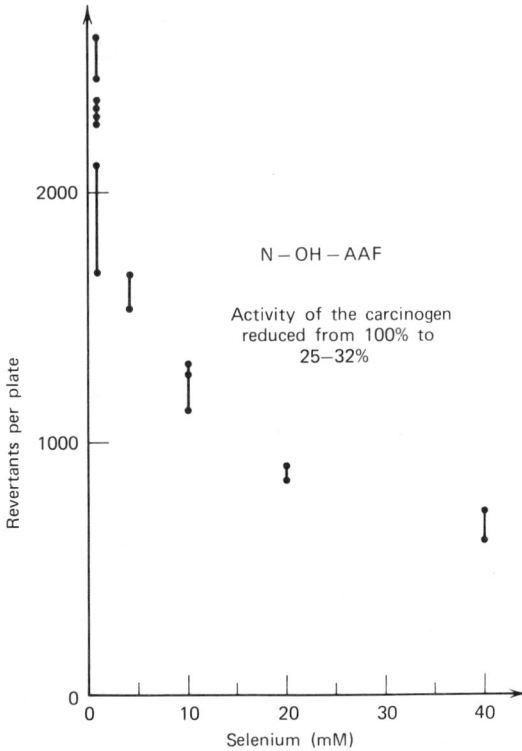

Figure 4-3. Se reduction of the mutagenicity of N-OH-AAF. [*Source.* Jacobs, M.M. (1977). Inhibitory effects of selenium on 1,2-dimethylhydrazine and methylazoxymethanol colon carcinogenesis. *Cancer* **40**:2557–2564.]

4-methylbenzene selenoic acid, while Schrauzer and Ishmael (1974) reported a decreased incidence of spontaneous mammary tumors in virgin female C_3H mice by the addition of selenium to drinking water.

In light of the above reported studies, it is evident that selenium may prevent the occurrence of cancer from several chemical agents in animal models. Whether this chemopreventive function occurs in humans is not yet known. However, ecologic-epidemiological studies do support the animal model research, but it should be clearly recognized that ecologic studies provide only associational and not causal relationships. Nevertheless, the combined findings in a wide range of animal model studies as well as human epidemiological investigations are quite consistent and should provide a strong impetus to further clarify the role of selenium as a chemopreventive agent in chemical carcinogenesis.

References

Clayton, C.C. and Baumann, C.A. (1949). Diet and azo dye tumors: effects of diet during a period when the dye is not fed. *Cancer Res.* **9**:575–582.

Fiala, E.S. (1977). Inhibition of the metabolism of the colon carcinogens 1,2-dimethylhydrazine and azoxymethane by disulfiram, carbon disulfide and related compounds. *Cancer* **40**:2436–2445.

Fiala, E.S.; Kulakis, C.; Bubotas, G.; and Weisburger, J.H. (1976). Brief communication—detection and estimation of azomethane in expired air of 1,2-dimethyl-hydrazine-treated rats. *J. Natl. Cancer Inst.* **56**:1271–1273.

Frost, D.V. (1972). The two faces of selenium—can selenophobia be cured? *CRC Crit. Rev. Toxicol.* **1**:467–514.

Harr, J.R.; Exon, J. H.; Weswig, P.H.; and Whanger, P.D. (1973). Relationship of dietary selenium concentration; chemical cancer induction; and tissue concentration of selenium in rats. *Clin. Toxicol.* **6**:487–495.

Harr, J.R.; Exon, J.H.; Weswig, P.H.; and Whanger, P.D. (1973a). Relationship of dietary selenium concentration; chemical cancer induction, and tissue concentration of selenium in rats. *Clin. Toxicol.* **6**:287–293.

Harr, J.R.; Exon, J.H.; Whanger, P.D.; and Weswig, P.H. (1972). Effect of dietary selenium on N-2 fluorenyl-acetamide (FAA)-induced cancer in vitamin E supplemented, selenium depleted rats. *Clin. Toxicol.* **5**(2):187–194.

Jacobs, B.; Jacobs, M.M.; and Griffin, A.C. (1978). Gastrointestinal cancer: epidemiology and experimental studies. In: *Inorganic and Nutritional Aspects of Cancer*, pp. 305–322. Edited by G.N. Schrauzer. Plenum Press, N.Y.

Jacobs, M.M. (1977). Inhibitory effects of selenium on 1,2-dimethylhydrazine and methylazoxymethanol colon carcinogenesis. *Cancer* **40**:2557–2564.

Jacobs, M.M.; Jansson, B.; and Griffin, A.C. (1977a). Inhibitory effects of selenium on 1,2-dimethylhydrazine and methylazoxymethanol acetate induction of colon tumors. *Cancer Letters* **2**:133–138.

Jacobs, M.M.; Matney, T.S.; and Griffin, A.C. (1977b). Inhibitory effects of selenium on the mutagenicity of 2-acetylaminofluorene (AAF) and AAF derivatives. *Cancer Letters* **2**:319–322.

Jansson, B. and Jacobs, M.M. (1976). Selenium—a possible inhibitor of colon and rectum cancer. I. Epidemiological aspects. B. Jansson. II. Biochemical aspects—M. Jacobs. Proc. Symp. on Selenium-Tellurium. Sponsored by the Industrial Health Foundation, Notre Dame, Pittsburgh, PA, pp. 326–337.

Jansson, B.; Malahy, M.A.; and Seibert, G.B. (1976). Geographical distribution of gastrointestinal cancer and breast cancer and its relation to selenium deficiency. Proc. Intern. Symposium Detection and Prevention of Cancer, N.Y., Marcel Dekker.

Jansson, B.; Seibert, B.; and Speer, J.F. (1975). Gastrointestinal cancer—its geographic distribution and correlation to breast cancer. *Cancer* **36**:2373–2384.

Riley, J.F. (1968). Mast cells, co-carcinogenesis and anticarcinogenesis in the skin of mice. *Experientia* **24**:1237.

Schrauzer, G.N. (1976). Selenium and cancer: a review. *Bio. Inorg. Chem.* **5**:275–281.

Schrauzer, G.N. (1978). Trace elements, nutrition and cancer: perspectives of prevention. In: *Inorganic and Nutritional Aspects of Cancer,* pp. 323–342. Edited by G.N. Schrauzer. Plenum Press, N.Y.

Schrauzer, G.N. and Ishmael, D. (1974). Effects of selenium and of arsenic on the genesis of spontaneous mammary tumors in inbred C_3H mice. *Ann. Clin. Lab. Sci.* **2**:441–447.

Shamberger, R.J. (1966). Protection against cocarcinogenesis by antioxidants. *Experientia* **22**:116.

Shamberger, R.J. (1969). *Proc. Am. Assoc. Cancer Res.* **10**:311.

Shamberger, R.J. (1970). Relationship of selenium to cancer. I. Inhibitory effect of selenium on carcinogenesis. *J. Natl. Cancer Inst.* **44**:931–936.

Shamberger, R.J.; Baughman, F.F.; Kalchert, S.L.; Willis, C.E.; and Hoffman, G.C. (1973). Carcinogen induced chromosomal breakage decreased by antioxidants. *Proc. Natl. Acad. Sci. USA* **70**(5):1461–1463.

Shamberger, R.J. and Rudolph, G. (1966). Protection against cocarcinogenesis by antioxidants. *Experientia* **22**:116.

Shamberger, R.J. and Willis, C.E. (1971). Selenium distribution and human cancer mortality. *CRC Crit. Rev. in Clin. Lab. Sci.* **2**:211–221.

Von Evler, V.H.; Hasselquist, H.; and Von Evler, B. (1956). Biologish verksame oligo Elemente in organischer Binding. *Arkiv. Kem.* **9**:583.

5. Dimethylnitrosamine

Dimethylnitrosamine (DMN) is well known for its hepatotoxic and carcinogenic effects in a variety of animal models (Magee and Barnes, 1967). Before it is able to exert its adverse effects, DMN requires bioactivation by the hepatic microsomal mixed-function oxidase system (Mizrahi and Emmelot, 1963; Kato et al., 1967) or some other independent enzymatic pathways (Lake et al., 1976).

Recently, it has been shown that the toxicity of DMN could be diminished by high doses of vitamin E (Dashman and Kamm, 1976). However, Skaare et al. (1977) revealed that the synthetic antioxidant ethoxyquin enhanced the toxicity of this compound. In an effort to obtain greater insight into the mechanisms by which the two antioxidants, vitamin E and ethoxyquin, divergently affect DMN hepatotoxicity, Skaare and Nafstad (1978) evaluated the influence of vitamin E and selenium on the acute hepatotoxicity of DMN in rats. With respect to selenium, it was found that 0.5 mg Se/kg administered IP 48 hours prior to DMN treatment enhanced the acute hepatotoxicity of DMBA as measured by an increased level of plasma asparagine-aminotransferase (AspAT) activity. However, morphological evaluation demonstrated no difference in DMN-induced hepatotoxicity between the two treatment groups. The mechanisms by which the three anti-oxidants tested affect DMN-induced hepatotoxicity remain to be determined. Skaare and Nafstad (1978) have offered several speculative mechanisms by which these compounds alter DMN toxicity. "All three compounds . . . influence drug metabolizing enzyme systems in the liver and may therefore generally interfere with DMN metabolism either by accelerating the DMN metabolism or by accelerating the DMN biotransformation by producing alternative pathways of metabolism leaving more or less toxic end products." In light of the ambivalent nature of their speculation, it is quite evident that further research is needed to clarify the mechanism(s) by which selenium (and other antioxidants) affect DMN toxicity.

References

Dashman, T. and Kamm, J.J. (1976). Effect of high doses of vitamin E on drug metabolism in the rat. *Pharmacologist* 18:154.

Kato, R.H.; Shoji, H.; and Takanaka, A. (1967). Metabolism of carcinogenic compounds. I. Effect of phenobarbital and methylcholanthrene on the activities of N-demethylation of carcinogenic compounds by liver microsomes of male and female rats. *Gann.* 58:467–469.

Lake, B.G.; Phillip, J.C.; Heading, C.E.; and Gangolli, S.D. (1976). Studies on the *in vitro* metabolism of dimethylnitrosamine by rat liver. *Toxicol.* 5:297–309.

Magee, P.N. and Barnes, J.M. (1967). Carcinogenic nitroso compounds. *Advan. Cancer Res.* 10:163–246.

Mizrahi, I.J. and Emmelot, P. (1963). Counteraction by sulfhydryl compounds of the enzymic conversion of and the metabolic lesions produced by two carcinogenic N-nitro compounds in rat liver. *Biochem. Pharm.* 12:55–63.

Skaare, J.U. and Nafstad, I. (1978). Interaction of vitamin E and selenium with the hepatotoxic agent dimethylnitrosamine. *Acta Pharmacol. Toxicol.* 43:119–128.

Skaare, J.U.; Nafstad, I.; and Dahle, H.K. (1977). Enhanced hepatotoxicity of dimethylnitrosamine by pretreatment of rats with the antioxidant ethoxyquin. *Toxicol. Appl. Pharmacol.* 42:19–31.

6. Herbicides: Paraquat

Paraquat has been widely employed as a broad-spectrum herbicide for several years. Various researchers have indicated that it may be toxic to both humans (Bullivant, 1966; Clark et al., 1966; Copland et al., 1974) and laboratory animals (Kimbrough and Gaines, 1970; Murray and Gibson, 1972). According to Bus et al. (1976), paraquat-induced toxicity may be described as a delayed development of pulmonary lesions that first appears as pulmonary edema and which subsequently develops into interstitial fibrosis (see Murray and Gibson, 1972; Toner et al., 1970). Electron microscopic studies of pulmonary lesions have indicated initial damage to type I pneumocytes, increased numbers of fibroblasts, and a subsequent proliferation of type II pneumocytes in both rats and mice (Kimbrough and Linder, 1973; Brook, 1971; Bus et al., 1976). That pulmonary lesions are a common feature of paraquat toxicity suggests that paraquat may be retained in lung tissue (Sharp et al., 1972; Murray and Gibson, 1974; Bus et al., 1975). In fact, Rose et al. (1974) have reported that rat lung slices accumulate paraquat via an active transport process.

In an effort to clarify the mechanisms of paraquat toxicity, Bus et al. (1976) proposed that paraquat undergo "a single electron reduction with NADPH as the source of electrons. Upon aerobic oxidation of reduced paraquat by molecular oxygen, superoxide radicals are formed which may nonenzymatically dismutate to singlet oxygen. Singlet oxygen then reacts with unsaturated lipids associated with cell membranes to produce lipid hydroperoxides, which spontaneously decompose in the presence of trace amounts of transition metal ions to lipid-free radicals (see Holman, 1954). The lipid free radicals then begin the

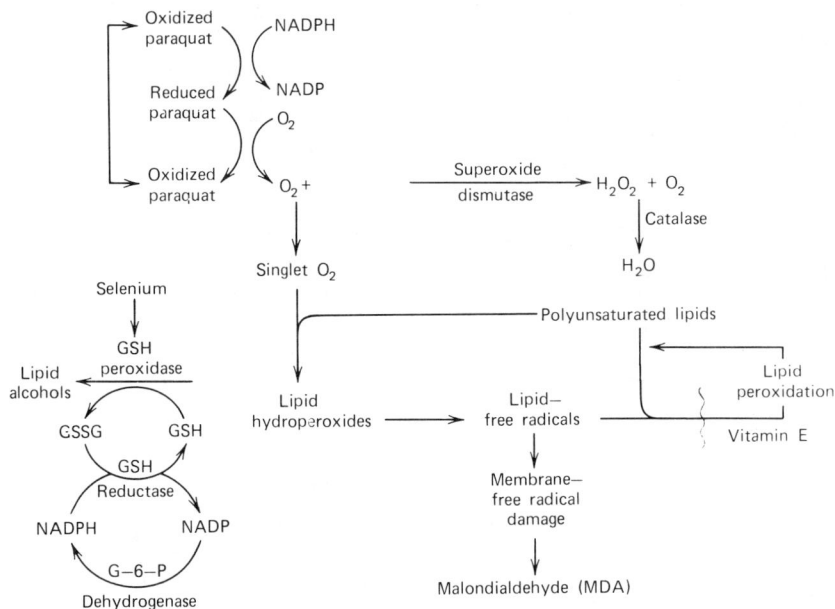

Figure 4-4. Proposed mechanism for paraquat toxicity. [*Source.* Bus et al. (1976).]

chain reaction process of lipid peroxidation which is damaging to cell membranes." This theory was based on research by Gage (1968), which indicated that (1) paraquat is reduced *in vitro* by rat liver microsomes, (2) superoxide radicals are formed from the cyclic reduction-oxidation of paraquat (Farrington, 1973), and (3) the transposition of the research model of Pederson and Aust (1973), which compared xanthine oxidase-induced lipid peroxidation to that of paraquat-induced lipid peroxidation. Figure 4-4 illustrates the proposed mechanism for paraquat toxicity, including possible means of biochemical adaptation and/or detoxification.

According to Bus et al. (1976), the three fundamental defense mechanisms against oxidant toxicity in mammalian systems are: (1) the scavenging of superoxide radicals via superoxide dismutase, (2) the role of endogenous vitamin E in preventing free-radical chain reactions of lipid peroxidation, and (3) the activity of GSH peroxidase in preventing the creation of free radicals via the reduction of unstable lipid peroxides to stable lipid alcohols.

Table 12. Alteration of Paraquat Single-Dose Seven-Day Intraperitoneal LD_{50} in Mice by Various Selenium or Vitamin E Diets and Diethyl Maleate Pretreatment

Treatment	Paraquat LD_{50}, mg/kg	95% Confidence Limits	Potency Ratio
Control	30.0	26.5–35.1	—
Selenium-deficient[a]	10.4	8.9–12.2	2.88[b]
Selenium, 0.1 ppm[c]	27.3	24.8–30.0	1.10
Selenium, 2.0 ppm[c]	25.5	22.2–29.3	1.18
Diethyl maleate[d]	9.4	6.5–13.5	3.20[b]
Vitamin E-deficient[a]	9.2	6.3–13.3	3.26[b]
Vitamin E, 1500 mg/kg[c]	29.0	23.8–35.4	1.03

[a] Deficient diet, 5-week exposure prior to paraquat treatment.
[b] Significantly different from control, $p < 0.05$.
[c] Basal deficient diet supplemented with selenium or vitamin E.
[d] 1.2 ml/kg, IP, 30 min before paraquat.

Source. Bus, J.S.; Aust, S.D.; and Gibson, J.E. (1976). Paraquat toxicity: proposed mechanism of action involving lipid peroxidation. *Environ. Health Perspect.* **16:**139–146.

Consequently, it logically follows that if one substantially reduced the amount of vitamin E ingested it would probably result in enhanced susceptibility to paraquat toxicity. The same reasoning would most likely hold true for dietary levels of selenium, since selenium is a component of GSH peroxidase (Rotruck et al., 1973; Tappel, 1965). In fact, Bus et al. (1975a) reported that mice deficient in either selenium (Table 12) or vitamin E exhibit enhanced susceptibility to paraquat toxicity as determined by single-dose seven-day intraperitoneal LD_{50}. Conversely, supplementation of the deficient diets with either selenium or vitamin E provided significant protection, as seen in Table 12. Thus, according to Bus et al. (1976), these data supported the hypothesized mechanism, since mice deficient in either selenium or vitamin E were at increased risk to paraquat toxicity.

References

Brook, R.E. (1971). Ultrastructure of lung lesions produced by ingested chemicals. I. Effect of the herbicide paraquat on mouse lung. *Lab. Invest.* **25**:536.

Bullivant, C.M. (1966). Accidental poisoning by paraquat: report of two cases in man. *Brit. Med. J.* **1**:1272.

Bus, J.S.; Aust, S.D.; and Gibson, J.E. (1975a). Lipid peroxidation: a possible mechanism for paraquat toxicity. *Res. Commun. Chem. Pharmacol.* **11**:31.

Bus, J.S.; Aust, S.D.; and Gibson, J.E. (1976). Paraquat toxicity: proposed mechanism of action involving lipid peroxidation. *Environ. Health Perspect.* **16**:139–146.

Bus, J.S.; Preache, M.M.; Cagen, S.Z.; Posner, H.S.; Eliason, B.C.; Sharp, C.W.; and Gibson, J.F. (1975). Fetal toxicity and distribution of paraquat and diquat in mice and rats. *Toxicol. Appl. Pharmacol.* **33**:450–460.

Clark, D.G.; McElligott, T.F.; and Hurst, E.W. (1966). The toxicity of paraquat. *Brit. J. Ind. Med.* **23**:126.

Copland, G.M.; Kalin, A.; and Shulman, H.S. (1974). Fatal pulmonary intraalveolar fibrosis after paraquat ingestion. *New Eng. J. Med.* **291**:290.

Farrington, J.A. (1973). Bipyridylium quarternary salts and related compounds. V. Pulse radiolysis studies of the reaction of paraquat radical with oxygen. Implications for the mode of action of bipyridyl herbicides. *Biochem. Biophys. Acta* **314**:372.

Gage, J.C. (1968). Actions of paraquat and diquat on liver cell fractions. *Biochem. J.* **109**:757.

Holman, R.T. (1954). Auto-oxidation of fats and related substances. In: *Progress in the Chemistry of Fats and Other Lipids*. Vol. 2. R.T. Holman, W.O. Lundberg, and T. Malbin, editors. Pergamon Press, Elmford, N.Y.

Kimbrough, R.D. and Gaines, T.B. (1970). Toxicity of paraquat to rat lungs. *Toxicol. Appl. Pharmacol.* **17**:679.

Kimbrough, R.D. and Linder, R.E. (1973). The ultrastructure of the paraquat lung lesion in the rat. *Environ. Res.* **6**:265.

Murray, R.E. and Gibson, J.E. (1972). A comparative study of paraquat intoxication in rats, guinea pigs, and monkeys. *Exptl. Molec. Pathol.* **17**:317.

Murray, R.E. and Gibson, J.E. (1974). Paraquat disposition in rats, guinea pigs, and monkeys. *Toxicol. Appl. Pharmacol.* **27**:283.

Pederson, T.C. and Aust, S.D. (1973). The role of superoxide and singlet oxygen in lipid peroxidation promoted by xanthine oxidase. *Biochem. Biophys. Res. Commun.* **52**:1071.

Rose, M.S.; Smith, L.L.; and Wyatt, I. (1974). Evidence for energy-dependent accumulation of paraquat into rat lung. *Nature* **252**:314.

Rotruck, J.T.; Pope, A.L.; Ganther, H.E.; Swanson, A.B.; Hafeman, D.G.; and Hoekstra, W.G. (1973). Selenium: biochemical role as a component of glutathione peroxidase. *Science* **179**:588.

Sharp, C.W.; Ottolenghi, A.; and Posner, H.S. (1972). Correlation of paraquat toxicity with tissue concentrations and weight of the rat. *Toxicol. Appl. Pharmacol.* **22**:241.

Tappel, A.L. (1965). Free radical lipid peroxidation and its inhibition by vitamin E and selenium. *Fed. Proc.* **24**:73.

Toner, P.G.; Vetters, J.M.; Spilg, W.G.S.; and Harland, W.A. (1970). Fine structure of the lung lesion in a case of paraquat poisoning. *J. Pathol.* **102**:182.

7.   PCBs

That exposure to polychlorinated biphenyls (PCBs) may affect selenium metabolism was first suggested by Combs et al. (1975) who observed that exposure of breeder hens to elevated levels of PCBs results in the occurrence of a selenium deficiency in their broiler-chick offspring. This casual field observation along with a report by Rehfield et al. (1971) that the PCB Aroclor 1254 produced what appeared to be exudative diathesis in chicks, led Combs et al. (1975) to speculate that PCB exposure may be a cause of either a selenium and/or vitamin-E deficiency in chickens.

This hypothesis was supported by observations of Siami et al. (1972) that inducers of hepatic microsomal mixed-function oxidases can affect selenium-induced growth functions of depleted rats, presumably by affecting their utilization. It was thus further reasoned by Combs et al. (1975) that because PCBs are strong inducers of liver microsomal enzymes, it is possible that they may be affecting an apparent selenium depletion in this manner. Experiments evaluating the hypothesis that PCBs do affect either selenium and/or vitamin E metabolism revealed that 10 ppm of Aroclor 1254 in the diet of breeding hens definitely enhanced susceptibility to exudative diathesis of offspring when those chicks were maintained on a vitamin E-deficient and marginally supplemented selenium diet.

While this study confirmed the previously noted hypothesis that PCB exposure enhances vitamin E and/or selenium requirements, it could not distinguish between the two nutrients. However, subsequent experiments by Combs and Scott (1975) did indicate that exposure of chicks to PCBs did not modify the protective function of vitamin E on membranes, but it did reduce the biological utilization of dietary selenium using several biochemical indicators of selenium function (e.g., glutathione peroxidase activity in plasma).

These authors concluded that "dietary PCBs interfere with the utilization of dietary selenium, increasing the chicks' requirement slightly but critically if the diet contains a marginal level and is low in vitamin E content. PCBs do not affect the physiological function of vitamin E in the protection of biological membranes but PCBs may interfere with the absorption and retention of this vitamin" (Combs and Scott, 1975). Finally they speculated that PCBs induce hepatic microsomal enzymes that alter the utilization of absorbed selenium by changing its oxidation status, thus reducing its incorporation into glutathione peroxidase and increasing its incorporation into selenium compounds of limited "usefulness."

The findings of Combs and his colleagues are of interest since they have clearly shown the PCBs in the diet alter normal selenium metabolism, thereby increasing its physiological requirements. In light of the fact that the animal model used was the chick and that the PCB levels were much higher than normal human exposure, it is not possible to assess the implications of these findings for man. However, continued research into this area, especially with other animal models, should be of interest.

References

Combs, G.F., Jr.; Cantor, A.H.; and Scott, M.L. (1975). Effects of dietary polychlorinated biphenyls on vitamin E and selenium nutrition in the chick. *Poult. Sci.* **54**(4):1143–1152.

Combs, G.F., Jr. and Scott, M.L. (1975). Polychlorinated biphenyl-stimulated selenium deficiency in the chick. *Poult. Sci.* **54**:1152–1158.

Rehfield, B.M.; Bradley, R.L., Jr.; and Sunde, M.L. (1971). Toxicity studies of polychlorinated biphenyls in the chick. I. Toxicity and symptoms. *Poult. Sci.* **50**:1090–1096.

Siami, G.; Schulbert, A.R.; and Neal, R.A. (1972). A possible role for the mixed function-oxidase enzyme system in the requirement for selenium in the rat. *J. Nutr.* **102**:857–862.

8. Tricresyl Phosphate

Tricresyl phosphate (Figure 4-5) is employed as a plasticizer for chlorinated rubber, vinyl plastics, polystyrene, polyacrylic, and polymetha-

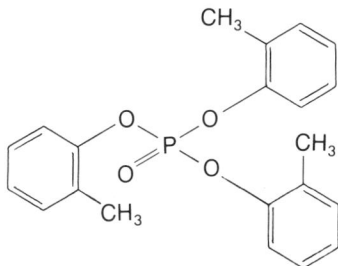

Figure 4-5. The chemical structure of tricresyl phosphate ortho-isomer.

crylic esters. In addition, it is used as an additive to synthetic lubricants and gasoline (Tabershaw et al., 1977). The tricresyl phosphates are found in several isomeric forms of which the ortho-isomer is the most toxic. The OSHA standard for the ortho-isomer is 0.1 mg/m^3, while there are no standards for the other isomers.

Exposure to tri-o-cresyl phosphate (TOCP) is known to cause a variety of adverse effects including neurological poisoning, muscular disorders, gastrointestinal symptoms including nausea, vomiting, diarrhea, liver necrosis, lung hemorrhage, and testicular atrophy (Shull and Cheeke, 1973; Tabershaw et al., 1977).

While treatment with vitamin E is known to reduce many of the symptoms of TOCP toxicity, it does not completely overcome TOCP-induced growth depression. In light of the capacity of vitamin E to effectively reduce many of the expressions of TOCP-induced toxicity as well as the known interrelationships of selenium with vitamin E including the mutual sparing effects of these nutrients, Shull and Cheeke (1973, 1975) evaluated how dietary selenium and vitamin E may affect TOCP toxicity. They reported that supplementation with either selenium (0.5 or 1.0 ppm) or vitamin E (100 IU/kg diet) overcomes the occurrence of TOCP-induced reduced growth rates and hemolysis in rats and quail, with selenium being the more effective of the two.

Since the selenium-TOCP interaction was the strongest, these researchers hypothesized that an antagonism of selenium by TOCP was taking place. It was speculated that (1) selenium may join with several possible phosphorus-containing excretory fractions of TOCP (i.e., diaryl phosphates, monoaryl phosphates, and phosphoric acid). Conceivably a selenophosphorus excretory compound could lead to a depletion of selenium reserves. (2) Selenium may also join with the nonphosphoric component of TOCP (i.e., o-cresol), forming an excretory compound which could also lead to a depletion of selenium stores as in the previously mentioned example. (3) Another degradation product of TOCP is o-hydroxybenzyl, which is excreted in part via an ethereal sulfate. Since selenium may be similarly excreted, it was speculated that selenium may be competing for the same conjugating agent.

These three speculative mechanisms of how selenium may affect the toxicity of TOCP are clearly in need of further investigation. In addition, epidemiologic studies concerning the role of dietary factors (i.e., selenium) in preventing TOCP toxicity should be initiated.

References

Shull, L.R. and Cheeke, P.R. (1973). Antiselenium activity of tri-o-cresyl phosphate in rats and Japanese quail. *J. Nutr.* **103**:560–568.

Shull, L.R. and Cheeke, P.R. (1975). Tri-o-cresyl phosphate interrelationships with selenium, vitamin E, and sulfur amino acids in the rat: growth, hemolysis, and glutathione peroxidase. *Nutr. Repts. Intern.* **11**(1):39–48.

Tabershaw, I.R.; Utidjian, H.M.D.; and Karahawa, B. (1977). Chemical hazards. In: *Occupational Diseases*. Edited by M.M. Key et al. NIOSH, Washington, D.C.

C. SELENIUM—POLLUTANT INTERACTIONS—A PERSPECTIVE

It has been shown that selenium may play an important role in reducing the toxicity, mutagenicity, and carcinogenicity of a variety of toxic substances encountered in the ambient and industrial environments. The types of compounds whose adverse effects are diminished by selenium are quite diverse and include several heavy metals such as cadmium, lead, mercury, and silver; a number of organic compounds such as benzene, CCl_4, and PCBs, the gaseous irritant ozone, and α-irradiation. Unlike nutrients such as ascorbic acid, research into the possibility that selenium may serve as a general detoxifying agent is relatively new. In fact, it is only within the past two decades that selenium has been recognized as an essential nutrient and not just a potentially toxic substance at high levels of exposure. With the exception of the arsenic-selenium interaction, all other interactions of selenium with the substances reviewed here are less than 20 years old, with the majority being less than a decade. In light of this new interest in the interaction of selenium with environmental pollutants, it would seem that new and potentially important interrelationships will be found within the near future.

The two most comprehensively studied interactions in which selenium protects against pollutant toxicity are with mercury and cadmium. There is certainly little question that dietary selenium reduces the toxicity of both inorganic and organic mercury as well as cadmium. However, despite the relatively large number of studies in which selenium offers protection from the adverse effects of these heavy metals, there is a total lack of human epidemiologic, experimental, and clinical investigations to verify these animal studies.

While the most studied interactions are with heavy metals, the newest area of potential value is that of the interaction of selenium with a variety of hydrocarbon carcinogens. A number of studies have appeared that have clearly shown that either dietary or topical administration of selenium compounds will reduce the occurrence of papillomas and colon tumors induced by several chemical carcinogenic compounds including BAP, DMBA, and DMH. Of further significance is that selenium compounds have also been shown to reduce the occurrence of chemically induced mutations via bacterial testing as well as in bioassays using human leucocytes (Shamberger, 1970, 1972, 1972a; Shamberger et al., 1973).

These findings, which clearly suggest the anticarcinogenic potential of selenium, have been supported by several epidemiological studies of an ecological nature in which the levels of selenium in the soil and food were inversely correlated with the occurrence of increased incidences of numerous types of cancer (Shamberger and Willis, 1971). While both the animal and epidemiological studies employed here support the hypothesis that certain selenium compounds may serve as chemopreventive substances, the findings considered singly or combined are not conclusive with respect to the role of selenium in affecting chemical carcinogenesis in humans. This is clearly a vital area of research in light of the widespread occurrence of low-selenium areas within the United States and other countries.

Of further interest along the same lines have been the recent European reports that suggest that benzene toxicity can be modified by selenium administration. While only a handful of reports are currently available, they do have a high degree of consistency. Such findings have important implications for the practice of industrial hygiene. It is certainly well known that there is a high degree of variability in the response of workers to exposure from toxic agents. Perhaps dietary factors such as selenium may play a role in the development of differential susceptibility to benzene. In light of the controversies surrounding the health risks associated with benzene exposure, further investigations of selenium-benzene interactions are warranted.

While it is important to evaluate critically the published literature for each selenium-pollutant interaction, it is also necessary to consider areas that have been generally ignored and yet which appear extremely promising. A prime example of this situation is the near dearth of information on the influence of selenium on ozone toxicity, especially to lung tissue and red blood cells. There is little question that animal and human cells respond to oxidant stress by increasing the activity of the hexose monophosphate shunt, including the activity of the selenium-dependent enzyme glutathione peroxidase. Bus et al. (1976) have shown that selenium-deficient rodents are at increased risk to the oxidizing activity of paraquat and there is a strong theoretical framework that a selenium deficiency may enhance ozone toxicity as well. In light of the widespread occurrence of elevated levels of ozone during spring and summer months, the EPA should adopt a research program designed to evaluate the influence of selenium on ozone toxicity. It is interesting to note that Los Angeles County has very high levels of ozone, while at the same time it also has a high level of selenium in its soil and therefore presumably in its locally grown food. Could the presence of high levels of selenium in the food of Los Angeles residents increase their adaptive capacity to ozone toxicity?

In addition to there being an almost total lack of published information on the influence of selenium on ozone toxicity either in animal models or epidemiologic investigations, there is a similar need for studies of an occupational epidemiologic nature on the relationship of dietary selenium ingestion and toxicity from silver, TOCP, and CCl_4, given the fact that selenium does reduce their toxicity in animal models.

The evidence presented here has established unequivocally that selenium reduces the toxicity and carcinogenicity of numerous environmental pollutants. Recognition of this evidence has understandably led to considerable interest within both the scientific and lay communities into the possibility that selenium is a general detoxifying agent with anticarcinogenic properties.

Despite the fact that selenium prevents the adverse effects of many toxic agents, it must be recognized that with the principal exception of correlational studies with human populations, the vast majority of research concerning selenium-pollutant interactions is with animal models. While there is good reason to assume that humans may respond in a comparable manner, there is still a high degree of uncertainty involved in extrapolating from animal models to humans.

Besides difficulties in extrapolation requiring caution in the development of policy concerning selenium ingestion, it must be recognized that selenium (1) has a long history of causing toxicity to a number of animal models at elevated levels of exposure, (2) has long been suspected of being a carcinogenic agent in rats, and (3) may enhance the toxicity of aflatoxin B_1 (Newberne and Conner, 1974).

Careful recognition of the claims of both the adverse as well as beneficial effects of selenium exposure is needed by our regulatory agencies. The irony of the present situation is that while the EPA has placed a 10-microgram-per-liter standard for selenium in drinking water, it is also permissible to purchase selenium dietary supplements (e.g., 50 microgram tablets) over the counter. Thus, while many in the general public have been led to believe that selenium is an anticancer agent, EPA assumes it may be a carcinogen. It is time for the federal government (EPA, FDA) to vigorously address this issue.

References

Bus, J.S.; Aust, S.D.; and Gibson, J.E. (1976). Paraquat toxicity: proposed mechanism of action involving lipid peroxidation. *Environ. Health Perspect.* **16**:139–146.

Newberne, P.M. and Conner, M.W. (1974). Effect of selenium on acute response to aflatoxin B_1. In: *Trace Substances in Environmental Health*, pp. 323–328. Edited by D.D. Hemphill. Univ. of Missouri at Columbia.

Shamberger, R.J. (1970). Relationship of selenium to cancer. I. Inhibitory effect of selenium on carcinogenesis. *J. Natl. Cancer Inst.* **44**:931–936.

Shamberger, R.J. (1972). Antioxidants and cancer. III. Selenium and other antioxidants decrease carcinogen-induced chromosome breakage. In: *Trace Element Metabolism in Animals* 2. Edited by W.G. Hoekstra, J.S. Suttie, W. Mertz. Univ. Park Press, Baltimore.

Shamberger, R.J. (1972a). Increase in peroxidation in carcinogenesis. *J. Natl. Cancer Inst.* **48**:1491–1497.

Shamberger, R.J.; Baughman, F.F.; Kalchert, S.L.; Willis, C.W.; and Hoffman, G.C. (1973). Carcinogen induced chromosomal breakage decreased by antioxidants. *Proc. Nat. Acad. Sci.* **70**:1461–1463.

Shamberger, R.J. and Willis, R.E. (1971). Selenium distribution and human cancer mortality. *CRC Crit. Rev. in Clin. Lab. Sci.* **2**:211–221.

Zinc

A. INORGANIC SUBSTANCES

1. Cadmium

The toxicity of cadmium has long been of concern to biomedical researchers. The range of toxic effects caused by cadmium is quite broad due to the fact that it is capable of disrupting the activity of a number of important enzyme systems. Of particular concern is that exposure to cadmium is known to result in damage to the kidneys and testes and may be a potential cause of hypertension and embryotoxic/teratogenic effects in rodents (Gunn et al., 1968).

Concomitant with research findings that have characterized the toxicity of cadmium on biochemical systems have been investigations of the interrelationships of cadmium with a number of essential nutrients. As has been shown elsewhere in this work, the toxicity of cadmium may be modified by dietary intakes of calcium, copper, iron (II), selenium, ascorbic acid, vitamin D, and protein. This section will evaluate the evidence of a further interaction of cadmium with an essential nutrient, zinc.

The first question, therefore, is why would researchers hypothesize that cadmium toxicity would be affected by the presence of Zn? This idea was suggested in the late 1950s by Parizek and Zahoe (1956). They were aware of a report of Elcoate et al. (1955), which revealed that a chronic nutritional deficiency of zinc resulted in testicular damage, and several studies (Alsberg and Schwartze, 1919; Schwartze and Alsberg, 1923) which revealed that cadmium also caused testicular damage in rats. In light of these findings, these two researchers speculated on the possibility of whether the same mechanism of testicular damage might be the cause of both toxic effects; that is, a depletion of essential zinc.

In evaluating this hypothesis, Parizek (1957) gave large amounts of zinc salts simultaneously with the cadmium to rats and noted complete morphologic protection of the testes for up to 10 days postinjection. Later findings by Gunn et al. (1961) revealed that the protection provided by zinc varied according to the breeding behavior; that is, immediate breeding after the cadmium-zinc exposure resulted in a 3–4 week duration of protection while a postponing of breeding of up to 8 weeks resulted in protection of up to 20 weeks after exposure. Presumably, there is a loss of zinc following ejaculation of sperm, thereby predisposing the development of cadmium toxicity.

Since the initial discoveries that zinc administration was capable of preventing cadmium-induced toxicity to testicular tissue, numerous researchers have not only verified this original finding (Gunn et al., 1961, 1963; Mason et al., 1964; Gunn et al., 1968b), but have shown that numerous other adverse effects caused by cadmium exposure may also be prevented by zinc administration (Table 1). In addition to the wide range of cadmium-induced adverse effects that zinc is able to prevent, it is also important to realize that these protective effects of zinc occur in a number of species including mice (Gunn et al., 1963), rats (Parizek, 1957; Banis et al., 1969; Mason et al., 1964; Schroeder, 1967; Schroeder and Buckman, 1967), turkey poults (Supplee, 1961), chicks (Supplee, 1963), hamsters (Ferm and Carpenter, 1967, 1968), lambs (Mills and Dalgarno, 1972), calves (Powell et al., 1964), and quail (Jacobs et al., 1969, 1978, 1978a) via oral and/or intraperitoneal routes of exposure.

The interaction of zinc with cadmium is such that the occurrence of low levels of zinc in the diet enhances cadmium toxicity, while supplementation in excess of amounts normally considered nutritionally adequate markedly reduces cadmium toxicity in turkey poults (Supplee, 1961). However, as important as this information is in developing a quantitative risk assessment concerning the cadmium-zinc interaction, very little research has specifically addressed this issue. More recently, Jacobs et al. (1978, 1978a) have reported that the consumption

Table 1.   Cadmium-Induced Toxic Effects Prevented by Zinc

Adverse Effect	Reference
Testicular damage	Parizek and Zahoe, 1956
	Parizek, 1957
	Gunn et al., 1961, 1962, 1963
	Mason et al., 1964
Epididymal damage	Gunn et al., 1963
Testicular vasculature damage	Gunn et al., 1963
Interstitial-cell tumors	Gunn et al., 1963a
Growth depression in chicks	Hill et al., 1963
Gizzard abnormality in chicks	Hill et al., 1963
Skin disorders in calves	Powell et al., 1964
Enlarged and sore joints in calves	Powell et al., 1964
Scrotal lesions in calves	Powell et al., 1964
Teratogenic/embryotoxic effects	Ferm and Carpenter, 1967, 1968
	Ahokas et al., 1979
Hypertension	Schroeder, 1967
	Schroeder and Buckman, 1967
Cytotoxic effects in mouse L cells	Petering, 1978
Lung/heart lesions in mice	Lal, 1976
	Petering, 1978

of diets by Japanese quail with about twice the necessary amounts of zinc, copper, and manganese reduced the quantity of dietary cadmium retained in tissue as compared to controls fed a basal diet. However, it was not possible to ascertain the specific contribution of zinc alone. Many studies not concerned with determining mechanisms of action have usually provided a large cadmium exposure either orally or by injection, along with varying degrees of zinc supplementation. Thus their general objective was to establish that zinc could actually prevent a rather striking adverse effect. This limited goal diminishes the opportunity of studying the influence of low-level chronic exposure to cadmium in animals given a diet with inadequate levels of zinc.

Mechanism of Protection.   The mechanism(s) by which zinc prevents cadmium toxicity has (have) been the source of considerable investigation. Does zinc reduce gastrointestinal absorption of Cd or enhance its excretion? Does zinc cause a redistribution of Cd within different tissues so that the cadmium does not reach the site of action in sufficient quantities to cause harm? Does zinc form a complex with

Cd? Does zinc outcompete Cd for reactive sites and thereby reduce the capacity of Cd to induce toxicity?

Following the finding that zinc administration prevented cadmium-induced testicular damage, Parizek (1957) speculated that a competitive interaction existed between these two elements. Other researchers have shown that there is evidence of interchange between zinc and Cd (Cotzias et al., 1961) as well as a lack of discrimination between these two metals by certain cell fractions (Cotzias et al., 1961a). This led to the hypothesis that Cd may be competing with zinc and to a certain extent replacing it in some organelles and at particular binding sites.

Other reports have indicated that Cd displaced the zinc of carboxypeptidase B, resulting in a change in catalytic specificity (Folk et al., 1962), while Coleman and Vallee (1961) noted the displacement of zinc by Cd and of Cd by zinc in carboxypeptidase A. In addition, Druyan and Vallee (1962) have reported that Cd can replace zinc in liver alcohol dehydrogenase and inactivate it. Hill et al. (1963) concluded that "in the presence of Cd, addition of zinc to the diet is required to restore the nutritional status of the animal to that of the controls not receiving Cd. This presumably takes place because the additional . . . zinc displaces the interfering Cd and restores normal metabolism."

Besides the apparent competition of zinc and cadmium for binding sites as a means to understand how zinc supplementation may reduce Cd toxicity, another important mechanism for protection has been suggested. Numerous reports have indicated that experimental exposure to Cd results in an increased synthesis of metal-binding protein molecules similar to or identical with metallothionein. Cadmium atoms aggressively bind to this protein, thereby resulting in a marked alteration in its toxicity and metabolism. The formation of metallothionein-like proteins in response to Cd exposure may actually be an adaptive response and has been suggested to explain the protective effect of pretreatment with small subtoxic quantities of Cd. Parizek (1976) has hypothesized that the "increased amounts of metal-binding proteins (able to sequester Cd) could well represent the main protective mechanism by which pretreatment with zinc alleviates Cd toxicity," since zinc salts are known to induce the synthesis of low-molecular-weight metal-binding proteins in a comparable manner with Cd (Webb, 1972; Parizek, 1976). Such a hypothesis would be consistent with the observation that zinc administration increases Cd retention in the body and "why the protective dose of zinc did not decrease but, on the contrary, increased Cd content in the liver of animals intoxicated by salts of this metal" (Parizek, 1976).

It appears that zinc may reduce or prevent Cd toxicity by outcompeting it for key binding sites as well as by enhancing the synthesis of metal-binding proteins to which Cd binds, thereby preventing Cd from reaching critical areas (at least temporarily). There is also evidence to suggest that Cd may diminish the gastrointestinal absorption of zinc (Roberts et al., 1973; Evans et al., 1974) and thus contribute to enhancing its (i.e., Cd) toxicity. Conversely, Hahn and Evans (1975) reported that low levels of zinc seem to slightly reduce the gastrointestinal uptake of Cd.

Discussion. It is quite evident that administration of zinc salts either in the diet or by injection prevents numerous toxic effects resulting from Cd exposure. Without exception, the levels of Cd employed in the zinc-Cd interaction studies cited here were far in excess of the level needed to cause toxicity in humans. In fact, nearly every study cited employed a level of Cd equivalent to an amount far greater than the estimated concentration that caused Itai Itai Byo disease (Jacobs et al., 1978). Future studies are needed to evaluate the influence of zinc on the development of the Cd body burden when exposure levels are within a normal range (i.e., the equivalent of 50 to 150 μg Cd/day) for a prolonged period of time (i.e., up to a year).

In addition, only one study has been reported where Cd toxicity via inhalation and a zinc interaction have been evaluated (Lal, 1976). Since industrial exposures are primarily via inhalation, this is an area that should be given further study.

The occurrence of a dietary zinc deficiency has been reported in the Middle East (Prasad, 1966; Sandstead et al., 1967), while several studies have indicated the presence of inadequate zinc status in children in the United States (Hambidge et al., 1976, Hambidge, 1977). Whether an inadequate dietary zinc intake enhances the toxicity of normally nontoxic levels of Cd remains to be determined.

References

Abe, T.; Itokawa, T.; and Inoue, K. (1972). Studies on experimental cadmium poisoning. I. Effect of pre-administration of heavy metals and vitamins on acute cadmium poisoning in mice. *Jap. J. Hyg.* **26**:498–504.

Ahokas, R.A.; Dilts, P.V., Jr.; and LaHaye, E.B. (1979). Cadmium-induced fetal growth retardation: Protective effect of excess dietary Zn. *Amer. J. Obstet. Gynecol.* (In press).

Alsberg, C.L. and Schwartze, E.W. (1919). Pharmacological actions of cadmium. *J. Pharm.* **13**:504–505.

Anonymous (1968). More clues in the cadmium and zinc puzzle. *Food and Cosmetics Tox.* 6:523.

Banis, R.J.; Pond, W.G.; Walker, E.F.; and O'Connor, J.R. (1969). Dietary cadmium, iron, and zinc interactions in the growing rat. *Proc. Soc. Exp. Biol. Med.* 130:802–806.

Bunn, C.R. and Matrone, G. (1966). *In vivo* interactions of cadmium, copper, zinc, and iron in the mouse and rat. *J. Nutr.* 90:395–399.

Campbell, J.K. and Mills, C.F. (1979). The toxicity of zinc to pregnant sheep. *Environ. Res.* 20:1–13.

Coleman, J.E. and Vallee, B. (1961). Metallocarboxypeptidases: stability constants and enzymatic characteristics. *J. Biol. Chem.* 236:2244–2249.

Cotzias, G.C.; Borg, D.C.; and Selleck, B. (1961). Specificity of zinc pathway in the rabbit: zinc-cadmium exchange. *Amer. J. Physiol.* 201:63–66.

Cotzias, G.C.; Borg, D.C.; and Selleck, B. (1961a). Virtual absence of turnover in cadmium metabolism: Cd^{109} studies in the mouse. *Amer. J. Physiol.* 201:927–930.

Druyan, R. and Vallee, B. (1962). Exchangeability of the zinc atoms in liver alcohol dehydrogenase. *Fed. Proc.* 21:247 (Abst.).

Elcoate, P.V.; Fischer, M.I.; Mawson, C.A.; and Millar, M.J. (1955). The effect of zinc deficiency on the male genital system. *J. Physiol.* 129:53P–54P.

Eli-gazzar, R.M.; Boyle, J.; and Peltung, H.G. (1977). Effect of cadmium ingestion on cadmium and zinc profile in male and female rat liver cytosol. Annual Report, Center for the Study of the Human Environment, Univ. of Cincinnati, p. 53.

Elinder, C.G.; Khellstrom, T.; Linnman, L.; and Pershagen, G. (1978). Urinary excretion of cadmium and zinc among persons from Sweden. *Environ. Res.* 15:473–484.

Evans, G.W.; Grace, C.I.; and Hahn, C. (1974). The effect of copper and cadmium on ^{65}Zn absorption in zinc-deficient and zinc-supplemented rat. *Bioinorg. Chem.* 3:115–120.

Eybl, V.; Sykora, J.; and Mertl, F. (1973). The influence of calcium and zinc complexes of aminopolycarbonic acids upon excretion and distribution of cadmium. *Acta Biol. Med. Germanica* 30:515–525.

Ferm, V.H. and Carpenter, S. (1967). Teratogenic effect of cadmium and its inhibition by zinc. *Nature* 216:1123.

Ferm, V.H. and Carpenter, S. (1968). The relationship of cadmium and zinc in experimental mammalian teratogenesis. *Lab. Invest.* 18(4):429–432.

Folk, J.E.; Wolff, E.C.; and Schirmer, C.W. (1962). The kinetics of carboxypeptidase B activity: II. Kinetic parameters of the cobalt and cadmium enzymes. *J. Biol. Chem.* 237:3100–3104.

Gale, T.F. (1973). The interaction of mercury with cadmium and zinc in mammalian embryonic development. *Environ. Res.* 6:95–105.

Gunn, S.A.; Gould, T.C.; and Anderson, W.A. (1961). Zinc protection against cadmium injury to rat testis. *Arch. Pathol.* 71:274–281.

Gunn, S.A.; Gould, T.C.; and Anderson, W.A.D. (1962). Interference with fecal excretion of Zn^{65} by cadmium. *Proc. Soc. Exp. Biol. Med.* 111:559–562.

Gunn, S.A.; Gould, T.C.; and Anderson, W.A.D. (1963). The selective injurious response of testicular and epididymal blood vessels to cadmium and its prevention by zinc. *Amer. J. Pathol.* 42:685–702.

Gunn, S.A.; Gould, T.C.; and Anderson, W.A.D. (1963a). Cadmium-induced interstitial cell tumors in rats and mice and their prevention by zinc. *J. Natl. Cancer Instit.* **31**(4):745–753.

Gunn, S.A.; Gould, T.C.; and Anderson, W.A.D. (1968). Mechanisms of zinc, cysteine, and selenium protection against cadmium-induced vascular injury to mouse testis. *J. Reprod. Fert.* **15**:65–70.

Gunn, S.A.; Gould, T.C.; and Anderson, W.A.D. (1968a). Selectivity of organ response to cadmium injury and various protective measures. *J. Path. and Bact.* **96**:89–96.

Gunn, S.A.; Gould, T.C.; and Anderson, W.A.D. (1968b). Specificity in protection against lethality and testicular toxicity from cadmium. *Proc. Soc. Exp. Biol. Med.* **128**:591–595.

Hahn, C.J. and Evans, G.W. (1975). Absorption of trace metals in the zinc deficient rat. *Amer. J. Physiol.* **228**(4):1020–1023.

Halsted, J.A.; Ronaghy, H.A.; Abadi, P.; Haghshenass, M.; Amirhakemi, G.H.; Barakat, R.M.; and Reinhold, J.G. (1972). Zinc deficiency in man: the Shiraz experiment. *Am. J. Med.* **53**:277–284.

Hambidge, K.M. (1977). The role of zinc and other trace metals in pediatric nutrition and health. *Pediat. Clin. N. Amer.* **24**:95.

Hambidge, K.M.; Hambidge, C.; Jacobs, M.; and Baum, J.D. (1972). Low levels of zinc in hair, anorexia, poor growth and hypogenersia in children. *Pediatr. Res.* **6**:868–874.

Hambidge, K.M.; Walravens, P.A.; Brown, R.M.; Webster, J.; White, S.; Anthony, M.; and Roth, M.L. (1976). Zinc nutrition of preschool children. *Am. J. Clin. Nutr.* **29**:734–738.

Hill, C.H.; Matrone, G.; Payne, W.L.; and Barber, C.W. (1963). *In vivo* interactions of cadmium with copper, zinc, and iron. *J. Nutr.* **80**:227–235.

Jacobs, R.M.; Fox, M.R.S.; Lee, A.O.; Harland, B.F.; and Fry, B.E., Jr. (1974). Increased duodenal and decreased hepatic and renal cadmium in Japanese quail fed supplements of zinc, manganese and copper. *Fed. Proc.* **33**:668.

Jacobs, R.M.; Jones, A.O.L.; Fry, B.E., Jr.; and Spivey-Fox, M.R. (1978). Decreased long-term retention of [115m]Cd in Japanese quail produced by a combined supplement of zinc, copper, and manganese. *J. Nutr.* **108**:901–910.

Jacobs, R.M.; Jones, A.O.L.; Spivey-Fox, M.R.; and Fry, B.E., Jr. (1978a). Retention of dietary cadmium and the ameliorative effect of zinc, copper, and manganese in Japanese quail. *J. Nutr.* **108**:22–32.

Jacobs, R.M.; Spivey-Fox, M.R.; and Aldridge, M.H. (1969). Changes in plasma proteins associated with the anemia produced by dietary cadmium in Japanese quail. *J. Nutr.* **99**:119–126.

Kar, A.B.; Das, R.P.; and Mukerji, F.N.I. (1960). Prevention of cadmium induced changes in the gonads of rat by zinc and selenium—a study in antagonism between metals in the biological system. *Proc. Natl. Instit. Sci. India* B 126, Suppl. 40.

Lal, J.B. (1976). The effect of low and high levels of dietary zinc on pathology in rats exposed to cadmium. Ph.D. dissertation, Univ. of Cinn., Cincinnati, OH.

Leber, A.P. and Miya, T.S. (1976). A mechanism for cadmium and zinc-induced tolerance to cadmium toxicity: involvement of metallothionein. *Toxicol. Appl. Pharmacol.* **37**:403–414.

Mason, K.E.; Young, J.O.; and Brown, J.E. (1964). Effectiveness of selenium and zinc in protecting against cadmium-induced injury of the rat testis. *Anat. Record* **148**:309.

A. Inorganic Substances 183

Mawson, C.A. and Fischer, M.I. (1951). Zinc content of the genital organs of the rat. *Nature* **167**:859.

Mills, C.F. and Dalgarno, A.C. (1972). Copper and zinc status of ewes and lambs receiving increased dietary concentrations of cadmium. *Nature* **239**:171–173.

Nordberg, M. (1978). Studies on metallothionein and cadmium. *Environ. Res.* **15**:381–404.

Oh, S.H.; Deagen, J.T.; Whanger, P.D.; and Weswig, P.H. (1978). Biological function of metallothionein. IV. Biosynthesis and degradation of liver and kidney metallothionein in rats fed diets containing zinc or cadmium. *Bioinorg. Chem.* **8**:245–254.

Ohanian, E.V.; Schaechtelin, G.; Brown, F.C.; and Iwai, J. (1977). Acute effects of intraarterial injections of cadmium, mercury and zinc on blood pressure and cardiovascular reactivity in Dahl rats. *Trace Substances in Environ. Health* **11**:272–279.

Parizek, J. (1957). The destructive effect of cadmium ion on testicular tissue and its prevention by zinc. *J. Endocrinol.* **15**:56–63.

Parizek, J. (1976). Interrelationships among trace elements. In: *Effects and dose-response relationships of toxic metals.* Edited by G.F. Nordberg. Elsevier Scientific Publishing Co., Amsterdam.

Parizek, J. and Zahoe, Z. (1956). Effect of cadmium salts on testicular tissue. *Nature* **177**:1036–1037.

Parzyck, D.C.; Shaw, S.M.; Kessler, W.V.; Vetter, R.J.; Van Sickle, D.C.; and Mayes, R.A. (1978). Fetal effects of cadmium in pregnant rats on normal and zinc deficient diets. *Bull. Environ. Contam. Toxicol.* **19**:206–214.

Petering, H.G. (1978). Some observations on the interaction of zinc, copper, and iron metabolism in lead and cadmium toxicity. *Environ. Health Perspect.* **25**:141–145.

Petering, H.G.; Johnson, M.A.; and Stemmer, K.L. (1969). Effect of cadmium on dose-response relationships of zinc in rats. *Fed. Proc.* **28**:691.

Petering, H.G.; Johnson, M.A.; and Stemmer, K.L. (1971). Studies of zinc metabolism in the rat. I. Dose-response effects of cadmium. *Arch. Environ. Health* **23**:93–101.

Powell, G.W.; Miller, W.J.; Morton, J.D.; and Clifton, C.M. (1964). Influence of dietary cadmium level and supplemental zinc on cadmium toxicity in the bovine. *J. Nutr.* **84**:205–214.

Prasad, A.S. (1966). Metabolism of zinc and its deficiency in human subjects. In: *Zinc Metabolism,* p. 250. Edited by A.S. Prasad. Charles C. Thomas, Springfield, IL.

Roberts, K.R.; Miller, W.J.; Stake, P.E.; Gentry, R.P.; and Neathery, M.W. (1973). High dietary cadmium on zinc absorption and metabolism in calves fed for comparable nitrogen balances. *Proc. Soc. Exp. Biol. Med.* **144**:906–908.

Rohrer, S.R.; Shaw, S.M.; Born, G.S.; and Vetter, R.J. (1978). The maternal distribution and placental transfer of cadmium in zinc deficient rats. *Bull. Environ. Contam. Toxicol.* **19**:556–563.

Sahagran, B.M.; Harding-Barlow, I.; and Perry, H.M., Jr. (1966). Uptakes of zinc, manganese, cadmium and mercury by intact strips of rat intestine. *J. Nutr.* **90**:259–267.

Sandstead, H.H.; Prasad, A.S.; Schulert, A.R.; Farid, Z.; Miale, A.; Bassilly, S.; and Darby, W.J. (1967). Human zinc deficiency, endocrine manifestations and responses to treatment. *Am. J. Clin. Nutr.* **20**:422–442.

Schroeder, H.A. (1967). Cadmium, chromium, and cardiovascular disease. *Circulation* **35**:570–582.

Schroeder, H.A. and Buckman, J. (1967). Cadmium hypertension. Its reversal in rats by a zinc chelate. *Arch. Environ. Health* **14**:693–697.

Schwartze, E.W. and Alsberg, C.L. (1923). Studies on the pharmacology of cadmium and zinc with particular reference to emesis. *J. Pharmacol.* **21**:1–22.

Shank, K.E. and Vetter, R.J. (1974). The effects of copper, mercury, and zinc on the uptake and distribution of cadmium 115m in the albino rat. *Environ. Letters* **6**(1):13–18.

Shank, K.E.; Vetter, R.J.; and Ziemer, P.C. (1974). Zinc-cadmium interrelationships and the kinetics of cadmium transport in a biological system. *Trace Sub. Environ. Health* **8**:395–402.

Stonard, M.D. and Webb, M. (1976). Influence of dietary cadmium on the distribution of the essential metals copper, zinc, and iron in tissues of the rat. *Chem. Biol. Interact.* **15**:349–363.

Stowe, H.D. (1976). Biliary excretion of cadmium by rats: effects of zinc, cadmium, and selenium pretreatments. *J. Toxicol. Environ. Health* **2**:45–53.

Supplee, W.C. (1961). Production of zinc deficiency in turkey poults by dietary cadmium. *Poult. Sci.* **40**:827–828.

Supplee, W.C. (1963). Antagonistic relationship between dietary cadmium and zinc. *Science* **139**:119–120.

Thind, G.S. and Biery, D.N. (1974). Antagonism of renal angiographic effects of cadmium by zinc. *Investigative Radiology* **9**(5):386–395.

Webb, M. (1971). Protection of zinc ions against the toxicity of cadmium ions. *Biochem. J.* **124**:17P–18P.

Webb, M. (1972). Protection by zinc against cadmium toxicity. *Biochem. Pharmacol.* **21**:2767–2771.

Webb, M. (1972a). Binding of cadmium ions by rat liver and kidney. *Biochem. Pharmacol.* **21**:2751–2765.

Webb, M. (1972b). Biochemical effects of Cd^{2+} injury in the rat and mouse testis. *J. Reproduct. Fert.* **30**:83–98.

Webb, M. and Verschoyle, R.D. (1976). An investigation of the role of metallothioneins in protection against the acute toxicity of the cadmium ion. *Biochem. Pharmacol.* **25**:673–679.

Winge, D.R.; Premakumar, R.; and Rajagopalan, K.V. (1978). Studies on the zinc content of Cd-induced thionein. *Arch. Biochem. Biophys.* **188**:466–475.

2. Copper

Toxicity resulting from chronic exposure to copper in the ambient air and drinking water is not thought to represent a serious environmental concern. In fact, in 1975, when the US EPA issued proposed primary drinking-water standards designed to protect human health, copper was not even included. Copper was actually given a secondary standard that is a nonenforceable limit concerned with aesthetic/taste considerations and not health issues.

Despite this low concern for the human health implications of ambient copper exposures, chronic copper poisoning of farm animals, particularly sheep, is widely recognized (Todd, 1969), resulting from the use of copper-containing fungicides as well as under natural grazing conditions via the influence of as yet poorly defined contributory nutritional factors.

Chronic copper poisoning is thought to be a two-phase process that includes (1) a passive accumulation of copper in the liver, followed by the (2) sudden release of the stored copper resulting in a hemolytic crisis (Bremmer, 1974). Presumably, the copper causes red cell lysis via the marked oxidation of glutathione, a tripeptide found in high concentrations in the cell membrane (Metz and Sagone, 1972).

It has been shown that copper-induced lipid peroxidation of membranes could be prevented by chelating agents and by Zn (Chvapil et al. 1972, 1972a). Furthermore, dietary zinc supplementation in lambs reared on high copper feeds prevented the expected copper-induced increase in serum aspartate amino transferase activity on starvation of the animals (Mills, 1974). Bremmer (1974) concluded that "zinc might provide some protection *in vivo* against liver degeneration and against the possible onset of the hemolytic crisis."

Other studies have revealed that zinc may prevent copper toxicity by reducing the absorption of copper in the rat (Van Campen and Scaiffe, 1967), as well as by effecting a redistribution of liver copper such that greater portions become bound to metallothionein.

These findings have been supported by a more recent report by Bremmer et al. (1976), which demonstrated that zinc supplementation within the diet (up to 220 mg/kg) provided striking protection against the development of copper-induced toxicity in sheep. These results led the authors to state that it is tempting to increase the level of zinc in the diet of sheep in order to prevent copper toxicosis. However, they indicated that elevated levels of zinc themselves (420 mg/kg) may cause a mild anemia in sheep and that pregnancy may further increase the susceptibility to zinc toxicosis. Therefore, it was concluded that their impressive findings of a zinc protection against copper toxicosis should be considered in view of the possible adverse effects of excess zinc supplementation.

References

Bremmer, I. (1974). Heavy metal toxicities. *Quart. Rev. Biophys.* 7(1):75–124.

Bremmer, I. and Marshall, R.B. (1974). Hepatic copper- and zinc-binding proteins in ruminants. 2. Relationship between Cu and Zn concentrations and the occurrence of a metallothionein-like fraction. *Brit. J. Nutr.* 32:293–300.

Bremmer, I.; Young, B.W.; and Mills, C.F. (1976). Protective effect of zinc supplementation against copper toxicosis in sheep. *Brit. J. Nutr.* **36**:551–561.

Chvapil, M.; Ryan, J.N.; and Zukoski, C.F. (1972). Effect of zinc on lipid peroxidation in liver microsomes and mitochondria. *Proc. Soc. Exp. Biol. Med.* **141**:150–153.

Chvapil, M.; Ryan, J.N.; and Zukoski, C.F. (1972a). Effect of zinc and other metals on the stability of lysosomes. *Proc. Soc. Exp. Biol. Med.* **140**:642–646.

Metz, E.N. and Sagone, A.L. (1972). The effect of copper on the erythrocyte hexose monophosphate shunt pathway. *J. Lab. Clin. Med.* **80**:405–413.

Mills, C.F. (1974). Trace element interactions: effects of dietary composition on the development of imbalance and toxicity. Proc. 2nd Inst. Symp. Trace Element Metabolism in Animals. Madison, WI.

Todd, J.R. (1969). Chronic copper toxicity of ruminants. *Proc. Nutr. Soc.* **28**:189–198.

Van Campen, D.R. and Scaiffe, P.V. (1967). Zinc interference with copper absorption in rats. *J. Nutr.* **91**:473–476.

3. Lead

That zinc may affect the toxicity of lead was first suggested by Willoughby et al. (1972, 1972a) who reviewed several earlier studies that noted the occurrence of intoxicated horses that grazed in the vicinity of lead-zinc smelters (see Hupka, 1955; Schmitt et al., 1971; Graham et al., 1940). These investigators were concerned with whether toxic levels of either zinc or lead would antagonize or enhance the occurrence of the adverse effects of the other. Experiments with a limited number of young horses suggested that toxic levels of zinc were able to prevent the occurrence of clinical signs of lead poisoning, despite enhancing the retention of lead in the liver and kidney cortex and medulla. In direct contrast to the findings of Willoughby et al. (1972, 1972a) was a study by Hsu et al. (1975), which revealed that zinc exaggerated the effects of lead toxicity in pigs.

These initial studies, while leading the way for future investigations of potential zinc-lead interactions (Cerklewski and Forbes, 1976; Papaioannov, 1978; Dilts and Ahokas, 1979), have little conceivable relevance to the human situation with respect to the influence of dietary zinc on lead toxicity. In fact, the levels of zinc employed in these respective studies were 5400 and 4000 ppm, while those for lead were 800 and 1000 ppm, respectively. In addition to the unrealistic nature of the exposure levels, it is well known that excess zinc can induce a trace-element imbalance involving copper and iron (Cox and Harris, 1960; Magee and Matrone, 1960).

Despite the lack of the human health relevance of these earlier studies, Cerklewski and Forbes (1976) indicated that from a conceptual perspective zinc and lead should interact within biological systems. They stated that divalent zinc and lead may exhibit similar chemical characteristics since both substances can have a coordination number of four and tetrahedral configuration (Vallee and Ulmer, 1972; Matrone, 1974) and similar affinities for several amino acids (Sillen and Martell, 1971; Sharma, 1967).

In testing their hypothesis, Cerklewski and Forbes (1976) demonstrated that increasing dietary zinc from 8 to 200 ppm in lead-intoxicated rats reduced lead levels in tissues (i.e., blood, liver, kidney, and tibias), urinary excretion of δ-aminolevulinic acid, and inhibition of δ-aminolevulinic acid dehydratase activity in the kidney. The magnitude of the protective effects of zinc was such that 200 ppm of Zn in the diet reduced the signs of lead toxicity at 200 ppm Pb to be equivalent to those effects caused by 50 ppm Pb in rats with 8 ppm zinc in the diet.

The ability of zinc supplements to reduce lead toxicity was speculated to result from its interference with lead absorption because zinc did not influence urinary lead excretion and injected zinc had no influence on lead toxicity. Despite this possibility, the effect of zinc on lead absorption due to the formation of a zinc-lead complex of low solubility was considered remote because zinc absorption is not affected by lead. More likely, however, is the possibility that zinc and lead competed for similar binding sites on a metallothionein-like protein transport in the intestinal tract.

In addition to the apparent ability of zinc to reduce the gastrointestinal absorption of lead and thereby reduce its toxicity, zinc also interacts with lead systemically. More specifically, the addition of zinc to *in vitro* and *in vivo* systems may activate the enzyme δ-aminolevulinic acid dehydratase and prevent inhibition of this enzyme by lead (Finelli et al., 1975; Haeger-Aronsen et al., 1976; Thomasino et al., 1977; Border et al., 1976). Border et al. (1976) expressed the concern that where industrial exposures to both zinc and lead are appreciable that the zinc might activate the enzyme sufficiently to hide the excessive body burden of lead.

Conclusion. The limited data available suggest that low levels of zinc in the diet enhance lead toxicity, while supplemental levels of zinc reduce lead toxicity (Cerklewski and Forbes, 1976). Since their findings were so impressive, the need to confirm this report is apparent. The findings of Papaioannov (1978) that zinc combined with vitamin C reduced Pb levels in human workers may offer potential implications for industrial hygiene professionals. Finally, it is interesting that Goyer and Cherian (1979) have recently noted that ascorbic acid is a very effective chelator of lead from the central nervous system of rats, especially in combination with EDTA.

References

Abdulla, M. and Haeger-Aronsen, B. (1971). ALA-dehydratase activation by zinc. *Enzyme* **12**:708–710.

Abdulla, M. and Haeger-Aronsen, B. (1973). Antagonistic effect of zinc in relatively high concentration on inhibition of ALA-dehydratase activity by heavy metals *in vitro*. *Intern. Res. Commun. Systems* (73-8)8-14-1.

Border, E.A.; Cantrell, A.C.; and Kilroe-Smith, T.A. (1976). The *in vitro* effect of zinc on the inhibition of human δ-aminolevulinic acid dehydratase by lead. *Brit. J. Indust. Med.* **33**:85–87.

Cerklewski, F. and Forbes, R.M. (1976). Influence of dietary zinc on lead toxicity in the rat. *J. Nutr.* **106**:689–696.

Cox, D.H. and Harris, D.L. (1960). Effects of excess zinc on iron and copper in the rat. *J. Nutr.* **70**:514–520.

Dilts, P.V. and Ahokas, R.A. (1979). Effects of dietary lead and zinc on pregnancy. *Amer. Jour. Obstet. Gynecol.* **135**:940–946.

Finelli, V.N.; Klauder, D.S.; Karaffa, M.A.; and Petering, H.G. (1975). Interaction of zinc and lead on δ-aminolevulinate dehydratase. *Biochem. Biophys. Res. Commun.* **65**(1):303–311.

Goyer, R.A. and Cherian, M.G. (1979). Ascorbic acid and EDTA treatment of lead toxicity in rats. *Life Sci.* **24**:433–438.

Graham, R.; Sampson, J.; and Hester, H.R. (1940). Results of feeding zinc to pregnant mares and to mares nursing foals. *J. Amer. Vet. Med. Assoc.* **97**:41–47.

Haeger-Aronsen, B.; Schutz, A.; and Abdulla, M. (1976). Antagonistic effect *in vivo* of zinc on inhibition of δ-aminolevulinic acid dehydratase by lead. *Arch. Environ. Health* **31**:215–220.

Hsu, F.S.; Krook, L.; Pond, W.G.; and Duncan, J.R. (1975). Interactions of dietary calcium with toxic levels of lead and zinc in pigs. *J. Nutr.* **105**:112–118.

Hupka, E. (1955). *Wien. Tierärztl. Mschr.* **42**:763.

Magee, A.C. and Matrone, G. (1960). Studies on growth, copper metabolism and iron metabolism of rats fed high levels of zinc. *J. Nutr.* **72**:233–242.

Matrone, G. (1974). Chemical parameters in trace element antagonisms. In: *Trace Element Metabolism in Animals—2*, pp. 91–103. Edited by W.G. Hoekstra, J.W. Suttie, H.E. Ganther, and W. Mertz. Univ. Park Press, Baltimore.

Papaioannov, R. (1978). Blood lead levels, zinc, and vitamin C. *J. Ortho. Molec. Psychiat.* **7**:94.

Schmitt, N.; Brown, G.; Devlin, E.L.; Larsen, A.A.; McCarsland, E.D.; and Saville, J.M. (1971). Lead poisoning in horses. *Arch. Environ. Health* **23**:185–195.

Sharma, V.S. (1967). The stability constants of metal ion complexes of serine and threonine. *Biochem. Biophys. Acta* **148**:37–41.

Sillen, L.G. and Martell, A.E. (1971). Stability instants of metal ion complexes. *Chem. Soc. Special Publication* #25, London.

Thomasino, J.A.; Zuroweste, E.; Brooks, S.M.; Petering, H.G.; Lerner, S.I.; and Finelli, V.N. (1977). Lead, zinc, and erythrocyte δ-aminolevulinic acid dehydratase: relationships in lead toxicity. *Arch. Environ. Health* **32**:244–247.

Vallee, B.I. and Ulmer, D.D. (1972). Biochemical effects of mercury, cadmium, and lead. *Ann. Rev. Biochem.* **41**:91–128.

Willoughby, R.A.; MacDonald, E.; McSherry, B.J.; and Brown, G. (1972). The interaction of toxic amounts of lead and zinc to young growing horses. *The Vet. Record* **91**:382–383.

Willoughby, R.A.; MacDonald, E.; McSherry, B.J.; and Brown, G. (1972a). Lead poisoning and the interaction between lead and zinc poisoning in the fowl. *Canad. J. Comp. Med.* **36**:348–359.

4. Mercury

Very little research has concerned any possible interactions of zinc with mercury. That zinc may affect mercury toxicity was inferred by analogy to the protective influence of zinc toward a variety of adverse effects caused by Cd. It was speculated by Yamane et al. (1976) that since zinc appears to reduce Cd toxicity via the synthesis of metallothionein, it may also similarly diminish the toxicity of mercury.

In evaluating this hypothesis, Yamane et al. (1976) administered subcutaneous injections of $HgCl_2$ (0.018 mM/kg/day) and oral doses of zinc acetate (30 mM/kg/day) simultaneously every day for 5 days in male Wistar rats. They reported that 9 of 10 rats given $HgCl_2$ alone died within 3 days, while 100% (10 of 10) died by the 4th day. In marked contrast, the conjoint treatment of mercury and zinc resulted in 0.0% (0 of 10) mortality by the 5th day. The unexposed zinc control also did not experience any mortality. In light of these findings, it appeared that zinc administration markedly reduced the toxicity of inorganic mercury.

Follow-up studies attempted to ascertain the mechanism by which zinc prevented mercury toxicity. Biochemical studies revealed that zinc treatment (but not mercury) resulted in a marked increase in the synthesis of metallothionein. This observation led the authors to "suggest that the biosynthesis of metallothionein by zinc is responsible for the suppressive effect of zinc on the toxicity of mercury."

In contract to this highly significant interaction of zinc with $HgCl_2$, Johnson and Pond (1974) were not able to discern any comparable protective action of dietary zinc to both dietary inorganic ($HgCl_2$) and organic (methyl and phenyl) mercury compounds in male weanling Sprague-Dawley rats after 4 weeks of the experiment.

The obvious discrepancy in the findings of these two studies certainly needs to be resolved. There were many differences in the experimental protocols of the two studies that may account for the differences in response. However, in light of the impressive protective function of zinc as shown by Yamane et al. (1976), further study of this interaction is necessary.

References

Johnson, S.L. and Pond, W.G. (1974). Inorganic vs organic Hg toxicity in growing rats: protection by dietary Se but not Zn. *Nutr. Rept. Intern.* **9**(2):135–147.

Yamane, Y.; Fukino, H.; and Imagawa, M. (1976). Suppressive effect of zinc on the toxicity of mercury. *Chem. Pharm. Bull.* **24**(4):836–837.

5. Ozone and Nitrogen Dioxide

Particular attention has been given to the capability of dietary antioxidants to reduce and/or prevent tissue and cellular damage caused by environmental oxidants such as O_3 and NO_2. In fact, Chapter 5 of *Nutrition and Environmental Health, Volume I, The Vitamins* devoted 20 pages to elucidating the interaction between vitamin E and O_3 and NO_2 on lung tissue and red blood cells. Since these environmental oxidants are known to proceed in part through lipid peroxidation of cellular membranes, Chvapil et al. (1972, 1973, 1974) have speculated that zinc nutritional status may modify oxidant toxicity because zinc has a stabilizing function with respect to cellular membranes. In fact, CCl_4-induced lipid peroxidation in the rat liver was markedly decreased via zinc pretreatments during *in vitro* and *in vivo* rat studies.

Subsequent experimentation evaluated the hypothesis that dietary levels of zinc affect NO_2 and O_3 toxicity. With regard to NO_2, Chvapil et al. (1974) demonstrated that pretreatment of female mice with a low dose of zinc [3 μM/kg body wt. by gavage for 3 days before NO_2 exposure (30 min at 35 ppm)] prevented the occurrence of NO_2-induced lung edema. However, in marked contrast, zinc supplementation did not offer protection of rats to acute ozone exposure (10 ppm) (Kang and Harnish, 1979).

Why zinc supplementation offered protection from NO_2-induced lung damage, but not from O_3-induced lethality, is unknown; Kang and Harnish (1979) have suggested that since zinc supplements resulted in higher zinc levels in the blood and liver but not the lungs, the lungs did not receive the "benefit" of the supplementation. Furthermore, since the lungs are the most critical tissue in acute O_3 toxicity, the results are not unexpected. However, their explanation ignored the protective effects of zinc with acute NO_2 toxicity—an acute toxicity also primarily of lung tissue. Clearly further research is needed to establish to what extent dietary zinc affects NO_2 toxicity.

References

Chvapil, M.; Ryan, J.N.; Elias, S.L.; and Peng, Y.H. (1973). Protective effect of zinc on CCl_4-induced liver injury in rats. *Exp. Mol. Pathol.* **19**:186.

Chvapil, M.; Ryan, J.N.; and Zukoski, C.F. (1972). Effect of zinc on lipid peroxidation in liver microsomes and mitochondria. *Proc. Soc. Exp. Biol. Med.* **141**:150–153.

Chvapil, M. and Zukoski, C.F. (1974). New concept on the mechanism(s) of the biological effect of zinc. In: *Clinical Application of Zinc Metabolism,* W.J. Pories, W. Strain, J. Hsu, and R. Woosley, (eds.) Charles C Thomas, Springfield, Il.

Kang, H.K. and Harnish, R.A. (1979). Zinc nutritional status and response to lethal level of ozone exposure in rats. *Bull. Environ. Contam. Toxicol.* **21**:206–212.

B. ORGANIC SUBSTANCES

1. Carbon Tetrachloride

There are numerous toxic agents in the industrial and community environments that cause oxidative damage to cellular membranes including ozone, nitrogen dioxide, and carbon tetrachloride (CCl_4). Lipid peroxidation of biomembranes produced by these environmental oxidants may be reduced in the presence of reducing agents such as cysteine and vitamin E as well as a variety of free radical scavengers.

Among those agents that are capable of reducing lipid peroxidation is the mineral zinc. Chvapil et al. (1972, 1973) have shown that the peroral administration of zinc to intact rats markedly diminished injected CCl_4-induced liver damage as reflected in part by the reduced level of lipid peroxides formed in liver microsomes, as well as enhancing the stability of lysosomes. In addition, the zinc administration reduced endogenous peroxidation resulting from normal metabolism without any exogenous source of oxidant stress. Previous studies by Saldeen (1969) are in fundamental agreement with the work of Chvapil et al. (1972, 1973).

The mechanism by which zinc may offer protection against oxidative stress is uncertain. Chvapil et al. (1972, 1973) have speculated that zinc may stabilize the lysosomal membranes, thereby preventing the rupture of such organelles and the release of oxidative enzymes within the cell. Based on these findings, Chvapil et al. speculated that the dietary status of zinc may affect the toxicity of other environmental oxidants including NO_2. Such experimentation with NO_2 is discussed in the previous section.

References

Chvapil, M.; Elias, S.L.; Ryan, J.N.; and Zukoski, C.F. (1973). Considerations on the biological effects of zinc. In *International Review of Neurobiology*, C.C. Pfeifer, ed., Academic Press, New York, Suppl. 1, pp. 115–173.

Chvapil, M.; Ryan, J.N.; and Zukoski, C.F. (1972). The effect of zinc and other metals on the stability of lysosomes. *Proc. Soc. Exp. Bio. Med.* **140**:642–646.

Chvapil, M.; Ryan, J.N.; and Zukoski, C.F. (1972a). Effect of zinc on lipid peroxidation in liver microsomes and mitochondria. *Proc. Soc. Exp. Biol. Med.* **141**:150–153.

Chvapil, M.; Ryan, J.N.; and Zukoski, C.F. (1974). New concept on the mechanism(s) of the biological effect of zinc. In *Clinical Applications of Zinc Metabolism,* W.J. Pories, W. Strain, J. Hsu, and R. Woosley, eds., Charles C Thomas, Springfield, Il., p. 187.

Saldeen, T. (1969). On the protective action of zinc against experimental liver damage due to choline free diet of CCl_4. *Z. Ges. Exp. Med.* **150**:251–259.

2. DDT

In 1972 Feaster et al. speculated that inadequate consumption of zinc may enhance the toxicity of DDT. This hypothesis was based on earlier observations that a zinc deficiency adversely affects growth and reproduction while a zinc excess also reduces growth, causes reproductive failure, and hypochromic anemia. Since both chlorinated hydrocarbon and organophosphate insecticides also adversely affect reproductive success, it was felt that evaluation of a zinc-pesticide interaction might be worthwhile.

In their study, female rats were given diets with low levels of DDT, parathion, or carbaryl for 4 months. These rats were permitted to become pregnant and to be exposed to either moderately low (8-10 ppm) or very high levels (4000 ppm) of zinc in the diet. The only pesticide and dietary treatment having any effect of note was the DDT-4000-ppm zinc group. The high-zinc diet resulted in an increase of DDT in maternal and fetal livers as compared to other comparison groups. In addition, hemoglobin levels in both maternal and fetal blood were not affected either by DDT or high-zinc treatments alone; however, they were diminished when DDT was fed with the high-zinc diets.

Reference

Feaster, J.P.; Van Middelem, C.H.; and Davis, G.K. (1972). Zinc-DDT interrelationships in growth and reproduction in the rat. *J. Nutr.* **102**:523–528.

3. Ethanol

Alcohol intoxication and alcoholism represent one of the most serious public health problems in the United States. Efforts to gain a greater understanding of alcohol abuse have attempted to deal with the many-faceted aspects of this problem including the social, legal, and psychological, as well as the physiological. One emerging area of physiological research concerns the influence of dietary status on ethanol intoxication. While considerable research has dealt with the interactions of B-vitamins with ethanol, it is also becoming recognized that dietary zinc levels may also influence the capacity of the body to detoxify ethanol. The subject of this section will be to evaluate the literature concerning any zinc-ethanol interrelationship, as well as indicate the potential biomedical relevance of these data.

That zinc levels in the diet may affect ethanol metabolism may be inferred by its presence as a metal component of alcohol dehydrogenase. Several studies, in fact, have demonstrated that hepatic alcohol dehydrogenase activity is reduced to about 60% of normal in zinc-deficient rats (Reinhold et al., 1970; Prasad et al., 1977). These findings suggest that low levels of dietary zinc may reduce the rate of ethanol degradation, thereby enhancing its (i.e., ethanol's) capacity for intoxification. Consistent with this hypothesis is the observation of abnormal zinc metabolism in patients with alcoholic cirrhosis so that those affected persons exhibited low serum zinc, diminished hepatic zinc, and hyperzincuria (Vallee et al., 1956, 1957). Several studies with animal models have also supported the idea that low body stores of zinc are associated with ethanol toxicity (Barak et al., 1967; Kahn and Ozeran, 1967; Kahn et al., 1968; Wang and Pierson, 1975).

In light of the above research, several groups of investigators have proposed that supplemental zinc may enhance ethanol metabolism by increasing hepatic activity of alcohol dehydrogenase and thus reduce ethanol toxicity (Yunice and Lindeman, 1977; Jamall et al., 1979). Results of their investigations indicated that zinc supplementation was able to reduce ethanol-induced acute toxicity in mice and rats. For example, mice given a 1 mM injection of Zn^{2+} one hour before 4.1 mM of ethanol were markedly protected from ethanol-induced mortality as measured 24 hours after ethanol exposure. The zinc-treated mice experienced a 23% mortality incidence (7 of 30 mice died), while the group of mice given only the ethanol treatment experienced an 86% mortality incidence (30 of 35 mice died). In addition, protection with zinc was enhanced when combined with l-lysine. Measurements of blood-ethanol levels in the zinc-lysine group were statistically significantly lower than controls at 0.5 and 1.0 hour after treatment (Jamall et al., 1979). Those on the zinc treatment alone (i.e., without the l-lysine) did not show a decrease in blood-ethanol levels until 2 hours after treatment. However, Yunice and Lindeman (1977) reported that blood-ethanol levels were significantly reduced 1 hour after ethanol treatment in animals pretreated with zinc.

These findings are certainly quite striking and require further extension with respect to the development of dose-response relationships and to the need to evaluate the potential of zinc to prevent chronic ethanol toxicity. Simultaneously, research should attempt to identify more precisely the mechanism(s) involved in the zinc protection and the nature of the zinc-l-lysine interaction.

References

Barak, A.J.; Harriet, C.B.; and Felix, J.K. (1967). Zinc and manganese levels in serum and liver after alcohol feeding and development of cirrhosis in rats. *Gut* 8:454.

Huber, A.M. and Gershoff, S.M. (1975). Effects of zinc deficiency on the oxidation of retinol and ethanol in rats. *J. Nutr.* 105:1486–1490.

Jamall, I.S.; Mignamo, J.E.; Lynch, V.D.; Bidanset, J.H.; Lau-Cam, C.; and Greening, M. (1979). Protective effects of zinc sulfate and L-lysine on acute ethanol toxicity in mice. *Environ. Res.* 19:112–120.

Kahn, A.M. and Ozeran, R.S. (1967). Liver and serum abnormalities in rats with cirrhosis. *Gastroenterology* 53(2):193.

Kahn, A.M.; Rizer, J.G.; Thomas, P.B.; and Gordon, H.E. (1968). Metabolism of zinc-65 in cirrhosis. *Surgery* 63(4):678.

Prasad, A.S.; Overleas, D.; Wolf, P.; and Horwitz, J.P. (1977). Studies on zinc deficiency: changes in trace elements and enzyme activities in tissues of zinc-deficient rats. *J. Clin. Invest.* 46(4):549.

Reinhold, J.G.; Pascoe, E.; Arscanian, M.; and Bitar, K. (1970). Relation of zinc metalloenzyme activities to zinc concentration in tissues. *Biochem. Biophys.* 215:430.

Vallee, B.L.; Wacker, W.E.C.; Batholomy, A.F.; and Hoch, F.L. (1957). Zinc metabolism in hepatic dysfunction: II. Correlation of metabolic patterns with biochemical findings. *New Engl. J. Med.* 257:1055–1065.

Vallee, B.L.; Wacker, W.E.C.; Bartholomy, A.F.; and Robin, E.D. (1956). Zinc metabolism in hepatic dysfunction: I. Serum zinc concentrations in Laennec's cirrhosis and their validation by sequential analysis. *New Engl. J. Med.* 255:403–408.

Wang, J. and Pierson, R.N. (1975). Distribution of zinc in skeletal muscle and liver tissue in normal and dietary controlled alcoholic rats. *J. Clin. Lab. Med.* **85**(1):50–58.

Yunice, A.A. and Lindeman, R.D. (1977). Effect of ascorbic acid and zinc sulfate on ethanol toxicity and metabolism. *Proc. Soc. Exp. Biol. Med.* **154**:146–150.

4. DMBA

Oral administration of zinc compounds (e.g., zinc sulfate) has been found to enhance the healing of wounds in young, healthy humans (Pories et al., 1967). Although the mechanism of how zinc enhances healing remains to be further assessed, Savlov et al. (1962) reported that zinc tends to accumulate in the healing tissues, achieving peak levels on the third day after insult. Based on these observations Poswillo and Cohen (1971) evaluated whether zinc supplementation to the drinking water (100 ppm) could affect susceptibility to DMBA-induced cancer. In pilot studies they reported that 13 of 15 Syrian golden hamsters given the control diet plus DMBA application (to the right cheek pouch in liquid paraffin three times weekly for 4 weeks) developed tumors by the ninth week after initiation. In contrast, only 1 of 9 animals given identical treatment plus 100 ppm zinc in the drinking water developed a tumor, and this appeared only after 25 weeks. As a result of these limited but striking findings, further research is necessary to evaluate more fully the hypothesis that zinc supplementation diminishes the occurrence of DMBA-induced cancer.

References

Pories, W.D.; Henzel, J.H.; Rob, C.E.; and Strain, W.H. (1967). *Lancet.* **1**:121.

Poswillo, D.E. and Cohen, B. (1971). Inhibition of carcinogenesis by dietary zinc. *Nature* **231**:447–448.

Savlov, E.D.; Strain, W.H.; and Huegin, F. (1962). *J. Surg. Res.* **2**:209.

5. Fungicide: Ethylenebisdithiocarbamate

Ethylenethiourea (ETU) is an animal teratogen and is thought to pose a possible risk to the public health because the fungicide ethylenebisdithiocarbamate can be transformed to residues of ETU in food (Khera, 1973; Khera and Shah, 1979). That nutritional status may affect the teratogenic potential of such fungicidal compounds was first illustrated by Larsson et al. (1976), who noted that the teratogenicity of manganese ethylenebisdithiocarbamate (Maneb) in the rat was diminished when zinc acetate and Maneb were simultaneously given by the oral route. It was speculated that the diminution of adverse effects caused by the zinc treatment resulted from an "interference with the gastrointestinal absorption of Maneb or an inhibition of the metabolic conversion of Maneb to ETU." However, follow-up studies by Khera and Shah (1979) were unable to demonstrate that zinc acetate was capable of preventing ETU induced fetal anomalies in rats thereby implying that zinc treatment affects the formation of ETU from Maneb but not the teratogenic effects of preformed ETU.

References

Khera, K.S. (1973). Ethylenethiourea: teratogenicity study in rats and rabbits. *Teratology* 7:243–252.

Khera, K.S. and Shah, B.G. (1979). Failure of zinc acetate to reduce ethylenethiourea-induced fetal anomalies in rats. *Toxicol. Appl. Pharm.* **48**:229–235.

Larsson, K.S.; Arnander, C.; Cekanova, E.; and Kjellberg, M. (1976). Studies of teratogenic effects of the dithiocarbamates Maneb, mancozeb and propineb. *Teratology* 14:171–184.

6. Microsomal Enzyme Detoxification

Very little research has been directed toward the influence of zinc dietary status on the function of the mixed-function oxidase (MFO) system. A review article by Campbell and Hayes (1974) has succinctly capsulized the relationship of dietary zinc to enzymatic detoxification via the liver microsomal enzymes.

Becking and Morrison (1970) have reported that a zinc deficiency can result in changes in the activity of certain microsomal MFO enzymes in rats, but only following a prolonged feeding. For instance, the metabolism of pentobarbital, aminopyrine, and p-nitrobenzoic acid was significantly decreased only after 37, 44, and 58 days, respectively. In contrast, even by the 58th day, no changes in the metabolism of aniline and zoxazolamine were noted as a result of the deficient diet.

While these changes in metabolism are quite modest, it would appear that further investigations of zinc dietary status on xenobiotic metabolism should be pursued. This could involve a wider range of xenobiotics and also the evaluation of the influence of a chronic marginal deficiency as well as a modest excess of zinc.

References

Becking, G.C. and Morrison, A.B. (1970). Hepatic drug metabolism in zinc-deficient rats. *Biochem. Pharm.* **19**:895–902.

Campbell, T.C. and Hayes, J.R. (1974). Role of nutrition in the drug-metabolizing enzyme system. *Pharmacol. Rev.* **26**:171–197.

7. Nitrosamines

Evidence that dietary zinc may influence the growth of tumors was first recognized in 1970, when a deficiency of this nutrient prevented the growth of Walker 256 carcinosarcoma in rats (McQuitty et al., 1970; DeWys et al., 1970). This finding was extended by DeWys and Pories (1972) and Pories et al. (1978) who reported that the tumor-inhibitory influence of zinc deficiency was of a more general nature; that is, the presence of a zinc deficiency was also able to inhibit the development of a spectrum of animal tumors, including Lewis lung carcinoma in mice and several ascites tumors in mice and rats. According to Pories et al. (1978), the inhibition of tumor growth may be caused by a deprivation of an essential nutrient. They cited several studies that indicated that several tumors [Walker 256 sarcomas in rats (Pories et al., 1978), prostatic tumors in rats (Hirayama, 1964), and breast tumors (Schwartz et al., 1974)] preferentially retain zinc, thereby inferring that a zinc deficiency may inhibit tumor growth.

While the findings of DeWys and his colleagues have clearly revealed that a dietary deficiency of zinc may inhibit the growth of a variety of tumors, a number of researchers have reported that a dietary deficiency of zinc enhances the occurrence of methylbenzylnitrosamine (MBN) (Fong et al., 1977, 1978) and MBN-and-alcohol-induced esophageal cancer (Gabrial and Newberne, 1979) in rats. The findings of Fong et al. (1978) also revealed that the zinc deficiency not only enhanced the incidence of esophageal cancer (Table 2), but also appeared to reduce markedly the latency period of tumor occurrence as compared to other published studies (Schmahl, 1976). A zinc-deficient diet also enhanced the occurrence of MBN-induced cancer over a broad range of MBN exposures, with the most striking differential incidence being at the lower levels of exposure.

These findings, which indicate that low levels of dietary zinc enhance MBN and alcohol-induced esophageal cancer, are consistent with epidemiological studies (Lin et al., 1977) showing that

Table 2. Incidence of Esophageal Tumors Induced by Low Doses of MBN in Male Charles River CD® Rats Fed Control and Zinc-Deficient Diets

Group	Diet	MBN[a] (mg/kg body wt)	Time to Killing from First Dose (days)[b]	Tumor Incidence[c]	Number of Tumors/Esophagus				Tumor Size, 2 × 2 mm
					1	2	3	>5	
III	Control, pair-fed	16	63	14/48 (29)	10/48	2/48	2/48	—	7/48
	Zinc-deficient, ad libitum	16	63	34/43 (79)	3/43	7/43	8/43	16/43	25/43
IV	Control, pair-fed	8	75	0/40 (0)	—	—	—	—	—
	Zinc-deficient, ad libitum	8	75	9/43 (21)	8/43	1/43	—	—	5/43

[a]Dose was 2 mg/kg body wt twice weekly.

[b]First dose was given at 7 weeks of age, 4 weeks after the rats were started on the experimental diet.

[c]Numbers in parentheses are percent incidence.

Source. Fong, L.Y.Y.; Sivak, A.; and Newberne, P.M. (1978). Zinc deficiency and methylbenzylnitrosamine-induced esophageal cancer in rats. *J. Natl. Cancer Instit.* **61**(1):145–150.

esophageal-cancer patients display lower zinc-tissue levels than do matched controls.

It is quite obvious that a dietary deficiency of zinc may enhance or inhibit the process of carcinogenesis, depending on the specific circumstances. While Pories et al. (1978) have provided a rationale for how a zinc deficiency may inhibit the growth of transplanted tumors, there has been no theoretical framework to explain how a zinc deficiency enhances MBN-plus-alcohol-induced cancer. Future studies should include an evaluation of the capacity of a zinc deficiency to alter the metabolism of precarcinogens to ultimate carcinogens. Also, there is an important need to explain more adequately the two-edged sword of zinc in the process of carcinogenesis.

References

DeWys, W. and Pories, W. (1972). Inhibition of a spectrum of animal tumors by dietary zinc deficiency. *J. Natl. Cancer Instit.* **48**:375–381.

DeWys, W.; Pories, W.; Richter, M.C.; and Strain, W.H. (1970). Inhibition of Walker 256 carcinosarcoma growth by dietary zinc deficiency. *Proc. Soc. Exp. Biol. Med.* **135**:17–22.

Duncan, J.R.; Dreosti, I.E.; and Albrecht, C.F. (1974). Zinc intake and growth of a transplanted hepatoma induced by 3-methyl-4-dimethylaminoazobenzene in rats. *J. Natl. Cancer Instit.* **53**:277.

Edward, M.B. (1976). Chemical carcinogenesis in the cheek pouch of Syrian hamsters receiving supplementary zinc. *Arch. Oral Biol.* **21**:133.

Fong, L.Y.Y.; Lin, H.J.; Chan, W.C.; and Newberne, P.M. (1977). Zinc and copper concentrations in tissues from esophageal cancer patients and animals. *Trace Substances in Environ. Health* **1**:184–192.

Fong, L.Y.Y.; Sivak, A.; and Newberne, P.M. (1978). Zinc deficiency and methylbenzylnitrosamine-induced esophageal cancer in rats. *J. Natl. Cancer Instit.* **61**(1):145–150.

Gabrial, G.N. and Newberne, P.M. (1979). Zinc deficiency, alcohol and esophageal cancer. Presented at the Trace Substances in Environ. Health Conf. Univ. of Missouri at Columbia, June.

Hirayama, M. (1964). Experimental studies of zinc metabolism in the prostatic gland. Part III. Experimental neoplasm of the prostatic gland. *Acta Urol.* (Japan) **10**:584.

Lin, H.J.; Chan, W.C.; Fong, Y.Y. et al. (1977). Zinc levels in serum, hair and tumors from patients with esophageal cancer. *Nutr. Rep. Intern.* **15**:635–643.

McQuitty, J.T., Jr.; DeWys, W.D.; Monaco, L.; et al. (1970). Inhibition of tumor growth by dietary zinc deficiency. *Cancer Res.* **30**:1387–1390.

Pories, W.J.; DeWys, W.D.; Flynn, A.; Mansour, E.G.; and Strain, W.H. (1978). Implications of the inhibition of animal tumors by dietary zinc deficiency. In: *Inorganic and Nutritional Aspects of Cancer,* pp. 243–257. Edited by G.N. Schrauzer. Plenum Press, N.Y.

Poswillo, D.E. and Cohen, B. (1971). Inhibition of carcinogenesis by dietary zinc. *Nature* **231**:447–448.

Schmahl, D. (1976). Investigations on esophageal carcinogenicity by methylphenyl nitrosamine and ethyl alcohol in rats. *Cancer Lett.* **1**:215–218.

Schwartz, A.E.; Ledicotte, G.W.; Fink, R.W.; and Friedman, E.W. (1974). Trace elements in normal and malignant human breast tissue. *Surgery* **76**:325.

C. ZINC—POLLUTANT INTERACTIONS—A PERSPECTIVE

It has been shown that low levels of zinc within the diet markedly enhance the toxicity of a number of heavy metals (e.g., cadmium, copper, lead, and mercury) and ethanol, as well as enhancing the carcinogenicity of nitrosamines. In addition, zinc supplementation seems to reduce CCl_4 and NO_2 toxicity as well as DMBA induced carcinogenicity.

Of great concern are surveys that indicate that less-than-adequate zinc intake and biochemical changes indicative of zinc deficiency occur in children from low-income groups (Owen and Lippman, 1977; Hambidge, 1977). How widespread dietary zinc deficiency may be is not well known. However, Mahaffey and Vanderveen (1979) have suggested that marginal zinc deficiency in adults may well be widespread based on dietary intake data.

Even though this chapter of zinc-pollutant interactions suggests that the large number of humans who are consuming diets inadequate in zinc are at enhanced risk to the above-mentioned pollutants, there is an almost total lack of data with human subjects. All risk assessments concerning zinc-pollutant interactions depend on findings derived from animal studies and as such have inherent limitations. The lack of human clinical and/or epidemiological findings concerning zinc-pollutant interactions is of serious concern. Epidemiologists must work with nutrition scientists in developing specific research hypotheses and study protocols in this area. Nutrient-pollutant epidemiological studies, especially those involved with carcinogenesis, present great difficulties to researchers in dealing with latency periods of 20-30 years and a past exposure to a multiplicity of carcinogenic agents. These and other difficulties can easily discourage the initiation of research in the entire broad area of nutrition and environmental cancer. Yet animal studies clearly suggest that dietary factors including zinc can profoundly affect the latency period and extent of cancer development. Therefore the challenge to initiate innovative epidemiological research approaches to evaluate the influence of zinc in modifying environmentally induced cancer in the human populations must be undertaken.

Lead. In light of the continuing problem of lead-paint poisoning in the United States, special consideration must be given to confirming and extending the singular findings of Cerklewski and Forbes (1976) that zinc supplementation markedly reduces lead toxicity.

Public health officials who are concerned with lead toxicity in children cannot overlook the importance of dietary factors in this problem. Unfortunately, children consuming diets low or inadequate in calcium, iron, and zinc are those most likely to be exposed to elevated levels of leaded paints. Preventive programs must include an elimination of the lead plus an improvement of the nutritional status. These goals are not mutually exclusive!

Ethanol. Perhaps the most well-founded of the zinc-pollutant interactions is the one with ethanol. In light of the magnitude of alcoholism within the United States and other countries, the findings that zinc supplementation can reduce alcohol toxicity are encouraging. However, biomedical findings of potential clinical significance are usually seen as only a small part of the complex picture of alcoholism.

Nitrosamines. Of recent interest has been the report of Fong et al. (1978) that a zinc deficiency enhances nitrosamine-induced esophageal cancer. Because of the widespread exposure to nitrosamines, these findings deserve attention.

Discussion. With the exception of the earlier investigations concerning a zinc-cadmium interaction, most articles studying zinc-pollutant interrelationships are less than 10 years old. The recent nature of these findings coupled with the striking protection that zinc has generally shown clearly suggest that the subsequent decades may yield major discoveries further extending the scope and biomedical relevance of zinc in modifying pollutant toxicity and carcinogenicity in animal models and humans.

Before concluding this section on zinc, it must be recognized that while zinc is an essential nutrient and is considered relatively nontoxic, its toxicity at elevated levels of exposure has been reported in sheep and cattle (Ott et al., 1966, 1966a) as well as rats (Ketcheson et al., 1969). With respect to sheep, toxicity occurred with a zinc intake of about 50 mg Zn/kg body weight/day, while at 240 mg/kg body weight/day, acute toxicity occurred. While the precise mechanisms by which zinc causes adverse effects remain to be determined, it is known that elevated levels of dietary zinc may induce copper deficiency in rats (Grant-Frost and Underwood, 1958; Cox and Harris, 1960; Campbell and Mills, 1974), as well as disrupt the metabolism of iron (Grant-Frost and Underwood, 1958).

The normal human-adult diet supplies about 12-15 mg Zn/day (Underwood, 1973). Despite the sensitivity of ruminants to excess zinc, Underwood (1973) has stated that "a wide margin of safety exists between normal intakes of zinc in food and those likely to produce deleterious effects in man, if the results of experiments with other monogastric animals can be safely extrapolated to the human species." However, cases of human intoxication by consumption of drinking water grossly contaminated with zinc (40 ppm) from galvanized pipes have been reported (Lawrence, 1958; Anonymous, 1957).

We are thus faced with a number of questions: How widespread are marginal zinc diets within the population? Does a marginal zinc diet enhance the toxicity of environmental agents? To what extent are these people at risk and to what agents? Would consumption of zinc in excess of the level normally ingested (12–15 mg/day) offer greater protection from pollutant toxicity? How much supplementation would offer the greatest degree of protection? At what point would the supplementary zinc begin to initiate deleterious metabolic changes such as alterations in copper and iron metabolism?

At the present time our knowledge of zinc-pollutant interactions does not permit satisfactory answers to these questions. Yet the available information clearly indicates that zinc nutritional status affects the toxicity and carcinogenicity of a range of substances. What is obviously needed is a vigorous and systematic research effort to further elucidate how zinc interacts with environmental agents and affects normal human metabolism so that the above-stated questions may be confidently answered.

References

Anonymous (1957). Outbreaks of food poisoning due to zinc, 1942-1956. *U.K. Min. Health Lab. Serv. Mon. Bull.*

Campbell, J.K. and Mills, C.F. (1974). Effects of dietary cadmium and zinc on rats maintained on diet low in copper. *Proc. Nutr. Soc.* **33**:15A–17A.

Cerklewski, F. and Forbes, R.M. (1976). Influence of dietary zinc on lead toxicity in the rat. *J. Nutrit.* **106**:689–696.

Cox, D.H. and Harris, D.L. (1960). Effects of excess zinc on iron and copper in the rat. *J. Nutrit.* **70**:514–520.

Fong, L.Y.Y.; Sivak, A.; and Newberne, P.M. (1978). Zinc deficiency and methyl-benzylnitrosamine-induced esophageal cancer in rats. *J. Natl. Cancer Instit.* **61**(1): 145–150.

Grant-Frost, D.R. and Underwood, E.J. (1958). Zinc toxicity in the rat and its interrelation with copper. *Aust. J. Exp. Biol. Med. Sci.* **36**:339–346.

Hambidge, K.M. (1977). The role of zinc and other trace metals in pediatric nutrition and health. *Pediat. Clin. North Amer.* **24**:95.

Ketcheson, M.R.; Barron, G.P.; and Cox, D.H. (1969). Relationship of maternal dietary zinc during gestation or lactation to development and zinc, iron and copper content of the postnatal rat. *J. Nutr.* **98**:303–311.

Lawrence, G. (1958). Zinc poisoning. *Brit. Med. J.* **1**:582.

Mahaffey, K.R. and Vanderveen, J.E. (1979). Nutrient-toxicant interactions: susceptible populations. *Environ. Health Perspect.* **29**:81–87.

Ott, E.A.; Smith, W.H.; Harrington, R.B.; and Beeson, W.M. (1966). Zinc toxicity in ruminants. I. Effect of high levels of dietary zinc on gains, feed consumption and feed efficiency of beef cattle. *J. Animal Sci.* **25**:414–418.

Ott, E.A.; Smith, W.H.; Harrington, R.B.; and Beeson, W.M. (1966a). Zinc toxicity in ruminants. II. Effect of high levels of dietary zinc on gains, feed consumption and feed efficiency of beef cattle. *J. Animal Sci.* **25**:419–423.

Owen, G. and Lippman, G. (1977). Nutritional status of infants and young children: USA. *Pediat. Clin. North Amer.* **24**:211.

Underwood, E.J. (1973). Trace elements. In: *Toxicants Occurring Naturally in Foods,* pp. 43–87. National Academy of Sciences, Washington, D.C.

Other Minerals

A. COBALT

1. Lead

The interaction of dietary cobalt with environmental stressor agents is generally unknown. However, limited Soviet studies suggest that dietary cobalt may significantly reduce symptoms of lead intoxication in animal models (Charka, 1968).

That cobalt may affect lead toxicity has been suggested by observations that cobalt supplementation enhances the formation of vitamin B_{12} (Skoropostizhnoja, 1958), a cobalt-containing vitamin that has been employed as a preventive treatment in experimental and clinical studies (Aldanozanov and Sabdenova, 1960). In addition, cobalt administration has been found to improve anemic conditions (Abrarov, 1963). In testing the hypothesis that cobalt supplementation may reduce lead toxicity, Charka (1968) exposed white rats to elevated levels of lead either by inhalation (120 days) or in food (90 days) and reared on either a basal diet adequate in all known aspects or a similar basal diet with 40 times the normal cobalt requirement. Charka (1968) found that cobalt supplementation was able to prevent the growth inhibitory action of lead. Interestingly, cobalt markedly increased the concentration of lead on the liver, which, according to Charka, may be a preliminary step leading to lead excretion in the bile.

While the study of Charka (1968) suggests that diets supplemented with cobalt may reduce some symptoms of lead toxicity, this study is clearly in need of replication. Of particular concern is whether the cobalt supplementation does in fact enhance biliary excretion of lead. Presently no evidence exists on whether a diet with marginal or inadequate cobalt levels affects lead toxicity. This would certainly seem to be an appropriate area of experimentation.

References

Abrarov, A. (1963). Vliianie kobal'ta i medi na gemopoez i sostav gemoglobina pri alimentarnoi anemii u belykh krys. *Voprosy Pitaniia* **22**:39–43.

Aldanozanov, A.T. and Sabdenova, Sh., S. (1960). Influence of vitamin B_{12} and folic acid on the development of lead intoxication in experimental animals. Kazakh SSR Acad. Sci., Inst. of Pathology. Alma-Ata. Vol. 8(15).

Charka, P.A. (1968). The effect of cobalt and copper salts in toxic action of lead on the animal organism. *Voprosy Pitaniia* **27**:29–33.

Skoropostizhnoja, A.S. (1958). Cobalt content in foodstuffs and its influence on animal organism. Ph.D. dissertation, Kiev.

B. IODINE

1. Polychlorinated Biphenyls (PCBs)

The interaction of iodine with environmental pollutants is almost totally unexplored. However, from a conceptual perspective, there appears to be ample opportunity for such interactions to occur. For instance, PCBs are active inducers of microsomal enzymes such as thyroxine-UDP glucuronyltransferase (Alvares et al., 1973; Kimbrough, 1974; Bastomsky and Murphy, 1976). Furthermore, thyroxine is excreted principally via the bile (Galton, 1968), with conjugation of thyroxine to glucuronic acid being rate-limiting (Bastomsky, 1973). In light of these findings, Bastomsky (1977) hypothesized that PCBs may be goitrogenic and that a low-iodine diet may enhance the goitrogenic potential of PCBs.

He reported that PCB exposure results in an enlargement of the thyroid gland in rats regardless of whether these animals are reared on a high- or low-iodine diet. However, as predicted, those rats reared on a low-iodine diet are more sensitive to the goitrogenic effects of PCBs. Consistent with the enlargement of the thyroid gland were the findings that rats reared on the low-iodine diet and exposed to PCBs had decreased thyroxine levels as well as increasing thyroid-stimulating hormone activity. These findings clearly suggest that PCB exposure disrupts normal iodine metabolism and that a diet low in iodine seems to enhance the goitrogenic effects of PCBs. Since these findings occurred following exposure to large quantities of PCBs (250 ppm) in the diet, it is not possible to predict the goitrogenic potential of PCB exposure at considerably lower levels. However, the recommendation of Bastomsky (1977) that thyroid function should be included in the health assessment of environmental accidents such as the poisoning of numerous Japanese in 1968 with PCB-contaminated cooking oil is well founded.

A potentially important aspect of this research is the apparent reduction of iodine stores in the PCB-treated rats. While this has extremely important implications for thyroid metabolism, it may also result in marked alterations of liver microsomal enzyme function. Table 1 illustrates the occurrence of sizable increases in enzymatic oxidative activities in liver homogenates from iodide-deficient mice. The rates of metabolism of type I and II substrates were increased by about two-fold, while 3,4-benzpyrene oxidation was increased by more than a factor of 10 (Catz et al., 1970).

Table 1. Effects of Iodide Deficiencies on Hepatic Drug Metabolic Activities of Propylthiouracil-Treated Mice[a]

	Specific Activity		
Substrates	Iodide-Supplemented	Iodide-Deficient	Change
			%
Aminopyrine	9.7 ± 1.5 (6)	18.8 ± 1.2 (6)	+94
Hexobarbital	14.7 ± 1.8 (6)	26.8 ± 3.3 (6)	+83
Aniline	2.5 ± 0.4 (6)	4.9 ± 0.6 (6)	+96
3,4-Benzpyrene	3.6 ± 0.3 (6)	37.0 ± 6.0 (6)	+1030
p-Nitrobenzoic acid	3.0 ± 0.4 (6)	2.2 ± 0.4 (6)	−27
o-Aminophenol	41.0 ± 16.0 (6)	107.0 ± 17.0 (6)	+161
p-Nitrophenol	37.0 ± 8.0 (6)	39.0 ± 11.0 (6)	+5

[a]Mice were kept on the specific diet for six months. Numbers in parentheses are the number of animals employed for each determination.

Source. Catz et al. (1970). *J. Pharm. Exper. Therap.* **174**(2):202.

These biochemical findings suggest that prolonged PCB exposure at levels sufficient to reduce body stores of iodine may alter the metabolic activity of the liver microsomal enzymes. This further suggests that PCB exposure may be expected to alter the toxicity and/or carcinogenicity of a number of xenobiotics presumably via inducing a change in the capacity of the microsomal enzymes to metabolize such compounds. While this is only theoretical, the biochemical foundations for this suggestion are sound and worthy of further study.

2. Polybrominated Biphenyls (PBBs)

That PBBs might interact with iodine was not as clearly conceived, at least biochemically, when compared to the rationale for the PCB-iodine interaction. However, interest in this possibility grew as a result of the well-known PBB contamination of livestock in Michigan and the suggestion by Norris et al. (1974) of a possible physiologic and pathologic response to competition between bromine and iodine. Furthermore, Michigan is considered part of the "goiter belt" and is known to have such low levels of iodine in the soil that it is often necessary to supplement livestock rations with iodine (Sleight et al., 1978). Thus the question was raised as to whether diets with highly variable levels of iodine may affect the occurrence of PBB toxicity.

In their study, Sleight et al. (1978) exposed young male rats to dietary PBBs (0, 1, 10, or 100 ppm). These animals were concomitantly reared on diets for 60 days that were iodine-deficient, iodine-adequate (0.2 ppm), or iodine excess (1000 ppm). As a result of these experimental exposures, a number of diet-PBB interactions occurred. Of greatest significance were the observations (1) that bile-duct proliferation occurred only in iodine-deficient fed rats exposed to 100 ppm PBB, and (2) that the iodine-excess diet plus 100 ppm PBB induced squamous metaplasia of respiratory bronchiolus epithelium.

While the significance of these findings is difficult to ascertain, it is evident that interactions between PBBs with iodine metabolism do occur. Further research is needed to elucidate this interaction.

References

Alvares, A.P.; Bickers, D.R.; and Kappas, A. (1973). Polychlorinated biphenyls: a new type of inducer of cytochrome P-448 in the liver. *Proc. Natl. Acad. Sci. USA* **70**:1321–1325.

Bastomsky, C.H. (1973). The biliary excretion of thyroxine and its glucuronic acid conjugate in normal and Gunn rats. *Endocrinology* **92**:35–40.

Bastomsky, C.H. (1977). Goitres in rats fed polychlorinated biphenyls. *Can. J. Physiol. Pharmacol.* **55**:288–292.

Bastomsky, C.H. and Murthy, P.V.M. (1976). Enhanced *in vitro* hepatic glucuronidation of thyroxine in rats following cutaneous application or ingestion of polychlorinated biphenyls. *Can. J. Physiol. Pharmacol.* **54**:23–26.

Catz, C.S.; Juchau, M.R.; and Yaffe, S.J. (1970). Effects of iron, riboflavin and iodide deficiencies on hepatic drug-metabolizing enzyme systems. *J. Pharm. Exper. Therap.* **174**:197–205.

Galton, V.A. (1968). The physiological role of thyroid hormone metabolism. In: *Recent Advances in Endocrinology,* pp. 181–206. 8th ed. Edited by V.H.T. James. J. and A. Churchill Ltd., London.

Kimbrough, R.D. (1974). The toxicity of polychlorinated polycyclic compounds and re-lated chemicals. *Crit. Rev. Toxicol.* **2**:445–498.

Norris, J.M.; et al. (1974). Toxicological and environmental factors involved in the selec-tion of decarbomodiphenyl oxide as a fire retardant chemical. *J. Fire Flammability/ Combustion Toxicol.* **1**:52. (Cited in Sleight et al., 1978.)

Sleight, S.D.; Mangkoewidjojo, S.; Akoso, B.T.; and Sanger, V.L. (1978). Polybrominated biphenyl toxicosis in rats fed an iodine-deficient, iodine-adequate, or iodine-excess diet. *Environ. Health Perspect.* **23**:341–346.

C. MAGNESIUM[1]

1. Fluoride

Information derived from research conducted on several animal species has indicated that dietary levels of Mg affect the toxicity of fluorides. For example, when very high levels of Mg and fluoride were fed to growing chicks, it caused noticeable leg weakness (Gardner et al., 1961) and reduced the mineral content of bone, but increased Mg content of bone. According to Marier (1968), commenting on Griffith et al. (1964), this condition of the bone implies a rachitic-like state that may be caused by a high-Mg low-citrate condition plus the presence of fluoride. Belanger et al. (1958) have noted that high fluoride sup-plements can produce a rachitic-like condition. Also, rachitic bone has an increased Mg content (Fourman and Morgan, 1962).

Animal studies with dogs and rats (Chiemchaiseri and Philips, 1963) revealed that in Mg-deficient dogs, fluoride supplements prevented soft-tissue calcification, but not the muscle weakness and convulsions. In rats, the dietary fluoride, while having no protective effect on soft-tissue calcification, aggravated the hypomagnesemia condition, which intensified the occurrence of convulsive seizures.

---

[1]See *Nutrition and Environmental Health,* Volume 1, chapter 2, for a discussion of how dietary magnesium affects the toxicity of ethylene glycol.

According to Marier et al. (1963), the symptoms of Mg deficiency are quite similar to those of fluoride intoxication (e.g., leg cramps, muscular twitching, tetaniform convulsions, optical neuritis, and bone exostoses or soft-tissue calcification). This is most probably due to a fluoride-induced increase in the uptake of Mg from plasma into bone. Marier (1968) notes that even small increases in bone Mg may be serious, since bone can contain up to 63% of body Mg whereas body fluids account for only about 1.0%.

Since Mg deficiency may influence the toxicity of fluoride, it is important to determine the dietary requirement for Mg. According to Seelig (1964), the assumption that the average daily intake of Mg is enough to maintain equilibrium in the normal adult is highly suspect. An analysis of metabolic data shows that the minimal dietary requirement is not 220-300 mg per day or even 5 mg/kg body wt./day as has also been suggested, but probably at least 6 mg/kg/day.

Seelig (1964) reports that clinical metabolic data indicate that with intakes below 6 mg/kg/day a negative Mg balance is likely to develop, especially in men. High protein, calcium, vitamin D, and alcohol ingestion function either to prevent retention or to increase the requirement of Mg, especially in individuals on low Mg intakes. The Western diet is calculated to supply an average of 250 to 300 mg of Mg daily, which is less than 5 mg/kg/day. Since the Western diet is usually rich in protein, calcium, vitamin D, and alcohol, Seelig (1964) suggests the optimal daily intake of magnesium should be between 7 and 10 mg/kg/day.

Although the data suggest that individuals living in the United States have less-than-sufficient Mg in the diet as well as having daily exposure to fluoride (when exposed to fluoridated drinking water at 1.0 ppm) via food and water of between 3.5 and 5.5 mg (Marier and Rose, 1966), the precise risk is difficult to ascertain because of the uncertainties of extrapolation from animal studies to man and the lack of supporting human epidemiologic data.

Finally, Schuck (1938) evaluated the influence of magnesium supplementation on the development of dental fluorosis in rats in a pilot study. The results revealed that the toxicity of fluoride was not affected by a doubling of the amount of dietary magnesium.

References

Belanger, L.F.; Visek, W.J.; Lotz, W.E.; and Comar, C.L. (1958). Rachitomimetic effects of fluoride feeding on the skeletal tissues of growing pigs. *Amer. J. Pathol.* **34**:25.

Chiemchaiseri, Y. and Philips, P.H. (1963). Effect of dietary fluoride upon magnesium calcinosis syndrome. *J. Nutr.* **81**:307–311.

Fourman, P. and Morgan, D.B. (1962). *Proc. Nutr. Soc.* **21**:34.

Gardner, E.E.; Rogler, J.C.; and Parker, H.E. (1961). Interrelationships between magnesium and fluoride in chicks. *J. Nutr.* **75**:270.

Marier, J.R. (1968). The importance of dietary magnesium with particular reference to humans. National Research Council of Canada, No. 10, 173.

Marier, J.R. and Rose, D. (1966). The fluoride content of some foods and beverages. *J. Fd. Sci.* **31**:941.

Marier, J.R.; Rose, D.; and Bovlet, M. (1963). Accumulation of skeletal fluoride and its implications. *Arch. Environ. Health* **6**:664–671.

Schuck, C. (1938). Study of the influence of magnesium and sodium on the activity of fluorides. *J. Nutr.* **17**:387–392.

Seelig, M.S. (1964). The requirement of magnesium by the normal adult. *Amer. J. Clin. Nutr.* **14**:342.

2. Lead

The influence of dietary magnesium on the intestinal absorption of lead has recently been addressed by Barltrop and Khoo (1975) and Fine et al. (1976). It was hypothesized that magnesium may interact with lead since it is a divalent cation known to affect the intestinal transport of calcium. Since low levels of dietary calcium are known to enhance the retention of lead, it was thought that any disruption of calcium transport may also affect the absorption and/or retention of lead (Fine et al., 1976).

In an experiment with beagle puppies, Fine et al. (1976) demonstrated that dogs, fed a magnesium-deficient diet for 15 days, absorbed ingested lead at a rate of 26.5%, while the magnesium-fed control group exhibited an absorption rate of 8.6%, a difference that was statistically significant at the 0.01 level.

These results are quite striking and certainly deserve further study. It should be pointed out that both control and experimental animals had diets devoid of calcium, while the experimental group obviously was without any magnesium as well. This type of situation is clearly not realistic in terms of the way humans eat. Thus the relevance of these results for humans is unknown. However, the findings of Fine et al. (1976) are in general agreement with an earlier report of Barltrop and Khoo (1975), which also revealed that a low-magnesium diet over 48 hours enhanced the retention of dietary lead in several tissues (blood 2.7, kidneys 1.6, femur 1.6, liver 1.7, and carcass 1.7) of rats. In this study there was no concomitant deficiency of calcium.

In light of these two studies, which indicate that low levels of magnesium in the diet enhance the intestinal absorption and tissue retention of lead, further research is necessary to develop more accurate quantitative relationships between highly variable levels of dietary magnesium and dietary lead with respect to tissue retention of lead and biochemical indicators of lead toxicity. Barltrop and Khoo (1975) have also shown that increases in lead absorption, because of a deficiency of separate minerals such as calcium, phosphate, and magnesium, do not add up to the total increased absorption of lead as compared to when all three minerals are simultaneously deficient, thereby suggesting a synergistic effect. Clearly, studies involving multiple marginal mineral deficiencies are necessary in order to establish a more realistic assessment of the influence of these dietary factors on lead toxicity.

Finally, a recent rat study by Singh et al. (1979) has revealed that dietary supplementation with magnesium enhances the mobilization of lead from bone, thereby leading to increasing blood and urinary lead levels. This may be of some significance since magnesium supplementation permits the once sequestered lead to move from the bone tissue where the lead was presumably innocuous to generally higher overall levels in the soft tissues including the brain.

References

Barltrop, D. and Khoo, H.E. (1975). The influence of nutritional factors on lead absorption. *Postgrad. Med. J.* **51**:795–800.

Fine, B.P.; Barth, A.; Sheffit, A.; and Lavenhar, A. (1976). Influence of magnesium on the intestinal absorption of lead. *Environ. Res.* **12**:224–227.

Singh, N.P.; Thind, I.S.; Vitale, L.F.; and Pawlow, M. (1979). Intake of magnesium and toxicity of lead: an experimental model. *Arch. Environ. Health.* May/June: 168–173.

3. Aspirin (Acetylsalicylic Acid)

The toxicity of acetylsalicylic acid has been found to be affected by several dietary components including the levels of protein, carbohydrate, and magnesium (West, 1964). He reported that a high-carbohydrate diet (sucrose 65%, casein 24%) markedly enhanced susceptibility to gastric ulceration in nonpregnant and pregnant female rats as compared to those given a high-protein diet (89% casein, 5% corn oil). In addition, the high-carbohydrate diet also enhanced the acute toxicity (i.e., death) of the fetus to acetylsalicylic acid. The adverse effects of acetylsalicylic acid to rats on either the high-protein or high-carbohydrate diet were markedly enhanced when combined with a magnesium deficiency (i.e., 1/10 of normal amount). The levels of acetylsalicylic acid used in this study were quite close to normal human intakes. In fact, in studies concerning fetal toxicity, the daily dose was 50 mg/kg or the equivalent of 3.5 grain tablets four times a day in man. These findings clearly imply the need for more adequate testing of drugs prior to their approval for use by the general public.

Reference

West, G.B. (1964). The influence of diet on the toxicity of acetylsalicylic acid. *J. Pharm. Pharmacol.* **16**:788–793.

4. Microsomal Enzyme Activity

Becking (1976) has clearly demonstrated that a magnesium deficiency significantly reduces the *in vitro* and *in vivo* metabolism of aniline. Further analyses revealed a lower level of cytochrome P-450 and cytochrome C-reductase activity in magnesium-deficient rats.

While these studies are of a very limited nature, they suggest that low levels of magnesium in the diet may markedly affect the detoxification and/or bioactivation of numerous xenobiotics. Further research directed toward identifying the role of magnesium on the functioning of the liver microsomal enzymes is to be encouraged.

Reference

Becking, G.C. (1976). Hepatic drug metabolism in iron-, magnesium- and potassium-deficient rats. *Fed. Proc.* **35**(13):2480–2485.

D. MANGANESE

1. Lead

The influence of dietary manganese (Mn) on the body burden and toxicity of lead has recently been addressed experimentally. Mylroie and Patterson (1980) first became interested in this relationship as a result of their study that revealed that rats reared on a purified, normal protein (NP) diet were more susceptible to the toxic effects of lead than rats fed stock diets such as purina rat chow. The NP diet was found to contain two times more fat than chow, no fiber, sucrose in place of starch, and lower levels of minerals (Ca, P) and essential trace metals (Fe, Cu, Zn, Mn, Cr, Co). In an effort to determine which missing factors in the purified diet enhanced lead toxicity, they initiated a systematic assessment of each separate component including Mn and its role in affecting lead toxicity. In their study it was found that by itself the addition of Mn to the NP diet resulted in no significant effects on tissue lead levels. In fact, neither did the combined addition of Fe, Zn, and Cu to unsupplemented NP diet have any significant effect on tissue levels of lead. However, the addition of Mn to the NP plus Fe, Zn, and Cu diet resulted in significantly decreased tissue lead levels in blood (43%), liver (67%), brain (38%), bone (22%), kidney (59%), and spleen (30%). Conversely, lead treatment was found to markedly reduce Mn levels in liver and kidney of rats reared on a NP diet and an NP plus Cu, Zn, and Fe diet.

According to Mylroie and Patterson (1980), the mechanism of the observed Pb-Mn interaction is not known. They suggested that Mn and Pb may compete (1) for absorption in the gastrointestinal tract, at the level of cellular transport and (2) at the level of storage in tissues. While the biomedical/public health significance of these findings remains to be assessed, such striking results should generate a vigorous research effort in this area. Finally, the fact that high levels of Ca and P impair the utilization of Mn (Mylroie and Patterson, 1980) suggests the critical need to evaluate the complex interrelationships of essential minerals amongst themselves and the heavy metals before recommending alterations in national dietary policies.

Reference

Mylroie, A.A. and Patterson, L. (1980). The influence of dietary manganese on tissue content and toxicity of ingested lead in the rat. *Trace Substances in Environmental Health*. University of Missouri, Columbia.

E. MOLYBDENUM

1. Bisulfite, Sulfite, and Sulfur Dioxide

It is certainly well known that persons with chronic respiratory disorders are at increased risk to the irritant effects of sulfur dioxide. However, it is also known that sulfur dioxide may affect systemic toxicity via the *in vivo* formation of sulfite. In addition to sulfite exposure indirectly from inhalation of sulfur dioxide, consumption of foods preserved with sulfite and/or bisulfite will provide additional exposure to such compounds.

Sulfite exposure is known to cause central nervous system toxicity (Wilkins et al., 1968) and immunological impairment as well as damage to DNA. Sulfite may be detoxified via the action of the enzyme sulfite oxidase, which oxidizes the toxicant to sulfate (Cohen et al., 1973).

It has recently been hypothesized that a deficiency of sulfite oxidase may result in an enhanced susceptibility to systemic sulfite, bisulfite, and sulfur dioxide toxicity (Anonymous, 1975; Hickey et al., 1976). Several cases of a total sulfite oxidase deficiency in humans have been reported (Mudd et al., 1967; Irreverre et al., 1967), as well as the occurrence of an apparent intermediate deficiency. However, the gene frequency of this condition in the human population is unknown but thought to be rare.

In addition to a sulfite oxidase deficiency being produced via the occurrence of a rare genetic disorder, it may also be produced via dietary manipulation involving the feeding of a low-molybdenum diet (30 μg per kg of diet) and consumption of drinking water supplemented with 100 ppm tungsten. The rationale for this treatment is that sulfite oxidase is a molybdenum-containing enzyme; thus, low levels of dietary molybdenum should diminish the synthesis of sulfite oxidase. As for the tungsten treatment, this element is a competitive antagonist of molybdenum in animal systems (Johnson et al., 1974; Higgins et al., 1956), thereby facilitating a reduction in sulfite oxidase synthesis.

In the testing of the hypothesis that a low level of sulfite oxidase enhances the toxicity of these oxidant stressor agents, Cohen et al. (1973) fed rats the above mentioned low-molybdenum high-tungsten combination. After three weeks of this diet, the sulfite oxidase level in the liver had been reduced to only 10% of the control rats given a low-molybdenum diet (without tungsten in drinking water). Importantly, with the exception of a tungsten-induced reduction in the activity of the molybdenum dependent enzyme xanthine oxidase, there appeared to be no sulfur dioxide or bisulfite pretreatment difference between the two groups of rats.

Subsequent exposure to sodium bisulfite in LD_{50} studies via intraperitoneal injection revealed that sulfite oxidase-deficient animals were clearly more susceptible to the bisulfite toxicity than the controls. The LD_{50} values for the sulfite oxidase-deficient group after 3 and 5 weeks were 271 and 181 mg/kg, respectively. In marked contrast, the control animals (i.e., given a low-molybdenum diet but no tungsten) had LD_{50} values after three weeks of 551 mg/kg and 475 mg/kg after 5 weeks. Of interest was that the animals appeared to be dying of bisulfite-induced neural toxicity. Presumably, the rats with the low levels of sulfite oxidase activity were not as able to convert bisulfite to sulfate.

Other studies revealed that rats deficient in sulfite oxidase were more susceptible to sulfur dioxide, as determined by a shorter survival at 925 ppm sulfur dioxide. Interestingly, the control animals displayed the well-known respiratory symptoms while the deficient rats exhibited central nervous system toxicity for the most part. However, when the levels of sulfur dioxide were reduced to 590 ppm, no differences between the groups were noted. Presumably, insufficient bisulfite is formed *in vivo* at the 590-ppm exposure to cause obvious central nervous system toxicity in the deficient animals, and both the deficient and control groups ultimately died from respiratory damage.

While these data clearly indicate that consumption of a low-molybdenum high-tungsten diet enhances the toxicity of bisulfite and sulfur dioxide, the relevance of these findings for humans is uncertain. Since only minute amounts of molybdenum are needed for enzyme function and tungsten may be present only in trace amounts in the diet, the chances for inducing a sulfite oxidase deficiency are probably exceedingly rare. In addition, the 925-ppm level of sulfur dioxide that was needed to cause enhanced toxicity in the deficient rats is nearly 200 times greater than levels only rarely approached (5 ppm) in urban centers (Anonymous, 1975).

References

Anonymous (1975). Bisulfite toxicity in molybdenum-deficient rats. *Nutr. Rev.* 33(6):185–186.

Cohen, H.J.; Drew, R.T.; Johnson, J.L.; and Rajagopalan, K.V. (1973). Molecular basis of the biological function of molybdenum. The relationship between sulfide oxidase and the acute toxicity of bisulfite and SO_2. *Proc. Natl. Acad. Sci. USA* 70:3655–3659.

Hickey, R.J.; Clelland, R.C.; Bower, E.J.; and Boyd, D.E. (1976). Health effects of atmospheric sulfur dioxide and dietary sulfite. *Arch. Environ. Health*, March/April, pp. 108–110.

Higgins, E.S.; Richert, D.A.; and Westerfeld, W.W. (1956). Molybdenum deficiency and tungstate inhibition studies. *J. Nutr.* 59:539–559.

Irreverre, F.; Mudd, S.H.; Heizer, W.D.; and Laster, L. (1967). Sulfite oxidase deficiency: studies of a patient with mental retardation, dislocated lenses and abnormal urinary excretion of S-sulfo-L-cysteine, sulfite, and thiosulfate. *Biochem. Med.* 1:187–217.

Johnson, J.L.; Cohen, J.J.; and Rajagopalan, K.V. (1974). Molecular basis of the biological function of molybdenum. Molybdenum-free sulfite oxidase from livers of tungsten-treated rats. *J. Biol. Chem.* 249:5046–5055.

Mudd, S.H.; Irreverre, F; and Laster, L. (1967). Sulfite oxidase deficiency in man: demonstration of the enzymatic defect. *Science* 156:1599–1602.

Wilkins, J.W.; Green, J.A., Jr.; and Weller, J.M. (1968). The toxicity of intraperitoneal bisulfite. *Clin. Pharm. Therap.* **9**:328–332.

F. PHOSPHORUS[2]

1. Cadmium

Considerable interest has been directed toward evaluating the influence of nutritional status on cadmium toxicity. While much of this interest has focused on the interactions of ascorbic acid, calcium, iron, and zinc with cadmium toxicity, little regard has been given toward potential interactions of phosphorus with cadmium. The first study suggesting that dietary phosphorus may modify the toxicity of cadmium was reported by Muto and Omori (1977). They noted the occurrence of renal damage resulting from long-term cadmium exposure to rats reared on a multinutritionally deficient diet, with low protein (10%), low calcium (0.05%), low phosphorus (0.14%), and no dietary fiber. Since it was not possible for these investigators to parcel out the contributions of each individual component, a follow-up study (Omori and Muto, 1977) attempted to evaluate the role of each of the above substances including phosphorus in affecting the absorption and retention of cadmium. In their study, which was of a one-month duration, it was found that diets low in calcium and phosphorus exhibited a highly significant retention of cadmium in the kidney and liver. In fact, of all the components tested, supplementation with these two minerals was most effective in reducing the tissue levels of cadmium.

While the study by Omori and Muto (1977) established that calcium and phosphorus deficiency enhanced cadmium retention in the kidney and liver, it did not differentiate between the influence of either mineral. However, a recent report by Koo et al. (1978) has clearly shown that separate deficiencies of calcium and phosphorus increase the duodenal absorption rate of labeled cadmium by approximately 79% for either mineral in chicks.

Further studies should attempt to replicate this finding in models other than the chick, as well as develop more quantitative dose-response relationships between the degree of phosphorus deficiency and the extent of enhanced cadmium absorption and retention.

[2]See Chapter 1 for the phosphate-lead interaction.

References

Koo, S.I.; Fullmer, C.S.; and Wasserman, R.H. (1978). Intestinal absorption and retention of ^{109}Cd: effects of cholecalciferol, calcium status and other variables. *J. Nutr.* **108**:1812–1822.

Muto, Y. and Omori, M. (1977). Nutritional influence on the onset of renal damage due to long-term administration of cadmium in young and adult rats. *J. Nutr. Sci. Vitaminol.* **23**:349–360.

Omori, M. and Muto, Y. (1977). Effects of dietary protein, calcium, phosphorus and fiber on renal accumulation of exogenous cadmium in young rats. *J. Nutr. Sci. Vitaminol.* **23**:361–373.

2. Fluoride

It has long been speculated that dietary factors may influence the incidence and severity of dental fluorosis. While the role of calcium has been the most studied nutrient in this regard, investigators have also made attempts to evaluate the potential influence of phosphorus. In essence, all attempts to assess the role of dietary phosphorus on dental fluorosis whether in animals (Smith, 1935–1936) or humans (Leverton and Smith, 1932), or enhanced fluoride retention or toxicity in animal models (Lawrenz and Mitchell, 1941; Gardiner et al., 1961), have not been able to demonstrate any effect directly attributable to the phosphorus. This has been particularly conclusive within the animal studies, in which a wide range of phosphorus concentrations were evaluated. Unfortunately, the only human studies were performed nearly 50 years ago and utilized a very small sample size, making it impossible to assess fairly the role of phosphorus on dental fluorosis.

References

Gardiner, E.E.: Rogler, J.C.; and Parker, H.E. (1961). Interrelationships between magnesium and fluoride in chicks. *J. Nutr.* **75**:270–274.

Lawrenz, M. and Mitchell, H.H. (1941). The effect of dietary calcium and phosphorus on the assimilation of dietary fluorine. *J. Nutr.* **22**:91–101.

Leverton, R.M. and Smith, M.C. (1932). The relation of calcium and phosphorus in the diet to the cause of mottled enamel of human teeth. *J. Home Economics* **24**:1091–1097.

Smith, M.C. (1935–1936). Dietary factors in relation to mottled enamel. *J. Dent. Res.* **15**:281–290.

G. POTASSIUM

1. Microsomal Enzymes

Becking (1976) has evaluated the influence of a dietary potassium deficiency on the metabolism of the liver microsomal enzymes. He

Table 2. Metabolism *in vivo* of Aminopyrine[a] in Potassium-Deficient Rats

Diet	Days on Test	Plasma Half-Life (min)	4-Amino-antipyrine[b] (μg/ml)
Deficient		122 $\pm$ 6[c]	12.9 $\pm$ 1.1
Control	38	80 $\pm$ 4	10.0 $\pm$ 0.9
Deficient + potassium		90 $\pm$ 7	9.8 $\pm$ 1.5
Control	38 + 18	84 $\pm$ 5	9.2 $\pm$ 1.1

[a]Administered as an intraperitoneal dose of 80 mg/kg to 6 groups of 5 rats. Results are expressed as the mean value $\pm$ SEM.

[b]Total 4-aminoantipyrine in plasma was determined 2 hr after drug administration to 6 rats on each diet.

[c]Significantly different from control values ($P < 0.05$).

Source.   Becking, G.C. (1976). Hepatic drug metabolism in iron-, magnesium-, and potassium-deficient rats. *Fed. Proc.* **35**(3):2480–2485.

Table 3. Effect of Potassium Depletion on Pentobarbital[a] Sleeping Times

Diet	Days on Test	Sleeping Time (min)
Deficient		142 $\pm$ 11[b]
Control	38	90 $\pm$ 8
Deficient + potassium		101 $\pm$ 12
Control	38 + 18	83 $\pm$ 7

[a]Administered as an i.p. dose of 40 mg/kg to groups of 20 rats. Results are expressed as the mean value $\pm$ SEM.

[b]Significantly different from control values ($P < 0.05$).

Source.   Becking, G.C. (1976). Hepatic drug metabolism in iron-, magnesium-, and potassium-deficient rats. *Fed. Proc.* **35**(3):2480–2485.

found that potassium depletion did not affect the occurrence of aniline hydroxylation or aminopyrine demethylation nor the reduction of nitrobenzoic acid *in vitro*. However, a potassium deficiency did enhance the *in vitro* activity of glucuronyl transferase. Other studies have shown that potassium-deficient diets significantly alter the *in vivo* plasma half-life of aminopyrine (Table 2) as well as prolonging the pentobarbital sleeping times in rats (Table 3). Such findings indicate that potassium dietary status affects the metabolism of a variety of xenobiotics. To what extent highly variable levels of potassium affect the susceptibility of humans to toxic and/or carcinogenic effects of environmental agents remains to be further studied.

Reference

Becking, G.C. (1976). Hepatic drug metabolism in iron-, magnesium- and potassium-deficient rats. *Fed. Proc.* **35**(3):2480–2485.

2. Sodium

That dietary potassium may affect sodium related increased blood pressure has a long history, going back to 1928 when Addison reported that "potassium salt regularly produced a decline in blood pressure, while sodium salt just as regularly produced a rise."

Evidence that dietary potassium reduces the magnitude of sodium-induced elevated blood pressure comes from a variety of sources including empirical observations of single individuals, clinical and epidemiological studies, and animal model experimentation. The capacity of short-term consumption of potassium supplements to reduce blood pressure has been reported in empirical (i.e., not experimental) studies by McQuarrie et al. (1936). They demonstrated that blood pressure was rapidly and markedly increased (i.e., by 20 mm Hg) in one patient (a 15-year-old diabetic female) with consumption of excess sodium and was similarly reduced when the sodium chloride intake was reduced to 4 gm/day. However, the blood pressure was even further diminished (i.e., by about 10 mm Hg) when supplemental potassium chloride was added to the diet. Additionally, supplementation with potassium chloride also reduced blood pressure in a 14-year-old diabetic female, even in the presence of continued consumption of excess dietary sodium chloride.

These findings are consistent with the observations of Sasaki et al. (1959, 1962) who reported a low incidence of apoplexy and comparatively low blood pressure among a Japanese population consuming a diet that was high in sodium chloride but also high in potassium. In addition, Bartorelli et al. (1966) reported that elevated blood pressure in hypertensive patients could be markedly reduced by an acute infusion of potassium. Experiments with rats have also demonstrated that potassium chloride supplementation reduces the adverse effects of elevated levels of dietary sodium (Meneely et al., 1957, 1961; Lemley-Stone et al., 1961). These researchers reported that administration of 5.6% NaCl in the diet of Sprague-Dawley rats produces hypertension. However, if a supplemental amount of potassium chloride is concomitantly provided throughout, the level of blood pressure is not significantly lowered by the potassium treatment, but the potassium-supplemented rats lived 7 months longer.

The mechanism(s) by which potassium reduces the adverse effects of sodium is (are) not known. Considerably more research with human subjects concerning the protective influence of potassium needs to be conducted. For despite the accumulation of data from empirical, clinical, epidemiological, and animal-model studies that indicate a protective role for potassium, there is need for a larger scale, double-blind clinical study to test this hypothesis. Finally, how potassium administration was able to prolong the lives of salt-free rats but not lower blood pressure is of importance to determine.

References

Addison, W. (1928). The use of sodium chloride, potassium chloride, sodium bromide and potassium bromide in cases of arterial hypertension which are amenable to potassium chloride. *Canad. Med. Assoc. J.* **18**:281–285.

Bartorelli, C.; Gargano, N.; and Leonett, G.C. (1966). Potassium replacement during long-term treatment in hypertension. In: *Antihypertensive Therapy. An International Symposium,* pp. 422–435. Edited by F. Gross. Berlin, Hiedelberg, N.Y., Springer-Verlag.

Dahl, L.K. (1972). Salt and hypertension. *Am. J. Clin. Nutr.* **25**:231–244.

Lemley-Stone, J.; Darby, W.J.; and Meneely, G.R. (1961). Effects of dietary sodium: potassium ratio on body content of sodium and potassium in rats. *Amer. J. Cardiol.* **8**:748–753.

McQuarrie, I.; Thompson, W.H.; and Anderson, J.A. (1936). Effects of excessive ingestion of sodium and potassium salts on carbohydrate metabolism and blood pressure in diabetic children. *J. Nutr.* **11**:77–101.

Meneely, G.R.; Ball, C.O.T.; and Youmans, J.B. (1957). Chronic sodium chloride toxicity: the protective effect of added potassium chloride. *Ann. Intern. Med.* **47**:263–273.

Meneely, G.R. and Battarbee, H.D. (1976). High sodium-low potassium environment and hypertension. *Amer. J. Cardiol.* **38**:768–785.

Meneely, G.R. and Battarbee, H.D. (1976a). Sodium and potassium. *Nutr. Rev.* **34**(8):225–235.

Meneely, G.R.; Lemley-Stone, J.; and Darby, W.J. (1961). Changes in blood pressure and body sodium of rats fed sodium and potassium chloride. *Amer. J. Cardiol.* **8**:527.

Odel, H.M. (1960). Chapter 26: Nutrition in cardiovascular disease. In: *Modern Nutrition in Health and Disease,* 2nd ed., pp. 758–760. Edited by M. Wohl and R. Goodhart.

Sasaki, N. (1962). High blood pressure and the salt intake of the Japanese. *Jap. Heart J.* **3**:313–324.

Sasaki, N.; Mitsuhashi, T.; and Fukushi, S. (1959). Effects of the ingestion of large amount of apples on blood pressure in farmers in Akita prefecture. *Igaku to Seibutsugaku* **51**:103–105.

H. SULFUR

1. Selenium

Toxicity to livestock as a result of ingestion of vegetation grown on soils with high levels of selenium in several Midwestern states became widely recognized in the 1930s (Franke, 1934, 1934a). As could be expected, investigators became interested in finding means to either reduce the uptake of selenium into vegetation prior to consumption by livestock or by an alteration in the diet that would reduce selenium toxicity.

Studies by Hurd-Karrer (1934, 1935) soon revealed that the amount of selenium absorbed by the plants could be diminished by increasing the sulfur level in the soil or nutrient solution. This of course led to the suggestion that the addition of excess sulfur to a selenized soil would probably diminish or even prevent the toxicity of wheat grown on it. This hypothesis was confirmed by Hurd-Karrer and Kennedy (1938) who showed that the addition of sulfur to selenium-treated soil prevented the occurrence of selenium-induced hepatic toxicity in white rats consuming wheat grown in the treated soil. Subsequent chemical analyses revealed that wheat grown on the selenium-treated soil exhibited an average selenium content of 12 ppm, while plants grown in soil to which both sulfur and selenium had been added had only 2 ppm of selenium. Presumably the sulfate inhibited the uptake of selenium by the wheat and thus reduced its toxicity.

Other investigators have also reported other sulfate-selenium interactions. For example, the influence of sulfate and sulfur compounds on the uptake of selenium by yeast (Fels and Cheldelin, 1949), *Chlorella* (Shrift, 1954), and *Aspergillus* (Weissman and Trelease, 1955) in selenate-containing media has been evaluated. In addition, Postgate (1952) has reported the occurrence of a competitive reversal by sulfate of selenate inhibition of sulfate reduction in *Desulfovibrio*.

Finally, several studies have also revealed that dietary sulfate supplementation may also reduce selenium-induced acute toxicity (Bonhorst and Palmer, 1957) and decreases in growth, but not liver damage in rats (Halverson and Monty, 1960).

The immediate implications of this study clearly suggested the possibility that sulfate application to soils may be employed as a possible control technique to prevent selenium intoxication. Interestingly, while the sulfate treatment may prevent excessive uptake of selenium in plants, it also follows that sulfate may prevent the uptake of adequate selenium in plants grown in low-selenium areas (Frost, 1972). Perhaps the combustion of high-sulfur fuels may lead to a disruption in the selenium cycle, resulting in a decrease of available selenium. In light of the enormous coal resources in the United States and their proposed extensive use as fuel in the future, the need to evaluate the potential impact of this energy utilization on selenium availability is of considerable potential concern.

References

Bonhorst, C.W. and Palmer, I.S. (1957). Metabolic interaction of selenate, sulfate, and phosphate. *Agric. and Food Chem.* **5**(12):931–933.

Fels, I.G. and Cheldelin, V.H. (1949). Selenate inhibition studies. III. The role of sulfate in selenate toxicity in yeast. *Arch. Biochem.* **22**:402–405.

Franke, K.W. (1934). A new toxicant occurring naturally in certain samples of plant foodstuffs. I. Results obtained in preliminary feeding trials. *J. Nutr.* **8**:597–608.

Franke, K.W. (1934a). A new toxicant occurring naturally in certain samples of plant foodstuffs. II. The occurrence of the toxicant in the protein fraction. *J. Nutr.* **8**:609–613.

Frost, D.V. (1972). The two faces of selenium—can selenophobia be cured? *CRC Crit. Rev. Toxicol.*, pp. 407–514.

Halverson, A.W. and Monty, K.J. (1960). An effect of dietary sulfate on selenium poisoning in the rat. *J. Nutr.* **70**:100–102.

Hurd-Karrer, A.M. (1934). Selenium injury to wheat plants and its inhibition of sulphur. *J. Agr. Res.* **49**:343–357.

Hurd-Karrer, A.M. (1935). Factors affecting the absorption of selenium from soils by plants. *J. Agr. Res.* **50**:413–427.

Hurd-Karrer, A.M. and Kennedy, M.H. (1938). Inhibiting effect of sulphur in selenized soil on toxicity of wheat to rats. *J. Agr. Res.* **52**(12):933–942.

Postgate, J.R. (1952). Competitive and noncompetitive inhibitors of bacterial sulphate reduction. *J. Gen. Microbiol.* **6**:128.

Shrift, A. (1954). Sulfur-selenium antagonism. I. Anti-metabolite action of selenate on the growth of *Chlorella vulgaris*. *Amer. J. Botany* **41**:223.

Weissman, G.S. and Trelease, S.F. (1955). Influence of sulfur on the toxicity of selenium to *Aspergillus*. *Amer. J. Botany* **42**:489.

7

Protein

A. INORGANIC SUBSTANCES

1. Arsenic

The use of arsenical therapy in the treatment of syphilis was widely practiced in the United States from the 1920s up to the 1940s. Although the arsenical compound arsphenamine was effective in treating syphilis, it also caused a variety of adverse side effects including mild-to-severe anaphylactic responses as well as liver damage (Abt, 1942; Messinger and Hawkins, 1940). The idea that arsenical-induced toxicity could be modified by nutrients was initially proposed in the early 1930s by Mayer and Sulzberger (1931), who suggested that adequate levels of ascorbic acid in the diet prevented or reduced the occurrence of arsenic-induced anaphylaxis. A number of researchers subsequently confirmed this initial report of an ascorbic acid-arsenic interaction (see Cormia, 1937; Dainow, 1937; Bise, 1938). (See Chapter 3 of *Nutrition and Environmental Health,* Volume 1, for a detailed discussion of the influence of ascorbic acid on arsenic toxicity as well as the chemical structure of arsphenamine and its metabolism.)

That dietary protein levels may affect the occurrence of arsphenamine-induced toxicity was also first recognized at about the same time as the ascorbic acid-arsenic interaction. However, in the initial report concerning the potential influence of dietary protein, Craven (1931) found diets high in either protein or carbohydrate to be noticeably inferior to a high-fat diet in preventing arsphenamine-induced atrophy of the liver in dogs. However, a subsequent report by Schifrin (1932) disagreed with the findings of Craven (1931) by noting that a high protein diet was more effective than a high fat diet in reducing arsphenamine injury in dogs. Although there has been little research following these two conflicting studies, a report by Messinger and Hawkins in 1940 clearly demonstrated that a high-meat diet (i.e., hamburger with a low-fat content) was very satisfactory in protecting against arsenical-induced toxicity. In addition, a high-carbohydrate diet was also protective against arsenic-induced toxicity but less than the meat, while a high-fat diet resulted in a marked sensitivity to the arsenical treatment.

Messinger and Hawkins (1940) suggested that the conclusions of the Craven (1931) report may not be contradictory with their study since he killed the dogs at the first sign of serum jaundice, while they followed their animals for up to a week after exposure and were able to develop a much more complete health assessment, including an icterex index as well as general clinical symptoms.

Why a high-protein diet provided greater protection from arsenical-induced toxicity than both high carbohydrate and fat diets was unknown. Messinger and Hawkins (1940) speculated that the high-fat diet may have enhanced toxicity because its metabolism facilitated a drain of carbohydrates followed by protein stores.

These findings are primarily of historical interest, especially in light of the elimination of arsenicals in the treatment of bacterial infections. Whether chronic arsenical poisoning within the occupational setting could be affected by the level of dietary protein, carbohydrates, and fats is not known. In fact, whether chronic arsenical poisoning caused liver damage is open to considerable debate (Tabershaw et al., 1977).

Finally, in 1961 the next and apparently most "recent" article on this subject appeared. Employing acute oral-toxicity (LD_{50}) studies with rats, Packman et al. (1961) reported that a diet high in fat was approximately 1.8 times *more* protective than a high protein diet, with a high-carbohydrate diet being intermediate. The authors suggested that the fat diet may reduce toxic symptoms by preventing the absorption of arsenic by coating the intestinal mucosa or by physically coating or chemically binding the arsenic compound. Since Messinger and Hawkins (1940) injected arsphenamine in their study, this may help explain the totally opposite findings of these two reports.

References

Abt, A.F. (1942). The human skin as an indicator of the detoxifying action of vitamin C (ascorbic acid) in reactions due to arsenicals used in anti-syphilitic therapy. *U.S. Naval Med. Bull.* **40**:291–303.

Bise, E. (1938). Grave erythroderma due to arsphenamine, case by ceritamic acid. *Rev. Med. de la Suisse Rom.* **58**:603 (cited by Abt, 1942).

Cormia, F.E. (1937). Experimental arsphenamine dermatitis: the influence of vitamin C in production of arsphenamine sensitiveness. *Canad. Med. Assoc. J.* **36**:392–396.

Craven, E.B. (1931). Importance of diet in preventing acute yellow atrophy during arsphenamine treatment. *Johns Hopkins Bull.* **48**:131–142.

Dainow, I. (1937). Intarance aux arsenobenzenes et vitamin C. *Presse Med.* **45**:1670–1672.

Mayer, R.L. and Sulzberger, M.B. (1931). Zur Frag der jahreszeitlichen schwankungen der kranheiten. Der Einfluss der kost auf experimentalle sensibilisierungen. *Archv. Fuer. Dermat. und syph.* **163**:245.

Messinger, W.J. and Hawkins, W.B. (1940). Arsphenamine liver injury modified by diet. Protein and carbohydrate protective, but fat injurious. *Amer. J. Med. Sci.* **199**:216.

Packman, E.W.; Abbott, D.D.; and Harrison, J.W.E. (1961). The acute oral toxicity in rats of several diet-arsenic trioxide mixtures. *Agricul. Food Chem.* **9**(4):271–272.

Schifrin, A. (1932). Der Einfluss qualitativ verschiender Ernährungsformen aut die durch Salvarsan hervorgenufenen Lebernekrosen. *Virchow's Arch.* **287**:175–202.

Tabershaw, I.R.; Utidjian, H.M.D.; and Kawahawa, B.L. (1977). Chemical hazards. In: *Occupational Diseases: A Guide to Their Recognition.* U.S. D. HEW, PHS, CDC, NIOSH. Washington, D.C.

2. Cadmium

Considerable interest has been directed toward elucidating the influence of various dietary factors on cadmium toxicity. Not only has significant research been conducted with several vitamins, especially ascorbic acid, but also with a number of minerals including calcium, iron, selenium, and zinc. Other investigations have broadened the perspective of nutrient-cadmium interactions to include dietary fiber and protein. The subsequent section will review the influence of dietary protein on cadmium toxicity.

Although there are only a handful of articles that have attempted to investigate the role of dietary protein in modifying the toxicity of cadmium, the first such study was published in 1941 by Fitzhugh and Meiller who demonstrated that a low-protein diet increased cadmium toxicity.

Despite this early report, it was not until 1973 that a follow-up study was published. In this case, Spivey-Fox et al. (1973) reported that the type of dietary protein in purified diets significantly affected the severity of cadmium-induced toxicity. For instance, when either casein gelatin or soy isolate was used as the source of dietary protein for Japanese quail given 75 ppm cadmium from 7 to 14 days of age, the animals developed anemia and low levels of liver iron, tibia zinc, and total ash. In contrast, when dried egg white was the protein source, cadmium toxicity was markedly reduced, presumably because of better utilization of dietary iron and zinc.

Based on these data, it was quite obvious that the quality of dietary protein markedly affected cadmium toxicity. As a follow-up, Spivey-Fox et al. (1979) compared the influence of several protein sources (i.e., soy isolate, casein gelatin) on the retention of cadmium in Japanese quail. Of great interest was that quail reared on the soy diet retained considerably more cadmium in the duodenum, jejunum-ileum, and liver but slightly less in the kidney. The overall cadmium retention was 14.7% for the casein-gelatin diet versus 48.0% for the quail on the soy-isolate diet.

While the quality of protein appears to affect tissue distribution and toxicity of cadmium as amply seen in the Spivey-Fox studies, the quantity of protein is also of significance as well. Omori and Muto (1977) have shown that a high-protein diet (25%) significantly reduced the level of cadmium retained in the kidneys of rats as compared to controls with a 10% level of dietary protein. These findings were consistent with those of Suzuki et al. (1969) who had noted earlier that a high-protein diet (40%) caused a marked decrease in labeled Cd retention, and also with a recent report of Gontzea and Popescu (1978) that revealed that rats reared on a low-protein (casein-8.8%) diet were more susceptible to the adverse effects (blood and liver enzyme parameters) of injected cadmium than controls given a diet with 17.8% casein. However, the mechanism by which protein reduces the retention and toxicity of cadmium remains obscure.

In contrast to these studies, which indicated that both quality and quantity of protein affect cadmium toxicity, was a recent report by Hill (1979) that noted that the toxicity of cadmium (i.e., as determined by growth and mortality) in chicks was not affected by increasing the level of protein (i.e., soybean meal) from 10 to 30% during short-term studies of up to several weeks. Such "apparent" discrepancies in reported findings clearly suggest a need to quantify the specific nutrients contained within the diet including the amount of those factors that are already known to influence cadmium toxicity, including vitamins C, D, and E, as well as Ca, Fe, P, Zn, fiber, and possibly others. Variations in any of these nutrients may result in a differential susceptibility to cadmium-induced toxicity, thereby introducing confounding variables.

References

Fitzhugh, O.G. and Meiller, F.H. (1941). The chronic toxicity of cadmium. *J. Pharm. Exper. Therapeut.* **72**:15.

Gontzea, I. and Popescu, F. (1978). The effect of body protein supply on resistance to cadmium. *Brit. J. Indus. Med.* **35**:154–160.

Hill, C.H. (1979). The effect of dietary protein levels on mineral toxicity in chicks. *J. Nutr.* **109**:501–507.

Omori, M. and Muto, Y. (1977). Effects of dietary protein, calcium, phosphorus and fiber on renal accumulation of exogenous cadmium in young rats. *J. Nutr. Sci. Vitaminol.* **23**:361–373.

Spivey-Fox, M.R. (1979). Nutritional influences on metal toxicity. Cadmium as a model toxic element. *Environ. Health Perspect.* **29**:95–104.

Spivey-Fox, M.R.; Jacobs, R.M.; Fry, B.E., Jr.; and Harland, B.F. (1973). Effect of protein source on response to cadmium. *Fed. Proc.* **32**:924.

Spivey-Fox, M.R.; Jacobs, R.M.; Jones, A.O.L.; and Fry, B.E., Jr. (1979). Effects of nutritional factors on metabolism of dietary cadmium at levels similar to those of man. *Environ. Health Perspect.* **28**:107–114.

Suzuki, S.; Taguchi, T.; and Yokohashi, G. (1969). Dietary factors influencing the retention rate of orally administered $^{115m}CdCl_2$ in mice with special reference to calcium and protein concentrations in diet. *Ind. Health* **7**:155–162.

3. Cyanide and Phenol

The toxicity of cyanide has been found to be affected by the dietary status of vitamin B_{12} (Mushett et al., 1952; Heaton et al., 1958; Chisholm et al., 1967), sulphur-containing amino acids (Calabrese, 1979), and possibly by ascorbic acid (Calabrese, 1979a), as well as carbohydrates and fats (Rothe Meyer, 1939). While the interactions of these specific nutrients with cyanide are addressed in their respective sections of this book, this section will consider the influence of dietary protein on cyanide toxicity.

Only one study has evaluated the influence of dietary protein on the toxicity of cyanide. In that experiment, Rothe Meyer (1939) exposed young rats to either a high-protein or normal stock diet, with both groups being given a series of subcutaneous injections of cyanide. No marked differences in toxicological responses between these two groups were noted.

In this same experiment, the influence of dietary protein on the toxicity of phenol was also evaluated, with testing protocol similar to the cyanide study. In contrast to the results of the cyanide study, the rats given the high-protein diet exhibited a somewhat lower mortality. In light of the extremely limited information concerning the influence of dietary protein on cyanide and phenol toxicity, no generalizations can be made with confidence.

References

Calabrese, E.J. (1979). Possible adverse side effects from treatment with laetrile. *Medical Hypotheses* **5**:1045–1049.

Calabrese, E.J. (1979a). Conjoint use of laetrile and megadoses of ascorbic acid in cancer treatment: possible side effects. *Medical Hypotheses.* **5**:995–997.

Chisholm, I.A.; Bronte-Stewart, J.; and Foulds, W.S. (1967). Hydroxocobalamin versus cyanocobalamin in the treatment of tobacco amblyopia. *Lancet* **2**:450–451.

Heaton, J.M.; McCormick, A.J.A.; and Freeman, A.G. (1958). Tobacco amblyopia: a clinical manifestation of vitamin B_{12} deficiency. *Lancet* **2**:286–290.

Mushett, C.W.; Kelley, K.L.; Boxer, G.E.; and Rickards, J.C. (1952). Antidotal efficacy of vitamin B_{12} (hydroxocobalamin) in experimental cyanide poisoning. *Proc. Soc. Exp. Biol. Med.* **81**:254–257.

Rothe Meyer, A. (1939). Influence of diet in intoxication with phenol and cyanide. *Proc. Soc. Exp. Biol. Med.* **41**:402–404.

4. Lead

Considerable interest has been directed toward identifying dietary factors that may affect the absorption, retention, and toxicity of lead. Within the decade of the 1970s, the greatest interest has focused on the influence of dietary calcium and iron (Mahaffey-Six and Goyer, 1970, 1972; Mahaffey, 1974; Mahaffey et al., 1977). However, a number of other nutrients are known to affect the occurrence of lead toxicity. These remaining nutrients include certain amino acids, various carbohydrates, fats, proteins, phosphorus, selenium, vitamins A, the B complex, C, D, and E (Levander, 1979; Stephens and Waldron, 1975). Since each of these nutrient-pollutant interactions is considered in its respective chapter, this section will critically assess only the role of dietary protein on the absorption, retention, and toxicity of lead.

The initial investigation concerning the influence of dietary protein on lead toxicity was published in 1942 by Baernstein and Grand of the Division of Industrial Hygiene of the U.S. Public Health Service. These researchers became interested in this area because previous investigators had demonstrated that dietary protein could modify the toxicity of hydrocarbons (White and White, 1939), cholic acid (White,

1935), iodoacetic acid (Stevenson and White, 1940), selenium compounds (Moxon, 1937; Smith and Stohlman, 1940), and sulfanilamide (Smith et al., 1941). Baernstein and Grand (1942) speculated that "protein protects through metabolic processes involving tissue repair rather than through more direct synthetic reaction resulting in detoxification because of the wide diversity of compounds involved and the general observation that animals fed high protein diets of good quality are usually healthier than those fed low protein diets of poor quality." In their study, the growth-inhibiting effects of diets with 1.5% lead chloride were enhanced by diets low in protein (6% casein) as compared to controls with 20% casein.

This initial study was subsequently supported by a number of investigators (MacDonald et al., 1953; Gontzea et al., 1964; Boyadzhiev, 1959, 1960). For instance, Gontzea et al. (1964) demonstrated that dietary protein increased the resistance of rats to the toxic effects of subcutaneously injected basic lead acetate. In addition, they reported that rats reared on a protein-deficient diet had a markedly greater retention of lead (40–73%) in the kidney, liver, spleen, and tibia than controls given adequate protein. Furthermore, several studies by Boyadzhiev (1959, 1960) revealed that rats reared on a low-protein, high-fat diet exhibited markedly enhanced symptoms of lead poisoning as compared to those given a high-protein, low-fat diet. Also, during this period of the 1950s several studies revealed that sulfur containing amino acids (i.e., methionine and cysteine) (Buckup et al., 1956; Niemoller, 1957) as well as serum albumin (Biondi, 1959; DeRenzi and Ricciardi-Pollini, 1952; Merli, 1957; Odeschalchi, 1956; Matsukubo, 1959), protected against the toxicity of lead.

Since 1970 there has been a renewed interest in the possible interactions of dietary protein and lead. This interest has stemmed primarily from the continuing widespread occurrence of lead intoxication in children, especially those of low socioeconomic background (Fine and Thomas, 1972; Lin-Fu, 1970, 1973, 1973a), among whom there is generally a high prevalence of inadequate nutrient intakes (Mahaffey, 1974).

The animal studies, which have been conducted exclusively with rats, have generally supported the hypothesis that low levels of dietary protein enhance the retention of lead in soft tissue (Milev et al., 1970; Gontzea et al., 1970; Der et al., 1974, 1974a; Fahim et al., 1975; Barltrop and Khoo, 1975). More specifically, Milev et al. (1970) provided 10 g of a semisynthetic diet with either 20 or 0% protein to rats for 8 consecutive days. At that time, the rats were administered 4

μCi Pb by stomach tube and then sacrificed 24 hours later. The investigators determined that the rats reared on a 0.0% protein diet retained 16.7% of the administered lead in the carcass while only 6.9% was retained in the carcass of the 20% group. Lead values in soft tissue including the blood, liver, and kidney, were greater in the deficient rats, while the lead levels in the femur were greater in the 20%-protein-fed rats.

Gontzea et al. (1970) reported that decreasing the protein level in the diet from 18 to 9% casein resulted in a greater retention of subcutaneously administered lead in a variety of tissues including the liver, kidney, blood, and tibia (on a μg/gm of dry wt). More recent studies by Der et al. (1974, 1974a) revealed that lead-exposed rats reared on a 4% casein diet retained markedly greater quantities of lead in whole blood (47 times greater than unexposed controls fed a 4% protein diet), liver (80×), brain (7.4×), bone (18×), and teeth (4×). Rats reared on normal protein diets (20%) and exposed to the same quantity of lead retained about 3 times more lead than the unexposed controls (20%), thereby indicating that a low-protein diet played an exceptional role in enhancing lead retention. The interpretation of the Der et al. (1974, 1974a) study has been the subject of some controversy (Mahaffey, 1977), since individual rats from both groups were given 100 μg of lead acetate daily regardless of body weight. This is of potential importance, since the rats receiving the low-protein diets had extreme growth retardation. Presumably, a better exposure scheme would have provided lead on a μg/kg body weight basis.

In 1975, Barltrop and Khoo not only reported that low levels of dietary protein (i.e., 0 and 5%) enhanced the retention of lead in the blood, kidney, femur, and liver compared to controls (at 20% casein), but that excessive protein (from 40% up to 80%) enhanced the retention of lead in the kidney and femur while diets with 10 and 15% protein had no effect relative to the 20% controls (Table 1).

While the general thrust of the recently discussed studies has supported the fundamental hypothesis that low levels of dietary protein enhance the retention of lead, Quarterman et al. (1978) reported on a variety of experiments that at times found that low levels of dietary protein enhanced the retention of lead, while other fundamentally similar experiments yielded opposite results. Despite the general ambivalent findings of the Quarterman et al. (1978) study, there did appear to be an enhanced retention of lead in the low-protein group with respect to the blood and liver, but the reverse was true for the kidney. Why these results differ from previously reported investigations is

Table 1.   Effects of Dietary Protein on Lead Absorption (Ratio of Mean Retention. Experimental:Control)

Diet (% protein)	Blood	Kidneys	Femur	Liver
0	5.1	2.5	2.8	2.2
5	2.2	2.8	3.3	3.0
10	1	1	1	1
15	1	1	1	1
20 control	1	1	1	1
40	1	2.0	1	1
50	1	1.9	1.3	1
60	1	3.7	2.6	1
80	1	2.5	1.5	1

Source.   Barltrop, D. and Khoo, H.E. (1975). The influence of nutritional factors on lead absorption. *Post-Grad. Med. J.* **51**:795–800.

not known. Possible reasons may be the use of a different strain of rats, different lengths of dietary exposure, differential protein levels, or other changes in research protocol.

In addition, Conrad and Barton (1978) reported that rats reared for three weeks on low-protein diets (0 and 5% protein) exhibited a slightly decreased lead absorption as compared to controls reared on a diet with 25% casein. Although the data of Conrad and Barton (1978) do not contradict the notion that low levels of protein in the diet enhance lead retention, they would suggest that any effect on enhanced retention would be through reducing the rate of lead excretion. Finally, one epidemiologic (i.e., a case-control) study was unable to find any significant differences in protein intake in lead-poisoned children compared to non-poisoned controls (Mooty et al., 1975).

Conclusions.   The question of whether differential dietary levels of protein affect the body burden of lead is still not resolved, especially in light of the ambivalent findings of Quarterman et al. (1978). Although most studies do indicate that a low-protein diet enhances the retention of lead, it must be emphasized that this hypothesis is not easy to evaluate experimentally. The prime reason is that voluntary consumption of food is diminished when the diet is low in protein. It is not known whether the reduction of food intake (i.e., simulation of starvation?) causes an increased retention or whether it is related to the low-protein content of the diet. While pair-feeding techniques have been used to circumvent this methodologic difficulty, Quarterman et al. (1978) stated that "there is no good basis on which to decide if experimental animals eating a low protein diet to appetite should be compared with animals eating the same quantity of a diet containing adequate protein (i.e., pair fed) or with animals eating a diet containing adequate protein to appetite."

In addition, in order to legitimately compare one study with another, one must be aware of the precise dietary levels of all other nutrients in the diet that may affect the uptake, retention, and excretion of lead.

Despite the methodologic problems inherent in this area it does represent a potentially important focus of toxicologic research. At present the results of no truly long-term studies have been published. Future studies should involve a wide range of protein quality and quantity (see Barltrop and Khoo, 1975, 1976) as well as lead levels. Lead exposure should be evaluated both via oral and respiratory routes of administration. Further research should also be directed toward the mechanism by which protein affects lead retention differentially according to tissue. Finally, this study hypothesis lends itself well to epidemiologic investigation as seen in the reports of Mooty et al. (1975) and Strehlow and Barltrop (1978) and should be pursued.

References

Baernstein, H.D. and Grand, J.A. (1942). The relation of protein intake to lead poisoning in rats. *J. Pharmacol. Exp. Therap.* **74**:18–24.

Barltrop, D. and Khoo, H.E. (1975). The influence of nutritional factors on lead absorption. *Post-Grad. Med. J.* **51**:795–800.

Barltrop, D. and Khoo, H.E. (1976). The influence of dietary minerals and fat on the absorption of lead. *The Sci. of the Total Environ.* **6**:265–273.

Biondi, S. (1959). Sull-imprego della sieroalbumine por la prevenzione del saturismo. *Folia. Med.* **42**:62.

Boyadzhiev, V. (1959). Effect of dietary factors on the development and cause of experimental and professional lead intoxication. *Cslka Gastroent Vyz.* **13**:328.

Boyadzhiev, V. (1960). Vlizanie na kraueto mlyako i maslo viskhu vuznikraneto i proichaneto na olovonoto otravyane mezhda akumulatomi rabotnitsi. *Nauchni Trud. Vissh. Med. Inst. Vulko Cheruenkov.* **39**:143.

Buckup, H.; Bohms, M.; Zimmerman, H.; Remy, R.; Portheine, F.U.; and Voss, C. (1956). Nahrungskomponenten und ihre bedutung fur die prophylaxie berufliches bleinergiftung (Experimentelle Untersuchungen am Kaninchen). *Zentbl. Arb. Med. Arb. Schutz.* **6**:29.

Conrad, M.E. and Barton, J.C. (1978). Factors affecting the absorption and excretion of lead in the rat. *Gastroenterology* **74**:731–740.

Der, R.; Fahim, Z.; Hilderbrand, D.; and Fahim, M. (1974). Combined effect of lead and low protein diet on growth, sexual development, and metabolism in female rats. *Res. Commun. Chem. Pathol. Pharmacol.* **9**:723–738.

Der, R.; Hilderbrand, D.; Fahim, Z.; Griffin, W.T.; and Fahim, M.S. (1974a). Combined effect of lead and low protein diet on growth, sexual development and metabolism in male rats. *Trace Substances Environ. Health* **8**:417–431.

De Renzi, S. and Ricciardi-Pollini, R. (1952). Sull'impiego di sero-albumina in compresse chertinzzate nella prevenzione delle intossieazonei da piomba. *Medna Lau.* **43**:276.

Fahim, M.S.; Der, R.; and Fahim, Z. (1975). Combined effect of lead and low protein diet on growth, sexual development, and metabolism. *Fed. Proc.* **34**:810.

Fine, P.R. and Thomas, C.W. (1972). Pediatric blood lead levels: study in 14 Illinois cities of intermediate population. *JAMA* **221**:1475–1479.

Gontzea, I.; Sutzesco, P.; Cocora, D.; and Lungu, D. (1964). Importance de l'apport de proteines sur la resistance de l'organisme a l'intoxication par le plomb. *Archs. Sci. Physiol.* **18**:211.

Gontzea, I.; Sutzesco, P.; Dumitracke, S.; and Bistriceanu, E. (1970). Recherches sur le role de l'apport proteique sur les moyens de defense de l'organisme envers quelque toxiques chimiques. *Arch. Mal. Prof. Med. Trav. Secur. Soc.* **31**:471–480.

Harper, H.A. (1971). *Reviews of Physiological Chemistry* 13th ed., p. 397. Blackwell, Oxford.

Johnson, N.E.; Alcantara, N.E.; and Linkswiler, H. (1970). Effect of level of protein intake on urinary and fecal calcium and calcium retention of young adult males. *J. Nutr.* **100**:1425–1430.

Levander, O.A. (1979). Lead toxicity and nutritional deficiencies. *Environ. Health Perspect.* **29**:115–125.

Lin-Fu, J.S. (1970). Lead poisoning in children. PHS Pub. No. 2180. Govt. Printing Office, Washington, D.C.

Lin-Fu, J.S. (1973). Vulnerability of children to lead exposure and toxicity. Part I. *The New Eng. J. Med.* **289**:1229–1232.

Lin-Fu, J.S. (1973a). Vulnerability of children to lead exposure and toxicity. *New Eng. J. Med.* **289**(24):1289–1293.

MacDonald, N.S. et al. (1953). Agents diminishing skeletal accumulation. *Arch. Ind. Hyg.* **7**:217.

Mahaffey, K.R. (1974). Nutritional factors in lead toxicity. *Environ. Health Perspect.* **7**:107.

Mahaffey, K.R. (1977). Quantities of lead producing health effects in humans: sources and bioavailability. *Environ. Health Perspect.* **19**:285–295.

Mahaffey, K.R.; Stone, C.L.; and Banks, T.A. (1977). Reduction in storage of lead in the rat by feeding diets with elevated iron concentrations. In: *Trace Element Metabolism—3. Proceedings, 3rd International Symposium on Trace Element Metabolism in Man and Animal,* Munich.

Mahaffey-Six, K.R. and Goyer, R.A. (1970). Experimental enhancement of lead toxicity by low dietary calcium. *J. Clin. Lab. Med.* **76**:933.

Mahaffey-Six, K.R. and Goyer, R.A. (1972). The influence of iron deficiency on tissue lead content and toxicity of ingested lead in the rat. *J. Lab. Clin. Med.* **79**:128–136.

Matsukubo, M. (1959). Binding lead with serum proteins. *Tokyo Jikeikai Ikadiagaku Zasshi* **74**:2484.

Merli, A. (1957). The use of serum albumin in the prophylaxis of lead poisoning. In: *Proceedings of XII International Congress on Occupational Health*, p. 294. Helsinki.

Milev, N.; Satler, E.L.U.; and Menden, N. (1970). Aufnahme und Einlaegerung von Glei im Korper unter verschiedenen Ernahrungshedingungen. *Medizin. Ennahr.* 11:29.

Mooty, J.; Ferrand, C.F.; and Harris, P. (1975). Relationship of diet to lead poisoning in children. *Pediatrics* 55(5):636–639.

Moxon, A.L. (1937). Alkali disease or selenium poisoning. *So. Dak. Agr. Exp. Sta. Bull.* 311:50.

Niemoller, H.K. (1957). Zur prophylaxie der bleivergiftung-inhalationsuersuche mit verschiedenen chemikalien. *Dt. Med. Wschr.* 82:738.

Odeschalchi, C.P. (1956). Richerche sulla preunzione medicumentosa del saturnismo. *Minerva Med.* 47:150.

Quarterman, J.; Morrison, E.; Morrison, J.N.; and Humphries, W.R. (1978). Dietary protein and lead retention. *Environ. Res.* 17:68–77.

Smith, M.I.; Lillie, R.D.; and Stohlman, E.F. (1941). The influence of dietary protein on the toxicity of sulfanilamide. *U.S. Pub. Health Repts.* 56:24–29.

Smith, M.I. and Stohlman, E.F. (1940). Further observations on the influence of dietary protein on the toxicity of selenium. *J. Pharm. Exp. Therap.* 40:270–278.

Stephens, R. and Waldron, H.A. (1975). The influence of milk and related dietary constituents on lead metabolism. *Fed. Cosmet. Toxicol.* 13:555–563.

Stevenson, E.S. and White, A. (1940). Influence of iodoacetic acid on sulfur metabolism. Growth studies in the young rat. *J. Biol. Chem.* 134:709–720.

Strehlow, C.D. and Barltrop, D. (1978). Nutritional status and lead exposure in a multiracial population. Presented at the Conference on *Trace Substances in Environmental Health.* University of Missouri, Columbia.

White, A. (1935). The production of a deficiency involving cystine and methionine by the administration of cholic acid. *J. Biol. Chem.* 112:503–509.

White, J. and White, A. (1939). Inhibition of growth of the rat by oral administration of methylcholanthrene, benzpyrene, or pyrene, and the effects of various dietary supplements. *J. Biol. Chem.* 131:149–161.

5. Oxygen

Exposure of patients to hyperbaric oxygen (i.e., oxygen under pressure) has been employed for a number of clinical conditions including carbon monoxide poisoning and thermal injuries. According to Hartz and Lemeshaw (1977), the principal impetus for the use of hyperbaric treatment for extensive burns derived from a study by Iwa (1966) who successfully treated 51 coal miners suffering from extensive thermal injury and carbon monoxide intoxication. Subsequently, numerous investigators replicated and extended the findings that hyperbaric oxygen treatment resulted in decreased mortality and infection as well as enhanced wound-healing (Hartz and Lemeshaw, 1977).

Despite the beneficial therapeutic effects of hyperbaric oxygen treatment, this therapy is not without its negative side effects such as convulsions and hemorrhage in patients and medical surgical personnel. As a result of the potential adverse health effects of hyperbaric oxygen exposure, Gupta and Abraham (1969) evaluated the influence of potential modifying factors such as age, sex, and diet on oxygen toxicity in rats. With respect to diet, these investigators evaluated the influence of 0%, 6%, and 15% (control) casein diets on 95% oxygen toxicity following exposure up to 168 continuous hours.

These investigators reported that rats reared on low-protein diets were markedly less susceptible to the oxygen toxicity. This was evidently based on an absence of toxic convulsions, fewer pathological alterations of the lungs, and longer life. It was speculated that the low-protein diets might have reduced susceptibility to oxygen indirectly via a decreased activity of the adrenal glands.

The relevance of these findings for humans remains to be determined. With so much interest in the use of hyperbaric oxygen in the treatment of burns, the potential for prolonged exposure to patients and workers is of serious concern. Consequently, a greater knowledge of how dietary factors may affect hyperbaric oxygen toxicity is clearly worthy of further investigation.

References

Gupta, S.R. and Abraham, S. (1969). Some factors that affect susceptibility to toxic effects of oxygen. *Ind. J. Med. Res.* **57**(4):739–746.

Hartz, S. and Lemeshaw, S. (1977). A clinical trial of hyperbaric oxygen in the treatment of burn injuries. A literature review and study protocol. Univ. of Mass., School of Public Health, Amherst, MA.

Iwa, T. (1966). *Proc. on the Third Int. Conf. on Hyperbaric Med.* Edited by I.W. Braum and B.G. Cox. *Natl. Acad. Sci.,* Washington, D.C.

6. Phosphorus

Industrial exposure to phosphorus compounds is widespread. Tabershaw et al. (1977) have revealed that "phosphorus is used in the manufacture of munitions, pyrotechnics, explosives, smoke bombs, and other incendiaries, in artificial fertilizers, rodenticides, phosphorbronze alloy, semiconductors, electroluminescent coating, and chemicals such as phosphoric acid and metallic acid . . . and numerous other products." Exposure to phosphorus compounds may result in the development of both adverse local (i.e., burns, irritation of mucous membranes) and systemic (i.e., kidney, pulmonary, jaw injury, dental problems) effects.

Several studies have revealed that diet may affect phosphorus toxicity. The effects of diet on phosphorus toxicity were evaluated because previous studies revealed that the hepatotoxic effects of chloroform could be modified by dietary protein levels (Opie and Alford, 1914), and since phosphorus was also a hepatotoxic agent, it was hypothesized that its toxicity may be similarly altered by dietary protein. In their testing procedure, white rats were fed on experimental diets (i.e., (a) oats and sugar, (b) pig's heart, or (c) beef-fat) 6 days before injection of phosphorus (Opie and Alford, 1914a). In contrast to their results with chloroform, Opie and Alford (1914) reported that the toxicity of phosphorus is enhanced in animals that were given a diet of meat as compared to those rats given diets with larger quantities of carbohydrates or fat. Such findings suggest that future epidemiologic studies concerning the hepatotoxic effects of phosphorus compounds should incorporate a dietary component as one of the variables that may affect the severity of phosphorus toxicity.

Other similarly designed studies revealed that white rats, given a diet rich in carbohydrates, are much less susceptible to nephritis produced by potassium chromate and uranium nitrate than animals reared on a diet of meat or fat (Opie and Alford, 1915).

References

Opie, E.L. and Alford, L.B. (1914). Influence of diet on the toxicity of substances which produce lesions of the liver or the kidney. *J. Amer. Med. Assoc.* **63**:136–137.

Opie, E.L. and Alford, L.B. (1914a). The influence of diet on hepatic necrosis and toxicity of chloroform. *J. Amer. Med. Assoc.* **63**:895.

Opie, E.L. and Alford, L.B. (1915). The influence of diet upon necrosis caused by hepatic and renal poisons. *J. Exp. Med.* **21**:1–21.

Tabershaw, I.R.; Utidjian, H.M.D.; and Kawahara, B. (1977). Chemical hazards. In: *Occupational Diseases: A Guide to Their Recognition.* U.S. DHEW, PHS, CDC, NIOSH. Washington, D.C.

7. Selenium

In contrast to metals such as cadmium, lead, and mercury, which are considered highly toxic agents without any known nutritional value, selenium is an essential nutrient at low levels of exposure in probably all animal species, but it also is a highly toxic as well as a potentially carcinogenic substance at elevated concentrations. Exposure to selenium is regulated in the United States by the EPA with respect to drinking water and by OSHA for occupational exposure. The present drinking water standard for selenium in the United States is 10 ppb and is designed to minimize to the extent feasible the possibility of selenium-induced cancer (EPA, 1975). With respect to occupational exposure, federal standards have been promulgated for several selenium compounds that vary somewhat in their toxicity. These standards are thought to be sufficient to prevent systemic toxicity while minimizing eye and respiratory irritation (Tabershaw et al., 1977; ACGIH, 1976).

Research concerning the influence of diet on selenium toxicity was initiated by Moxon (1937), who was interested in determining if dietary factor(s) could prevent or diminish the toxicity of seleniferous rations to livestock. In studies with rats, Moxon (1937) reported that increasing the calcium and phosphorus content (from 2.8% to 11.2% tri-calcium phosphate) and changing the Ca:P ratio of the ration (1:2 to 1:6) had no beneficial influence. Similarly, it was shown that vitamins A and D did not seem to affect selenium toxicity, as determined by being fed a ration of up to 4% cod-liver oil.

In contrast to the inability of calcium, phosphorus, and vitamins A and D to modify the toxicity of selenium, research began to emerge at about the same time that suggested that dietary protein levels may have a profound influence on the extent and course of selenium toxicity. The first such observation of a protein-selenium interaction was provided by Lewis and Gortner (1937) who noted rats reared on a diet with 30% casein were considerably less susceptible to the adverse health effects (i.e., slowed growth, decreased life span) of added sodium selenite than other rats fed on a diet with only 6% casein.

In that same year, Moxon (1937) also demonstrated that high-protein diets protected rats against selenium-induced toxicity as compared to controls reared on lower-protein diets. For instance, when rats were fed diets containing 10, 20, and 55% of casein along with 37.5 ppm of selenium as sodium selenite, growth was directly related to the level of dietary protein. These initial studies set the stage for subsequent research on the protein-selenium interaction.

In the research that followed, investigators also generally found that animals reared on low levels of protein (e.g., casein) in the diet were much more susceptible to selenium toxicity (Smith, 1939; Gortner, 1940; Smith and Stohlman, 1940; Lewis et al., 1940; Anderson et al., 1941; Moxon, 1941; Moxon and Rhian, 1943; Rosenfeld and Beath, 1946). While most of this research utilized young rats (4–6 weeks old) as the animal model (Smith, 1939; Gortner, 1940; Smith and Stohlman, 1940; Lewis et al., 1940; Moxon, 1937), other models including dogs (Moxon and Rhian, 1943), sheep (Rosenfeld and Beath, 1946), and chicks (Anderson et al., 1941) were used. The type of selenium employed usually involved that naturally occurring in food (i.e., sodium selenite) (Smith, 1939; Smith and Stohlman, 1940) at a concentration of 10 ppm (Moxon, 1937; Gortner, 1940; Lewis and Gortner, 1937; Lewis et al., 1940; Smith and Stohlman, 1940), as well as organic selenium ranging from 15 to 55 ppm (Rosenfeld and Beath, 1946).

Not only did the level of protein (as casein) affect the susceptibility of the animal models to selenium-induced toxicity, so did the type of protein employed (Gortner, 1940; Smith and Stohlman, 1940). Smith and Stohlman (1940) revealed that other proteins (i.e., lactalbumin, ovalbumin, gelatin, and proteins derived from wheat-dried brewer's yeast and desiccated liver), in addition to casein, were also very effective in preventing the occurrence of toxicity from selenium found naturally in food. In partial contrast, Gortner (1940) reported that gelatin (and edestin) were unable to protect against selenium toxicity. Since these various researchers utilized somewhat different study protocols [i.e., each used the gelatin to supplement a different protein base (e.g., either casein or wheat protein)], it is possible that this dietary difference may contribute to these "apparent" conflicting results.

In light of the data showing that not only does the level of protein in the diet but also the quality of protein affect selenium toxicity, researchers decided to evaluate the influence of specific amino acids such as cystine and methionine (Smith and Stohlman, 1940; Klug et al., 1952; Lewis et al., 1940; Gortner, 1940). Since this book is organized according to nutrient, the interaction of specific amino acids such as cystine and methionine will be assessed in the chapter on amino acids. The relevance of the amino acid-selenium interaction is worthy of considerable interest, for it will be there that the mechanisms of how protein detoxifies selenium will be more completely understood. Finally, a recent report by Hill (1979) has indicated that the toxicity (i.e., growth and mortality) of selenium in chicks was not influenced by the protein level in the diet.

References

ACGIH (1976). *Documentation of the Threshold Limit Values*. American Conference of Governmental Industrial Hygienists, Cincinnati, OH.

Anderson, H.D.; Poley, W.E.; and Moxon, A.L. (1941). The effect of dietary protein supplements on the toxicity of seleniferous grains for the chick. *Poult. Sci.* **20**:454.

EPA (1975). Rationale for Drinking Water Standards. Washington, D.C.

Gortner, R.A. Jr. (1940). Chronic selenium poisoning of rats as influenced by dietary protein. *J. Nutr.* **19**(2):105–112.

Hill, C.H. (1979). The effect of dietary protein levels on mineral toxicity in chicks. *J. Nutr.* **109**:501–507.

Klug, H.L.; Harshfield, R.D.; Pengra, R.M.; and Moxon, A.L. (1952). Methionine and selenium. *J. Nutr.* **48**:409–420.

Lewis, H.B. and Gortner, R.A., Jr. (1937). Unpublished data. (Cited in Gortner, 1940).

Lewis, H.B.; Schultz, J.; and Gortner, R.A., Jr. (1940). Dietary protein and the toxicity of sodium selenite in the white rat. *J. Pharm. Exper. Therap.* **68**:292–299.

Moxon, A.L. (1937). Alkali disease or selenium poisoning. *So. Dak. Agr. Exp. Sta. Bull.* **311**:50.

Moxon, A.L. (1941). Some factors influencing the toxicity of selenium. Ph.D. dissertation. Univ. of Wisconsin.

Moxon, A.L. and Rhian, M. (1943). Selenium poisoning. *Physiol. Rev.* **23**:305–337.

Rosenfeld, I. and Beath, O.A. (1946). The influence of protein diets on selenium poisoning. I. *Am. J. Vet. Res.* **7**:52–56.

Schultz, J. and Lewis, H.B. (1940). The excretion of volatile selenium compounds after the administration of sodium selenite to white rats. *J. Biol. Chem.* **133**:199.

Smith, M.I. (1939). The influence of diet on the chronic toxicity of selenium. *Pub. Health Repts.* **54**:1441–1453.

Smith, M.I. and Stohlman, E.F. (1940). Further observations on the influence of dietary protein on the toxicity of selenium. *J. Pharm. Exp. Therap.* **40**:270–278.

Tabershaw, I.R.; Utidjian, H.M.D.; and Kawahara, B.L. (1977). Chemical hazards. In: *Occupational Diseases: A Guide to Their Recognition.* Edited by M. Key et al. U.S. DHEW, NIOSH, Washington, D.C.

B. ORGANIC SUBSTANCES

1. Aflatoxin

An important public health problem that was first recognized in the early 1960s is the presence of fungal contamination on many grains (e.g., peanuts, corn) that are consumed in large quantities by millions of people. Of principal concern is contamination of these grains by *Aspergillus flavus* since the metabolites of this fungus, which are generally termed aflatoxin, are potent hepatotoxic and carcinogenic agents in numerous species (Wogan and Newberne, 1967; Miller, 1973; Newberne, 1974).

Considerable interest has been directed toward identifying dietary factors that may modify the expression of aflatoxin-induced toxicity and carcinogenicity. Some important dietary influences include vitamin A (Newberne and Rogers, 1972; Reddy et al., 1973) and lipotropes (Newberne et al., 1966; Rogers and Newberne, 1969, 1971), as well as protein (Madhavan et al., 1965; Temcharoen et al., 1978).

That dietary protein levels may affect the toxicity of aflatoxin was first reported in 1965 by Madhavan and Gopalan in research with weanling male rats. In a short-term study lasting 20 days these investigators evaluated the influence of a very low level of dietary protein (i.e., 4% casein) on the hepatotoxic effects of aflatoxin (50 μg/day) as compared to similarly exposed controls given a 20%-casein diet. Their study revealed that the low-protein-fed rats developed severe liver lesions while only mild alterations were found in the livers of the controls. However, while the liver changes in the high-protein-fed group were mild, they included vacuolation and atypical cells that suggested the appearance of a precancerous condition.

Since this initial study, researchers have evaluated the influence of dietary protein on aflatoxin toxicity in a variety of species including the rat (McLean and McLean, 1967; Hsu and Tung, 1969), chicks (Marcos and Lebshtein, 1963; Smith et al., 1971), swine (Sisk and Carlton, 1972), and the monkey (Madhavan et al., 1965a), as well as carcinogenicity in rats (Madhavan and Gopalan, 1968) and fish (Leew et al., 1978). In general, the hypothesis that low levels of dietary protein enhance the toxicity of aflatoxin has been confirmed. In contrast, the research of Madhavan and Gapalan (1968) supported their earlier (1965) suspicion that normal levels of dietary protein (in contrast to low levels) enhance the development of aflatoxin-induced hepatomas and tumors of other organs.

A number of studies have revealed that the parent aflatoxin compound is transformed by liver enzymes to its ultimate carcinogenic state, presumably the 2,3-epoxide (AFB-epox) metabolite (Garner et al., 1971, 1972; Garner, 1973, 1973a; Garner and Wright, 1973; Swenson et al., 1973, 1974). In theory, the formation of the "ultimate carcinogen" may be diminished in animal models by consumption of low-protein diets. In fact, Preston et al. (1976) have reported that the proportion of a labeled aflatoxin dose that covalently binds to rat liver nuclear DNA is markedly diminished in rats reared on low-protein diets. Other studies have also supported this perspective by revealing a marked decrease of hepatic mixed-function oxidase activities in rats given a 5%-casein diet for only two weeks.

Thus, when animals are fed a low-protein diet, the parent compound that is more toxic than its metabolites is metabolized more slowly than would occur in animals reared on a higher-protein diet. This may explain why animals reared on a low-protein diet exhibit enhanced susceptibility to the hepatotoxic effects of aflatoxin. In contrast, since the ultimate carcinogen of aflatoxin is a metabolite, then the process of carcinogenesis is dependent on the conversion of the parent compound to the metabolites via the action of the mixed-function oxidase system. Since sufficient protein levels are needed to sustain the activity of these liver enzymes, it follows that animals with adequate dietary protein will be at greater risk to the carcinogenic effects of aflatoxin.

Despite the apparent consistency of the pathological and biochemical investigations for explaining the reasons why low dietary protein enhances aflatoxin-induced toxicity but protects against the aflatoxin-induced carcinogenicity, Adekunle et al. (1978) have partially challenged this position. For instance, "phenobarbitone pretreatment of rats induces mixed function oxidase activity and cytochrome P-450, which have increased abilities to produce aflatoxin epoxide" (Guengerich, 1977), but depresses the binding of aflatoxin epoxide to DNA and tumor formation (Swenson et al., 1977; McLean and Marshall, 1971). Thus, other reaction mechanisms are suggested under certain experimental conditions.

Conclusions. It has been abundantly demonstrated that low levels of dietary protein enhance the hepatotoxicity of aflatoxin; however, that normal levels of protein, sufficient to sustain the activity of the mixed-function oxidase enzymes, enhance the carcinogenicity of AFB, remains to be further evaluated, especially since the only study that specifically demonstrated this was that of Madhavan and Gopalan (1968). Assuming that these findings accurately reflect the influence of dietary protein on the adverse effects of aflatoxin, it appears that dietary manipulation to reduce the adverse effect of aflatoxin would only substitute toxicity for carcinogenicity, or the reverse. While it is true that the present data base is inadequate especially with respect to the influence of excessive supplementation of protein (as well as human epidemiological studies), the only appropriate course of action is to minimize exposure to this potent hepatotoxic and carcinogenic agent.

References

Adekunle, A.A.; Hayes, J.R.; and Campbell, T.C. (1978). Interrelationships of dietary protein levels, aflatoxin B_1 metabolism, and hepatic microsomal epoxide hydrase activity. *Life Sciences* **21**:1785–1792.

Allen-Hoffman, B. and Campbell, T.C. (1977). The relationship between hepatic glutathione levels and the formation of aflatoxin B_1-DNA adducts as influenced by dietary protein intake. *Fed. Proc.* **36**:1116.

Campbell, T.C. and Hayes, J.R. (1976). The role of aflatoxin metabolism in its toxic lesion. *Toxicol. Appl. Pharmacol.* **35**:199–222.

Drill, V.A. and Loomis, T.A. (1946). Effect of methionine on hepatic injury produced by carbon tetrachloride. *Science* **103**:199–201.

Garner, R.C. (1973). Microsome-dependent binding of aflatoxin B_1 to DNA, RNA, polyribonucleotides and protein *in vitro*. *Chem-Biol. Interactions* **6**:125–129.

Garner, R.C. (1973a). Chemical evidence for the formation of a reactive aflatoxin B_1 metabolite, by hamster liver microsomes. *FEBS Letters* **36**:261–264.

Garner, R.C.; Miller, E.C.; and Miller, J.A. (1972). Liver microsomal metabolism of aflatoxin B_1 to reactive derivative toxic to *Salmonella typhimurium* TA 1530. *Cancer Res.* **32**:2058–2066.

Garner, R.C.; Miller, E.C.; Miller, J.A.; Garner, J.V.; and Hanson, R.C. (1971). Formation of a factor lethal for *S. typhimurium* TA 1530 on incubation of aflatoxin B_1 with rat liver microsomes. *Biochem. Biophys. Res. Comm.* **45**:774–780.

Garner, R.C. and Wright, C.M. (1973). Induction of mutations in DNA-repair deficient bacteria by a liver microsomal metabolite of aflatoxin B_1. *Brit. J. Cancer* **28**:544.

Guengerich, F.P. (1977). Separation and purification of multiple forms of microsomal cytochrome P-450. *J. Biol. Chem.* **252**:3970–3979.

Gyorgy, P.; Seifter, J.; Tomarelli, R.M.; and Goldblatt, H. (1946). Influence of dietary factors and sex in toxicity of carbon tetrachloride in rats. *J. Exp. Med.* **83**:449–462.

Hayes, J.R. and Campbell, T.C. (1974). Effect of protein deficiency on the inducibility of the hepatic microsomal drug-metabolizing enzyme system. III. Effect of 3-methylcholanthrene induction on activity and binding kinetics. *Biochem. Pharmacol.* **23**:1721–1731.

Hayes, J.R.; Mgbodile, M.V.K.; and Campbell, T.C. (1973). Effect of protein deficiency on the inducibility of the hepatic microsomal drug-metabolizing enzyme system. I. Effect on substrate interaction with cytochrome P-450. *Biochem. Pharmacol.* **22**:1005–1014.

Hsu, L.C. and Tung, T. (1969). Effects of a low protein diet on aflatoxin toxicity in rats. *Med. Assoc. of Formosa J.* **68**:468–477.

Leew, D.J.; Sinnhuber, R.O.; Wales, J.H.; and Putman, G.B. (1978). Effect of dietary protein on the response of rainbow trout (*Salmo gairdneri*) to aflatoxin B_1. *J. Natl. Can. Inst.* **60**:317–320.

Madhavan, T.V. and Gopalan, C. (1965). Effect of dietary protein on aflatoxin liver injury in weanling rats. *Arch. Pathol.* **80**:123–126.

Madhavan, T.V. and Gopalan, C. (1968). The effect of dietary protein on carcinogenesis of aflatoxin. *Arch. Path.* **85**:133–137.

Madhavan, T.V.; Suryanarayanarao Rao, K.; and Tutpule, P.G. (1965a). Effect of dietary protein level on susceptibility of monkeys to aflatoxin liver injury. *Ind. J. Med. Res.* **53**(10): 984–989.

Madhavan, T.V.; Tulpule, P.G.; and Gopalan, C. (1965). Aflatoxin-induced hepatic fibrosis in Rhesus monkeys. *Arch. Pathol.* **79**:466–469.

Marcos, S.R. and Lebshtein, A.K. (1963). Proteins and toxicity: the effect of different dietary levels of protein in the changes produced by the "groundnut toxin" in chicks. *Arab. Vet. Med. Assoc. J.* **24**:375–380.

McLean, A.E.M. and Marshall, A. (1971). Reduced carcinogenic effects of aflatoxin in rats given phenobarbitone. *Brit. J. Exp. Pathol.* **52**:322–329.

McLean, A.E.M. and McLean, E.K. (1967). Protein depletion and toxic liver injury due to carbon tetrachloride and aflatoxin. *Proc. Nutr. Soc.* **26**:13.

Mgbodile, M.V.K. and Campbell, T.C. (1972). Effect of protein deprivation of male weanling rats on the kinetics of hepatic microsomal enzyme activity. *J. Nutr.* **102**:52–60.

Mgbodile, M.V.K.; Hayes, J.R.; and Campbell, T.C. (1973). Effect of protein deficiency on the inducibility of the hepatic microsomal drug metabolizing enzyme system—II. Effect on enzyme kinetics and electron transport system. *Biochem. Pharmacol.* **22**:1125–1132.

Miller, J.A. (1973). Naturally occurring substances that can induce tumors. In: *Toxicants—Occurring Naturally in Foods*, pp. 508–549. 2nd ed. National Academy of Science.

Miller, L.C. and Whipple, G.H. (1923). Liver injury, liver protection, and sulfur metabolism. *J. Exp. Med.* **76**:421–435.

Newberne, P.M. (1974). Mycotoxins: toxicity, carcinogenicity, and the influence of various nutritional conditions. *Environ. Health Perspect.* **9**:1–32.

Newberne, P.M.; Harrington, D.H.; and Wogen, G.N. (1966). Effects of cirrhosis and other liver insults on induction of liver tumors by aflatoxin in rats. *Lab. Invest.* **15**:962.

Newberne, P.M. and Rogers, A.E. (1972). Vitamin A, liver and colon carcinoma in rats fed low levels of aflatoxin. *Toxicol. Appl. Pharmacol.* **22**:280.

Newberne, P.M. and Rogers, A.E. (1973). Rat colon carcinomas associated with aflatoxin and marginal vitamin A. *J. Natl. Cancer Inst.* **50**:439–448.

Nutr. Rev. (1967). Effect of dietary protein level on aflatoxin liver injury. *Nutrition Reviews* **25**(1):26–28.

Preston, R.S.; Hayes, J.R.; and Campbell, T.C. (1976). The effect of protein deficiency on the *in vivo* binding of aflatoxin B_1 to rat liver macromolecules. *Life Sci.* **19**:1191–1197.

Reddy, G.R.; Tilak, T.B.K.; and Krishnamurthi, D. (1973). Susceptibility of vitamin A-deficient rats to aflatoxin. *Fd. Cosmet. Toxicol.* **11**:467–470.

Rogers, A.E. and Newberne, P.M. (1969). Aflatoxin B_1 carcinogenesis in lipotrope-deficient rats. *Cancer Res.* **29**:1965.

Rogers, A.E. and Newberne, P.M. (1971). Nutrition and aflatoxin carcinogenesis. *Nature* **229**:62.

Sisk, D.B. and Carlton, W.W. (1972). Effect of dietary protein concentration on response on miniature swine to aflatoxins. *Amer. J. Vet. Res.* **33**:107–114.

Smith, J.W.; Hill, C.H.; and Hamilton, P.B. (1971). The effect of dietary modifications on aflatoxicosis in the broiler chicken. *Poult. Sci.* **50**:768–774.

Sriramachari, S. (1958). Nutritional factors in the pathogenesis of hepatic fibrosis. Part II. Effect of low protein diet on mesenchymal response in CCl_4 induced cirrhosis. *Ind. J. Path. Bact.* **1**:35–44.

Swenson, D.H.; Lin, J.K.; Miller, E.C.; and Miller, J.A. (1977). Aflatoxin B_1-2,3-oxide as a probable intermediate in covalent binding of aflatoxins B_1 and B_2 to rat liver DNA and ribosomal RNA *in vivo*. *Cancer Res.* **37**:172–181.

Swenson, D.H.; Miller, J.A.; and Miller, E.C. (1973). 2,3-dihydro-2,3-dihydroxy-aflatoxin B_1: an acid hydrolysis product of an RNA-aflatoxin B_1 adduct formed by hamster and rat liver microsomes *in vitro*. *Biochem. Biophys. Res. Commun.* **53**:1260–1267.

Swenson, D.H.; Miller, J.A.; and Miller, E.C. (1973a). 2,3-dihydro-aflatoxin B_1 adduct formed by hamster and rat liver microsomes *in vitro*. *Biochem. Biophys. Res. Commun.* **53**:1260–1267.

Swenson, D.H.; Miller, J.A.; and Miller, E.C. (1974). Aflatoxin B_1-2,3-oxide: evidence for its formation in rat liver *in vivo* and by human liver microsomes *in vitro*. *Biochem. Biophys. Res. Commun.* **60**:1036–1043.

Temcharoen, P.; Anukaraharonta, T.; and Bhamarapravat, N. (1978). Influence of dietary protein and vitamin B_{12} on the toxicity and carcinogenicity of aflatoxin in rat liver. *Cancer Res.* **38**:2185–2190.

Wogan, G.N. and Newberne, P.M. (1967). Dose-response characteristics of aflatoxin B_1 carcinogenesis in the rat. *Cancer Res.* **12**:50.

2. Azo Dyes

For many years p-dimethylaminoazobenzene (DAB) was used as a dye and as a coloring agent in margarine and butter and had acquired the nickname of "butter yellow." However, the use of DAB as a food additive has long been banned because toxicological/pathological investigations have clearly demonstrated its carcinogenic properties. Today DAB is found exclusively in research laboratories and is employed only for experimental purposes. Thus, exposure of the general public to DAB in food has been eliminated and the industrial use of DAB is regulated by the Occupational Safety and Health Administration (OSHA) (Tabershaw et al., 1977).

While there is very little health-related research associated with DAB today, there were extensive investigations into its toxicological and carcinogenic properties during the 1930s and 1940s. An important component in this health-related research has been a collectively strong attempt to evaluate the influence of nutritional status on the occurrence of tumors caused by exposure to DAB. Readers interested in the influence of vitamins (especially those of the B complex) on the carcinogenicity of DAB should consult *Nutrition and Environmental Health*, volume 1.

That the protein nutritional status of the individual could affect the expression of azo dye-induced tumors was first demonstrated in 1941 by Kensler et al., and Miller et al. Their interest in a possible protein-DAB relationship evolved out of earlier research, which attempted to assess the role of riboflavin in the occurrence of DAB-induced tumors.

While earlier research suggested that inadequate levels of dietary riboflavin enhanced the carcinogenicity of DAB (Kinosita, 1937), subsequent findings of Kensler et al. (1941) revealed that the picture was much more complex. Even though dietary levels of riboflavin were clearly a critical factor affecting susceptibility to DAB-induced tumors, these researchers demonstrated that other dietary factors, including nicotinic acid and casein levels, were also important. In addition, they noted that for riboflavin to be a very effective agent in assisting in the prevention of carcinogenesis, it appeared to require the concomitant presence of casein in sufficient quantity.

Other observations have also confirmed the earlier report of Kensler et al. (1941) that both dietary casein and riboflavin work in concert to help prevent the occurrence of DAB-induced tumors (Harris et al., 1947; Kensler, 1947). While the interaction of sufficient levels of both of these nutrients is necessary to maximize the protective effects, progressive increases of only casein or riboflavin are not effective in reducing azo dye-induced tumors (Griffin et al., 1949; Kensler et al., 1941; Nakahara et al., 1939). Not only does dietary protein interact with riboflavin to reduce the incidence of DAB-induced tumors, it also interacts with the B-vitamin pyridoxine to affect the incidence of DAB-induced tumors. While there were no obvious differences in the incidence of DAB-induced tumors (80 to 90%) between groups of rats given either 48 or 12% casein in the diet along with 2.5 mg/kg of pyridoxine, lowering of the pyridoxine content to only 0.2 mg/kg in both groups resulted in a dramatic decrease in the tumor incidence to "only" 50 and 19% in the low- and high-casein dietary groups, respectively (Miller et al., 1945).

How does dietary protein interact with riboflavin and pyridoxine to prevent DAB-induced cancer? With respect to riboflavin, Serett and Perlzweig (1943) reported that dietary casein and methionine facilitated the retention of riboflavin in the liver of rats administered azo dyes. Several subsequent studies have confirmed the Serett and Perlzweig (1943) report in that the addition of methionine to diets enhanced the storage of riboflavin in the liver (Riesen et al., 1946; Unna et al., 1944; Czaczkes and Guggenheim, 1946; Serett et al., 1942; Serett and Perlzweig, 1943; Griffin et al., 1949; Miller et al., 1948).

As for pyridoxine, it is known to affect protein metabolism in rodents. For example, the nutritional needs of mice for this vitamin are approximately 3 to 4 times greater when there is 60% casein in the diet as compared to only 20% casein (Miller and Baumann, 1945). According to Miller et al. (1945) the metabolism of large quantities of casein seems to facilitate a rapid decrease of the pyridoxal stores in rats. Thus, rats reared on the high-casein (48%), low-pyridoxine (0.2 mg/kg) diet were probably more deficient in pyridoxine than those on the low-casein, low-pyridoxine diet, thereby explaining the greater weight loss and less healthy condition of the rats on the high-protein, low-pyridoxine diet. They concluded that "after the animals reach a certain state of deficiency they may be unable to utilize a sufficient amount of one or more amino acid for the synthesis of protein. In such a situation, the synthesis of protein in both normal and neoplastic tissue could not proceed, which would account for the loss in weight and for the failure of tumor induction and growth."

Conclusions. It is evident that dietary protein does affect the occurrence of DAB-induced tumors in animal models primarily via its interaction with the B-vitamins riboflavin and pyridoxine. In light of the extreme restrictions on the use of azo dyes, such as DAB, the importance of these interesting findings is of more historical than public health interest. However, in light of the widespread exposure to DAB in foods prior to its restriction, one can only speculate as to whether persons exposed to DAB 40 years ago may yet experience DAB-induced tumors and whether the dietary status of protein and B-vitamins may have a role in affecting the expression of such tumorigenesis.

References

Clayton, C.C. and Baumann, C.A. (1949). Diet and azo dye tumors: effect of diet during a period when the dye is not fed. *Cancer Res.* **9**:575–582.

Czaczkes, J.W. and Guggenheim, K.J. (1946). The influence of diet on the riboflavin metabolism of the rat. *J. Biol. Chem.* **162**:267.

Griffin, A.C.; Clayton, C.C.; and Baumann, C.A. (1949). The effects of casein and methionine on the retention of hepatic riboflavin and on the development of liver tumors in rats fed certain azo dyes. *Cancer Res.* **9**:82–87.

Harris, P.N. (1947). The effect of diet containing dried egg albumin upon p-dimethylaminoazobenzene carcinogenesis. *Cancer Res.* **7**:178–179.

Harris, P.N.; Krahl, M.E.; and Clowes, G.H.A. (1947). P-dimethylaminoazobenzene carcinogenesis with purified diets varying in content of cysteine, cystine, liver extract, protein, riboflavin, and other factors. *Cancer Res.* **7**:162–175.

Kensler, C.J. (1947). Effect of diet on the production of liver tumors in the rat by N,N-dimethyl-p-aminoazobenzene. *Ann. New York Acad. Sci.* **49**:29–40.

Kensler, C.J.; Sugiura, K.; Young, N.F.; Halter, C.R.; and Rhoads, C.P. (1941). Partial protection of rats by riboflavin with casein against liver cancer caused by dimethylaminoazobenzene. *Science* **93**:308–310.

Kinosita, R. (1937). Studies on the cancerogenic chemical substances. *Trans. Soc. Path. Jap.* **27**:665–727.

Lepkovsky, S.; Roboz, E.; and Haagen-Smit, A.J. (1943). Xanthurenic acid and its role in the tryptophane metabolism of pyridoxine-deficient rats. *J. Biol. Chem.* **149**:195–201.

Miller, E.C. and Baumann, C.A. (1945). Relative effects of casein and tryptophane on the health and xanthurenic acid excretion of pyridoxine-deficient mice. *J. Biol. Chem.* **157**:551–562.

Miller, E.C. and Baumann, C.A. (1945a). Further factors affecting the excretion of xanthurenic acid. *J. Biol. Chem.* **159**:173–183.

Miller, E.C.; Baumann, C.A.; and Rusch, H.P. (1945). Certain effects of dietary pyridoxine and casein on the carcinogenicity of p-dimethylaminoazobenzene. *Can. Res.* **5**:713–716.

Miller, E.C.; Miller, J.A.; Kline, B.E.; and Rusch, H.P. (1948). Correlation of the level of hepatic riboflavin with the appearance of liver tumors in rats fed aminoazo dyes. *J. Exp. Med.* **88**:89–98.

Miller, J.A.; Miner, D.L.; Rusch, H.P.; and Baumann, C.A. (1941). Diet and hepatic tumor formation. *Can. Res.* **9**:699.

Nakahara, W.; Mori, K.; and Fujiwara, T. (1939). Inhibition of experimental production of liver cancer by liver feeding: a study in nutrition. *Gann.* **33**:406–428.

Riesen, W.H.; Schweisert, B.S.; and Elvehjem, C.A. (1946). The effect of the level of casein, cystine, and methionine intake on riboflavin retention and protein utilization by the rat. *Arch. Biochem.* **10**:387–395.

Schaefer, A.E.; Copeland, D.H.; Salmon, W.D.; and Hale, O.M. (1950). The influence of riboflavin, pyridoxine, inositol, and protein depletion-repletion upon choline deficiency induced neoplasms. *Cancer Res.* **10**:239.

Serett, H.P.; Klein, J.R.; and Perlzweig, W.A. (1942). The effect of the level of protein upon the urinary excretion of riboflavin and nicotinic acid in dogs and rats. *J. Nutr.* **24**:295.

Serett, H.P. and Perlzweig, W.A. (1943). The effect of protein and B-vitamin levels of the diet upon the tissue content and balance of riboflavin and nicotinic acid in rats. *J. Nutr.* **25**:173–183.

Smith, M.I.; Lillie, R.D.; and Stohlman, E.F. (1943). The toxicity and histopathology of some azo compounds as influenced by dietary protein. *Pub. Hlth. Repts.* **58**:304–317.

Tabershaw, I.R.; Utidjian, H.M.D.; and Kawahara, B. (1977). Chemical hazards. In: *Occupational Diseases: A Guide to Their Recognition.* Edited by M.M. Key et al. U.S. DHEW. NIOSH, Washington, D.C.

Westerfield, W.W.; Richert, D.A.; and Hilfinger, M.F. (1950). Studies on xanthine oxidase during carcinogenesis by p-dimethylaminoazobenzene. *Cancer Res.* **10**:486–494.

White, J.; Hein, R.; and White, F.R. (1950). The influence of certain diets on the formation of hepatomas in rats. *Cancer Res.* **10**:249.

Unna, K.; Singher, H.O.; Kensler, C.J.; Taylor, H.C.; and Rhoads, C.P. (1944). Effect of dietary protein on liver riboflavin levels and on inactivation of estradiol. *Proc. Soc. Exper. Biol. Med.* **55**:254–256.

3. Benzene

That benzene toxicity could be modified by dietary factors has been the subject of numerous experiments, especially in the 1930s and 1940s. Particular interest was directed toward the possible interactions of ascorbic acid and benzene, presumably because of the similarities between some of the hemorrhagic manifestations seen in severe benzene poisoning and those of advanced scurvy (Greenburg et al., 1939; Cathala et al., 1936; Castrovilli, 1937; Meyer, 1937; Friemann, 1936, 1938; Bormann, 1938; Hagen, 1938, 1939; Roubinent, 1939; Poumeau-Delille, 1941; Libowitkzy and Seyfried, 1940; Forssman and Frykholm, 1947; Shils and Goldwater, 1949). In addition, several

B-vitamins such as folic acid, pyridoxine, and riboflavin have also been evaluated to a limited degree with respect to their ability to reduce benzene toxicity (Platt et al., 1946; Knutson et al., 1946; Huff and Perlzweig, 1944). In similar fashion, research interest concerning the capacity of dietary protein to affect benzene toxicity was also conducted in the 1940s.

According to Li et al. (1945), dogs reared on an adequate-stock diet are quite resistant to chronic benzene poisoning (see Hough et al., 1944). This observation led them to speculate that the protein level in the diet as well as the functional state of the liver are of major importance in determining the ability to detoxify benzene. Consequently, Li and Freeman (1945, 1947; Li et al., 1945) initiated a series of studies designed to evaluate this hypothesis, using dogs and rats as their animal models.

In the initial study, dogs were exposed for 42 hours each week to benzene vapors (90% C_6H_6) at 600 ppm until they died, or for a maximum of one year for those surviving. Four dietary patterns were followed in this study. They included (1) high protein (21%)-low fat (15%), (2) high protein (25%)-high fat (33%), (3) low protein (8.5%)-low fat (15%), and (4) low protein (10%)-high fat (33%). Among the health parameters considered were: survival time, hematological characteristics, liver function, and urine-sulfate partition.

The results of this investigation indicated that consumption of low-protein diets markedly enhanced benzene toxicity. More specifically, benzene-exposed dogs reared on the low-protein diets exhibited a strikingly lower survival time (5–27 days) as compared to benzene-exposed dogs given a high-protein diet (i.e., greater than 43 days) and dogs reared on a low-protein diet but not exposed to benzene (i.e., survival for at least 42 days).

Modifying the fat levels of the diet while maintaining the protein at a constant level did not produce any significant difference in susceptibility to benzene. In addition, the benzene treatment caused earlier and larger reductions in hepatic-dye clearance and more enhanced leukopenia, thrombopenia, and anemia in dogs consuming the low-protein diets as compared to the unexposed control dogs given a similar low-protein diet and in exposed dogs reared on a high-protein diet.

With respect to their rat study, Li and Freeman (1945) altered the level of protein, fats, and carbohydrates in a way comparable to that described in the dog-exposure studies. In this case the rats reared on the low-protein diets (9 to 11%) and exposed to the same level of benzene in the dog studies (i.e., 600 ppm, 42 hours/week/12 weeks) displayed markedly poorer growth than those maintained on a high-protein diet (30 to 36%) and identically exposed to benzene or than the unexposed controls reared on the low-protein diet. In similar fashion to the dog study, the benzene treatment induced a more marked leukopenia in rats on the low-protein diets. The authors concluded by stating that ". . . a high protein intake supplies more abundantly elements such as sulfur that are necessary for the mechanism of detoxification."

In the evaluation of this hypothesis, Li and Freeman (1947) added enough methionine to produce a sulfur intake equivalent to that of a 30%-casein diet and exposed rats to benzene for the same duration and concentration as in the previous rat study. The incidence of leukopenia among rats that were poisoned with benzene and received methionine was significantly less than it was among rats identically exposed to benzene but whose diet lacked the methionine supplementation, but neither a supplemental intake of methionine nor a 30%-protein diet (Li and Freeman, 1945) totally prevented leukopenia in those groups of rats that were exposed to the benzene.

It is unfortunate that these striking findings of Li and Freeman have not been followed up by other researchers. This is especially true in light of the fact that chronic exposure to benzene is thought to be a cause of leukemia in certain workers (NIOSH, 1976). Is it possible that these individuals consumed diets with lower-than-adequate levels of dietary protein? Could their protein intake not have been of sufficient quality to offset the adverse effect of benzene on leukocytes? Unfortunately, the answers to such questions are not yet known. However, in light of the widespread use of benzene within industry a vigorous effort should be made to more precisely identify and quantify the influence of dietary factors in benzene toxicity and carcinogenicity.

References

Bormann, G. (1938). Zur Diagnose und therapie der chronischen Benzolvergiftung. *Arch. f. Gewerbepath. u. Gewerbehyg.* **8**:194.

Castrovilli, G. (1937). Contributo alla terapia della intossicazione da benzolo (la vitamina C) nel benzolismo specimentale. *Med. d. lavoro* **28**:106.

Cathala, J.; Bolgert, M.; and Grenet, P. (1936). Scorbut chez un sujet soumis a une intoxication benzolique professionelle. *Bull. et mem. soc. med. d. hop. de Paris* **52**:1648.

Drill, V.A. (1952). Hepatotoxic agents: mechanism of action and dietary interrelationship. *Pharm. Rev.* **4**:1–41.

Forssman, S. and Frykholm, K.O. (1947). Benzene poisoning: II. Explanation of workers exposed to benzene with reference to the presence of estersulfate, muconic acid, urochrome A and polyphenols in the urine together with vitamin C deficiency; prophylactic measures. *Acta Med. Scandinav.* **128**:256.

Friemann, W. (1936). Zur Diagnose der chronischen benzolvengiftung. *Arch. f. Gewerbepath. V.* **7**:278.

Friemann, W. (1938). Ueber Verhutung und Neilung der chronischen Benzolvergiftung. *Reichsarbeitsblatt. Arbeitsschutz.* pt. 3, vol. 14, p. 5.

Greenburg, L.; Mayers, M.R.; Goldwater, L.J.; and Smith, A.R. (1939). Benzene (Benzol) poisoning in the rotogravure printing industry in New York City. *J. Indus. Hyg. and Toxicol.* **21**:395.

Hagen, J. (1938). Vitamin C: Stoffruechsel und chronische benzolvergiftung. *Arch. f. Gewerbepath. u. Gewerbehyg.* **8**:541.

Hagen, J. (1939). Erfolge mit vitamin C: Behandlung chronischer benzolschadigungen bei tiefdruckern. *Arch. f. Gewerbepath u. Gewerbehyg.* **9**:698.

Hough, V.H.; Gunn, F.D.; and Freeman, S. (1944). Studies of toxicity of commercial benzene and of mixture of benzene, toluene and xylene. *J. Indus. Hyg. Toxicol.* **26**:296–306.

Huff, I.W. and Perlzweig, W.A. (1944). A product of oxidative metabolism of pyridoxine, 2-methyl-3-hydroxy-4-carboxy-5-hydroxy methyl pyridene. *J. Biol. Chem.* **155**:345.

Knutson, D.; Oldfelt, C.O.; and Wising, P. (1946). The treatment of leukopenia and granulocytopenia with pyridoxine (vitamin B_6). *Acta Med. Scandinav.* **125**:326.

Li, T.W. and Freeman, S. (1945). The effect of protein and fat content of the diet upon the toxicity of benzene for rats. *Amer. J. Physiol.* **145**:158–165.

Li, T.W. and Freeman, S. (1947). The effect of methionine on protein-deficient rats exposed to benzene. *Amer. J. Physiol.* **148**:358–364.

Li, T.W.; Freeman, S.; Hough, V.H.; and Gunn, F.D. (1945). The increased susceptibility of protein-deficient dogs to benzene poisoning. *Amer. J. Physiol.* **145**:166–176.

Libowitkzy, O. and Seyfried, H. (1940). Bedeutung des vitamin C fur benzolarbeiter. *Wien Klin. Wschnschr.* **53**:543.

Meyer, A. (1937). Chronische benzolvergiftung und vitamin C. *Ztschr. f. vitamin forsch.* 6:83, 1937; benzene poisoning. *JAMA* **108**:911.

NIOSH (1976). Criteria document, benzene. National Institute for Occupational Safety and Health. Washington, D.C.

Platt, W.R.; Bluestein, S.G.; and Sisson, R.G. (1946). The effect of liver extract and methylacetamide with p-chlorxylol on artificially induced leukopenia in rats. *Yale J. Biol. Med.* **18**:275.

Poumeau-Delille, G. (1941). Taux de l'acide ascorbique surrenal, hypophysaire et hepatique au cours de l'intoxication benzenique subarque du cobage. *Compt. rend. Soc. de Biol.* **135**:1276.

Roubinent, R. (1939). Le benzolisme professionel. Thesis, Paris. T. Peyrannet.

Shils, M.E. and Goldwater, C.J. (1949). Nutritional factors affecting the toxicity of some aromatic hydrocarbons with special reference to benzene and nitrobenzene compounds: a review. *J. Indust. Hyg. Toxicol.* **31**(4):175–189.

4. Carbon Tetrachloride

Exposure to carbon tetrachloride (CCl_4) is widespread in many industrial settings, as a consequence of its use as a solvent for oils, fats, lacquers, varnishes, rubber, waxes, and resins (Tabershaw et al.,

1977). Industrial exposures to CCl_4 are known to cause irritation to the mucous membranes and depression of the central nervous system, as well as injury to kidneys and especially the liver (ACGIH, 1976). Chronic exposure to as little as 10 ppm CCl_4 will cause liver damage in laboratory animals (Adams et al., 1952). With respect to humans, industrial exposures as low as 25 ppm (but not 10 ppm) are known to result in adverse subjective symptoms including upset stomach, nausea, headache, and dizziness. In light of these data on humans, the ACGIH (1976) proposed a TLV of 10 ppm (65 mg/m³), a value that was adopted by OSHA as the present permissible exposure level in industry.

Toxicity resulting from exposure to CCl_4 has been long known to be affected by dietary factors including several B-vitamins (vitamin B_{12} [Popper et al., 1949; Hove and Hardin, 1951] and nicotinic acid [Gallagher and Simmonds, 1959] and vitamin E [Hove, 1948; Hove and Hardin, 1951; Gallagher, 1961, 1962]), as well as dietary protein. The intention of this section is to critically assess the influence of dietary protein on the toxicity of CCl_4 and to comment on the possible role of such knowledge in industrial hygiene policy.

That the level of dietary protein may affect the expression of CCl_4-induced toxicity was first suggested by Davis in 1924. He was concerned with CCl_4 in light of the then current medical interest in its use as an antihelminthic agent. From his research, Davis clearly demonstrated that diet affected oral CCl_4 toxicity in dogs, with a high-carbohydrate diet being very protective and a high-fat diet enhancing the toxicity. High-protein levels in the diet were generally protective, but not to the extent of the high-carbohydrate diet. While Bollman (1943) confirmed these earlier findings of Davis (1924), Gyorgy et al. (1946) became interested in this topic because the influence of dietary protein on chloroform and CCl_4 toxicity differed. That is, while protein was a very important factor affecting the toxicity of chloroform, it seemed less important with respect to CCl_4.

The results of Gyorgy et al. (1946), while supporting the earlier reports of Davis (1924) and Bollman (1943) that high levels of carbohydrates protect against CCl_4-induced liver and especially renal toxicity and that high dietary fat enhances CCl_4 toxicity, reported that the experimental animals (i.e., rats) fed a low-protein diet (8% casein) exhibited a noticeably greater susceptibility to develop necrotizing nephrosis and liver damage (such as hydropic degeneration, necrosis, and cirrhosis) than those on an 18%-casein diet when exposed to 300 ppm CCl_4 in air for 5 months. In fact, the influence of the protein level in the diet was more important than that of carbohydrate. In addition, they reported that supplements of methionine could successfully replace the protein. In light of their findings, Gyorgy et al. (1946) suggested that "supplements of methionine and of methionine containing protein appear to be the most suitable dietary directions, especially with regard to the renal changes. Nephrosis is often the leading symptom in acute or more protracted exposure to CCl_4 in man (Smetana, 1939). Its possible management by dietary means is worthy of consideration." Other studies by Hove (1948) with male rats supported the Gyorgy et al. (1946) study in that rats reared on a 10%-casein diet were more susceptible to an IP dose of CCl_4 than rats reared on a 14%-casein diet.

Since it seemed that a diet low in protein enhanced the toxicity of CCl_4 (Hove, 1948; Gyorgy et al., 1946) [see Campbell and Kosterlitz (1948) and Sriramachari (1958) for exceptions to this perspective] and that other researchers also seemed to agree that animals reared on a diet deficient in protein were quite susceptible to poisons affecting the liver (Drill, 1952; Rouiller, 1964; McLean et al., 1965), it is difficult to understand why the impressive findings, especially of Gyorgy et al. (1946), were not actively pursued. However, that brief period of apparent quiescence ended in the mid-1960s when McLean and McLean (1965, 1966) reported that rats reared on a protein-free diet as compared to those on a 30%-casein diet were unusually resistant to the adverse effects of CCl_4 as indicated by LD_{50} values and several biochemical and histological-pathological parameters. These investigators originally uncovered this relationship in studies dealing with reno-occlusive disease of the liver, in which CCl_4 was provided to rats reared on a low-protein diet. To their surprise, the rats were found to be quite resistant to the CCl_4, thereby providing the stimulation for further study in this area. Since the enhanced resistance to CCl_4 in the rats fed protein-deficient diets could be markedly reduced by treatment with microsomal enzyme inducers such as DDT (McLean and McLean, 1965, 1966, 1969; Seawright and McLean, 1967), it was speculated that CCl_4 is metabolized by microsomal enzymes resulting in a biointoxification of CCl_4. More recent work by Deo et al. (1975) supported these findings by noting that rhesus monkeys reared on a diet with only 2% casein for 6 weeks were protected from CCl_4-induced hepatotoxicity.

Despite what appears to be a conflict concerning whether or not low levels of dietary protein enhance the toxicity of CCl_4, the problem up to this point seems only to be what is meant by a "low level" of dietary protein. For instance, Gyorgy et al. (1946) and Hove (1948) used 8% and 10% casein as their "low" levels while McLean and associates have employed levels from 0–6% as their "low" levels. Thus, these differences may be more apparent than real. In addition, variation in the levels of vitamins like B_{12} and E may also contribute to differences between reported research findings.

While the preceding explanation has attempted to reconcile the findings of several apparently conflicting studies concerning the influence of dietary protein on CCl_4 toxicity, a number of more recent reports have made this reconciliation quite difficult. Several studies have revealed that a protein-free diet did not reduce the hepatotoxicity of CCl_4 and that an assessment of the hepatocyte ultrastructure of rats reared on a protein-free diet suggested that these cells were more susceptible to damage (Nayak et al., 1970; Chopra et al., 1972, 1972a). A subsequent report by Korsrud et al. (1976) also revealed that rats fed on a diet with 0 or 3% protein were more susceptible to CCl_4-induced hepatotoxicity than those given diets with 10 and 20% casein. In addition, a very high level of protein (i.e., 40%) also enhanced CCl_4 toxicity.

It is difficult to resolve the conflicts between the reports of McLean and associates (1965, 1965a, 1966, 1969) and those of Korsrud et al. (1976). However, Korsrud et al. (1976) have attempted to speculate as to what may have brought about these divergent findings.

"Differences in the design of the experiment might explain the difference between our conclusions regarding a protein-free diet and that made by McLean and McLean (1966). In many of their studies the diets were fed for 4 days. In our study the diet was fed for 14 days. Campbell and Kosterlitz (1948) indicated that the protective effect of a protein-free diet applied only to short-term studies. Another possible cause for the discrepancy could be that McLean and McLean used nonfasted rats. In the present study the rats were fasted for 24 hours before they were killed. However, with the large dose of CCl_4 (2.5 ml/kg) given by McLean and McLean, food consumption would have been considerably reduced. Also, the larger rats used in the present study might have been more resistant to the effects of a protein-free diet."

Conclusions. It has been shown that dietary protein levels markedly affect the toxicity of CCl_4 in ways that are dependent on the degree of deficiency and the extent of excess supplementation, as well as the duration of the dietary regimen prior to CCl_4 exposure. While it is clear from the McLean and McLean (1966) study that 0-to-3%-casein diets markedly enhance resistance to large oral doses of CCl_4, the application of this type of study design for developing extrapolative risk assessments for the industrial worker is exceptionally limited. This is because of (1) the oral route of their exposures versus respiratory, as would customarily occur in industry; (2) the extremely high dosage 2.5

ml/kg, whereas the U.S. federal standard of 10 ppm as a time-weighted average (65 mg/m³) is much lower; and (3) the consumption of diets very low in protein for a prolonged period (i.e., beyond several days) would not be commonly encountered in a normal working population.

The most relevant study with respect to industrial hygiene implications is that of Gyorgy et al. (1946) who employed an inhalation exposure of 300 ppm CCl_4 for up to 5 months (7 hours/day, 5 days/week). The diets of the experimental animals (i.e., male and female rats) were more realistic in that the "low" protein group was given 8% casein as compared to 18% in the controls. Of significance is that the rats fed the low-protein diet exhibited considerably greater susceptibility to the CCl_4 toxicity. While the 300 ppm exposure exceeds the industrial standard by a factor of 30, the study design was remarkably appropriate to the problem at hand. It would certainly be of great relevance to replicate the fundamental approach of this study today, employing a variety of CCl_4-exposure groups (e.g., 0, 5, 10, 25, 50, 100 ppm) for between 12- to 18-months duration with variable levels of protein in the diet. The diets should contain normal, moderately deficient, and moderately excessive intakes of protein in a greater effort to simulate realistic situations. In addition, special consideration must be given to the levels of vitamins B_{12} and E, since they affect protein utilization and CCl_4 toxicity. Finally, the quality of the protein must be quantitatively assessed since diets with differential levels of the sulfur-containing amino acid methionine may result in an altered susceptibility to CCl_4. This is especially important because methionine is thought to be a critical component of protein, which affects CCl_4 toxicity.

References

ACGIH (1976). Documentation of Threshold Limit Values. American Conference of Government Industrial Hygienists. Cincinnati, OH.

Adams, E.M.; Spencer, H.C.; Rowe, V.K.; McCollister, D.D.; and Irish, D.C. (1952). Vapor toxicity of carbon tetrachloride determined by experiments on laboratory animals. *Arch. Ind. Hyg. Occ. Med.* **6**:50–66.

Blendermann, E.M. and Friedman, L. (1968). Influence of carbon tetrachloride, vitamin E, and protein upon liver slice respiratory activity. *Proc. Soc. Exp. Biol. Med.* **129**:831–836.

Bollman, J.L. (1943). Protective value of foods in experimental cirrhosis. *JAMA* **121**:1413.

Campbell, R.M. and Kosterlitz, H.W. (1948). The effects of short-term changes in dietary protein on the response of the liver to carbon tetrachloride injury. *Brit. J. Exp. Path.* **29**:149–159.

Chopra, P.; Roy, S.; Ramalingaswami, V.; and Nayak, N.C. (1972). Mechanism of carbon tetrachloride hepatotoxicity. An *in vivo* study of its molecular basis in rats and monkeys. *Lab. Invest.* **26**:716–725.

Chopra, P.; Roy, S.; Ramalingaswami, V.; and Nayak, N.C. (1972a). Effect of protein-free diet on the ultrastructure of rat liver. *Ind. J. Pathol. Bacteriol.* **15**:1–4.

Davis, N.C. (1924). The influence of diet upon the liver injury produced by carbon tetrachloride. *J. Med. Res.* **44**:601–614.

Deo, M.G.; Roy, H.; and Ramalingaswami, V. (1975). Protein deficiency in carbon tetrachloride-induced hepatic lesions. *Arch. Pathol.* **99**:147–151.

Drill, V.A. (1952). Hepatotoxic agents: mechanism of action and dietary interrelationship. *Pharmacol. Rev.* **4**:1–41.

Gallagher, C.H. (1961). Protection by antioxidants against lethal doses of carbon tetrachloride. *Nature* **192**:881–882.

Gallagher, C.H. (1962). The effect of antioxidants on poisoning by carbon tetrachloride. *Austral. J. Exp. Biol.* **40**:241–254.

Gallagher, C.H. and Simmonds, R.A. (1959). Prophylaxis of poisoning by carbon tetrachloride. *Nature* **184**:1407–1408.

Gyorgy, P.; Seifter, J.; Tomarelli, R.M.; and Goldblatt, H. (1946). Influence of dietary factors and sex on the toxicity of carbon tetrachloride in rats. *J. Exp. Med.* **83**:449–462.

Hove, E.L. (1948). Interrelation between α-tocopherol and protein metabolism. III. The protective effect of vitamin E and certain nitrogenous compounds against CCl_4 poisoning in rats. *Arch. Biochem. Biophys.* **17**:467–474.

Hove, E.L. and Hardin, J.O. (1951). Effect of vitamin E, B_{12}, and folacin on CCl_4 toxicity and protein utilization in rats. *Proc. Soc. Exp. Biol. Med.* **77**:502–505.

Korsrud, G.O.; Kuiper-Goodman, T.; Hasselager, E.; Grice, H.C.; and McLaughlan, J.M. (1976). Effects of dietary protein level on carbon tetrachloride-induced liver damage in rats. *Toxicol. Appl. Pharmacol.* **37**:1–12.

McLean, A.E.M. (1967). The effect of diet and vitamin E on liver injury due to carbon tetrachloride. *Brit. J. Exp. Path.* **48**:632–636.

McLean, A.E.M. and McLean, E.K. (1965). Diet, microsomal enzymes and carbon tetrachloride toxicity. *Biochem. J.* **97**:31p.

McLean, A.E.M. and McLean, E.K. (1966). The effect of diet and 1,1,1-trichloro-2,2-bis-(p-chlorophenyl) ethane (DDT) on microsomal hydroxylating enzymes and on sensitivity of rats to carbon tetrachloride poisoning. *Biochem. J.* **100**:564–571.

McLean, A.E.M. and McLean, E.K. (1969). Diet and toxicity. *Brit. Med. Bull.* **25**:278–281.

McLean, A.E.M.; McLean, E.K.; and Judah, J.D. (1965). Cellular necrosis in the liver induced and modified by drugs. *Intern. Rev. Exp. Pathol.* **4**:127–157.

McLean, E.K.; Bras, G.; and McLean, A.E.M. (1965a). Venous occlusions in the liver following dimethylnitrosamine. *Brit. J. Exp. Path.* **46**:367–369.

Nayak, N.C.; Chopra, P.; and Ramalingaswami, V. (1970). The role of liver cell endoplasmic reticulum and microsomal enzymes in carbon tetrachloride toxicity. An *in vivo* study. *Life Sci.* **9**:1431–1439.

Popper, N.; Koch-Weser, D.; and Szanto, P.B. (1949). Protective effect of vitamin B_{12} upon hepatic injury produced by carbon tetrachloride. *Proc. Soc. Exp. Bio. Med.* **71**:688–690.

Rouiller, C. (1964). In: *The Liver,* Vol. 2, p. 335. Edited by C. Rouiller. Academic Press, N.Y. and London.

Seawright, A.A. and McLean, A.E.M. (1967). The effect of diet on carbon tetrachloride metabolism. *Biochem. J.* **105**:1055–1060.

Smetana, H. (1939). Nephrosis due to carbon tetrachloride. *Arch. Int. Med.* **63**:760–777.

Sriramachari, S. (1958). Nutritional factors in the pathogenesis of hepatic fibrosis: Part II. Effect of low protein diet on mesenchymal response in CCl₄ induced cirrhosis. *Ind. J. Path. Bact.* **1**:35–44.

Tabershaw, J.R.; Utidjian, H.M.D.; and Kawahara, B. (1977). *Chemical hazards.* In: *Occupational Diseases: A Guide to Their Recognition.* Edited by M.M. Key et al. U.S., DHEW, NIOSH, Washington, D.C.

5. Chloroform

Chloroform ($CHCl_3$) is a broadly used solvent in many industries. Of particular importance is its usage in the lacquer industry, in the manufacture of certain pharmaceuticals such as penicillin, as well as in the synthesis of artificial silk, plastics, floor polishes, and fluorocarbons (Tabershaw et al., 1977). The Occupational Safety and Health Administration has established a federal standard of 50 ppm, while in 1976 the ACGIH recommended a TLV of only 25 ppm. Prolonged industrial exposure is known to result in liver and kidney damage. As expected, alcoholics are at particularly high risk to developing chloroform-induced liver damage. More recently, the EPA has been especially concerned over the inadvertent formation of chloroform resulting from the treatment of drinking water with chlorine for disinfection purposes (NAS, 1977). Widespread exposure of the general public to even low levels of chloroform (i.e., between 50–200 ppb) in drinking water is of concern since animal experimentation suggests that chloroform may be a carcinogen (NCI, 1976). To what extent exposure to chloroform in drinking water may present a cancer hazard is highly debatable (Stokinger, 1977; NAS, 1977).

That dietary status may affect the toxicity of chloroform has long been known. In fact, as far back as 1914, Opie and Alford reported on the influence of various diets on acute chloroform toxicity. These researchers tested the hypothesis that dietary protein levels may affect the extent of chloroform toxicity based on the research of Strassmann/Salkowski and Howland/Richards, who reported that chloroform increased the excretion of sulfur and nitrogen (Opie and Alford, 1914, 1915). Their results indicated that white rats reared for 4 days on a diet of oats and sugar were markedly more resistant to the acutely toxic effects of chloroform than rats reared on either meats (i.e., pig's heart) or fat (of beef), with those on the fat diet being exceptionally more susceptible.

Based on these findings and several subsequent reports (Davis and Whipple, 1919; Moise and Smith, 1924; Smith and Moise, 1924; Goldschmidt et al., 1939; Miller and Whipple, 1940, 1942; Campbell and Kosterlitz, 1948), Miller (1948) concluded that a high-fat diet enhances the storage of chloroform in the liver, thereby enhancing toxicity, while a diet high in carbohydrates and/or protein protects against the destruction of body proteins.

High-protein diets are thought to provide protection against liver damage because of the presence of specific factors in the protein. This conclusion is based on reports that consumption of diets low in protein increase resistance to liver damage if there are adequate levels of lipotropes (e.g., methionine), vitamins (e.g., vitamin E), and certain trace elements (e.g., selenium) (Campbell and Kosterlitz, 1948; McLean et al., 1965).

In marked contrast to these very consistent findings was the more recent study of McLean and McLean (1969) that noted that protein depletion did not markedly affect the toxicity of chloroform given as a single oral dose. According to McLean and McLean (1969), it is difficult to resolve the apparent disagreement between their studies and those of the previously cited researchers. However, they suggested that "factors . . . which might account for the difference includes larger numbers of animals, quantitative assessment of liver damage, oral administration of chloroform instead of by inhalation, and highly purified diets."

In light of the findings of McLean and McLean (1969), it is not very clear how low levels of protein may affect the toxicity of chloroform. It is also unclear as to the public health significance of chronic low-level exposure to chloroform. While there is currently a flurry of epidemiologic studies being sponsored by the EPA on the possible association of chloroform in drinking water with cancer of the gastrointestinal tract, kidney, and liver, it would seem that toxicological research designed to establish more firmly the animal cancer findings should include an evaluation of the possible enhancing (or protective) effects of different levels of dietary protein, including specific amino acids such as methionine.

References

ACGIH (1976). Documentation of the Threshold Limit Values for Substances in Workroom Air. *Amer. Conf. Govern. Indus. Hyg.*, Cincinnati, OH., 3rd ed.

Campbell, R.M. and Kosterlitz, H.W. (1948). The effects of short-term changes in dietary protein on the response of the liver to carbon tetrachloride injury. *Brit. J. Exp. Path.* **29**:149.

Davis, N.C. and Whipple, G.H. (1919). The influence of fasting and various diets on the liver injury effected by chloroform anaesthesia. *Arch. Int. Med.* **23**:612.

Goldschmidt, S.; Vars, H.M.; and Raudin, I.S. (1939). The influence of the foodstuffs upon the susceptibility of the liver to injury by chloroform, and the probable mechanism of their action. *J. Clin. Invest.* **18**:277–289.

McLean, A.E.M. and McLean, E.K. (1969). Diet and toxicity. *Brit. Med. Bull.* **25**:278–281.

McLean, A.E.M.; McLean, E.K.; and Judah, J.D. (1965). Cellular necrosis in the liver induced and modified by drugs. *Inter. Rev. Exp. Path.* **4**:127–157.

Miller, L.L. (1948). Nutritional factors affecting the toxicity of halogenated hydrocarbons. *Occup. Med.* **5**:194–209.

Miller, L.L. and Whipple, G.H. (1940). Chloroform liver injury increases versus protein stores decrease. Studies in nitrogen metabolism in these dogs. *Amer. J. Med. Sci.* **19**:204–225.

Miller, L.L. and Whipple, G.H. (1942). Liver injury, liver protection, and sulfur metabolism. *J. Exper. Med.* **76**:421–435.

Moise, T.S. and Smith, A.H. (1924). The regeneration of liver tissue on various adequate diets. *J. Exper. Med.* **40**:13.

NAS (1977). *Drinking Water and Health.* The National Research Council, National Academy of Engineering, National Academy of Science, Washington, D.C.

NCI (1976). Report on the carcinogenesis bioassay of chloroform. National Cancer Institute, Bethesda, MD.

Opie, E.L. and Alford, L.B. (1914). The influence of diet on hepatic necrosis and toxicity of chloroform. *J. Amer. Med. Assoc.* **62**:895–896.

Opie, E.L. and Alford, L.B. (1915). The influence of diet upon necrosis caused by hepatic and renal poisons. *J. Exper. Med.* **21**:1–21.

Smith, A.H. and Moise, T.S. (1924). The regeneration of liver tissue during nutrition on inadequate diets and fasting. *J. Exper. Med.* **40**:209.

Stokinger, H.E. (1977). Toxicology and drinking water contaminants. *AWWA J.* **399**:402.

Tabershaw, I.R.; Utidjian, H.M.D.; and Kawahara, B. (1977). Chemical hazards. In: *Occupational Diseases: A Guide to Their Recognition.* Edited by Key, M.M. et al. U.S. DHEW, NIOSH, Washington, D.C.

6. 1,2-Dichloroethane

Occupational exposure to 1,2-dichloroethane ($ClCH_2CH_2Cl$) is commonly found today as a result of its widespread use in the manufacture of a number of products including ethyl glycol, diaminoethylene, chlorocholine chloride, polyvinyl chloride, nylon, viscose rayon, styrene-butadiene rubber, and certain plastics. In addition, it is employed as a solvent for resins, asphalt, bitumen, rubber, cellulose acetate ester, and paint; other uses include being a degreaser in the engineering, textile, and petroleum industries, an extracting agent for soybean oil and caffeine, an antiknock agent in gasoline, a pickling agent, fumigant and dry-cleaning agent, as well as being used in photography, xerography, water softening and in the production of adhesives, cosmetics, pharmaceuticals, and varnishes (Tabershaw et al., 1977). With that list of possible industrial uses, it is not unexpected that numerous occupations will ultimately provide exposure to this agent.

Research on the toxicological effects of 1,2-dichloroethane is not very extensive. However, a number of studies with animal models have revealed it to cause liver and kidney damage following prolonged exposure (Heppel et al., 1946; Spencer et al., 1951). Several instances of human fatalities resulting from accidental ingestion and/or inhalation also resulted in liver, kidney, and pulmonary damage (Spencer et al., 1951). Based on chronic animal exposure studies at 100 ppm for 6 months (Spencer et al., 1951) and industrial monitoring that suggested that levels between 25 to 50 ppm were safe for prolonged exposure (Fassett, 1962), the ACGIH (1976) recommended a TLV of 50 ppm; this value was adopted by OSHA for the federal standard as well.

Since only a few studies have investigated the toxicity of 1,2-dichloroethane, it is not unexpected that research concerning the influence of dietary status on the toxicity of this compound is also minimal (Heppel et al., 1945, 1946). However, in the one study that considered the influence of protein dietary status on the toxicity of 1,2-dichloroethane, the researchers did find that protein status could play a major role. In short-term exposure studies of up to 43 days, Heppel et al. (1945) reported that a low-casein diet (4%) markedly enhanced the toxicity (i.e., mortality incidence, pathological studies) of inhaled 1,2-dichloroethane at 400 and 1000 ppm as compared to controls given 20% casein. The combination of a low-casein-plus-high-fat (40%) diet further enhanced the toxicity.

The relevance of these studies remains to be more properly assessed. It may be legitimately argued that the exposures of 400 and 1000 ppm were greatly in excess of the present TLV of 50 ppm and therefore quite unrealistic; in addition, while high-fat diets may be common, a consistently inadequate protein intake by workers is probably the exception.

These results therefore indicate that rats reared on either low-protein or low-protein, high-fat diets are at increased risk to 1,2-dichloroethane toxicity. In order to make these interesting findings more relevant, they must be followed up with studies that involve exposure and diets that reflect those of workers. In light of the findings of Heppel et al. (1945) and the widespread industrial exposure to 1,2-dichloroethane (Tabershaw et al., 1977), it would seem that further research in this area would be of value.

References

ACGIH (1976). Documentation of the Threshold Limit Values for Substances in Workroom Air. Amer. Conf. Govern. Indust. Hygienists, Cincinnati, OH. 3rd edition, pp. 79–80.

Fassett, D. (1962). Private communication (cited in ACGIH, 1976).

Heppel, L.A.; Neal, P.A.; Perrin, T.L.; Endicott, K.M.; and Porterfield, V.T. (1945). The toxicity of 1,2-dichloroethane (ethylene) (III). Its acute toxicity and the effect of protective agents. *J. Pharm. Exp. Therap.* **84**:53.

Heppel, L.A.; Neal, P.A.; Perrin, T.L.; and Porterfield, V.T. (1946). Toxicology of 1,2-dichloroethane (ethylene dichloride); influence of dietary factors on toxicity of dichloropropane. *J. Indust. Hyg. Tox.* **28**:113–120.

Spencer, H.C.; Rowe, V.K.; Adams, E.M.; McCollister, D.D.; and Irish, D.D. (1951). Vapor of ethylene dichloride determined by experiments on laboratory animals. *Arch. Indust. Hyg. Occ. Med.* **4**:482.

Tabershaw, I.R.; Utidjian, H.M.D.; and Kawahara, B.L. (1977). Chemical hazards. In: *Occupational Diseases. A Guide to Their Recognition.* Edited by M.M. Key et al. U.S. DHEW, NIOSH, pp. 199–201.

7. 1,2-Dichloropropane

1,2-Dichloropropane (propylene dichloride) ($CH_3CHClCH_2Cl$) is quite similar to 1,2-dichloroethane with regard to structure as well as industrial functions, some of which include its use for degreasing and dry cleaning, in the manufacture of cellulose plastics, rubber, waxes, and numerous organics, as well as being a soil fumigant (Tabershaw et al., 1977).

Prolonged exposure to elevated levels (1000 ppm) resulted in death and liver damage to dogs, guinea pigs, and rats (Heppel et al., 1946). Studies by Heppel et al. (1948) reported that long-term exposure studies (about 6 months) at 400 ppm/7 hours/day/5 days/week caused no adverse histological changes in several species of animals. However, a mouse of the C_3H strain died from such exposure, while survivors developed hepatomas. Although these data should have generated considerable concern, the ACGIH (1976) apparently was not convinced that it was a carcinogen and established 75 ppm as its TLV.

That diet (i.e., protein status) can modify the toxicity of propylene dichloride has been the subject of only one study. Using an experimental protocol similar to their earlier studies with 1,2-dichloroethane, Heppel et al. (1946a) exposed weanling rats via inhalation to 1000 ppm or 1500 ppm propylene dichloride for 7 hours/days/5 days/week. Animals reared on a low-protein diet (8%) were markedly more susceptible as judged by mortality and liver pathology as compared to the controls (25%). In light of the limited data, it is not possible to extrapolate such findings to humans with confidence. However, such findings do suggest a need for further research in this area.

References

ACGIH (1976). Documentation of the Threshold Limit Values for Workroom Air. Amer. Conf. Gov. Indus. Hygienists. 3rd edition.

Heppel, L.A.; Highman, B.; and Peake, E.G. (1948). Toxicology of 1,2-dichloropropane (propylene dichloride); effects of repeated exposures to low concentration of vapor. *J. Ind. Hyg. Tox.* **30**:189–191.

Heppel, L.A.; Highman, B.; and Porterfield, V.T. (1946a). Toxicology of 1,2-dichloropropane (propylene dichloride). *J. Pharmacol. Exp. Therapy.* **87**:11–17.

Heppel, L.A.; Neal, P.A.; Highman, B.; and Porterfield, V.T. (1946). Toxicology of 1,2-dichloropropane (propylene dichloride): studies on effects of daily inhalations. *J. Ind. Hyg. and Tox.* **28**:1–8.

Tabershaw, I.R.; Utidjian, H.M.; and Kawahawa, B.L. (1977). Chemical hazards. In: *Occupational Diseases: A Guide to Their Recognition.* Edited by M.M. Key et al. U.S. DHEW, NIOSH, Washington, D.C.

8. Dimethylbenz[a]anthracene (DMBA)

Using DMBA as a chemical model, Clinton et al. (1979) attempted to evaluate the influence of dietary protein levels (7.5, 15, and 45%) on chemical carcinogenesis in the rat. They reported that when rats were fed the above mentioned percentages of dietary protein for 4 weeks prior to initiation by DMBA, followed by placing all animals on an identical 15% protein diet, an inverse relationship between protein levels and cancer incidence occurred. In addition, when the dietary pattern was reversed so that all diets were identical prior to initiation but with different protein levels (7.5, 15, and 45%) after initiation for an additional 25 weeks, no effect of diet on cancer outcome was found.

The authors concluded by stating that the evidence supports the hypothesis that dietary protein level affects the initiation but not the promotion phase of carcinogenesis.

Reference

Clinton, S.L.; Truex, C.R.; and Visek, W.J. (1979). Dietary protein, aryl hydrocarbon hydroxylase and chemical carcinogenesis in rats. *J. Nutr.* **109**:55–62.

9. 1,2-Dimethylhydrazine

A growing number of epidemiologic studies has associated the distribution of large-bowel cancer with dietary habits, especially those that involve the consumption of large quantities of fat and beef (Wynder et al., 1968; Doll, 1969; Stemmermann, 1970; Haenszel et al., 1973; Armstrong and Doll, 1975), use of refined sugar, and deficiency of fiber (Burkitt, 1975). While these epidemiological studies have been of enormous value in the identification of potential-risk factors, there is considerable need to isolate potential-risk factors and evaluate them in a vigorously controlled experimental fashion via the use of appropriate animal models. In light of the fact that several teams of investigators have developed animal models to induce colon cancer via the administration of dimethylhydrazine (DMH), Reddy et al. (1976) decided to investigate the influence of high-protein (beef or soybean protein) and high-fat (beef fat or corn oil) diets on DMH-induced colon tumors in rats. Their results indicated that rats fed on a diet high in protein and fat and administered DMH (sc) exhibited a statistically significant higher incidence of colon tumors than DMH-exposed rats reared on a diet with normal levels of protein and fat. Of particular interest was that the protein or fat source (i.e., whether it was of plant or animal origin) had no major influence on the incidence of colon cancer (Reddy et al., 1976a).

Considerable research has been conducted in order to establish a biochemical explanation of how elevated levels of protein and/or fat may enhance the occurrence of chemical carcinogenesis. It has been speculated that diets with high quantities of fat alter the level of the intraluminal bile acids and neutral steroids (Hill et al., 1971; Wynder and Reddy, 1975; Reddy et al., 1976). That bile salts may be implicated in the promotion of colon cancer in animal models has also been supported by other investigations as well (Narisawa et al., 1974; Reddy et al., 1974, 1976b; Nigro et al., 1973; Chomchai et al., 1974).

Although there are many uncertainties still to be resolved with respect to the role of dietary protein in chemical carcinogenesis, the research by Reddy and co-workers has helped to open up an important area of biomedical research. For not only may elevated levels of protein and/or fat be factors in colon cancer but they may also serve to promote the occurrence of cancer that has been initiated from exposure to certain industrial carcinogens.

References

Armstrong, B. and Doll, R. (1975). Environmental factors and the incidence and mortality from cancer in different countries with special reference to dietary practices. *Int. J. Cancer* **15**:617–631.

Burkitt, D.P. (1975). Large-bowel cancer: an epidemiological jigsaw puzzle. *J. Natl. Cancer Instit.* **54**:3–6.

Chomchai, C.; Bhadrachari, N.; and Nigro, N.D. (1974). The effect of bile on the induction of experimental tumors in rats. *Dis. Colon Rectum* **17**:310–312.

Doll, R. (1969). The geographic distribution of cancer. *Brit. J. Cancer* **23**:1–8.

Haenszel, W.; Berg, J.W.; Segi, M.; et al. (1973). Large-bowel cancer in Hawaiian Japanese. *J. Natl. Cancer Instit.* **51**:1756–1799.

Hill, M.J.; Crowther, J.S.; Drasar, B.S.; Hawksworth, G.; Aries, V.; and Williams, R.E.O. (1971). Bacteria and aetiology of cancer of the large bowel. *Lancet* **1**:95–100.

Narisawa, T.; Magadia, N.E.; Weisburger, J.H.; et al. (1974). Promoting effect of bile acids on colon carcinogenesis after intrarectal instillation of N-methyl-n-nitro-n-nitrosoguanidine in rats. *J. Natl. Cancer Instit.* **53**:1093–1097.

Nigro, N.D.; Bhadrachari, N.; and Chomchai, C.A. (1973). Rat model for studying colonic cancer: effect of cholestyramine on induced tumors. *Dis. Colon Rectum* **16**:438–443.

Reddy, B.S.; Narisawa, T.; Vukusich, D.; Weisburger, J.H.; and Wynder, E.L. (1976). Effect of quality and quantity of dietary fat and dimethylhydrazine in colon carcinogenesis in rats. *Proc. Soc. Exp. Biol. Med.* **151**:237–239.

Reddy, B.S.; Narisawa, T.; and Weisburger, J.H. (1976a). Effect of a diet with high levels of protein and fat on colon carcinogenesis in F344 rats treated with 1,2-dimethylhydrazine. *J. Natl. Cancer Instit.* **57**:567–569.

Reddy, B.S.; Narisawa, T.; Weisburger, J.H.; et al. (1976b). Promoting effect of deoxycholate on colon adenocarcinomas in germfree rats. *J. Natl. Cancer Instit.* **56**:441–442.

Reddy, B.S.; Weisburger, J.H.; and Wynder, E.L. (1974). Effect of dietary fat level and dimethylhydrazine on fecal acid and neutral sterol excretion and colon carcinogenesis. *J. Natl. Cancer Instit.* **52**:507–511.

Stemmermann, G.N. (1970). Patterns of disease among Japanese living in Hawaii. *Arch. Environ. Health* **20**:266–273.

Wynder, E.L.; Kajitani, T.; Ishikawa, S.; Dodo, H.; and Takano, A. (1968). Environmental factors of cancer of the colon and rectum. II. Japanese epidemiological data. *Cancer* **23**:1210–1220.

Wynder, E.L. and Reddy, B.S. (1975). Dietary fat and colon cancer. *J. Natl. Cancer Instit.* **54**:7–10.

10. Microsomal Enzyme Detoxification

The role of liver microsomal enzymes in environmental toxicology is truly immense. For while the detoxification and excretion of xenobiotic compounds is exceptionally complex and multifaceted, no clear understanding and genuine appreciation of this process is complete without defining the role of the microsomal enzymes. Indeed, not only are these enzymes involved in the process of detoxification but also with biointoxication, as a result of which many compounds are made more toxic and/or carcinogenic than the parent compound.

Considerable interest has been directed toward clarifying the influence of nutritional status on drug metabolism (Campbell et al., 1979). According to Basu and Dickerson (1974), several important issues must be addressed in this regard. Can dietary deficiencies disrupt or diminish detoxification mechanisms? Can the process of detoxification result in a specific nutrient deficiency? If inadequate nutrition reduces the efficiency of the detoxification process, can it then be hypothesized that adverse effects from pollutant exposure would be more frequent in poorly nourished individuals?

The role of dietary protein on the function of microsomal enzymes has been studied to a limited extent (Kato et al., 1962, 1968; Saggers et al., 1970; Mgbodile and Campbell, 1972; Marshall and McLean, 1969; Weatherholtz et al., 1969; Campbell et al., 1979). Kato et al. (1968) have reported that the toxicities of a number of xenobiotics (including pentobarbital, aminopyrine, and aniline) in young rats of both sexes reared on diets with variable levels of protein for two weeks are highly correlated with the rate of drug metabolism by liver microsomal enzymes, and that the activities of these enzymes are likewise highly correlated to the levels of dietary protein ingested. These findings have been supported by other workers such as Marshall and McLean (1969), who have demonstrated that giving a 3%-casein diet to adult male rats for 14 days reduces the level of cytochrome P-450 per gram of liver tissue to approximately 1/3 of the control values.

Numerous examples can be given that demonstrate that a low-protein diet affects the ability of the body to form toxicologically active metabolites, presumably by reducing the activity of the microsomal enzymes (Basu and Dickerson, 1974; Czygan et al., 1974, 1974a; Kleihues et al., 1976). For instance, McLean and Verschuuren (1969) demonstrated that a protein-free diet protects young male rats from the lethal and hepatotoxic effects of dimethylnitrosamine (DMN), possibly via preventing or reducing the formation of a toxic product, diazomethone, a potent methylating agent (Magee and Vandekar, 1958; Magee and Lee, 1964). Other research with DMN has revealed that its metabolism, that is, its biointoxication to a bacterial mutagen, depends on cytochrome P-450, the terminal oxidase of the microsomal biotransformation system (Czygan et al., 1973, 1974; Popper et al.,

1973). Other studies by Czygan et al. (1974a) revealed that the activation of DMN was decreased in mice by protein- and protein-choline-deficient diets (Figure 7-1) and that this reduction coincided with a reduction in microsomal cytochrome P-450 levels. Similarly, the chlorinated hydrocarbon insecticide heptachlor is considerably less toxic (i.e., by a factor of 3) in rats reared on a low-protein diet (5% casein for 10 days) as compared to pair-fed controls given 20% or 40% dietary casein (Weatherholtz et al., 1969), presumably due to the lack of ability to form the toxic metabolite heptachlor epoxide (Wong and Terriere, 1965; Weatherholtz and Webb, 1971).

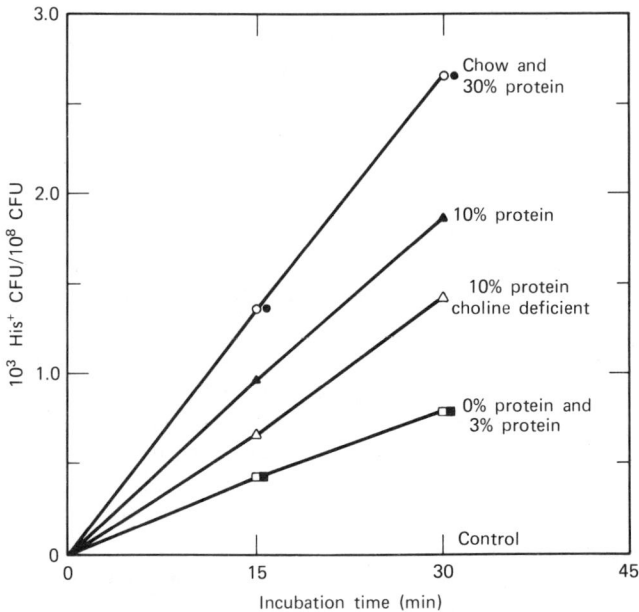

Figure 7-1. Influence of microsomes isolated from mice fed different diets on the frequency of DMN induced *his** colony-forming units *((CFU)* of *S. typhimurium* TA 1535 (generously provided by Professor B. N. Ames, Department of Biochemistry, University of California at Berkley). The incubation mixture contained 15 mg microsomal protein, an NADPH-generating system, 6 to 9 × 10^3 *his* colony-forming units, and 100 mM DMN in 2.75 ml 0.1 M phosphate buffer, pH 7.4, and was incubated at 37°. In the controls either the microsomes or NADPH-generating system or DMN were omitted. [*Source.* Czygan, P.; Greim, H.; Garro, A.; Schaffner, F.; and Popper, H. (1974). The effect of dietary deficiency on the ability of isolated hepatic microsomes to alter the mutagenicity of a primary and a secondary carcinogen. *Cancer Res.* **34:**119–123.]

In contrast to these examples where a low-protein diet resulted in a diminution of either toxicity or mutagenicity is the response of N-methyl-N-nitro-N-nitrosoguanidine (MNNG). Presumably, MNNG is a primary mutagen whose metabolism results in the formation of fewer mutagenic metabolites. In this case, a low-protein diet would maximize the adverse effect, while the situation is reversed when DMN is considered (Czygan et al., 1974).

Not only does the quantity of protein in the diet affect the capacity of microsomal enzymes to metabolize xenobiotic compounds, the quality of protein does so as well. Miranda and Webb (1973) were able to demonstrate that rats given either casein (18%) or gluten (18%) in the diet have markedly different capacities to metabolize a number of xenobiotics, including ethylmorphine, aniline, and phenobarbital. The reduced capacity of the gluten-treated rats to metabolize the xenobiotics to as great an extent as those given a similar percentage of casein in the diet was speculated as resulting from the "imbalance and/or deficiency of amino acids in gluten. Either amino acid imbalance or deficiency or both might be hindering the *de novo* synthesis of microsomal enzymes or of some factors or components of the mixed function oxidase system for drug metabolism."

The above discussion clearly demonstrates that the quantity and quality of dietary protein can markedly influence the ability of the liver microsomal enzymes to metabolize a wide variety of foreign compounds. Depending on the specific compounds, this altered metabolism may result in greater or less toxicologic and carcinogenic capabilities than the parent compound. Thus the presence of low protein does not necessarily result in an adverse response. Even though these findings have provided a greater understanding of nutrient-pollutant interactions, there are insufficient data upon which to infer with confidence the potential role of protein dietary status in environmental carcinogenesis. However, these data are sufficiently impressive to lead one to recognize that the quality and quantity of dietary protein may play an important role in the body's capacity to detoxify or toxify foreign compounds. Future research should be directed to elucidate further the complexity of this important area, especially with respect to the influence of animal-vs.-plant protein sources.

While previously discussed studies evaluated the influence of dietary protein on microsomal enzyme metabolism of xenobiotics in either bacterial or rodent models, Alvares et al. (1976) studied the interaction of nutritional factors (i.e., dietary protein and carbohydrate levels) with drug metabolism in human volunteers. Three normal volunteers were provided a low-carbohydrate, high-protein diet for 14 days, followed by a high-carbohydrate, low-protein diet for the next 14 days. At the end of each two-week testing period, the plasma-elimination rates of antipyrene and theophylline were assessed. The data revealed that the type of diet markedly altered the metabolism of both drugs, with the plasma half-life being considerably longer for the high-carbohydrate, low-protein dietary treatment with both antipyrene (17.5 hr vs. 9.2 hr) and theophylline (8.9 hr vs. 5.9 hr). These findings are consistent with published studies with animals in which a high-protein diet enhanced the MFO activity and diminished the action of drugs (Kato et al., 1968), and with reports indicating that consumption of high-carbohydrate diets reduces the MFO activity (Strother et al., 1971; Jansson and Schenkman, 1975). In recent investigations with human volunteers, Anderson et al. (1979) have supported and extended the original findings of Alvares et al. (1976) by revealing that a high-protein diet markedly reduces the mean plasma half life of antipyrine and theophylline as compared to high carbohydrate and fat diets. In addition, the degree of saturation of the dietary fat did not affect the metabolic rate of these two drugs.

What are the biomedical implications of these findings? According to Alvares et al. (1976), the nutritional-pharmacological interactions observed in these studies in man have considerable importance in relation to the biological effect of drugs ingested in individuals suffering from protein malnutrition, in debilitated chronically ill patients, in postoperative patients receiving glucose, and especially among the large segment of the normal population among whom dietary manipulations (e.g., a decrease in carbohydrate intake), are carried out in weight-reducing regimens. These striking findings clearly have just touched the tip of the iceberg and suggest that important advances will be forthcoming in this critical area of nutritional status and drug/pollutant metabolism.

References

Alvares, A.P.; Anderson, K.E.; Conney, A.; and Kappas, A. (1976). Interactions between nutritional factors and drug biotransformations in man. *Proc. Natl. Acad. USA* **73**(7):2501–2504.

Anderson, K.E.; Conney, A.H.; and Kappas, A. (1979). Nutrition and oxidative drug metabolism in man: Relative influence of dietary lipids, carbohydrate, and protein. *Clin. Pharm. Therap.* **26**:493–501.

Basu, T.K. and Dickerson, J.W.T. (1974). Inter-relationships of nutrition and the metabolism of drugs. *Chem-Biol. Interactions* **8**:193–206.

Campbell, T.C.; Hayes, J.R.; Merrill, A.H. Jr.; Maso, M.; and Goethchius, M. (1979). The influence of dietary factors on drug metabolism in animals. *Drug Metabolism Rev.* **9**:173–184.

Czygan, P.; Greim, H.; Garro, A.J.; Hutterer, F.; Rudick, J.; Schaffner, F.; and Popper, H. (1974a). Cytochrome-P-450 content and the ability of liver microsomes from patients undergoing abdominal surgery to alter the mutagenicity of a primary carcinogen and a secondary one. *J. Natl. Cancer Instit.* (Cited in *Cancer Res.* **34**:119–123, 1974).

Czygan, P.; Greim, H.; Garro, A.J.; Hutterer, F.; Schaffner, F.; Popper, H.; Rosenthal, O.; and Cooper, D.Y. (1973). Microsomal metabolism of dimethylnitrosamine and the cytochrome P-450 dependency of its activation to a mutagen. *Cancer Res.* **33**:2983–2986.

Czygan, P.; Greim, H.; Garro, A.J.; Schaffner, F.; and Popper, H. (1974). The effect of dietary deficiency on the ability of isolated hepatic microsomes to alter the mutagenicity of a primary and a secondary carcinogen. *Cancer Res.* **34**:119–123.

Jansson, I. and Schenkman, J.B. (1975). Studies on three microsomal electron transfer enzyme systems. *Mol. Pharmacol.* **11**:450–461.

Kato, R.; Chiesara, E.; and Vassanelli, P. (1962). Factors influencing induction of hepatic microsomal drug-metabolizing enzymes. *Biochem. Pharmacol.* **11**:211–220.

Kato, R.; Oshima, T.; and Tumizawa, S. (1968). Toxicity and metabolism of drugs in relation to dietary protein. *Jap. J. Pharmacol.* **18**:356–366.

Kleihues, P.; Kolar, G.F.; and Margison, G.P. (1976). Interaction of the carcinogen 3,3-dimethyl-l-phenyl-triazene with nucleic acids of various rat tissues and the effect of a protein-free diet. *Cancer Res.* **36**:2189–2193.

Magee, P.N. and Lee, K.Y. (1964). Cellular injury and carcinogenesis. *Biochem. J.* **91**:35–42.

Magee, P.N. and Vandekar, M. (1958). Toxicity of liver injury: the metabolism of dimethylnitrosamine *in vitro. Biochem. J.* **70**:600–605.

Marshall, W.J. and McLean, A.E.M. (1969). The effect of oral phenobarbitone on hepatic microsomal cytochrome P-450 and demethylation activity in rats fed normal and low protein diets. *Biochem. Pharmacol.* **18**:158.

McLean, A.E.M. and Verschuuren, H.G. (1969). Effects of diet and microsomal enzyme induction on the toxicity of dimethylnitrosamine. *Brit. J. Exptl. Pathol.* **50**:22–25.

Mgbodile, M.V.K. and Campbell, T.C. (1972). Effect of protein deprivation of male weanling rats on the kinetics of hepatic microsomal enzyme activity. *J. Nutr.* **102**:53–60.

Miranda, C.L. and Webb, R.E. (1973). Effect of dietary protein quality on drug metabolism in the rat. *J. Nutr.* **103**:1425–1430.

Popper, H.; Czygan, P.; Greim, H.; Schaffner, F.; and Garro, A.J. (1973). Mutagenicity of primary and secondary carcinogens altered by normal and induced hepatic microsomes. *Proc. Soc. Exptl. Biol. Med.* **142**:727–729.

Saggers, V.H.; Harirathnajothi, N.; and McLean, A.E.M. (1970). The effect of diet and phenobarbitone on quinine metabolism in the rat and in man. *Biochem. Pharmacol.* **19**:499–503.

Strother, A.; Throckmorton, J.K.; and Herzer, C. (1971). The influence of high sugar consumption by mice on the duration of action of barbiturates and *in vitro* metabolism of barbiturates, aniline and p-nitroanisole. *J. Pharmacol. Exp. Therap.* **179**:490–498.

Weatherholtz, W.M.; Campbell, T.C.; and Webb, R.E. (1969). Effect of dietary protein levels on the toxicity and metabolism of heptachlor. *J. Nutr.* **98**:90–94.

Weatherholtz, W.M. and Webb, R.E. (1971). Influence of dietary protein on the activity of microsomal epoxidase in the growing rat. *J. Nutr.* **101**:9–12.

Wong, D.T. and Terriere, L.C. (1965). Epoxidation of aldrin, isodrin and heptachlor by
    rat liver microsomes. *Biochem. Pharmacol.* **14**:375–377.

11. MOCA—4,4′-methylene-bis (2-chloroaniline):
An Aromatic Amine

MOCA (Figure 7-2) is an aromatic diamine that is employed as a
curing agent for epoxy resins. Linch et al. (1971) have reported that
Dupont initiated the production of MOCA in 1954 with full-scale commercial manufacture in 1962. While MOCA displays typical toxicity
characteristics of aromatic amines, the main concern with MOCA is
whether it is a human carcinogen.

This concern surfaced in 1969 when Steinhoff and Grundmann reported that MOCA was carcinogenic to rats. In the years that followed
MOCA has repeatedly been shown to induce cancerous growths in a
variety of tissues in mice (Russfield et al., 1975), rats (Steinhoff and
Grundmann, 1969; Stula et al., 1975; Kommineni et al., 1979) and dogs
(Stula et al., 1977). However, epidemiological evidence of MOCA's carcinogenicity in humans has not yet been demonstrated, perhaps due to
the lack of a sufficient latency period and/or population size.

Although it is not known whether MOCA is a human carcinogen,
there is evidence that dietary protein may affect the occurrence of
MOCA-induced cancer in rats. In fact, the original studies of Steinhoff
and Grundmann (1969, 1971) demonstrating the capability of MOCA
to induce tumors in rats utilized low protein diets (i.e., about 7% protein) based on a review by Badger and Lewis (1952), which suggested
that dietary protein status affected azo dye-induced carcinogenicity.
However, no comparison with the influence of a normal protein diet on
MOCA carcinogenicity was carried out. Later studies by Steinhoff and
Grundmann (1971) revealed that consumption of a low-protein diet
reduced the latency period of MOCA-induced liver cancer as compared
to rats fed an adequate diet. Unfortunately, a detailed presentation of
the research methodology was not given.

More recent findings by Kommineni et al. (1979) have revealed that
a low-protein diet enhanced the occurrence of MOCA-induced heman-

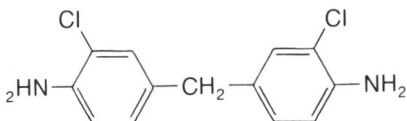

Figure 7-2. Chemical structure of
MOCA.

giosarcomas as well as liver and zymbol gland cancer at 500 ppm compared to protein adequate rats. In contrast, rats fed on a protein-adequate diet developed a higher incidence of lung and mammary tumors than the low-protein groups at MOCA levels of 250 and 500 ppm. Since the low-protein-fed rats weighed approximately 20% less than the protein-adequate group at adulthood, possible differential caloric intake may be a confounding factor. This is of potential importance since consumption of low caloric diets diminishes cancer risk (Tannenbaum, 1940, 1942, 1944, 1945; Carroll, 1975).

In conclusion, MOCA has been clearly established as a carcinogen in three animal species, the mouse, rat, and dog. Evidence indicates that a low-protein dietary intake may enhance the occurrence of MOCA-induced liver and zymbol gland cancer as well as hemangiosarcomas at 500 ppm but not at lower exposures in rats (Kommineni et al., 1979). Finally, while the original MOCA carcinogenicity studies of Steinhoff and Grundmann (1969) utilized low-protein diets, since this was thought to be a condition that enhanced azo dye-induced carcinogenicity, the principal point of the Badger and Lewis (1952) study was that low riboflavin consumption may enhance azo dye-induced cancer. Perhaps future studies should evaluate whether riboflavin levels affect MOCA induced carcinogenicity.

References

Badger, G.M. and Lewis, G.E. (1952). The carcinogenic azo-compounds: Chemical constitution and carcinogenic activity. *Brit. J. Cancer* **6**:270–292.

Carroll, K.K. (1975). Experimental evidence of dietary factors and hormone-dependent cancers. *Cancer Research* **35**:3374–3383.

Grundmann, E. and Steinhoff, D. (1970). Liver and lung tumors due to 3,3'-dichloro-4,4'diamino-diphenylmethane in rats. *Z. Krebsforsch.* **74**:28–39.

Kommineni, C.; Groth, D.H.; Frockt, I.J.; Voelker, R.W.; and Stanovick, R.P. (1979). Determination of the tumorigenic potential of methylene-bis-orthochloroaniline. *J. Environ. Pathol. Toxicol.* **2**:149–171.

Linch, A.L.; O'Connor, G.B.; Barnes, J.R.; Killian, A.S., Jr.; and Neeld, W.E. (1971). Methylene-bis-ortho-chloroaniline (MOCA): Evaluation of the hazards and exposure control. *Amer. Ind. Hyg. Assoc. J.* **32**:802–819.

Russfield, A.B.; Homburger, F.; Boger, E.; Van Dongen, L.G.; Weisburger, E.K.; and Weisburger, J.H. (1975). The carcinogenic effect of 4,4'-methylene bis (2-chloroaniline) in mice and rats. *Toxicol. Appl. Pharmacol.* **31**:47–54.

Steinhoff, D. and Grundmann, E. (1969). Carcerogene wirking von 3,3'-dichlor-4,4'-diaminodiphenylmethan bei Ratten. *Naturwissenschaften* **56**:215–216.

Steinhoff, D. and Grundmann, E. (1971). Zur cancerogenen wirking von 3,3'-dichlor-4,4'-diaminodiphenylmethan bei Ratten. *Naturwissenschaften* **58**:578.

Stula, E.F.; Barnes, J.R.; Sherman, H.; Reinhardt, C.F.; and Zapp, J.A., Jr. (1977). Urinary bladder tumors in dogs from 4,4'-methylene-bis (2-chloroaniline) (MOCA). *J. Environ. Pathol. Toxicol.* 1:31–50.

Stula, E.F.; Sherman, H.; Zapp, J.A., Jr.; and Clayton, J.W., Jr. (1975). Experimental neoplasia in rats from oral administration of 3,3'-dichlorobenzidine, 4,4'methylene-bis (2-chloroaniline), and 4,4'-methylene-bis (2-methylaniline). *Toxicol. Appl. Pharmacol.* 31:159–176.

Tannenbaum, A. (1940). The initiation and growth of tumors. Introduction. I. Effects of underfeeding. *Amer. J. Cancer* 38:335–350.

Tannenbaum, A. (1942). The genesis and growth of tumors. II. Effects of caloric restriction per se. *Cancer Res.* 2:460–467.

Tannenbaum, A. (1944). The dependence of the genesis of induced skin tumors on the caloric intake during different stages of carcinogenesis. *Cancer Res.* 4:673–677.

Tannenbaum, A. (1945). The dependence of tumor formation on the composition of the calorie-restricted diet as well as on the degree of restriction. *Cancer Res.* 5:616–625.

12. Nitrosamines

The toxicity of a variety of compounds is known to be affected by the level of protein in the diet. For instance, rats reared on a protein-free diet are more resistant to carbon tetrachloride (McLean and McLean, 1965, 1966). Presumably, the lack of adequate protein in the diet markedly reduces the activity of liver microsomal enzymes, which are needed to transform the carbon tetrachloride to a more toxic state. In fact, administering potent microsomal enzyme inducers such as phenobarbitone or DDT to rats reared on a protein-deficient diet results in enhanced susceptibility to the toxic effects of carbon tetrachloride. Since dimethylnitrosamine (DMN) is hypothesized to cause its acute toxic as well as carcinogenic effects following its conversion to a toxic metabolite via action of liver microsomal enzymes in a comparable fashion to the carbon tetrachloride scheme, McLean and Verschuuren (1969) suggested that the toxicity of nitrosamines may also be modified by dietary levels of protein.

Subsequent experimentation confirmed their hypothesis, in that rats reared on a protein-free diet were protected from the lethal (LD_{50} studies) and hepatotoxic (plasma isocitric dehydrogenase and bilirubin levels) effects of DMN. However, in contrast to studies with carbon tetrachloride, the protection could not be reversed by treatments that restore microsomal enzyme activity (phenobarbital or DDT treatment). That a protein-deficient diet offered protection against the acute toxic effects of DMN was subsequently verified by McLean and Magee (1970), but this dietary treatment enhanced the production of kidney tumors (McLean and Magee, 1970; Swann and McLean, 1968, 1971). Correlated with the enhanced renal carcinogenesis of the protein deficiency was the recognition that "the methylation by DMN of guanine in kidney nucleic acids of these rats was three times that in the rats fed on a normal diet." The enhanced susceptibility of the kidney to DMN-induced tumors in rats reared on a protein-deficient diet results presumably because this animal model can only metabolize a small percentage of the original dose of DMN in the liver, leaving more to be metabolized in the kidney.

While the studies of McLean and associates have revealed that a protein-deficient diet enhanced renal carcinogenicity in DMN-treated rats, Czygan et al. (1974) have noted that a protein deficiency in mice led to a significantly reduced capacity of isolated microsomes to produce DMN-induced mutations in bacteria. Since most carcinogens are known to be mutagens, this suggests that a protein deficiency may reduce the carcinogenicity of DMN. Yet the data on carcinogenic responses with the rat model revealed just the opposite. Such findings, while not in direct conflict with each other, do illustrate the potential complexity of nutrient-pollutant-species interactions (see the microsomal enzyme section in this chapter).

References

Czygan, P.; Greim, H.; Garro, A.; Schaffner, F.; and Popper, H. (1974). The effect of dietary protein deficiency on the ability of isolated hepatic microsomes to alter the mutagenicity of a primary and a secondary carcinogen. *Cancer Res.* 34:119–123.

McLean, A.E.M. and Magee, P.N. (1970). Increased renal carcinogenesis by dimethylnitrosamine in protein deficient rats. *Brit. J. Exptl. Path.* 51:587–590.

McLean, A.E.M. and McLean, E.K. (1965). Diet, microsomal enzymes and carbon tetrachloride toxicity. *Biochem. J.* 97:31P.

McLean, A.E.M. and McLean, E.K. (1966). The effect of diet and 1,1,1-trichloro-2,2-bis-(p-chlorophenyl) ethane (DDT) on microsomal hydroxylating enzymes and on sensitivity of rats to carbon tetrachloride poisoning. *Biochem. J.* 100:564–571.

McLean, A.E.M. and Vershuuren, H.G. (1969). Effects of diet and microsomal enzyme induction on the toxicity of dimethylnitrosamine. *Brit. J. Exptl. Path.* 50:22–25.

Swann, P.F. and McLean, A.E.M. (1968). The effect of diet on the toxic and carcinogenic action of dimethylnitrosamine. *Biochem. J.* 107:14P–15P.

Swann, P.F. and McLean, A.E.M. (1971). Cellular injury and carcinogenesis. The effect of a protein-free, high-carbohydrate diet on the metabolism of dimethylnitrosamine in the rat. *Biochem. J.* 124:283–288.

13. Pesticides

Introduction. Volumes have been written about pesticides, including their synthesis, mechanisms of action, and ecological and human health effects. Not only is the technical literature extensive, but a considerable number of books concerning pesticides have been written in order to increase the awareness of the general public to the environmental health considerations of widespread pesticide use.

While the predominant emphasis in the toxicological research area has focused on the relationship of molecular structure and the toxicity of the specific pesticide, there has been interest in identifying biological factors that may affect pesticide toxicity (Calabrese, 1978, 1979). While limited investigations have suggested that certain developmental, genetic, and disease conditions may enhance pesticide toxicity, the notion that nutritional status may affect pesticide toxicity has been the most widely studied of these biological predispositions. One of the earliest nutritional factors identified as influencing pesticide toxicity is the level of dietary protein. This section will review the relationship between dietary protein and pesticide toxicity, with particular emphasis on its public health significance.

Initial Investigations.   There has been considerable interest concerning the effects of dietary protein status on the toxicity of chlorinated hydrocarbon pesticides. The first such study was published by Lee et al. in 1964 and evaluated the hypothesis that several of the hepatotoxic manifestations of chlorinated hydrocarbon insecticide exposure (i.e., fatty infiltration, hydropic degeneration, and focal necrosis [Durham et al., 1963; Treon and Cleveland, 1955; Laug et al., 1950]) could be modified by a variable level of dietary protein. Male rats were maintained on either a low- (10%) or high- (25%) protein diet for up to one month and exposed to variable levels of dieldrin (0 to 200 ppm), depending on the specific treatment. The rats were compared for a range of parameters including weight gain, body composition, mortality, organ weights, certain liver enzyme activities (i.e., glucose-6-phosphate dehydrogenase, α-ketoglutarate-phenylalanine transaminase, α-ketoglutarate-aspartate transaminase, and pyruvic-phenylalanine transaminase), vitamin A metabolism, liver histology, and resistance to swimming stress as measured by the length of time the animal could remain afloat in a cylinder of water with a 5 gm weight attached to the tail. The results indicated that at both levels of dietary protein a decrease in weight gain occurred over 1 month as the concentration of dieldrin increased. However, statistical significance at the .01 level occurred only in the low-protein group exposed to 200 ppm dieldrin. Dieldrin-enhanced mortality occurred in both the high- and low-protein-fed rats consuming 200 ppm of dieldrin but only among the low-protein-fed rats consuming 150 ppm dieldrin. In addition, only in dieldrin-exposed rats reared on the low-protein diets was there an increase in liver lipids. Vitamin A per gram of liver was also diminished in all dieldrin-treated groups on either diet, while the total liver-vitamin A levels were reduced in the low-protein groups at 150 and 200 ppm and only at the 200 ppm level for rats maintained on the high-protein diet. Finally, the livers of rats on either the high- or low-protein diets exhibited dieldrin-induced cellular edema and fatty infiltration. These changes were more marked in the rats maintained on the low-protein diets. As a result of the above findings, the authors concluded that the protein content of the diet confers some protection with respect to weight gain and hepatic injury. However, the differential level of protein in the diet did not seem to significantly affect other changes including vitamin-A metabolism, liver-enzyme activities, and response to swimming stress. It should be pointed out that the food was given ad libitum and not in a pair-fed arrangement. Since these data indicated that at elevated levels of dieldrin exposure (e.g., 200 ppm) the diet appeared sufficiently unpalatable to the rats, the decrease in weight gain was not necessarily a function of dieldrin toxicity and/or protein content of the diet. This type of methodological limitation is an important consideration, since it introduces an important confounding variable.

Low Levels of Dietary Protein. Following the original publication by Lee et al. (1964), a series of articles was published by Eldon Boyd and his colleagues concerning the influence of dietary protein on pesticide toxicity (see Boyd, 1969, for a review). The prime public health focus was the concern that in many undeveloped countries the levels of protein in the diet may be very inadequate and consequently may predispose individuals to become susceptible to pesticide-induced toxicity.

In 1968, DeCastro and Boyd reported that the growth of weanling albino rats was diminished by 50% when they were reared for one month on a diet containing 8% casein, 75% starch, 14% hydrogenated vegetable oils, 3% salt mix, and adequate vitamin supplements as compared to rats given Purina laboratory chow. However, there was a slight decrease in growth rate when the level of casein was increased to 27% and the starch reduced to 56% when compared to the growth of such rats given the Purina laboratory chow. In that same year, Liu and Boyd reported that intragastrically administered starch in doses of 100 g/kg of body weight/day did not reduce growth to as great an extent as the low-protein diets in young albino rats. Consequently, Liu and Boyd (1967) suggested that the predominate explanation for the stunted growth in the DeCastro and Boyd (1968) study could not be the influence of the starch (at 75%), but most likely was the low-protein (8%) content of their diet.

Based on the assumption that the low-protein diet not only affected an impaired growth but also may cause a decreased capacity to detoxify drugs, Boyd and DeCastro (1968) reasoned that individuals who consume diets low in protein may have an enhanced risk to experience pesticide-induced toxicity. Of particular interest in evaluating this hypothesis was that DeCastro and Boyd (1968) reported that an animal model (i.e., weanling rats) could be made to develop a kwashiorkor-like condition when fed a protein-deficient diet (8%) for 28 days, or 3% of their life span. DeCastro and Boyd (1968) stated that this 28-day time period is equivalent to 2–3 years of a human life and it is during this time after weaning that kwashiorkor is most prevalent. In fact, clinical symptoms of the experimental rats are comparable to those of kwashiorkor in infants (see Trowell et al., 1964), except for the absence of anorexia, edema, diarrhea, a generalized dermatitis, and a very high death rate.[1] Certain gross and microscopic pathological changes (i.e., fatty livers and degenerative changes in the gastrointestinal tract, salivary glands, kidneys, thymus and adrenal glands) that were seen in human infants with kwashiorkor were not found in the rat model (Trowell et al., 1964; DeCastro and Boyd, 1968).

During the rearing of the weanling rats on the low-protein diets there was little or no growth during the first week, with the concomitant development of symptoms of kwashiorkor. The rats seemed to adapt to the diet from week 2 through week 4 and usually exhibited a growth approximately one-third of that of the rats fed the normal diet. Consequently, the initial toxicologic studies of Boyd and his associates compared the responses of the weanling male rats on the low-protein diet (8%) for 28 days to similar rats given a diet with 27% casein and 56% starch, with all other conditions being identical (Boyd, 1969).

In the initial two studies the influence of the low-protein diets was evaluated with respect to DDT (Boyd and DeCastro, 1968) and carbaryl[2] toxicity (Boyd and Boulanger, 1968). Under the experimental conditions it was reported that both DDT and carbaryl toxicity were enhanced in the low-protein groups as indicated by decreased LD_{50} values (481 mg/kg to 345 mg/kg for DDT; 575 mg/kg to 506 mg/kg for carbaryl). Although these increases in toxicity were statistically sig-

---

[1]However, anorexia did occur in the kwashiorkoric rats just before death, while the dermatitis in human infants begins as zones of depigmentation that would not appear in the rat model.

[2]Carbaryl (1-naphthyl-N-methylcarbamate) is a carbamate insecticide acting via an anticholinesterase mechanism.

nificant, the authors did not feel that degree of enhancement was of particular public health importance. This conclusion was based not just on the LD_{50} values but on a variety of clinical symptoms (i.e., immediate lacrimation, salivation, tremors, convulsive movement, anorexia, aciduria, hematuria, glycosuria, proteinuria, and respiratory failure) that were generally similar between the two groups.

Following these two initial studies, Boyd (1969) reported that the 8%-casein diet that had been used for the low-protein regimen was removed from the commercial market. Thus they adopted a new low-protein diet[3] that contained 3.5% casein instead of 8%. In addition, the "normal" protein diet was also changed from 27 to 26% casein, from 56 to 59% cornstarch, with the remainder being identical to that of the low diet. Interestingly, under this new diet the weanling male rats reared on the low-protein diet were 2 times more susceptible to the acute oral toxic effects of lindane than the controls; that is, the LD_{50} was 95 mg/kg for the rats on the low-protein diet and 184 mg/kg for those on the control diet. Based on these findings, Boyd and Chen (1968) suggested that the proposed lethal dose in humans for lindane of 150 mg/kg (WHO, 1967) may be reduced for populations with low-protein diets. In a similar fashion, Boyd and Krijnen (1968) reported that the LD_{50} of captan in rats fed the 3.5%-casein diet was only 1/26th of the controls.

In light of the rather striking augmentation of lindane and captan toxicity in weanling rats given a low-protein diet of 3.5% casein, the original conclusion of Boyd and DeCastro (based on studies in which the low-protein diet was 8% casein) that "DDT is no more dangerous as a pesticide in countries where the diet is low in protein and high in carbohydrate than in countries where the intake of these foods is adequate" may not be appropriate.

Consequently, Boyd and Krijnen (1969) evaluated the acute oral toxicity of DDT in albino rats fed for 28 days from weaning on diets containing from 0 to 81% of protein as casein. The results indicated that at 0%, 3%, and 9% casein in the diet there was an 83%, 64%, and 32% decrease in the LD_{50}, respectively, compared to controls on a 21% casein diet, thereby forcing a change in the original conclusion on DDT toxicity as stated above. Similarly, Boyd and DeCastro (1970) administered DDT orally in a dose of 350 mg/kg of body weight to albino rats that had been fed for 28 days from weaning on the same types of diets

---

[3]The new low-protein diet consisted of 3.5% casein, 81.5% cornstarch, 8% of hydrogenated cottonseed oil, 4% of salt mix, and 3% of an all-vitamin mixture prepared from the formula of Hegsted and Chang, 1965.

with 0%, 3%, 9%, 27%, or 81% as casein. Rats reared on 0%, 3%, and 9% casein demonstrated docility, pallor, food-spilling, piloerection, a scaly dermatitis over the tail, a normal or augmented food intake per kg of body weight, and an inclination toward oliguria and hypothermia. Animals fed an 0%-casein diet did not grow, while growth in rats fed 9% casein was at about one-third the rate as rats fed 27% casein. The death rate from DDT toxicity in rats fed 0%- and 3%-casein diets was significantly higher than in rats fed a diet containing 27% casein.

With the newly acquired recognition that the toxicity of several insecticides (e.g., carbaryl, DDT, lindane) became markedly enhanced as the level of protein in the diet was reduced from 8–9% to 0–3.5%, it became necessary to reevaluate this phenomenon on an expanded number of insecticides (Boyd, 1969). When weanling albino rats were reared for 4 weeks on a diet with 8–9% casein, they also exhibited statistically insignificant increased susceptibility to the acute oral toxic effects of two herbicides, chlorpropham (isopropyl-N-[3-chlorophenyl] carbamate), and monuron (N-P-chlorophenyl-N, N-dimethylurea). However, the acute LD_{50} values of a variety of insecticides and herbicides could be remarkably reduced in weanling albino rats reared for 28 days on diets with 0% to 3.5% casein. Although the effects of the pesticides on the rats reared on the 0%-protein diets may have been unduly caused by the confounding of starvation, the animals given the 3% to 3.5% casein did not exhibit any enhanced predisposition to starvation. Thus the adoption of the 3.5%-casein diet became standard for testing a protein deficiency (Boyd, 1969).

A summarization of the effects of the 3.5%-casein diet on insecticide and herbicide toxicity has been presented by Boyd (1969). Animals consuming diets with 26% casein served as controls and a minimum of 100 rats were employed to calculate each LD_{50} via linear regression. Table 2 illustrates that all insecticides and herbicides exhibited an enhanced toxicity to the weanling rats reared on the low-protein diets with the exception of dimethoate, which was no more toxic to rats fed a protein-deficient diet than for adequately fed controls. Of particular significance is the potential magnitude of the enhanced toxicity. For example, the toxicity of captan was increased from 17.8 to 39.8 times the controls with an average of 26.3 times. It also appears that it is difficult to generalize toxicity to a pesticide type (at least with respect to organophosphates) since diazinon and malathion are organophosphate insecticides that had their toxicity enhanced by 1.9 and 2.3, respectively, while parathion (see Casterline and Williams, 1969), another organophosphate, had its toxicity increased by a factor of 7.6. In contrast to the results presented in Table 2, Weatherholtz et al.

Table 2. Comparison of Enhanced Toxicities (as Measured by LD$_{50}$) of Pesticides in Protein-Deficient Rats

Pesticide/ Herbicide	LD$_{50}$ Low Protein Diet[b] (mg/kg)	LD$_{50}$ Normal Protein Diet[a] (mg/kg)	Increased Toxicity[c]	Reference
Dimethoate	147	152	1.0	Boyd and Muis, 1970
Lindane	95	184	1.9	Boyd and Chen, 1968
Diazinon	215	415	1.9	Boyd and Carsky, 1969
Chlordane	137	267	2.0	Boyd and Taylor, 1969
Malathion	599	1401	2.3	Boyd and Tanikella, 1969
Endrin	6.7	16.6	2.5	Boyd and Stefec, 1969
DDT	165	481	2.9	Boyd and Krijnen, 1969a
Monuron	950	2880	3.0	Boyd and Dobos, 1969a
Demeton	2.1	7.6	3.6	Boyd and Krupa, 1969
Toxaphene	80	293	3.6	Boyd and Taylor, 1971
Chlorpropham	2590	10390	4.0	Boyd and Carsky, 1969a
Endosulfan	24	102	4.3	Boyd and Dobos, 1969b
Diuron	437	2390	5.4	Boyd and Krupa, 1970
Carbaryl	89	575	6.5	Boyd and Krijnen, 1969
Parathion	4.9	37	7.6	Boyd et al. (1969)
Captan	480	12600	26.3	Boyd and Krijnen, 1968

[a]Containing 26% of protein as casein.
[b]Containing 3.5% of protein as casein.
[c]Calculated rate of the LD$_{50}$ in rats fed protein test diet-normal divided by the LD$_{50}$ in rats fed protein test diet-low.

Source. Boyd, E.M. (1969). Dietary protein and pesticide toxicity in male weanling rats. *Bull. Wld. Health Org.* **40**:803.

(1969) reported that male weanling rats reared on a 5%-casein diet exhibited a threefold tolerance to heptachlor as compared to pair-fed rats reared on either 20%- or 40%-casein diets. Presumably the rats reared on 20%- and 40%-casein diets produced the highly toxic metabolite heptachlor epoxide at a faster rate than those fed the 5%-casein diet.

High Levels of Dietary Protein. According to Boyd (1969), experiments on the effects of feeding for 28 days from weaning on a high-casein diet were conducted incidentally "to the research on protein-deficient diets." Boyd and DeCastro (1970) evaluated the influence of diets with highly variable levels of casein and cornstarch (i.e., 0% protein and 85% cornstarch; 3% and 82%; 9% and 76%; 27% and 58%; 81% and 4%). Animals reared on the high-casein diet (81%) exhibited a renal overload (i.e., renal congestion and hypertrophy diuresis, proteinuria, and polydipsia) and had an enhanced susceptibility to DDT toxic effects, including a death rate greater than twice that in rats given 27% casein (i.e., normal levels). Other studies by Boyd and Krijnen (1969) were in agreement with those of Boyd and DeCastro (1970), in that the oral LD_{50} value for weanling male rats fed for 28 days on diets with 27% casein was 481 ± 13 mg/kg, while similar rats maintained on a diet with 81% casein had an LD_{50} value of 130 ± 41 mg/kg. Krijnen and Boyd (1971) considerably extended the earlier two studies by Boyd and DeCastro (1968) and Boyd and Krijnen (1969) by determining the LD_{50} values for nine pesticides (including DDT) on male weanling rats raised on diets ranging in casein values from 0 to 81%. Table 3 indicates the increase in toxicity of the nine pesticides according to the percentages of dietary protein. Of particular interest are the values from the 81%-casein treatment. The results indicated several of the pesticides, including diazinon, malathion, and especially DDT were more toxic to weanling rats fed the high-protein diet than to the controls.

Other Factors Affecting Pesticide Toxicity. The age of rats when given a high-protein diet is also an important factor affecting the influence of diet on toxicity indices. For instance, Peters (1967) reported that male rats (133 g and 2–3 weeks past weaning) given a diet containing 80% casein grew as well as the controls given a typical laboratory diet.

Finally, Boyd et al. (1969) considered not only the amount but also the nature of dietary proteins as modifying factors in pesticide toxicity. They gave albino weanling rats diets containing either 0%, 3%, 9%,

Table 3. Increase in Toxicity of Pesticides in Rats Fed Varying Percentages of Dietary Protein[a]

	0	3.5	9.0	81
Captan	2100.0	26.3	1.2	2.4
Carbaryl	8.6	6.5	1.1	1.0
Chlorpropham	8.7	4.0	1.7	—
Diazinon	7.4	1.9	1.8	2.0
Dicophane (DDT)	4.0	2.9	1.5	3.7
Endosulfan	20.0	4.3	1.8	1.0
Lindane	12.3	1.9	1.0	1.8
Malathion	2.6	2.3	1.8	2.2
Monuron	11.5	3.0	1.8	—

[a]Increase in toxicity is expressed as the LD_{50} in rats fed a normal (26%) casein diet, divided by that in rats fed the percentages of casein specified.

Source. Krijnen, C.J. and Boyd, E.M. (1971). The influence of diets containing from 0 to 81% of protein and tolerated doses of pesticide. *Compar. Gen. Pharmacol.* **2**:374.

27%, or 81% of casein or 26% of lactalbumin or 26% of soy protein, with the balance of up to 85% as cornstarch and with 8% of hydrogenated cottonseed oil,.4% salt mix, and 3% of an all-vitamin mixture (see Hegsted and Chang, 1965). They found that the acute oral toxicity of phenacetin was similar in the 9% and 27% casein and the 26% lactalbumin and the standard laboratory chow fed rats. However, the mortality index and clinical indications of toxicity were markedly enhanced in rats given 0%, 3%, and 81% casein and in animals fed 26% soybean.

Conclusions. It is difficult to accurately assess the public health significance of the influence of low or excessive levels of dietary protein on pesticide and/or herbicide toxicity. It may be generally accepted (with at least a few exceptions) that a very marked reduction in protein (as casein) in the diet (13% of normal) appears to substantially enhance the acute toxicity of most agents tested. In addition, it would appear that moderate to fairly extensive reductions (to 33% of normal) in the diet would not be an important predisposing factor to acute pesticide toxicity. However, the research of Boyd and his associates does imply that in cases where protein intake is severely reduced as in children with kwashiorkor, the toxicity from many pesticides may be markedly enhanced.

Since the occurrence of grossly inadequate diets with respect to protein levels is a genuine problem in certain areas of the world and since pesticide use in those areas may presumably be indiscriminate at times, the possibility of a "high risk" kwashiorkoric-appearing person being exposed to high levels of pesticide may not be infrequent. Therein seems to be the prime significance of Boyd's research. There are several problems that emerge, however. First, the primary focus of the research has been on acute toxicity. Almost nothing is known about the influence of a moderately low-protein intake on the response to chronic, low-level pesticide exposure. Similarly, it is not known how a grossly inadequate intake of protein (3.5% casein) may affect chronic exposure toxicity. Secondly, if a person is consuming a diet inadequate in protein, it is probable that several other nutrients may also be inadequately supplied. The influence of multiple interactive factors may represent an important health problem. Thirdly, the adequacy of extrapolating from rat to human must always be viewed with some caution. Yet most of the research presented was performed with the weanling male rat. Fourth, in the United States and other developed countries it is not unlikely to have a large number of persons who consume levels of protein far in excess of what is needed for growth and maintenance. Since the research of Boyd and associates indicates that consumption of very high levels of dietary protein enhances the toxicity of certain pesticides, these individuals may also bear important consideration as a potential high-risk group. Fifth, the complexity of the issue makes generalizations difficult. Thus, the recognition of the influence of not only the amount of protein but also its quality is an important case in point. This area has just been superficially touched. Also, the influence of age on the response to diet-pesticide interactions has been examined only in the most limited fashion.

Clearly, the research of Boyd and associates has repeatedly pointed out that inadequate dietary protein may enhance pesticide toxicity and that children with severe protein shortages are at highest risk. But what can be done about this from a policy perspective? Boyd has repeatedly suggested that their data implied that certain pesticides such as captan should not be used in countries where kwashiorkor occurs. This makes sense since a low-protein diet markedly enhances the toxicity of captan. Their data can therefore be used to select which insecticides may be used. This knowledge should also alert people in responsible positions as to the protective as well as growth and maintenance functions of protein. The implications of Boyd's research should help to create a stronger effort to eliminate world hunger. It seems ludicrous to wait for human epidemiological tragedies to prove that Boyd's rat model was reasonably accurate. Yet continued research in the above-noted areas has important public health implications and should be initiated again.

References

Boyd, E.M. (1969). Dietary protein and pesticide toxicity in male weanling rats. *Bull. World Health Org.* **40**:801–805.

Boyd, E.M. and Boulanger, M. (1968). Insecticide toxicology: augmented susceptibility to carbaryl toxicity in albino rats fed purified casein diets. *J. Agr. Food Chem.* **16**(5):834.

Boyd, E.M.; Boulanger, M.; and DeCastro, E.S. (1969). *Pharmacol. Res. Commun.* (cited in Boyd, 1969).

Boyd, E.M. and Carsky, E. (1969). Kwashiorkorigenic diet and diazinon toxicity. *Acta Pharmacol. et Toxicol.* **27**:284–294.

Boyd, E.M. and Carsky, E. (1969a). The acute oral toxicity of the herbicide chlorpropham in albino rats: effect of diets containing varying amounts of protein. *Arch. Environ. Health* **19**:621–627.

Boyd, E.M. and Chen, C.P. (1968). Lindane toxicity and protein-deficient diet. *Arch. Environ. Health* **17**:156–163.

Boyd, E.M.; Chen, C.P.; and Liu, S.J. (1969). The acute oral toxicity of parathion in relation to dietary protein. *Archiv. fuer Toxikologie* **25**:238–253.

Boyd, E.M. and DeCastro, E.S. (1968). Protein-deficient diet and DDT toxicity. *Bull. World Health Org.* **38**:141–150.

Boyd, E.M. and DeCastro, E.S. (1970). Toxicity of dicophane (DDT) in relation to dietary protein intake. *Indus. Med.* **39**(5):53–60.

Boyd, E.M. and Dobos, I. (1969a). Protein deficiency and tolerated oral doses of endosulfan. *Arch. Int. Pharmacodyn.* **178**:152–165.

Boyd, E.M. and Dobos, I. (1969b). Acute oral toxicity of monuron in albino rat fed from weaning on different diets. *J. Agr. Food Chem.* **17**(6):1213–1216.

Boyd, E.M. and Krijnen, C.J. (1968). Toxicity of captan and protein-deficient diet. *J. Clin. Pharmacol.* **8**:225–234.

Boyd, E.M. and Krijnen, C.J. (1969). Dietary protein and DDT toxicity. *Bull. Environ. Contam. Toxicol.* **4**(5):256–261.

Boyd, E.M. and Krijnen, C.J. (1969a). The influence of protein intake on the acute oral toxicity of carbaryl. *J. Clin. Pharmacol.* **9**:292–297.

Boyd, E.M. and Krupa, V. (1969). The acute oral toxicity of demeton in albino rats fed from weaning on diets of varying protein content. *Canad. J. Pharmaceut. Sc.* **4**:35–40.

Boyd, E.M. and Krupa, V. (1970). Protein-deficient diet and kiuron toxicity. *J. Agr. Food Chem.* **18**(6):1104–1107.

Boyd, E.M. and Muis, L.F. (1970). Acute oral toxicity of dimethoate in albino rats fed a protein-deficient diet. *J. Pharmaceut. Sci.* **59**:1098–1102.

Boyd, E.M. and Stefec, J. (1969). Dietary protein and pesticide toxicity: with particular reference to endrin. *Canad. Med. Assoc. J.* **101**:335–339.

Boyd, E.M. and Tanikella, T.K. (1969). The acute oral toxicity of malathion in relation to dietary protein. *Arch. f. Toxikol.* **24**:292–303.

Boyd, E.M. and Taylor, F.I. (1969). The acute oral toxicity of chlordane in albino rats fed for 28 days from weaning on a protein-deficient diet. *Indus. Med.* **38**(12):42–49.

Boyd, E.M. and Taylor, F.I. (1971). Toxaphene toxicity in protein-deficient rats. *Toxicol. Appl. Pharmacol.* **18**:158–161.

Calabrese, E.J. (1978). *Pollutants and High Risk Groups: The Biological Basis of Increased Human Susceptibility to Environmental and Occupational Pollutants.* Wiley–Interscience, N.Y.

Calabrese, E.J. (1979). Nutritional factors affecting pesticide toxicity. Proceedings of Conference on Pesticides and Human Health. Society for Occupational and Environmental Health.

Casterline, J.L., Jr. and Williams, C.H. (1969). Effect of pesticide administration upon esterase activities in serum and tissues of rats fed variable casein diets. *Toxicol. Appl. Pharmacol.* **14**:266–275.

Chapman, R.A. (1967). *Tolerances for residues of pesticides chemicals.* T.I.L. No. 20 Food and drug directorate, Dept. of National Health and Welfare, Ottawa.

DeCastro, E.S. and Boyd, E.M. (1968). Organ weights and water content of rats fed protein-deficient diets. *Bull. World Health Org.* **38**:971–977.

Durham, W.F.; Ortega, P.; and Hayes, W.J. (1963). The effect of various levels of DDT on liver function, cell morphology, and DDT storage in the Rhesus monkey. *Arch. Int. Pharm. Therap.* **141**:111.

Hegsted, D.M. and Chang, Y.O. (1965). Protein utilization in growing rats: I. Relative growth index as a bioassay procedure. *J. Nutr.* **85**:159–168.

Krijnen, C.J. and Boyd, E.M. (1971). The influence of diets containing from 0 to 81 percent of protein on tolerated doses of pesticides. *Compar. Gen. Pharmacol.* **2**:373–376.

Laug, E.P.; Nelson, A.A.; Fitzhugh, O.G.; and Kunze, F.M. (1950). Liver cell alteration and DDT storage in the fat of the rat induced by dietary levels of 1 to 50 ppm DDT. *J. Pharmacol. Exp. Therap.* **98**:268.

Lee, M.; Harris, K.; and Trowbridge, H. (1964). Effect of the level of dietary protein on the toxicity of dieldrin for the laboratory rat. *J. Nutr.* **84**:136–144.

Liu, S.J. and Boyd, E.M. (1967). *Proc. Canad. Fed. Biol. Soc.* **10**:49–50.

Peters, J.M. (1967). A separation of the direct toxic effects of dietary raw egg white powder from its action in producing biotin deficiency. *Brit. J. Nutr.* **21**:801–809.

Treon, J.F. and Cleveland, F.P. (1955). Toxicity of certain chlorinated hydrocarbon insecticides of laboratory animals with special reference to aldrin and dieldrin. *J. Agr. Food Chem.* **3**:402.

Trowell, H.C.; Davies, J.N.P.; and Dean, R.F.A. (1964). *Kwashiorkor.* London: Arnold.

Weatherholtz, W.M.; Campbell, T.C.; and Webb, R.E. (1969). Effect of dietary protein levels on the toxicity and metabolism of heptachlor. *J. Nutr.* **98**:90–94.

WHO (1967). Report of the Joint Meeting of the FAO working party and the WHO expert committee on pesticide residues: Evaluation of some pesticide residues in food. Report FAO PL:CP/15 of the Food and Agriculture Organization and WHO/Food/Atd/67:32 of WHO, United Nations, Geneva, pp. 126–147.

14. TNT and DNT

That dietary factors could influence the toxicity of trinitrotoluene
(TNT) was suggested as far back as 1917 by Viscount Chetwynd, who
reported that the manager of a large ordnance plant in England initiated a dietary improvement program for female employees because of
a greater incidence of gastrointestinal disorders concomitant with a
generally poorer diet in women than men. After only four months of
the nutrition improvement program, there was a marked reduction in
the occurrence of gastrointestinal disorders, from 11.6% to only 0.7%.
In that same year, O'Reilly (1917) recommended that British munition
workers protect themselves from the adverse health effects of prolonged TNT exposure by consuming a diet that included milk, fruit,
and vegetables.

Based on these and other experiences with TNT during World War I,
Voegtlin et al. (1920, 1921–1922, 1921–1922a) evaluated the influence
of diet on dogs that were exposed to TNT, since they displayed many of
the same toxicological responses of humans to TNT. The influence of
three different diets were compared. The diets consisted of the following: Diet 1—bread and milk; Diet 2—meat; Diet 3—a mixed diet of
white bread, milk, and medium-fat beef. While the findings were not
conclusive, they did suggest that the mixed and meat diets offered
greater protection (i.e., less anemia and longer survival), presumably
because of their higher protein levels. Because of the lack of standardization among the diets, variations in the levels of proteins, carbohydrates, fats, vitamins, and minerals existed, thereby precluding any
definitive conclusions.

As expected, interest in the adverse effects of TNT on human health
nearly disappeared once World War I ended. The next big flurry of
research activity predictably occurred in the early 1940s during World
War II, when the need for explosives dramatically increased. During
the Second World War, a number of investigators recommended certain dietary schemes as preventive or therapeutic measures for workers in the munitions industries (Holmes, 1942; Foulgar, 1943; Hilton
and Swanston, 1941; McCausland and Hawkins, 1944; Watson, 1941;
Williams and Thomson, 1941; Evans, 1941). These recommendations
frequently included high-carbohydrate diets, and large quantities of
ascorbic acid, calcium, milk, and meats. As pointed out in Chapter 3 of
volume 1, despite the general lack of experimental studies supporting
these recommendations, numerous ammunitions plants within the
United States and Europe did adopt certain dietary regimens to protect

workers against TNT toxicity (Holmes, 1942; Cowgill, 1943). The subsequent section will review the literature concerning the influence of dietary protein in modifying TNT toxicity.

The first major research effort in this area since those of Voegtlin et al. (1920, 1921–1922, 1921–1922a) was published in 1942 by Himsworth and Glynn. They evaluated how three different diets, each with either elevated protein, fat, or carbohydrate, and each containing variable quantities of bread and casein, 5 to 6% of yeast, and supplemented with cod-liver oil, affected the toxicity of dietary TNT (0.15 gm/kg of body weight/day in rats). They reported that rats reared on the high-fat diet developed severe symptoms of TNT poisoning, while those on the high-carbohydrate diet exhibited slight adverse effects. The rats given the high-protein diet were not affected.

Further investigation of the specific diets used in this study of Himsworth and Glynn (1942) revealed the high-fat diet was also low in protein (about 9% of the dietary calories), while the high-carbohydrate diet had an adequate protein level (i.e., 23% of the dietary calories). Thus, Shils and Goldwater (1949, 1950) hypothesized that the increased toxicity in those rats reared on the high-fat diet may also have been related to the low-protein intake. Further, susceptibility to TNT toxicity is markedly decreased in rats reared on a diet low in fat, high in carbohydrate, and adequate in protein. In addition, a further increase in protein intake (up to 75% of dietary calories), along with a low level of dietary fat, resulted in an even greater reduction in susceptibility.

Since the study of Himsworth and Glynn (1942) did not differentiate between the influence of high levels of dietary fat and low levels of protein on TNT toxicity in rats, Shils and Goldwater (1950) attempted to fill this gap. Unfortunately, the results of their study are not in concert with those of Himsworth and Glynn (1942), primarily because only minor differences were found between the effects of fat and protein on the toxicity of TNT. Although there were several methodological differences between the two studies that could possibly account for the differences in the findings, Shils and Goldwater (1950) were forced to conclude that "a high fat intake does not appear to increase susceptibility to TNT to any marked degree . . . [while dietary] protein exerts no specific detoxifying effect on TNT."

The only other study that attempted to evaluate the influence of dietary protein on TNT toxicity was published in 1943 by Smith et al., who noted that as one increased the level of dietary casein from 5 to 18 to 37% there was a diminution in the TNT toxicity indices (i.e., liver-function test, hemoglobin levels, weight change). However, no unexposed controls at these higher casein levels were tested, thereby diminishing the strength of these tentative conclusions.

While no further studies concerning a protein-TNT interaction are available, several investigators have revealed that dietary protein levels may affect the toxicity of an analogue of TNT, that is, 2-4-dinitrotoluene (DNT). Clayton and Baumann (1944) observed that mice exhibited greater resistance to DNT when reared on a high-fat (30% by weight) diet as compared to those mice on a no-fat (0%) diet. Furthermore, an increase in the level of protein in the diet from 4 to 8% and to 50% improved growth whether DNT was employed as a treatment or not. However, the authors did note that the growth of the mice given the DNT was greater on the diet high in fat than on the high-protein diet.

In contrast to the previous study in which the DNT was added to all the diets as a percentage of weight, Clayton and Baumann (1948) decided to evaluate the influence of these nutrient parameters when the DNT was provided on an equicaloric basis; that is, the quantity of DNT ingested was kept constant for each calorie consumed, even though fat and carbohydrate varied. Despite this change in experimental procedure, the hypothesis that a high-fat diet protects against DNT toxicity was supported. These researchers speculated that the mice given the higher-fat diets were more capable of detoxifying the DNT to less toxic derivatives. Subsequent research by Shils and Goldwater (1949) also revealed that a high-fat intake markedly reduced the toxicity of injected DNT in rats while only having a slight effect on DNT- (or TNT) induced growth retardation.

Summary. It is clear that dietary levels of protein, fats, and carbohydrates may influence the toxicity of TNT and its analogue DNT. In addition, volume 1 of this study also revealed that several vitamins including ascorbic acid may play a role in affecting susceptibility to TNT toxicity. However, a careful consideration of the present studies reveals a general inadequacy of the data base from which reliable conclusions can be drawn. While numerous investigators made sweeping dietary recommendations to workers in the two world wars to prevent the occurrence of TNT toxicity, their foundations in the scientific literature are quite meager. This is not to say that certain diet practices could not play an important role both prophylactically and therapeutically. Clearly the findings of Smith et al. (1943) and Shils and Goldwater (1949) support such a possibility. The point is that nothing has been published in the last three decades on the subject. Animal-model and epidemiological studies in this area would seem to be highly relevant, especially in light of the opportunity to incorporate more standard nutrition-research techniques, including greater standardization of diets, pair-feeding techniques, and greater diversity of biochemical indicators of toxicity.

References

Barger, G. and Tutin, F. (1918). Carrosine, constitution and synthesis. *Biochem. J.* **12**:402–407.

Clayton, C.C. and Baumann, C.A. (1944). Some effects of diet on the resistance of mice toward 2,4-dinitrotoluene. *Arch. Biochem.* **5**:115.

Clayton, C.C. and Baumann, C.A. (1948). Effect of fat and calories on the resistance of mice to 2,4-dinitrotoluene. *Arch. Biochem.* **16**:415.

Cowgill, G.R. (1943). Current nutritional activity in industry: a review and appraisal. *JAMA* **121**(11):817–820.

Davie, T.B. (1942). Discussion on trinitrotoluene. *Proc. Roy. Soc. Med.* **35**:558–559.

Eddy, J.H., Jr. (1945). Methionine in the treatment of toxic hepatitis. *Amer. J. Med. Sci.* **210**:374–380.

Eddy, J.H., Jr. (1945a). Carbon tetrachloride poisoning, a preliminary report on the use of methionine in hepatitis. *J. Amer. Med. Assoc.* **128**:994–996.

Evans, R.M. (1941). TNT jaundice. *Lancet* **2**:552.

Foulgar, J.H. Quoted by Cowgill, G.R. (1943). Nutrition: a factor important for industrial hygiene. *Amer. J. Pub. Health* **34**:630.

Goldwater, C.J. and Shils, M.E. (1949a). Some relationships of nutrition to detoxification. *Amer. Ind. Hyg. Assoc. J.* **10**:17–20.

Hilton, J. and Swanston, C.N. (1941). Clinical manifestation of tetryl and trinitrotoluene. *Brit. Med. J.* **2**:509.

Himsworth, H.P. and Glynn, L.E. (1942). Experimental trinitrotoluene poisoning; the effect of diet. *Clin. Sci.* **4**:421–443.

Holmes, H.N. (1942). Vitamin C in the war. *Science* **96**:348.

Lane, R.E. (1942). Discussion on trinitrotoluene poisoning. *Proc. Roy. Soc. Med.* **35**:556–557.

McCausland, A. and Hawkins, R.F. (1944). Toxicity of trinitrotoluene. *Virginia Med. Monthly* **71**:242.

O'Reilly, P.S. (1917). In a symposium. The origin, symptoms, pathology, treatment and prophylaxis of toxic jaundice observed in munitions workers. *Proc. Roy. Soc. Med.* **10**:91.

Panton, P.N. and Bates, H.E. (1921). Summary of an experimental investigation into TNT poisoning. *Med. Res. Coun.* (Lond.) Special Rept. Series. No. 58, pp. 62–71.

Shils, M.E. and Goldwater, L.J. (1949). Influence of dietary protein and fat on the toxicities of trinitrotoluene (TNT and 2,4-dinitrotoluene [DNT]) for the rat. *Fed. Proc.* **8**:397.

Shils, M.E. and Goldwater, L.J. (1950). The effect of diet on the susceptibility of rats to poisoning by 2,4,6-trinitrotoluene (TNT). *J. Nutr.* **41**:239–305.

Smith, M.I.; Westfall, B.B.; and Stohlman, E.F. (1943). Experimental trinitrotoluene poisoning with attempts at detoxification. *J. Indus. Hyg. Toxicol.* **25**:391–395.

Swanston, C. (1942). Discussion on trinitrotoluene poisoning. *Proc. Roy. Soc. Med.* **35**:553–555.

Viscount Chetwynd (1917). In discussion on the origin, symptoms, pathology, treatment, and prophylaxis of toxic jaundice observed in munitions workers. *Proc. Roy. Soc. Med.* **10**:6.

Voegtlin, C.; Hooper, C.W.; and Johnson, J.M. (1920). Trinitrotoluene poisoning. Hygiene Laboratory Bulletin. 126. *U.S. Public Health Repts.* **34**:1307–1311.

Voegtlin, C.; Hooper, C.W.; and Johnson, J.M. (1921–1922). Trinitrotoluene poisoning—its nature, diagnosis and prevention. *J. Indus. Hyg.* **3**:239–254.

Voegtlin, C.; Hooper, C.W.; and Johnson, J.M. (1921–1922a). Trinitrotoluene poisoning—its nature, diagnosis and prevention (cont'd). *J. Indus. Hyg.* **3**:280–292.

Watson, J.H. (1941). Clinical manifestation of exposure to tetryl and TNT. *Brit. Med. J.* **2**:593.

Williams, E.K. and Thomson, G.H. (1941). Clinical manifestations of exposure to tetryl and TNT. *Brit. Med. J.* **2**:593.

C. PROTEIN—POLLUTANT INTERACTIONS—A PERSPECTIVE

It has been demonstrated that dietary protein intake can markedly influence the toxicity and carcinogenicity of numerous toxic substances. These toxic substances comprise a very diverse and seemingly unrelated group of agents, including at least 10 heavy metals and over twenty organic chemicals representing several different classifications of organic molecules. Evidence does exist that suggests that the amount and quality of dietary protein consumed can modify the toxic and carcinogenic properties of agents of extreme societal concern including arsenic, cadmium, lead, mercury, aflatoxin, benzene, nitrosamines, and others (Tables 4 and 5).

For the most part, investigators have evaluated whether diets inadequate in protein enhance toxicity of the agents under investigation. The animal model employed with by far the greatest frequency has been the rat. Generally, the researchers have assumed that the levels of dietary protein (i.e., casein) considered normal or adequate for control groups is between 18 to 30% of the diet, while low-protein diets range from 0.0 to 10%. From these ranges it is clear that animals reared on the low-protein regime have usually been consuming diets with less than 50% of the level of protein found in the control group. In numerous instances, especially those in the pesticide section, the level of protein in the low group was consistently 3.5% casein, or only 13% of

Table 4. Summary—Rating the Importance of Protein-Heavy Metal Interactions

Substance	Comment
Arsenic	Not recent[a]; biomedical relevance uncertain
Cadmium	Very recent; limited data base; supported hypothesis that protein quality influences cadmium toxicity
Cobalt	Very recent; limited data base; biomedical relevance uncertain
Cyanide	Not recent; very limited data; biomedical relevance uncertain
Lead	Quite recent; sizable data base; although all studies not in agreement, they generally support the hypothesis that low levels of dietary protein enhance lead toxicity
Mercury	Recent; limited data base; biomedical relevance uncertain
Nickel	Very recent; limited data base; biomedical relevance uncertain
Phosphorus	Not recent; limited data base; biomedical relevance uncertain
Potassium chromate	Not recent; limited data base; biomedical relevance uncertain
Selenium	Not recent; considerable amount of published data supports hypothesis that a low-protein diet enhances selenium toxicity
Uranium nitrate	Not recent; limited data base; biochemical relevance uncertain
Vanadium	Very recent; limited data base; biomedical relevance uncertain

Note. While these heavy metals have been shown to be more toxic in animal models reared on low-protein diets (as compared to controls), qualitative distinctions between the different metals are needed.

[a] Whether the data are listed as recent or not is a qualitative judgment of the author, but "not recent" means that the majority of the articles upon which the risk assessments are made are at least 20 years old, while "recent" is within 5–20 years old and "very recent" is within 5 years old.

the controls. The question naturally arises as to whom these low-protein-fed animals represent with respect to human extrapolation. Since the research of Boyd and his associates with the 3.5%-casein diets was expressly designed to simulate the response of infants with kwashiorkor, the use of a very low quantity of casein seems very appropriate. Also, studies with aflatoxin in which the low-protein level was 4 and 5% casein may also be appropriate if one was concerned with children in certain developing countries. However, the use of 4-to-5%-casein diets in studies with TNT, lead, 1,2-dichloroethane, and several other industrial toxicants most likely represents a greatly exaggerated deficiency state for workers and is therefore not too realistic.

Only in exceptional experiments have investigators (Barltrop and Khoo, 1975) evaluated the influence of graded levels of protein in the diet (0, 5, 10, 15, and 20%), including only a marginal (15%) and therefore more realistic deficiency condition. Perhaps the reason for the emphasis of researchers to evaluate very low protein diets (i.e., 3–6% casein) as compared to controls with 20–25% casein instead of a 15%-vs.-20% comparison is to ensure a greater chance of an adverse effect occurring. This is analogous to research concerned with the toxicity and/or carcinogenicity of agents in which investigators utilized exposure levels far in excess of realistic values in order to evoke an easily interpretable response. Such types of studies have the advantage of being able to be conducted over a short time span and virtually eliminate the problem of competing causes of injury and/or death. Unfortunately, these experimental conditions leave little similarity to realistic human exposures. With but few exceptions, research concerned with the influence of protein deficiency on pollutant toxicity has not considered the influence of chronic, marginal protein-deficiency conditions. This is clearly an area where future research should be directed.

Not only are marginal-deficiency conditions of concern but also whether an excess of protein in the diet affects toxicity as well. While there is little information upon which to provide rational judgments, Boyd (1969) has clearly shown that a diet with 81% casein markedly enhances pesticide toxicity. On the other hand, levels of 37% and 55% casein in the diet offered greater protection to animal models given TNT (Smith et al., 1943) and selenium (Moxon, 1937), respectively, as compared to similarly exposed controls reared on diets with approximately 18-to-20% casein. In light of the not too uncommon situation in the United States of people consuming much greater than the RDA for protein, the question of how excessive protein intake influences pollutant toxicity and/or carcinogenicity is of practical concern.

One of the major relevant problems, especially with the early studies

Table 5. Summary—Rating the Importance of Protein Interactions with Toxic Chemicals of an Organic Nature

Substance	Comment
Aflatoxin	Recent; data indicate that low-protein diets enhance aflatoxin toxicity but reduce the carcinogenic response
Azo dyes	Not recent; while low dietary protein intake is a factor enhancing carcinogenicity of azo dyes, these carcinogenic dyes have only a very restricted usage today; thus, they have a low public health importance
Benzene (and Bromobenzene)	Not recent; important initial findings have unfortunately not been followed up
Carbon tetrachloride	Recent; contradictory findings need to be resolved
Chloroform	Recent; limited and controversial findings; need for further study in light of widespread presence of chloroform in drinking water
1,2-dichloroethane	Not recent; limited data base; biomedical relevance uncertain
1,2-dimethyl-hydrazine	Very recent; limited but potentially very important findings; studies indicate that a high-protein-and-fat diet of either animal or plant origin enhances carcinogenicity
DNT	While the results are not recent and quite limited, they are very consistent that a high-fat diet protects against DNT toxicity
Ethanol	Recent; limited data base; biomedical relevance uncertain
Heptachlor	Recent; low levels of protein protect against toxicity
Methyl chloride	Not recent; very limited data base; biochemical relevance uncertain
N-Nitroso Compounds a. Dimethylnitrosamine (DMN)	Very recent; very limited data base; however, results strongly suggest that dietary protein affects DMN-induced carcinogenicity
b. MNNG (N-methyl-N-Nitro-N-Nitroso-guanidine)	Very recent; a low-protein diet enhances mutagenicity in bacterial systems
Pesticides (including a variety of insecticides and herbicides)	Recent; with few exceptions (see heptachlor), very low levels of protein in the diet markedly enhance the acute toxicity of a variety of insecticides and herbicides

292

Table 5. (Continued)

Substance	Comment
Phenol	Not recent; very limited data base; biomedical relevance uncertain
Polychlorinated biphenyls	Recent; very limited data base; biomedical relevance uncertain
Propylene dichloride	Not recent; very limited data base; biomedical relevance uncertain
Pyridine	Not recent; very limited data base; biomedical relevance uncertain
TNT	Not recent; results from published studies not sufficiently consistent to draw general conclusions

on protein-pollutant interactions, has been the placing of up to 5 and 6 rats per cage and the lack of pair-feeding/isocaloric dietary techniques. This has often led to difficulty in distinguishing effects of protein-pollutant interactions vs. the influence of starvation. Several researchers have attempted to circumvent this problem by comparing food consumption on the aggregate level, but this clearly prevents any interpretation on individuals on which the toxicological data are taken. Fortunately, it is now common practice to employ pair-feeding in studies with highly variable levels of dietary protein.

The data from which any conclusions can be drawn in the area of protein-pollutant interaction are almost exclusively those of animal-model toxicological investigations. Only two potential protein-pollutant interactions have any data dealing with human responses. These include lead (Barltrop and Khoo, 1975) and TNT (Viscount Chetwynd, 1917). Unfortunately, neither offer any help in developing a more quantifiable risk assessment. Such a paucity of information on human responses clearly suggests the need for environmental/occupational health epidemiologists to initiate research efforts to further elucidate any potential protein-pollutant interactions.

In light of the available data it is possible to conclude with some confidence that low levels of dietary protein can enhance the toxicity of selenium, aflatoxin, and a variety of pesticides in animal models. Suggestive evidence reveals that low-protein levels enhance the toxicity of benzene, 1,2-dichloroethane, methyl chloride, pyridine, and propylene dichloride. All of the substances of this grouping have an interesting but inadequate data base and require further documenta-

Table 6. The Influence of Dietary Protein on Toxic Agents—Selected Examples Where Data are Quite Limited

Source	Comment	Reference
Arsenic	Depletion of protein stores enhances arsenic toxicity	Goodell et al., 1944 Messinger and Hawkins, 1940
Atabrine	Rats reared on a high-protein, low-fat diet were re-sistant to the hepatotoxic effects of atabrine, com-pared to controls reared on either a low-protein or high-fat diet	Scudi and Hamlin, 1944
Bromobenzene	Low levels of casein in the diet (6%) enhance the toxicity of bromobenzene. Supplements of cystine or methionine offset the effects of this compound	White and Jackson, 1935
Butylated hydroxytoluene (BHT)	The LD_{50} values of BHT were inversely related to the levels of protein in the diet. Thus the acute oral LD_{50}s were 3900, 2150, and 1350 mg/kg in rats reared on diets with 24%, 8%, and 4% protein	Nikonorow and Karlowski, 1973
Cobalt	Low levels of dietary protein (11.88%) enhanced the toxicity of cobalt in chicks when compared to those on diets with normal-protein levels (24.6%)	Olson and Kienholz, 1968 Hill, 1979
Ethanol	Toxicity affected by level and type of dietary protein	Lucas et al., 1968
Mercury	Resistance to mercury toxicity is enhanced in hypoproteinemic dogs presumably due to in-creased extracellular volume and, more significantly, a relatively small binding of Hg^{++} by protein, thereby allowing more rapid excretion and reduced cell susceptibility	Martin and Reid, 1951 (also see Larkin et al., 1965)
Methyl chloride	The toxicity of inhaled methyl chloride as measured by survival is decreased by diets low in protein. Supplements of cystine and methionine increased survival time	Smith, 1946

Nickel	Toxicity (i.e., depressed growth) of nickel in chicks was decreased by increased dietary protein	Hill, 1979
Polychlorinated biphenyls (PCBs)	Variations in protein and fat levels in diet did not influence the adverse effects of PCBs on chickens	Hansen et al., 1976
Pyridine	Animals reared on a low-protein diet (10% casein) are at markedly enhanced risk to pyridine as determined by growth when compared to controls reared on a diet with 20% casein	Baxter, 1947
Radiation	Adequate dietary protein offsets radiation-induced toxicity	Hugon and Bounous, 1973 Egorova and Perepelkin, 1970
Sulfanilamide	Low-protein diets increase the susceptibility of rats to this compound as determined by a greater mortality rate and a higher incidence of anemia	Kapnick et al., 1942 Smith, 1941
Temperature	Rats exposed to prolonged cold had their survival diminished when diet was low in protein	Beaton, 1963, 1967 Lang and Grab, 1944; see Giaga and Gelineo, 1934, and Rixon and Stevenson (1957) for an opposing viewpoint
Tyrosine	Low levels of dietary protein (6%) enhance the toxicity of tyrosine (3%) in rats; increased levels of protein markedly reduce tyrosine toxicity	Ip and Harper, 1974
Vanadium	Increasing dietary protein levels diminished the toxicity of vanadium in chicks as determined by growth; while 6 ppm V noticeably depressed growth when given a 10%-protein diet, no depression occurred when protein levels were 20 or 30% of the diet	Hill, 1979. (See Hafez and Kratzer, 1976; Berg, 1966)

tion. Other protein-pollutant interactions including CCl_4, chloroform, TNT, and lead need further study with standard research protocols to resolve what appears to be conflicting reports of different investigators.

While the majority of investigations have focused on the expression of toxicity, it is important to realize that dietary protein levels have been found to modify the occurrence of chemically induced mutagenicity and carcinogenicity involving such agents as aflatoxin, azo dyes, 1,2-dimethylhydrazine, DMN, and MNNG. Since protein status is known to have an important effect on liver microsomal oxidase enzymes, this widespread influence on the expression of mutagenicity and/or carcinogenicity should not be unexpected. Whether the level of protein enhances or reduces the expression of an adverse effect is dependent to a large degree on whether the chemical in question requires bioactivation. The type of research represented in the mutagenicity and/or carcinogenicity studies also shares some of the same fundamental limitations as those mentioned earlier, in the sense that future efforts must be made to simulate human exposures more closely with respect to dietary protein and pollutant levels.

The derivation of the RDA for protein is based on growth and development requirements. Whether subsequent studies of interactions of dietary protein with ubiquitous pollutants will lead nutritionists to modify the RDA for protein remains to be seen. Certainly, the present evidence does not suggest any modification in the RDA. However, future discoveries may change that stance and the scientific community should be opened to that possibility.

While the data are limited on the importance of protein quality on pollutant toxicity (see Table 6), sufficient evidence has emerged demonstrating that the toxicity of substances such as cadmium (Fox et al., 1973) and selenium (Smith and Stohlman, 1940), among others, can be markedly altered by the type of protein. This is an area of considerable potential importance that has generally not been emphasized in the protein-pollutant research. Of potential importance in this regard would be future studies concerning the potential differential impact of a vegetarian life-style on pollutant toxicity/carcinogenicity.

Finally, how serious a problem within the general population of the United States is the consumption of diets with less than the RDA for protein? According to Bogert et al. (1973), 30% of women and 10% of men aged 30 to 60 years ingest less than two-thirds of the RDA for protein. These figures clearly suggest that the presence of dietary inadequacy with respect to protein ingestion is quite sizable in the United States. Further breakdown of these data by race, education, social class, and so on, would most likely reveal that these percentages would be much higher among the poorer segments of society. Whether the persons consuming diets with inadequate levels of protein are also being exposed to elevated levels of pollutants whose toxicity is enhanced by low-protein diets remains to be investigated. Also, whether a consumption of only two-thirds of the RDA predisposes such individuals to the adverse effects of certain pollutants discussed herein is not known either. As can clearly be seen from this discussion, our knowledge and understanding of how protein nutritional status affects the adverse effects of numerous toxic substances needs to be strengthened to a considerable degree so that accurate risk assessments and policy directions can be derived.

References

Barltrop, D. and Khoo, H.E. (1975). The influence of nutritional factors on lead absorption. *Post Grad. Med. J.* **51**:795–800.

Baxter, J.H. (1947). Studies of the mechanisms of liver and kidney injury. III. Methionine protects against damage produced in rat by diets containing pyridine. *J. Pharmacol. Exp. Therap.* **91**:345–349.

Beaton, J.R. (1963). Previous dietary protein level and survival of starving rats in the cold. *Canad. J. Biochem. Physiol.* **41**:171–178.

Beaton, J.R. (1967). Vitamin C metabolism in rats fed a low-protein diet and exposed to cold. *Canad. J. Physiol. Pharmacol.* **45**:335–342.

Berg, L.R. (1966). Effect of diet composition on vanadium toxicity for the chick. *Poult. Sci.* **45**:1346–1352.

Bogert, L.J.; Briggs, G.M.; and Calloway, D.H. (1973). *Nutrition and Physical Fitness.* 9th ed. Saunders, Phila.

Boyd, E.M. (1969). Dietary protein and pesticide toxicity in male weanling rats. *Bull. World Health Org.* **40**:801–805.

Egorova, N.D. and Perepelkin, S.R. (1970). Disturbance of the excretion of riboflavin and ascorbic acid in radiation sickness against a background of qualitatively different protein nutrition. *Radiobiologia* **11**:271–274.

Fox, M.R.S.; Jacobs, R.M.; Fry, B.E., Jr.; and Harland, B.F. (1973). Effect of protein source on response to cadmium. *Fed. Proc.* **32**:924.

Giaga, J. and Gelineo, S. (1934). Alimentation et resistance au froid. *Compt. Rend.* **198**:2277–2278.

Goodell, J.P.B.; Hanson, P.C.; and Hawkins, W.B. (1944). Methionine protects against mapharsen liver injury in protein-depleted dogs. *J. Exp. Med.* **79**:625–632.

Hafez, Y.S.M. and Kratzer, F.H. (1976). The effect of diet on the toxicity of vanadium. *Poult. Sci.* **55**:918–922.

Hansen, L.G.; Beamer, P.D.; Wilson, D.W.; and Metcalf, R.L. (1976). Effects of feeding polychlorinated biphenyls to broiler cockerels in three dietary regimens. *Poult. Sci.* **55**(3):1084–1088.

Hill, C.H. (1979). The effect of dietary protein levels on mineral toxicity in chicks. *J. Nutr.* **109**:501–507.

Hugon, J.S. and Bounous, G. (1973). Protective effect of an elemental diet on radiation enteropathy in the mouse. *Strehentherapie* **146**:701–712.

Ip, C.C.Y. and Harper, A.E. (1974). Effects of dietary protein content and glucagon administration on tyrosine metabolism and tyrosine toxicity in the cat. *J. Nutr.* **103**:1594–1607.

Kapnick, I.; Lyons, C.; and Stewart, J.D. (1942). Influence of diet on sulfanilamide toxicity. *J. Pharmacol. Exp. Therap.* **74**:284–289.

Lang, K. and Grab, W. (1944). *Klin. Wochschr.* **21**:226.

Larkin, D.V.; Miller, V.L.; Bearse, G.E.; and Hamilton, C.M. (1965). Effects of starvation and protein depletion on mercury retention in two strains of chickens. *Nature* **208**:706–707.

Lucas, C.C.; Ridout, J.H.; and Lumchick, G.L. (1968). Dietary protein and chronic intoxication with ethanol. *Canad. J. Biochem. Phys.* **46**:475–485.

Martin, H.F. and Reid, N.H. (1951). Hypoproteinemia on protection in mercuric chloride poisoning. *Proc. Soc. Exp. Biol. Med.* **78**:863–865.

Messinger, W.J. and Hawkins, W.B. (1940). Arsphenamine liver injury modified by diet. Protein and carbohydrate protective, but fat injurious. *Am. J. Med. Sci.* **199**:216.

Moxon, A.L. (1937). Alkali disease or selenium poisoning. *So. Dak. Agr. Exp. Sta. Bull.* **311**:50.

Nikonorow, M. and Karlowski, K. (1973). Protein-deficient diets. II. Toxicity of butylated hydroxytoluene. *Toxicol.* **1**:277–287.

Olson, J.D. and Kienholz, E.W. (1968). Cobalt and vitamin C for chicks. *Poult. Sci.* **47**:1709.

Rixon, R.H. and Stevenson, J.A.F. (1957). Factors influencing survival of rats in fasting metabolic rate and body weight loss. *Amer. J. Physiol.* **188**:332–336.

Scudi, J.V. and Hamlin, M.T. (1944). Biochemical aspects of the toxicity of atabrine. II. The influence of the diet upon the effects produced by repeated doses of the drug. *J. Pharmacol. Exp. Therap.* **80**:150–159.

Smith, M.I. (1941). The influence of dietary protein on the toxicity of sulfanilamide. *U.S. Pub. Hlth. Repts.* **56**:24–29.

Smith, M.I. and Stohlman, E.F. (1940). Further observations on the influence of dietary protein on the toxicity of selenium. *J. Pharmacol. Exp. Therap.* **40**:270–278.

Smith, M.I.; Westfall, B.B.; and Stohlman, E.F. (1943). Experimental trinitrotoluene poisoning with attempts at detoxification. *J. Indus. Hyg. Toxicol.* **25**:391–395.

Smith, W.W. (1946). The protective action of cystine and methionine in rats exposed to methyl chloride. *Fed. Proc.* **5**:97.

Viscount Chetwynd (1917). In discussion on the origin, symptoms, pathology, treatment, and prophylaxis of toxic jaundice observed in munition workers. *Proc. Roy. Soc. Med.* **10**:6.

White, A. and Jackson, R.W. (1935). The effect of bromobenzene on utilization of cystine and methionine by the growing rat. *J. Biol. Chem.* **111**:507.

Amino Acids

A. INORGANIC SUBSTANCES

1. Arsenic

Observations by Miller and Whipple in 1942 that methionine could prevent the occurrence of chloroform-induced liver damage led Beattie and Marshall (1944) to hypothesize that infective hepatitis and the incidence of post-arsphenamine jaundice was possibly related to a suboptimal protein (i.e., methionine) intake.

Experiments testing this hypothesis with 450 patients revealed that liver damage caused by arsenical treatment could be prevented or reduced by methionine treatment or by the use of casein diets high in methionine and cystine. More specifically, the methionine treatment resulted in markedly reduced hospitalization periods as well as being particularly effective in facilitating the recovery of extremely ill patients who had previously shown no beneficial response to other treatments. Subsequent clinical reports by Peters et al. (1944, 1945) supported the notion that methionine administration would be of use in treating the occurrence of jaundice by demonstrating that methionine (2.5 or 5.0 gm/day) treatments reduced the mean number of days required for serum bilirubin to return to a more normal

299

level, as compared to an untreated control group and to groups given dietary casein (60 gm/day) and cysteine (2 gm/day), even though these final two treatments were somewhat protective.

Finally, Goodell et al. (1944) reported that methionine protected against Mapharsen-induced liver injury in protein-depleted dogs. All dogs were fasted for one week and then given a diet with practically no protein for various time intervals (5 to 10 weeks) before the Marpharsen treatment. Methionine was given either orally or intravenously 24 hours or immediately before the arsenic treatment, respectively.

In light of the fact that arsenical medications are no longer employed, the relevance of these findings to present-day medical problems is difficult to discern, especially since the hypothesis that chronic arsenic exposure is a cause of liver damage is still unresolved (Tabershaw et al., 1977). However, these data do suggest that low levels of methionine (or cystine) in the diet may enhance arsenic-induced liver damage, and since the data are primarily derived from human subjects, it should not be dismissed without further investigation.

References

Beattie, J. and Marshall, J. (1944). Methionine in the treatment of liver damage. *Nature* **153**(3887):525–526.

Drill, V.A. (1952). Hepatotoxic agents: mechanism of action and dietary interrelationship. *Pharmacol. Rev.* **4**:1–41.

Goodell, J.P.B.; Hanson, P.C.; and Hawkins, W.B. (1944). Methionine protects against mapharsen liver injury in protein-depleted dogs. *J. Exp. Med.* **79**:625–632.

Miller, L.L. and Whipple, G.H. (1942). Liver injury, liver protection, and sulfur metabolism. Methionine protects against chloroform liver injury even when given after anesthesia. *J. Exp. Med.* **76**:421–435.

Peters, R.A.; Thompson, R.H.S.; King, A.J.; Williams, D.I.; and Nicol, C. (1944). Sulphur-containing amino-acids and jaundice. *Nature* **153**(3895):773.

Peters, R.A.; Thompson, R.H.S.; King, A.J.; Williams, D.I.; and Nicol, C. (1945). The treatment of postarsphenamine jaundice with sulphur-containing amino acids. *Quart. J. Med.* **14**:35–56.

Tabershaw, I.R.; Utidjian, H.M.B.; and Kawahara, B. (1977). Chemical hazards. In: *Occupational Diseases: A Guide to Their Recognition.* U.S. DHEW, PHS, CDC, NIOSH. Washington, D.C.

2. Cadmium

That certain nutrients may reduce the toxicity of cadmium was first reported in 1957 by Parizek, who reported that zinc administration prevented cadmium-induced damage to the testes of mice and rats. This led to the testing of a variety of nutrients in hopes that they too might be able to reduce cadmium toxicity. Among the nutrients included for evaluation was the sulfur-containing amino acid cysteine. In 1966, Gunn et al. first reported that cysteine was able to reduce cadmium-induced testicular damage in rodents. This finding was subsequently confirmed two years later by the same research group (Gunn et al., 1968). However, the relative effectiveness of cysteine to prevent cadmium damage to testes was quite minimal as compared to other such protective agents, including selenium, zinc, and cobalt. In fact, a 500-to-1 ratio of cysteine to cadmium was required to prevent damage, while only a 2:1 ratio was needed for selenium to be effective (Gunn et al., 1968).

Efforts to determine if cysteine protected the testis from cadmium damage by reducing cadmium-tissue levels proved to be quite surprising. Not only did cysteine not reduce cadmium levels in the testis, it actually increased them (Gunn et al., 1968a). The question still remains as to how cysteine may reduce cadmium-induced testicle damage.

In marked contrast to the protective effects of cysteine on testicular tissue, Gunn et al. (1968) reported that cysteine enhanced cadmium lethality. In fact, they noted that "doses of cadmium one-fifth of the LD_{50}, when administered with cysteine are fatal by causing acute devastation of renal proximal convoluted tubules." Unfortunately, further research into the manner of interaction between cysteine and cadmium has not continued.

References

Gunn, S.A.; Gould, T.C.; and Anderson, W.A.D. (1966). Protective effect of thiol compounds against cadmium-induced damage to testis. *Proc. Soc. Exp. Biol. Med.* **122**:1036.

Gunn, S.A.; Gould, T.C.; and Anderson, W.A.D. (1968). Mechanism of zinc, cysteine and selenium protection against cadmium-induced vascular injury to mouse testis. *J. Reprod. Fert.* **15**:65–70.

Gunn, S.A.; Gould, T.C.; and Anderson, W.A.D. (1968a). Specificity in protection against lethality and testicular toxicity from cadmium. *Proc. Soc. Exp. Biol. Med.* **128**:591–595.

Parizek, J. (1957). The destructive effect of cadmium on testicular tissue and its prevention by zinc. *J. Endocrinol.* **15**:56.

3. Cobalt and Nickel

Exposure to potentially toxic levels of cobalt may occur in workers involved with the manufacture of nickel, aluminum, copper, beryllium, chromium, and molybdenum alloys that are used in the electrical, automobile, and aircraft industries (Tabershaw et al., 1977). Industrial cobalt exposure usually results in skin or eye irritation, allergic responses, and a variety of respiratory disorders. Ingestion of cobalt within the industrial sphere is not common according to Tabershaw et al. (1977). While exposure to cobalt is regulated by a standard of 0.1 mg/m³ by OSHA, there is no ambient air or drinking-water standard for cobalt in the United States.

There are a few studies that indicate that the dietary status of cystine, cysteine, and methionine may reduce the toxicity of elevated levels of cobalt in rats (Griffith et al., 1942) and calves (Dunn et al., 1952). For instance, Griffith et al. (1942) demonstrated that these S-containing amino acids diminished cobalt toxicity (i.e., lacrimation, salivation, dysporea, incoordination, defecation, and urination) in rats when the cobalt and the specific amino acid were given jointly, either orally or intraperitoneally. They speculated that the amino acids and cobalt form a complex in the blood and that the newly formed complex has a diminished toxicity compared to the cobalt alone.

While the idea that adequate levels of these amino acids in the diet help to prevent the systemic toxicity of cobalt as has been demonstrated in rats and calves, its relevance for humans is probably quite minimal, since exposure to excessive levels of cobalt is infrequent. However, if it is true that cystine, cysteine, and/or methionine form complexes with cobalt, it is interesting to evaluate what influence a diet very high in methionine may have on normal cobalt metabolism, especially its functioning in cobalamin. Finally, similar experiments also revealed that cysteine administration markedly reduced the acute toxicity of nickel in rats. That cysteine may detoxify the nickel is an interesting finding that should be further evaluated, especially with respect to chronic toxicology and possible carcinogenicity studies.

References

Dunn, K.M.; Ely, R.E.; and Huffman, C.F. (1952). Alleviation of cobalt toxicity in calves by methionine administration. *J. Animal Sci.* **11**:326–331.

Griffith, W.H.; Paucek, P.L.; and Mulford, D.J. (1942). The relation of the sulphur amino acids to the toxicity of cobalt and nickel in the rat. *J. Nutr.* **23**:603–612.

Michaelis, L. (1929). Oxidation-reduction systems of biological significance. VI. The mechanism of the catalytic effect of iron on the oxidation of cysteine. *J. Biol. Chem.* **87**:777.

Michaelis, L. and Yamaguchi, S. (1929). Oxidation reduction systems of biological significance. V. The composition of the oxidized cobalt complex of cysteine. A colorimetric method for the micro analysis of cobalt. *J. Biol. Chem.* **83**:307.

Schmidt, C.L.A. (1945). *Chemistry of the Amino Acids and Proteins.* Thomas Book Co., Springfield, IL., p. 769.

Tabershaw, I.R.; Utidjian, H.M.B.; and Kawahara, B. (1977). Chemical hazards. In: *Occupational Diseases: A Guide to Their Recognition.* Edited by M.M. Key et al. U.S. DHEW, PHS, CDC, NIOSH. Washington, D.C.

Vickery, H.B. and Leavenworth, C.S. (1930). The behavior of cystine with silver salts. *J. Biol. Chem.* **86**:129.

4. Copper

Despite the fact that copper is an essential nutrient in animal and human systems, it is also highly toxic at elevated levels of exposure. In fact, Wilson's disease (hepatolenticular degeneration) in humans is characterized by an accumulation of potentially toxic levels of copper in both the liver and brain (NAS, 1977). Furthermore, Underwood (1971) has noted that sheep experience adverse effects from copper at levels of less than 100 ppm within the diet. Since elevated levels of dietary copper may result in adverse health effects and since 100 to 250 ppm of copper is customarily added to the diets of poultry and swine as an antifungal agent and/or a growth enhancer, it is of more than theoretical importance that a review of dietary factors affecting the toxicity of copper is in order. Even though the literature is not replete with articles concerning dietary factors influencing the occurrence of copper-induced adverse health effects, there are sufficient data available to indicate that dietary status may significantly alter copper toxicity. For instance, Bunch et al. (1963) reported that pigs reared on diets marginal in iron and zinc tolerated much less copper than controls given diets with considerably higher levels of these two elements. Waibel et al. (1964) noted that turkey poults reared on a purified diet were very susceptible to 50 ppm of dietary copper, while 800 ppm of dietary copper only minimally affected similar poults given a diet composed of common feedstuffs. More recently, Jensen (1975) reported that adding 800 ppm copper to a diet marginal in selenium induced exudative diathesis and muscular dystrophy in chicks.

Jensen and Maurice (1979) suggested that copper may disrupt normal sulfur amino acid metabolism. This suggestion was based on the earlier noted observation that copper toxicity induced muscular dystrophy in chicks and that cystine, a sulfur containing amino acid, is known to help prevent this myopathy in chicks (see Hathcock et al., 1968).

With respect to the sulfur-containing amino acids methionine and L-cystine, Jensen and Maurice (1979, 1979a) have clearly established that diets marginal in these nutrients cause chicks to be at enhanced risk to copper toxicity, while dietary supplementation markedly diminishes copper toxicity in this species. More specifically, they reported that the addition of as low as 500 ppm copper to a diet deficient or marginally adequate in sulfur containing amino acids resulted in a statistically significant reduced growth rate and efficiency of food utilization in chicks. However, the addition of 0.4% of DL methionine to the diet, a level that provided a quantity of this amino acid in excess of known physiological requirements, prevented the two previously stated adverse health effects when copper levels were 500 ppm. However, with a copper exposure of 750 ppm, this level of methionine supplementation prevented only the copper-induced reduction in food utilization efficiency. Other beneficial effects of the methionine treatment included a reduction in the level of copper in the liver, plasma, and spleen. However, methionine treatment did not affect the copper levels of the kidney. Other studies revealed that the addition of 0.332% L-cystine to a diet adequate in sulfur amino acids markedly prevented copper-induced (500 ppm) growth depression as well as significantly reducing copper levels in the blood plasma, spleen, and bile, as well as the kidney (but to a lesser extent).

In attempting to understand how L-cystine and methionine may affect the toxicity of copper, Jensen and Maurice (1979) hypothesized that these amino acids may (1) diminish the absorption of copper, (2) form a complex with copper in vivo, (3) enhance the synthesis of copper-binding proteins, and (4) increase the biliary excretion of copper. In addition, they speculated that high levels of dietary copper may diminish the availability of sulfur-containing amino acids for normal developmental and maintenance requirements, thereby increasing the dietary needs of this amino acid.

Since the viability of each of these potential explanations needs to be evaluated, further research in this particular area should prove to be of considerable toxicological interest. While copper toxicosis is not considered an important problem for humans, it may be a practical issue for farmers who raise cattle and especially sheep. In light of the influence of L-cystine and methionine on copper toxicity, further investigations should be directed toward developing a more quantitative assessment of this interaction as well as the influence of variable levels of multiple nutrients such as zinc, iron, molybdenum, and sulfate, along with S-containing amino acids, on the toxicity of copper.

References

Bunch, R.J.; Speer, V.C.; Hays, V.W.; and McCall, J.T. (1963). Effects of high levels of copper and chlortetracyline on performance of pigs. *J. Anim. Sci.* **22**:56–60.

Hathcock, J.N.; Hull, S.J.; and Scott, M.L. (1968). Derivatives and analogs of cysteine and selected sulfhydryl compounds in nutritional muscular dystrophy in chicks. *J. Nutr.* **94**:147–150.

Jensen, L.S. (1975). Precipitation of a selenium deficiency by high dietary levels of copper and zinc. *Proc. Soc. Exp. Biol. Med.* **149**:113–116.

Jensen, L.S. and Maurice, D.V. (1979). Influence of sulfur amino acids on copper toxicity in chicks. *J. Nutr.* **109**:91–97.

Jensen, L.S. and Maurice, D.V. (1979a). Effect of methionine on copper-induced growth depression and gizzard erosion. *Poult. Sci.* (in press).

NAS (1977). Copper. The National Academy of Sciences, Washington, D.C.

Underwood, E.J. (1971). In *Trace Elements in Human and Animal Nutrition.* Academic Press, New York, p. 543.

Waibel, P.E.; Snetsinger, C.C.; Ball, R.A.; and Sautter, J.H. (1964). Variation in tolerance of turkeys to dietary copper. *Poult. Sci.* **43**:504–506.

5. Cyanide

Introduction. With the exception of the attempt of the U.S. Food and Drug Administration (FDA) to ban the widespread use of saccharin within American society, no other biomedical issue has recently seemed to cause as much commotion as whether laetrile should be allowed as a possible treatment for cancer patients. Various state legislatures, in fact, have bypassed the authority of the FDA to legalize the usage of laetrile within their jurisdiction. Controversy has engulfed the claims of proponents and opponents concerning the effectiveness of laetrile to the extent that at the Sloan-Kettering Institute, where research on laetrile has been proceeding for several years, a group of workers challenging "official" conclusions has issue a series of opposing newsletters entitled "Second Opinion." In light of this present controversy and notoriety, it is quite likely that the use of laetrile, at least over the next several years, will dramatically increase until it rises or falls on its patients' outcomes.

Always an important issue in the treatment of cancer patients is the potential problem of adverse side effects. Yet this has been one component of the laetrile debate that has been largely ignored. Since the extent and nature of possible side effects can significantly affect the utility of anticancer drugs, it is necessary that investigations into possible side effects be rigorously pursued. The purpose of this section is to identify dietary factors (i.e., the sulfur-containing amino acids cysteine and methionine) that may affect a predisposition to the development of side effects from laetrile treatment.

Laetrile: Background Information. According to its proponents, the active ingredient in laetrile is called amygdalin, or vitamin B_{17} (Richardson and Griffin, 1977). Natural sources of amygdalin include oil of bitter almonds and apricot and peach pits (Richardson and

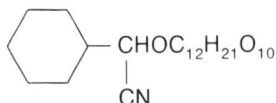

Figure 8-1. Chemical structure of amygdalin.

Griffin, 1977; Hall, 1973). Amygdalin is a glucoside that contains cyanide (Hall, 1973); its chemical structure is represented in Figure 8-1. When amygdalin is acted upon by certain hydrolytic enzymes, hydrogen cyanide may be liberated (Hall, 1973; Corn, 1973). According to Richardson and Griffin (1977), amygdalin acts as an anticancer agent via the toxic action of cyanide on the cancerous tissue. Richardson and Griffin (1977) stated that the enzyme rhodanese, which readily converts cyanide to the relatively nontoxic thiocyanate,[1] is not found in cancerous tissue but is generally prevalent elsewhere throughout bodily tissue. More specifically, rhodanese exhibits considerable activity in liver, kidney, thyroid, adrenal, and pancreas tissue, but somewhat lower activity in heart, brain, alimentary tract, and elsewhere (Rosenthal, 1948). Based on this information, it has been suggested that amygdalin destroys cancer cells in a very selective manner, whereas normal tissue is afforded extra protection from cyanide via the detoxifying activity of rhodanese.

The question now arises as to what happens to individuals who are receiving amygdalin treatment and who also may experience a decreased capacity to convert cyanide to thiocyanate. What is the likelihood of such an occurrence and what would be the toxic effects, if any? There are several dietary conditions that may exacerbate the toxicity of cyanide, including diets low in sulfur-containing amino acids and vitamin B_{12}.

Dietary Factors Affecting Cyanide Toxicity. The occurrence of cyanogenetic glucosides has been reported in a number of common plants, including lima beans, cassava, sweet potato, maize, and sorghum. In fact, numerous cases of human poisoning have been reported following consumption of cassava and lima beans (Corn, 1973; Anonymous, 1969). Furthermore, importation of lima beans into the United States is limited to those varieties with less than 20 mg HCN/ 100 g of seeds (Corn, 1973).

[1]According to Williams (1963) and Parke (1968), the inorganic cyanide ion is conjugated with sulfur to form thiocyanate via the enzyme rhodanese. Thiocyanate conjugation represents a striking detoxification reaction that is accompanied by a 200-fold decrease of toxicity.

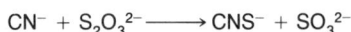

$$CN^- + S_2O_3^{2-} \longrightarrow CNS^- + SO_3^{2-}$$

Osuntokun has reported a rather widespread "tropical neuropathy" in association with the consumption of cassava, a tuber whose outer integument has high levels of the cyanogenetic glycoside linamarin (Wilson, 1965). Those affected with this "tropical neuropathy" had diets low in cysteine and other sulfur-containing amino acids.

The detoxification of cyanide occurs via the conjugation of cyanide with cysteine, resulting in the formation of 2-iminothiazolidine-4-carboxylic acid.

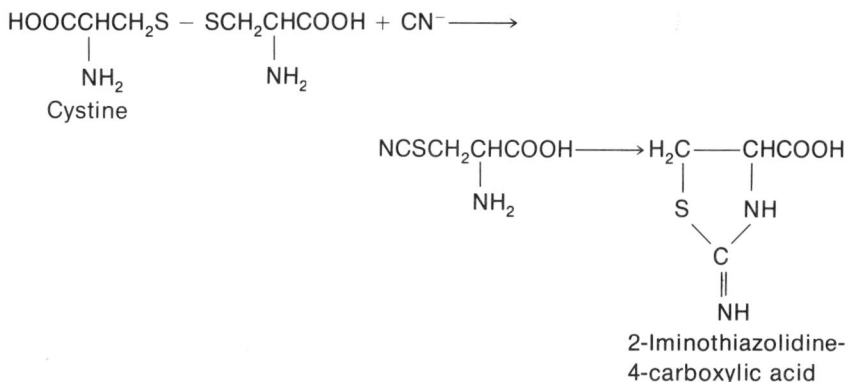

$$\underset{\substack{| \\ NH_2 \\ \text{Cystine}}}{HOOCCHCH_2S} - \underset{\substack{| \\ NH_2}}{SCH_2CHCOOH} + CN^- \longrightarrow$$

$$\underset{\substack{| \\ NH_2}}{NCSCH_2CHCOOH} \longrightarrow H_2C-CHCOOH$$

2-Iminothiazolidine-
4-carboxylic acid

It was thought that the synergistic interaction of low dietary levels of these sulfur-containing amino acids and their increased use for the detoxification of cyanide may have resulted in extremely depleted levels of plasma cysteine and methionine in these patients (Anonymous, 1969).

Conclusion. Patients receiving laetrile treatment should be closely examined for the occurrence of adverse side effects resulting from the cyanide toxicity. Individuals with reduced metabolic capacity to detoxify cyanide to thiocyanate as a result of dietary factors such as low levels of the sulfur-containing amino acids methionine and cysteine would be at increased risk to the development of such side effects.

References

Anonymous. (1969). Chronic cyanide neurotoxicity. *Lancet* 11:962.

Corn, E.E. (1973). Cyanogenetic glycosides. In: *Toxicants Occurring Naturally in Foods,* 2nd ed., pp. 299–308. National Academy of Sciences, Washington, D.C.

Hall, R.L. (1973). Toxicants occurring naturally in spices and flowers. In: *Toxicants Occurring Naturally in Foods,* 2nd ed., pp. 449–451. National Academy of Sciences, Washington, D.C.

Parke, D.V. (1968). *The Biochemistry of Foreign Compounds*. Pergamon Press, N.Y., p. 97.

Richardson, J.A. and Griffin, P. (1977). *Laetrile: case histories*. Bantam Books, New York.

Rosenthal, O. (1948). The distribution of rhodanese. *Fed. Proc.* **7**:181–182.

Williams, R.T. (1963). Metabolic fate of foreign compounds. *Arch. Environ. Health* **7**:612–620.

Wilson, J. (1965). Leber's hereditary optic atrophy: a possible defect of cyanide metabolism. *Clin. Sci.* **29**:505–515.

6. Lead

Within recent years there has been a growing concern over the notion that dietary factors may play an important role in either facilitating or preventing the gastrointestinal absorption of lead (Mahaffey, 1974). While much research has been directed toward the interactions of lead with minerals such as calcium and iron and certain vitamins including ascorbic acid and α-tocopherol, much less emphasis has been given to specific amino acids. In this section, the influence of the sulfur-containing amino acids cysteine, cystine, and methionine on lead uptake, retention, and toxicity will be reviewed.

The initial report was published in 1942 by Baernstein and Grand, who noted that cystine or methionine supplementation to a 6%-casein diet reduced the degree of lead-induced decreases in hemoglobin levels and red blood cell counts in pair-fed experiments. They suggested that these dietary supplements were most likely not enhancing the detoxification and excretion of lead, but probably enhancing the efficiency of casein utilization for hemoglobin synthesis and general growth. Occasional reports were subsequently published on the general topic of the potential protective influence of S-containing amino acids on lead intoxication. For example, in 1956, Buckup et al. reported that rabbits given methionine and cysteine exhibited enhanced resistance to lead intoxication, while Niemöller (1957) reported on the use of methionine as an inhalant prophylactic with some apparent success. In addition, Uzbekov (1960) noted that the joint treatment of ascorbic acid and cysteine reduced the toxicity of lead and facilitated its excretion.

A more recent study by Mylorie et al. (1977) has supported the original findings that supplementation of the diet with S-containing amino acids reduces the risk of lead intoxication. In their study, young male rats were placed on diets that consisted of either (1) normal protein (NP) (27% casein); (2) low protein (LP) (8% casein) plus 1% alanine; (3)

LP + 1% cystine (LP + cys); and (4) LP + 1% methionine (LP + meth). With the exception of the unexposed NP controls all rat treatments were exposed to 1 μg Pb/ml of drinking water ad libitum for 5 weeks, at which time the study was terminated. While there were no marked differences in the total exposure to lead among the various treatments, these groups did exhibit significantly different degrees of lead retention with the LP + Pb group having markedly higher values for lead in the blood, spleen, and liver (Table 1). Both LP + cystine and LP + methionine treatments were effective in preventing the retention of lead in the blood, spleen, and liver. However, they were not able to prevent accumulation in bone and kidney. Cystine and methionine treatments also prevented, to a limited degree, the adverse effects of lead on the hematopoietic system. For instance, the blood parameters (i.e., RBC, Hgb, Hct) of lead-exposed rats given methionine or cystine supplements were only slightly decreased (i.e., 5 to 8%) as compared to controls, while there was a 24–27% decrease of these values in the rats given the LP diet. In addition, ALA values were reduced in the LP + cystine and LP + methionine groups as compared to the LP group, thereby providing further evidence of protection. These authors concluded that "the sulfur-containing amino acids appear to protect rats against lead induced anemia. Since they did not prevent the accumulation of lead in the bones and kidney, the 'protection' may be of dubious value."

In apparent conflict with these findings of Mylorie et al. (1977), Conrad and Barton (1978) showed that cystine, cysteine, tyrosine, arginine, and methionine enhanced the solubility of lead at neutral pH, thereby enhancing the absorption of lead by approximately 15–50% in experiments involving labeled lead with the isolated duodenal-loop technique (Figure 8-2). Another experiment that measured the percentage of radioactive lead in the carcass 4 hours after the test dose revealed that methionine enhanced the percentage of lead absorbed by nearly 100% when given along with the lead dose. Thus the methionine-treated group exhibited a 17.82% lead-absorption rate, compared to 9.84% of the controls. However, when methionine and ferric chloride were given together, the influence of methionine was nearly completely abrogated.

While the findings of Mylorie et al. (1977) and Conrad and Barton (1978) do not necessarily contradict each other, they do appear inconsistent. Future efforts should be directed toward resolving this issue. Finally, the striking findings reported by Mylorie et al. (1977) are of considerable interest, especially when considered along with other nutrients that may affect lead toxicity. Not only are their experiments

Table 1. Concentration of Lead in Blood and Tissues of Rats Ingesting Different Diets and Consuming Lead in Their Drinking Water[a]

Diet		Blood	Bone	Kidney	Spleen	Liver
NP + Pb	(20)	61 ± 4[b]	384 ± 20[b]	50 ± 1	3.8 ± 0.2[b]	4.4 ± 0.5
LP + Pb	(20)	369 ± 39	243 ± 26	37 ± 6	8.9 ± 1.9	5.4 ± 0.4
LP + Cys + Pb	(20)	46 ± 3[b]	259 ± 21	40 ± 5	1.5 ± 0.3[b]	2.1 ± 0.2[b]
LP + Meth + Pb	(20)	65 ± 11[b]	205 ± 18	32 ± 6	2.4 ± 0.5[b]	1.8 ± 0.2[b]
NP[c]	(20)	<0.1	<0.5	<0.1	<0.1	<0.1

[a]Data are expressed as micrograms of Pb per 100 ml of blood or micrograms of Pb per gram wet weight of tissue. Values are given as the mean ± SE of the number of determinations in parentheses.

[b]Significantly different ($p < 0.01$) from animals receiving a low-protein diet.

[c]Blood-lead concentration of rats not given lead acetate did not vary significantly with the type of diet.

Source. Mylorie, A.A.; Moore, L.; and Erogbogbo, V. (1977). Influence of dietary factors on blood and tissue-lead concentrations and lead toxicity. *Toxicol. Appl. Pharmacol.* **41**:364.

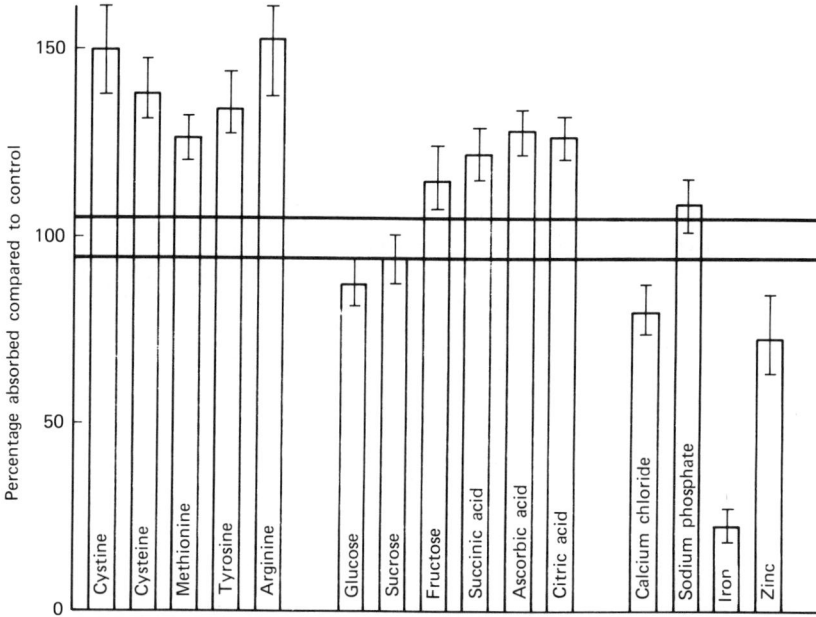

Figure 8-2. Effect of millimolar concentrations of various compounds upon the absorption of a test dose of ^{203}Pb from an isolated duodenal loop is shown. Values are expressed as a percentage of that absorbed from a comparable test dose administered to rats in distilled water on the same day because there is a significant daily variation in absorption among control animals. The mean ± SEM for control animals is shown in the *horizontal crosshatched area.* The addition of amino acids with sulfhydryl groups and certain reducing substances seemed to increase lead absorption, whereas calcium, iron, and zinc decreased absorption. [*Source.* Conrad, M.E. and Barton, J.C. (1978). Factors affecting the absorption and excretion of lead in the rat. *Gastroenterology* **74**:736.]

in need of replication but also of considerable extension, including interactive studies with calcium and iron.

References

Baernstein, H.D. and Grand, J.A. (1942). The relationship of protein intake to lead poisoning in rats. *J. Pharm. Exper. Therap.* **74**:18–24.

Buckup, H.; Böhm, M.; Zimmerman, H.; Remy, R.; Portheine, F.U.; and Voss, C. (1956). Nahrungskomponenten und ihre Bedeutung fur die Prophylaxie beiflicher Bleivergiftung (Experimentelle Untersuchungen am Kaninchen). *Zentbl. ArbMed. ArbSchut* **6**:29.

Conrad, M.E. and Barton, J.C. (1978). Factors affecting the absorption and excretion of lead in the rat. *Gastroenterology* **74**:731–740.

Mahaffey, K.R. (1974). Nutritional factors in lead toxicity. *Environ. Health Perspect.* **7**:107.

Mylorie, A.A.; Moore, L.; and Erogbogbo, V. (1977). Influence of dietary factors in blood and tissue lead concentrations and lead toxicity. *Toxicol. Appl. Pharmacol.* **41**:361–367.

Niemöller, H.K. (1957). Zur Prophylaxie der Bleivergiftung. Inhalationsversuche mit verschiedenen Chemikalien. *Dt. Med. Wschr.* **82**:738.

Uzbekov, G.A. (1960). The role of ascorbic acid and cysteine as detoxicants in lead poisoning. *Voprosy Medisinskoi* **6**:183–187.

7. Mercury

There has been considerable research designed to evaluate the influence of nutrients on mercury toxicity. The most studied of these interactions is that of selenium with mercury. That cystine may also affect the toxicity of mercury was conceived following the initial reports of Parizek and Ostadalova (1967) and Parizek et al. (1971) concerning the interaction of selenium and mercury, but also in recognition of the observation that mercury exposure significantly reduces the number of free sulfhydryl groups in various tissues including the brain (Perkanen and Sandholm, 1971).

In a series of experiments with rats (Stillings et al., 1972, 1974), it was shown that diets with cystine supplements provided a striking protective influence on methylmercury toxicity as measured by increased growth and survival time. Cystine did not reduce methylmercury toxicity by increasing its excretion via urine and feces. In addition, only small changes attributable to cystine were found in the tissue distribution patterns of mercury, with the exception of one experiment in which those rats given cystine supplements also had significantly lower kidney-mercury values. While the manner by which cystine reduces mercury toxicity is unknown, it was suggested that (1) cystine offers sulfur-binding sites in proteins that complex with mercury, or (2) cystine enhances the conversion of methylmercury to a less toxic form. In partial support of this latter possibility, Norseth and Clarkson (1970) reported that inorganic mercury was released from methylmercuric chloride when placed in a buffered solution containing 0.1 M cysteine. In the absence of cysteine, no inorganic mercury was released.

Finally, an abstract published by El-Begearmi et al. (1974) revealed that cystine (0.3%) supplementation provided only a very slight protection against methylmercury-induced (10 ppm) lethality in Japanese quail. Methionine supplementation at 0.3% likewise did not affect methylmercury toxicity. However, the joint treatment of selenium, arsenic, and methionine did provide nearly complete protection from mercury-induced lethality, a finding not predicted by the individual effects of the three test compounds.

References

El-Begearmi, M.; Ganther, H.E.; and Sunde, M.L. (1974). Effect of some sulfur amino acids, selenium and arsenic on mercury toxicity using Japanese quail. *Poult. Sci.* **53**:1921.

Norseth, T. and Clarkson, W.T. (1970). Studies on the biotransformation of [203]Hg labeled methyl mercury chloride in rats. *Arch. Environ. Health* **21**:717–727.

Parizek, J. and Ostadalova, T. (1967). Protective effect of small amounts of selenite in sublimate intoxication. *Experientia* **23**:142–143.

Parizek, J.; Ostadalova, T.; Kalouskova, T.; Babicky, A.; Pavlik, L.; and Bibr, B.C. (1971). Effect of mercuric compounds on the maternal transmission of selenium in the pregnant and lactating rat. *J. Reprod. Fert.* **25**:157–170.

Perkanen, T. and Sandholm, M. (1971). The effect of experimental methyl mercury poisoning on the number of sulfhydryl (SH) groups in the brain, liver, and muscle of rats. *Acta Vet. Scand.* **12**:551–559.

Stillings, B.R.; Lagally, H.; Baversfeld, P.; and Soares, J. (1974). Effect of cystine, selenium and fish protein on the toxicity and metabolism of methylmercury in rats. *Toxicol. Appl. Pharmacol.* **30**:243–254.

Stillings, B.R.; Lagally, H.; Soares, J.; and Miller, D. (1972). Effect of cystine and selenium on the toxicological effects of methyl mercury in rats. In: *Proceedings of the IX International Congress of Nutrition,* p. 206. Summaria, Mexico City.

8. Nitrate—Nitrite

There is considerable public health concern over the capability of nitrate and nitrite in particular, to cause methemoglobin formation, especially among infants (PHS, 1962). In fact, the present EPA drinking water standard of 10 mg NO_3 as N/L is designed to prevent infants from nitrate-induced methemoglobinemia (Calabrese, 1978).

Over the years it has become generally recognized that a number of biological and dietary factors either enhance or retard the formation of nitrate/nitrite-induced methemoglobinemia. For instance, infants are at particularly high risk as a result of their reduced enzymatic capacity to reduce methemoglobin to hemoglobin and the presence of nitrate-reducing bacteria in their stomachs (Calabrese, 1978). As for dietary factors that may affect the formation of methemoglobin, the most thoroughly studied is ascorbic acid (see Volume 1—ascorbic acid). This section will address the influence of methionine and its interaction with ascorbic acid in preventing the formation of nitrite-induced methemoglobin.

While the first indication that dietary levels of methionine may affect nitrite-induced methemoglobin formation was published by Mortensen in 1953, it was not until 20 years later that a detailed assessment of this hypothesis was published (Stoewsand et al., 1973). They found that neither ascorbic acid nor methionine (both up to 1% of the diet) given separately reduced the occurrence of nitrite-induced (7.6 mg/kg) methemoglobin formation (approximately 11%). There was no apparent protection even when both substances were provided, with only one substance being as high as 1.0% in the diet. However, when both compounds were given at a level of 1.0% in the diet, a reduction of greater than 50% of the methemoglobin levels occurred. Further supplementation of ascorbic acid and methionine up to 2.0% of the diet for each substance resulted in only a slight further decrease in methemoglobin levels.

This striking synergistic interaction of ascorbic acid and methionine in reducing nitrite-induced methemoglobin levels is worthy of consideration from a theoretical perspective. However, since such elevated levels are needed to cause a reduction in methemoglobin levels, the prophylactic use of ascorbic acid-methionine supplements do not appear practical. Therapeutic uses of such a supplementation may be worthy of further study.

References

Calabrese, E.J. (1978). *Methodological Approaches to Deriving Environmental and Occupational Health Standards*. Wiley, New York.

Mortensen, R.B. (1953). The effect of diet on methemoglobin levels of nitrite-injected rats. *Arch. Bioch. Biophys.* **46**:241.

PHS (1962). Drinking Water Standards. Washington, D.C.

Stoewsand, G.S.: Anderson, J.L.; and Lee, C.Y. (1973). Nitrite-induced methemoglobinemia in guinea pigs: influence of diets containing beets with varying amounts of nitrate, and the effect of ascorbic acid and methionine. *J. Nutr.* **103**:419–424.

9. Selenium

In the chapter on the interaction of dietary protein with various toxicants, it was demonstrated that a high-protein diet provides greater protection against selenium toxicity in laboratory animals (i.e., rats) than a diet low in protein content (Moxon, 1937; Smith, 1939; Smith and Stohlman, 1940; Gortner, 1940; Lewis et al., 1940; Rosenfeld and Beath, 1946). Not only does the level of protein in the diet offset selenium toxicity but also the type of protein as well (Moxon, 1941; Anderson et al., 1941). The next question, of course, is what particular protein constituent or group of constituents are needed for this enhanced protection from selenium toxicity?

One of the leading contenders in attempting to explain, at least in part, the protective nature of dietary protein is the presence of sulfur-containing amino acids, particularly methionine. Despite the fact that methionine is thought to affect selenium intoxication, its role, especially in the early investigations into this problem, was very equivocal. In fact, the first attempt to evaluate the possible protective role of methionine supplementation in preventing selenium intoxication was not supportive (Smith, 1939). In this experiment, rats were reared on a low-protein (10% wheat protein, 0% commercial casein), high-carbohydrate (75%) diet with 10 ppm of naturally occurring selenium and 0.8% methionine added to the diet.

In apparent contrast to the findings of Smith (1939), Lewis et al. (1940) reported that methionine supplementation (0.45 to 0.89%) to a diet with 6% casein resulted in a degree of protection from selenium intoxication equivalent to a 30%-casein diet. Furthermore, they noted that a methionine-supplemented 15% arachin[2] diet provided reduced susceptibility to selenium toxicity relative to a plain arachin diet.

While the findings of Lewis et al. (1940) are strikingly different from those of Smith (1939), it is difficult to directly compare their divergent findings since Lewis et al. (1940) (1) used casein as a protein source; in contrast to Smith, (2) had higher selenium concentrations (i.e., 25 to 50 ppm vs. only 10 ppm); (3) added sodium selenite as the selenium source in contrast to naturally occurring seleniferous grains; and (4) employed lower levels of carbohydrate and higher levels of fat in the diet. In any case, these divergent findings with respect to the role of methionine in preventing the toxicity of selenium encouraged further research to attempt to resolve the issue.

Since 1940, a number of investigators have attempted to evaluate the interaction of methionine with toxic levels of selenium (Smith and Stohlman, 1940; Moxon and Rhian, 1943; Fels and Cheldelin, 1948; Sellers et al., 1950; Klug et al., 1952; Drill, 1952; Olson et al., 1958; Whitting and Horwitt, 1964; and Levander and Morris, 1970). While several of these researchers continued to find little or no protective

[2]A protein deficient in methionine.

action for methionine (Smith and Stohlman, 1940; Klug et al., 1952), as well as cystine (Smith and Stohlman, 1940; Schneider, 1936), other investigators noted a beneficial influence of methionine against selenium in tocopherol-deficient rats fed 1.25 ppm selenium (Whitting and Horwitt, 1964), or when given along with 0.05% α-tocopherol acetate at a selenite level of 20 ppm (Sellers et al., 1950). More recent studies by Levander and Morris (1970) supported the findings of Sellers et al. (1950), in that methionine (0.5%) supplements were only protective against selenium (10 ppm) intoxication when adequate vitamin E (0.05%) was present in the diet. These authors specifically stated "that methionine can be of value in protecting the livers of rats against damage caused by diets containing toxic levels of selenium as long as sufficient vitamin E or fat soluble antioxidants are present in the diet. This beneficial effect of methionine against selenium poisoning could be explained by an increased excretion of selenium either via the lungs or urine. Animals challenged with subacute doses of selenium form volatile methylated selenide derivatives as detoxification products which are eliminated via the lungs (Ganther et al., 1966), and S-adenosyl-L-methionine has been shown to be the probable methyl donor in this process (Ganther, 1966). In chronic selenium poisoning, on the other hand, trimethyl selenide has been shown to be a major selenium metabolite in the urine (Byard, 1969; Palmer et al., 1969). If the availability of methionine for the biosynthesis of either of these two selenium metabolites were the limiting factor in the detoxification of selenium, this would account for the ability of methionine and the failure of cysteine or betaine to counteract selenium toxicity. Any antagonism of guanidacetic acid against the protective effect of methionine could also be explained, since this compound would utilize methyl groups needed for selenium detoxification."

As for the role of vitamin E in the process, Levander and Morris (1970), commenting on Sukharevskaya and Shtutman (1968), suggested that vitamin E may facilitate the availability of methyl groups from methionine for the detoxification of selenium.

References

Anderson, H.D.; Poley, W.E.; and Moxon, A.L. (1941). The effect of dietary protein supplements on the toxicity of seleniferous grains for the chick. *Poult. Sci.* **20**:454.

Byard, J.L. (1969). Trimethyl selenide. A urinary metabolite of selenite. *Arch. Biochem. Biophys.* **130**:556.

Drill, V.A. (1952). Hepatotoxic agents: mechanism of action and dietary interrelationship. *Pharmacol. Rev.* **4**:1–41.

Fels, I.G. and Cheldelin, V.H. (1948). Methionine in selenium poisoning. *J. Biol. Chem.* **176**:819–828.

Ganther, H.E. (1966). Enzymatic synthesis of dimethyl selenide from sodium selenite in mouse liver extracts. *Biochem.* **5**:1089.

Ganther, H.E.; Levander, O.A.; and Baumann, C.A. (1966). Dietary control of selenium volatilization in the rat. *J. Nutr.* **88**:55.

Gortner, R.A., Jr. (1940). Chronic selenium poisoning of rats as influenced by dietary protein. *J. Nutr.* **19**:105–112.

Klug, H.C.; Harshfield, R.D.; Pengra, R.M.; and Moxon, A.L. (1952). Methionine and selenium toxicity. *J. Nutr.* **48**:409–420.

Levander, O.A. and Morris, V.C. (1970). Interactions of methionine, vitamin E, and antioxidants in selenium toxicity in the rat. *J. Nutr.* **100**:1111–1118.

Lewis, H.B.; Schultz, J.; and Gortner, R.A., Jr. (1940). Dietary protein and the toxicity of sodium selenite in the white rat. *J. Pharmacol. Exp. Therap.* **68**:292.

Moxon, A.L. (1937). Alkali disease or selenium poisoning. *So. Dakota Agric. Expt. Sta. Bull.* No. 311, pp. 1–91.

Moxon, A.L. (1941). Alkali disease. Ph.D. dissertation, Univ. of Wisconsin, Madison.

Moxon, A.L. and Rhian, M. (1943). Selenium poisoning. *Physiol. Rev.* **23**:305–337.

Olson, O.E.; Carlson, C.W.; and Leitis, E. (1958). Methionine and related compounds and selenium poisoning. Tech. Bull. No. 20, S. Dakota Agr. Exp. Sta., College Station, Brookings, S.D.

Palmer, I.S.; Fischer, D.D.; Halverson, A.W.; and Olson, O.E. (1969). Identification of a major selenium excretory product in rat urine. *Biochim. Biophys. Acta* **177**:336.

Rosenfeld, I. and Beath, O.A. (1946). The influence of protein diets on selenium poisoning. *Am J. Vet. Res.* **7**:52.

Schneider, H.A. (1936). Selenium in nutrition. *Science* **83**:32.

Sellers, E.A.; Yon, R.W.; and Lucas, C.C. (1950). Lipotropic agents in liver damage produced by selenium on carbon tetrachloride. *Proc. Soc. Exp. Biol. Med.* **75**:118–121.

Smith, M.I. (1939). The influence of diet on the chronic toxicity of selenium. *Pub. Health Repts.* **54**:1441–1453.

Smith, M.I. and Stohlman, E.F. (1940). Further observations on the influence of dietary protein on the toxicity of selenium. *J. Pharmacol. Exp. Therap.* **70**:270–278.

Sukharevskaya, A.M. and Shtutman, M. (1968). Relations among vitamin E, selenium and sulfur-containing amino acids. *Vop. Pitan.* **27**:13.

Whitting, L.A. and Horwitt, M.K. (1964). Effects of dietary selenium, methionine, fat level and tocopherol on rat growth. *J. Nutr.* **84**:351.

10. Silver

Exposure to silver is primarily an industrial hygiene concern since it is employed in many manufacturing processes, including the formation of silverware, jewelry, scientific instruments, automobile bearings, grids in storage batteries, and numerous other products (Tabershaw et al., 1977). The Occupational Safety and Health Administration (OSHA) has promulgated a federal standard for occupational exposure to silver metal and soluble compounds at 0.01 mg/m^3, an exposure limit that should prevent the development of generalized argyria following a lifetime of work exposure (ACGIH, 1976). While industrial exposure to silver is not regarded as a high or even moderate priority, elevated levels of silver salts have been reported to cause dystrophic lesions, necrotic degeneration of the liver, and high mortality in rats reared on a vitamin-E-deficient diet (Shaver and Mason, 1951), presumably by increasing the physiological requirement for this vitamin. In an effort to further explore the nature of silver toxicity, Diplock et al. (1967) evaluated the interaction of several nutrients including methionine on the toxicity of silver.

In their study, weanling vitamin-E-deficient rats were exposed to silver acetate (0.05% w/v) in distilled water and compared to a similarly exposed group whose diet was supplemented with methionine. Their findings revealed that the methionine-supplemented rats were somewhat more resistant to the hepatotoxic effects of silver, but this treatment did not affect the length of survival.

While this study does indicate a protective influence of methionine from silver toxicity, its biomedical relevance is uncertain. This is especially true since (1) the level of silver employed was exceptionally high, and (2) liver toxicity from silver exposure is not anticipated (or known) to be a problem in the industrial setting (Tabershaw et al., 1977; ACGIH, 1976). Before serious concern is directed toward the findings that diets inadequate in methionine enhance the toxicity of silver, it would be necessary to replicate the original study at realistic exposure levels using pair-feeding techniques, and to evaluate the influence of variable levels of dietary methionine on liver toxicity when vitamin E levels are adequate.

References

ACGIH (1976). Documentation of TLVs. American Conference of Governmental Industrial Hygienists. Cincinnati, OH.

Diplock, A.T.; Green, J.; Bunyan, J.; McHale, D.; and Muthy, I.R. (1967). Vitamin E and stress. The metabolism of D-α-tocopherol in the rat under dietary stress with silver. *Brit. J. Nutr.* **21**:115–125.

Shaver, S.L. and Mason, K.E. (1951). Impaired tolerance to silver in vitamin E deficient rats. *Anat. Rec.* **109**:382.

Tabershaw, I.R.; Utidjian, H.M.D.; and Kawahara, B. (1977). Chemical hazards. In: *Occupational Diseases: A Guide to Their Recognition.* Edited by M.M. Key et al. U.S. DHEW, PHS, CDC, NIOSH, Washington, D.C.

11. Thallium

Thallium, which is a soft, heavy metal, is considered to be one of the more toxic elements with respect to acute and chronic toxicity (Patty, 1963). Thallium intoxication may be characterized by loss of hair (alopecia) and various neurological symptoms such as lack of coordination and limb pain. More acute intoxication, which usually results from ingestion, involves gastrointestinal symptoms, abdominal colic, impaired renal function, and rapid alopecia, among other symptoms (Tabershaw et al., 1977).

Exposure to thallium occurs in workers in a number of occupations, since thallium and its compounds are employed "as rodenticides, fungicides, insecticides, catalysts in certain reactions, and phosphor activators, in bromoiodide crystals for lenses, plates, and prisms in infrared optical instruments, in photoelectric cells, in mineralogical analysis, alloyed with mercury in low temperature thermometers, switches and closures, in high-density liquids, in dyes and pigments, and in the manufacture of optical lenses, fireworks, and imitation precious jewelry. It forms a stainless alloy with silver and a corrosion-resistant alloy with lead."

The occurrence of human intoxication by thallium compounds is well known. Nearly 800 cases of thallium poisoning were reported by Heyroth (1947) in his review of the literature, with nearly 50 of these cases being fatalities. These intoxications resulted for the most part from the ingestion of thallium salts. Later studies by Reed et al. (1963) resulted in a continued documentation of thallium poisonings, especially in children, from the ingestion of thallium pesticides. Occupational exposures have also resulted in human intoxication (abdominal pain, fatigue, irritability, loss of hair, pains in legs), usually in association with the production of pesticides (Richeson, 1958; Anonymous, 1955, 1962). According to the ACGIH (1976), the TLV of 0.1 mg/m³ is "based largely on analogy with other highly toxic heavy metals" and is thought to prevent systemic effects.

That thallium toxicity may be influenced by nutritional status was first suggested by Buschke et al. (1939–1940) who stated that "nutrition plays a certain role in relation to the toxicity as well as the pilotropic effect of thallium." They also mentioned studies by Leukovich and Hoffman that revealed a differential susceptibility of sheep to thallium toxicity, depending on whether they were fed hay, fresh fodder, or grass. After this initial recognition of a diet-thallium relationship came a report by Bietti (1941), which noted that thallium-induced cataract formation and alopecia could be prevented by the addition of 10–15% brewer's yeast to the diet.

In light of these initial reports in the literature and the recognition that several of the toxic manifestations of thallium exposure such as diffuse alopecia, cataracts, hyperplasma of the forestomach, and rickets are known to be caused by nutritional deficiencies as well, Gross et al. (1948) speculated that specific nutritional deficiencies or excesses could modify the course of thallium intoxication. The nutrients evaluated as potential modifying agents of thallium toxicity included (1) levels of protein in the diet; (2) presence of several amino acids such as cystine, methionine, and tryptophane; and (3) several B-vitamins such as pyridoxine, thiamine, pathothenic acid, nicotinic acid, and para-aminobenzoic acid.

With respect to the sulfur-containing amino acid methionine, Gross et al. (1948) decided to include it for study after another sulfur-containing amino acid, cystine, had been found to markedly prevent thallium toxicity. Since methionine provides sulfur during the synthesis of cysteine and cystine, it was "thought that differences in its action from that of cystine might throw further light on the mechanism of thallium poisoning."

In their study with rats, Gross et al. (1948) found that providing 2% methionine in the daily diet did not give any noticeable protection from thallium-induced mortality. However, the methionine treatment did cause some delay in the occurrence of thallium-related deaths. In addition, this treatment reduced the incidence of thallium-induced alopecia relative to the controls.

Why dietary supplementation with methionine was much less efficient than cystine in preventing the toxicity of thallium is the obvious question. According to Gross et al. (1948), it is logical to hypothesize, based on the known mechanisms of catalytic responses of metals on sulfhydryl compounds, that thallium joins with l-homocysteine and l-cysteine, forming a compound that cannot be converted to cystine. This results in a cystine deficiency that leads to the occurrence of alopecia, especially since the synthesis of hair has a high cystine requirement. This theoretical scheme provides a consistent explanation for why cystine supplementation is so successful in combating thallium toxicity, while methionine supplementation is only marginally prophylactic.

The findings of Gross et al. (1948) are of great interest, since they provide not only novel insights into elucidating the dietary interaction with thallium but also for establishing a conceptual framework for understanding, in part, a mechanism for some of the toxicity attributed to thallium. Whether these findings have relevance for the occupational setting is difficult to ascertain in light of the limited scope of the studies and the paucity of supporting data in this area. Despite the limited information, the findings of Gross et al. (1948) are clearly impressive and do suggest that further research concerning the role of sulfur-containing amino acids (especially cystine) in preventing thallium toxicosis should be undertaken.

References

ACGIH (1976). Documentation for TLVs. American Conference of Governmental Industrial Hygienists, Cincinnati, OH.

Anonymous (1955). Foreign Letters section: Brief note on thallium poisoning. *J. Am. Med. Assoc.* **159**:510.

Anonymous (1962). Thallium poisoning. *Pub. Health Repts.* **77**:518.

Bietti, G. (1941). Sulla possibilita di influenzare, mediante vitamine del gruppo B, il decorso di alcune forme di cataratta speimentale, con ponticalare riguardo a quella da tallio. *Med. Sper. Arch. Ital.* **7**:3.

Buschke, A. and Peiser, B. (1939–1940). Biologische und klinische Ausblicke der neuern Thallium Forschung mit besonderer Beziehung zu den Haarpilz-Kranheiten. *Mycopathologia* **2**:204.

Gross, P.; Runne, E; and Wilson, J.W. (1948). Studies on the effect of thallium on poisoning of the rat. The influence of cystine and methionine on alopecia and survival periods. *J. Invest. Derm.* **10**:119–134.

Heyroth, F.E. (1947). *Pub. Health Repts.* Suppl. 197.

Patty, F.A. (1963). *Industrial Hygiene and Toxicology.* Vol. II, 2nd ed. Interscience, N.Y., pp. 1138–1143.

Reed, D.; Crawley, J.; Faro, S.N.; Pieper, S.J.; and Kurland, L.T. (1963). Thallotoxicosis: acute manifestations and sequelae. *JAMA* **183**:516–522.

Richeson, E.M. (1958). Industrial thallium intoxication. *Ind. Med. Surg.* **27**:607–619.

Tabershaw, I.R.; Utidjian, H.M.B.; and Kawahara, B. (1977). Chemical hazards. In: *Occupational Diseases: A Guide to Their Recognition.* Edited by M.M. Key et al. U.S. DHEW, PHS, CDC, NIOSH, Washington, D.C.

B. ORGANIC SUBSTANCES

1. Acetaldehyde and Ethanol

L-cysteine. Sprince et al. (1974, 1974a, 1975) have identified acetaldehyde as an important toxicant that results from both alcohol consumption and cigarette smoking. It is an intermediary metabolite of ethyl alcohol and is more toxic than ethanol. Heavy drinkers (James et al., 1970; Majchrowicz and Mendelson, 1970) and heavy cigarette smokers (Egle, 1970; Rylander, 1973) have been reported to have elevated body levels of acetaldehyde even though it is quickly metabolized. In fact, in 1970, James et al. suggested that some of the adverse health effects associated with both drinking and smoking may be related to acetaldehyde. In their excellent literature review, Sprince et al. (1975) noted that acetaldehyde exposure was associated with a variety of adverse health effects including alcoholic cardiomyopathy (Schreiber et al., 1974; James and Bear, 1967, 1968), alcohol addiction (Davis and Walsh, 1970; Cohen and Collins, 1970), in ethnic sensitivity to alcohol (Ewing et al., 1974), and others. In addition, Sprince et al. (1975) noted that acetaldehyde exposure from heavy cigarette smoking has been related to heart (Schreiber et al., 1974; James and Bear, 1967, 1968) and pulmonary disease via an inhibitory effect on cilia (Guillerm et al., 1961). As a result of such adverse effects resulting from acetaldehyde via excessive drinking and cigarette smoking, Sprince et al. (1975, 1975a, 1976, 1977, 1978) suggested that it is important to investigate the influence of chemical compounds that may protect against its adverse health effects. Among those compounds tested for their protective action against the anesthetic and lethal effects of acetaldehyde in male white rats are L-ascorbic acid and a variety of sulfur compounds.

According to Sprince et al. (1975), L-cysteine was thought to be a good potential prophylactic agent since it had been found to protect rats against thiourea-induced lethal pulmonary edema (Sprince et al., 1974), and acetaldehyde (Akabane, 1970). Other sulfur-containing compounds as well as L-ascorbic acid were also compared for their capacity to diminish acetaldehyde toxicity. The administration of L-cysteine (2 mM/kg) offered marked protection in mice against both the anesthetic and lethal effects of acetaldehyde (Sprince et al., 1975). While the control groups exhibited 54 and 90% death after 3 and 24 hours, respectively, the L-cysteine-treated groups had only 8 and 20% lethality following similar respective time periods. A comparable protective effect against acetaldehyde-induced anesthesia was noted in the L-cysteine-treated group. For comparative purposes the L-cysteine treatment was more effective than L-ascorbic acid (2 mM/kg), DL-homocysteine (2 mM/kg), but less effective than L-glutathione (2 mM/kg) and N-acetyl-L-cysteine (2 mM/kg), with zero out of 20 mice dying after 72 hours in the later group. Furthermore, a combined treatment with L-ascorbic acid (2.0 mM/kg), L-cysteine (1.0 mM/kg), and thiamin HCl (0.3 mM/kg) totally prevented the occurrence of mortality in mice while controls exhibited 90% mortality.

Sprince et al. (1975) have speculated on a mechanism by which L-cysteine protects against the toxicity of acetaldehyde. They stated that

L-cysteine joins with acetaldehyde to form a new compound called L-2-methylthiazolidine-4-carboxylic acid (L-MTCA). Presumably the L-MTCA may act as a nontoxic metabolic detoxification product and a "protectant by generating free intracellular (-SH) groups to complex with acetaldehyde more effectively (Debey et al., 1958). Biochemically, it has already been suggested that cysteine can protect Coenzyme A against acetaldehyde inhibition by complexing preferentially with acetaldehyde (Martin et al., 1966). Presumably, reduced glutathione, homocysteine, and N-acetyl-cysteine could also complex with acetaldehyde by virtue of their free (-SH) groups" (Friedman, 1973). While these findings are impressive, their relevance to the human condition remains to be further explored. Future research should be directed to chronic exposure studies in appropriate animal models.

Research into the efficacy of other amino acids in preventing or reducing the toxicity of ethanol and/or acetaldehyde has also been reported (Ward et al., 1972; Breglia et al., 1973). The specific amino acids evaluated were L-lysine, L-arginine, L-ornithine, and glycine.

In their rationale for such investigations, Breglia et al. (1973) described the extent to which these amino acids had been previously reported to affect ethanol metabolism and/or toxicity. For instance, Schiller et al. (1958, 1959) reported that an IV-administered amino acid-dextrose mixture given along with 120 ml p.o. of ethanol (50% v/v) to chronic alcoholics with hepatic dysfunction or nutritional deficiency enhanced the metabolism of ethanol. Follow-up investigations of this amino acid-dextrose mixture revealed its ability to enhance rat-liver slices to metabolize ethanol confirming previous observations in humans. While the specific amino acids responsible for this apparent enhanced metabolism of ethanol could not be specifically determined, studies did reveal that they were composed of four carbon atoms or less.

Other Amino Acids. Studies with specific amino acids including glycine or alanine revealed that administration of both of these amino acids to dogs resulted in lower blood-ethanol levels than appropriate controls, presumably by preventing the absorption (Widmark, 1933) and/or via an enhanced metabolism of ethanol via the Krebs cycle. This later explanation is more appropriate for the influence of alanine since it can be converted to pyruvate, which functions as a Krebs cycle intermediate (Westerfeld et al., 1942; LeBreton, 1934).

Other investigators have reported the protective influence of DL-threonine, L-methionine, and DL-glutamine against ethanol-induced changes in behavioral performance of rats (Mueller et al., 1971). Administration of L-lysine caused a marked reduction in the depressant and hypnotic effects of ethanol (Ward et al., 1972). Furthermore, acetaldehyde combines in an efficient manner with certain amino acids. The magnitude of reaction between amino acids and acetaldehyde is dependent on the nature of the amino acid and the pH of the medium (Robert and Penaranda, 1954; Greenstein and Winitz, 1961). Reactive carbonyl groups, as occur in acetaldehyde, have been theorized to combine with the undissociated amino groups of the amino acid, with lysine having the highest degree of amino groups in the undissociated form of all the essential amino acids that could react with acetaldehyde (Greenstein and Winitz, 1961).

In their evaluation of the hypothesis that administration of selected amino acids (L-lysine, L-arginine, L-ornithine, and glycine) could diminish the toxicity of ethanol, Breglia et al. (1973) utilized male and female rats with a variety of experimental conditions, including pretreatment and simultaneous exposure with amino acid(s) and ethanol as well as a consideration of a number of toxicity indices including acute toxicity ataxia and sleeping time. The results of this study indicated that amino acid treatment prolonged the start of ataxia, diminished the length of sleeping time, and reduced the number of animals losing the righting reflex, but it did not affect the LD_{50} values. According to the authors, the reason why the LD_{50} values were not affected by the amino acid treatments was probably because the dosage was so high and the G.I. absorption so fast as to mask any detoxicant effect apparent at lower concentrations.

It is of interest to note that the protective effects of the various amino acids were generally much greater at the highest concentrations of the amino acids employed. Since values as high as 2.5 g/kg of L-lysine were successfully employed to diminish ethanol toxicity, one can speculate on the possibility of these amino acids being toxic themselves at such elevated levels. However, the authors specifically stated that no toxicity was seen at the amino acid doses administered in this study. Yet they pointed out that amino acid toxicity resulting from excessive exposure is a concern and may result in an increase of ammonia, urea, and other nitrogen acceptors (McLean and McLean, 1969; Gullino et al., 1956). Finally, these findings, along with those of Sprince and his associates, clearly indicate that a variety of amino acids given in excess of nutritional needs, helps to prevent a range of toxicity indices associated with excess ethanol ingestion. These findings suggest that clinical research investigations should be initiated to establish the role of amino acid nutritional status in preventing the toxicity of acetaldehyde, especially in alcoholics.

References

Akabane, J. (1970). Aldehydes and related compounds. In *International Encyclopedia of Pharmacology and Therapeutics*. Vol. II., pp. 523–560. Edited by J. Tremolieres. Pergamon Press, New York.

Breglia, R.J.; Ward, C.O.; and Jarowski, C.I. (1973). Effect of selected amino acids on ethanol toxicity in rats. *J. Pharm. Sci.* **62**(1):49–55.

Cohen, G. and Collins, M. (1970). Alkaloids from catecholamines in adrenal tissue: possible role in alcoholism. *Science* **167**:1749–1751.

Davis, V.E. and Walsh, M.J. (1970). Alcohol, amines, and alkaloids: a possible biochemical basis for alcohol addiction. *Science* **167**:1005–1007.

Debey, H.J.; MacKenzie, J.B.; and MacKenzie, C.G. (1958). The replacement by thiazolidinecarboxylic acid of exogenous cystine and cysteine. *J. Nutr.* **66**:607–619.

Egle, J.L., Jr. (1970). Retention of inhaled acetaldehyde in man. *J. Pharmacol. Exp. Ther.* **174**:14–19.

Ewing, J.A.; Rouse, B.A.; and Pellizzari, E.D. (1974). Alcohol sensitivity and ethnic background. *Am. J. Psychiat.* **131**:200–210.

Friedman, M. (1973). *The Chemistry and Biochemistry of the Sulfhydryl Group in Amino Acids, Peptides and Proteins*. Pergamon Press, N.Y., pp. 88–90, 92–95.

Greenstein, J.P. and Winitz, M. (1961). *Chemistry of the Amino Acids*. Wiley, N.Y., pp. 448–449.

Guillerm, R.; Badre, R.; and Bignon, B. (1961). Effets inhibiteurs de la fumie de tabac sur l'activite ciliaire de l'epithelium respiratoire et nature des composants responsables. *Bull. Acad. Nat. Med.* **145**:416–423.

Gullino, P.; Winitz, M.; Birnbaum, S.M.; Cornfield, J.; Otey, M.C.; and Greenstein, J.P. (1956). Studies on the metabolism of amino acids and related compounds *in vivo*. I. Toxicity of essential amino acids, individually and in mixtures, and the protective effect of L-arginine. *Arch. Biochem. Biophys.* **64**:319–332.

Horton, A.D. and Guerin, M.R. (1974). Determination of acetaldehyde and acrolein in the gas phase of cigarette smoke using cryothermal gas chromatography. *Tobacco* **176**(4):45–48.

James, T.N. and Bear, E.S. (1967). Effects of ethanol and acetaldehyde on the heart. *Am. Heart J.* **74**:243–255.

James, T.N. and Bear, E.S. (1968). Cardiac effects of some simple aliphatic aldehydes. *J. Pharmacol. Exp. Ther.* **163**:300–308.

James, T.N.; Bear, E.S.; Lange, K.F.; Green, E.W.; and Winkler, H.H. (1970). Adrenergic mechanisms in the sinus node. *Arch. Int. Med.* **125**:512–547.

LeBreton, E. (1934). Influence de la nature de l'aliment brule la vitesse d'oxydation de l'alcool dans l'organisme. *Compt. Rend. Soc. Biol.* **117**:709–712.

Majchrowicz, E. and Mendelson, J.H. (1970). Blood concentrations of acetaldehyde and ethanol in chronic alcoholics. *Science* **168**:1100–1102.

Martin, G.J.; Moss, J.N.; Smyth, R.D.; and Beck, H. (1966). The effect of cysteine in modifying the action of ethanol given chronically in rats. *Life Sci.* **5**:2357–2362.

McLean, A.E.M. and McLean, E.K. (1969). Diet and toxicity. *Brit. Med. Bull.* **25**:278–281.

Mueller, A.J.; Kissel, J.W.; and McKinney, G.R. (1971). A method to measure interactions of various agents and ethanol on behavioral performance in rats. *Proc. Soc. Exp. Biol. Med.* **136**:203–206.

Robert, L. and Penaranda, F.S. (1954). Studies on aldehyde protein interaction. I. Reactions of amino acids with lower aldehydes. *J. Polymer Sci.* **12**:337–350.

Rylander, R. (1973). Toxicity of cigarette smoke components: free lung cell response in acute exposures. *Am. Rev. Resp. Dis.* **108**:1279–1282.

Schiller, J.; Peck, R.E.; and Goldberg, M.A. (1958). The effect of dextrose, fat emulsion and amino acids on the rate of disappearance of alcohol in the blood. *Amer. J. Psychiat.* **115**:365–366.

Schiller, J.; Peck, R.E.; and Goldberg, M.A. (1959). Studies in alcoholism: effects of amino acids on rate of disappearance of alcohol from blood. *Arch. Neurol.* **1**:127–132.

Schreiber, S.S.; Oratz, M.; Rothschild, M.A.; Reff, F.; and Evans, C. (1974). Alcoholic cardiomyopathy. II. The inhibition of cardiac microsomal protein synthesis by acetaldehyde. *J. Mole. Cell. Cardiol.* **6**:207–213.

Sprince, H.; Parker, C.M.; and Smith, G.G. (1977). L-ascorbic acid in alcoholism and smoking: protection against acetaldehyde toxicity as an experimental model. *Internat. J. Vit. Nut. Res.* **47** (Suppl. 16) (cited in Sprince, H., et al., *Nutr. Repts. Internat.* **17**(4):441–455, 1978).

Sprince, H.; Parker, C.M.; and Smith, G.G. (1978). Acetaldehyde, ascorbic acid, and catecholamine-regulating drugs: data and hypothesis in relation to alcoholism and smoking. *Nutr. Repts. Internat.* **17**(4):441–455.

Sprince, H.; Parker, C.M.; Smith, G.G.; and Gonzales, L.J. (1974). Protection against acetaldehyde toxicity in the rat by L-cysteine, thiamin, and L-2-methyl-thiazalidine-4-carboxylic acid. *Agents and Actions* **4**:125–130.

Sprince, H.; Parker, C.M.; Smith, G.G.; and Gonzales, L.J. (1974a). Protectants against acetaldehyde toxicity, sulfhydryl compounds and ascorbic acid. *Fed. Proc. Am. Soc. Exp. Biol.* 33, No. 3, part 1, 233, Abstract No. 172.

Sprince, H.; Parker, C.M.; Smith, G.G.; and Gonzales, L.J. (1975). Protective action of ascorbic acid and sulfur compounds against acetaldehyde toxicity: implications in alcoholism and smoking. *Agents and Actions* **5**(2):164–173.

Sprince, H.; Parker, C.M.; Smith, G.G.; and Gonzales, L.J. (1975a). Protection against acetaldehyde toxicity by ascorbic acid plus reserpine or atropine. *Fed. Proc. Am. Soc. Exp. Biol.* **34**(3):277. (Abst. No. 51)

Sprince, H.; Parker, C.M.; Smith, G.G.; and Gonzales, L.J. (1976). Protection against acetaldehyde toxicity by ascorbic acid plus propranolol or phenoxybenzamine. *Fed. Proc. Am. Soc. Exp. Biol.* **35**(3):707. (Abst. No. 2758)

Truitt, E.B., Jr.; and Walsh, M.J. (1971). The role of acetaldehyde in the actions of ethanol. In *The Biology of Alcoholism*, vol. 1. B. Kissin and H. Begleiter, eds. Plenum Press, New York, pp. 161–195.

Ward, C.O.; Lau Cam, C.A.; Tang, A.S.M.; Breglia, R.J.; and Jarowski, C.I. (1972). Effect of lysine on toxicity and depressant effects of ethanol in rats. *Toxicol. Appl. Pharmacol.* **22**:422–426.

Westerfeld, W.W.; Stotz, E.; and Berg, R.L. (1942). The role of pyruvate in the metabolism of ethyl alcohol. *J. Biol. Chem.* **144**:657–665.

Widmark, E.M.P. (1933). Uber die Einwirkung von Aminosauren auf den Alkoholgehalt des Blutes. *Biochem. Z.* **265**:237–240.

2. Aflatoxin

a. Methionine

While aflatoxin B_1 (AFB_1) is widely recognized as a potent hepatotoxin and carcinogen, it is also toxic to a variety of other tissues including the kidney. This knowledge, coupled with the observation that a diet marginal in lipotropes (i.e., 0.1% choline, 0.3% methionine, and no cystine or vitamin B_{12}), while not causing a morphological irregularity of liver tissue, did result in considerable degenerative lesions of the proximal convoluted tubules of the kidney (Newberne and Young, 1966) similar to an AFB_1-induced renal damage (Newberne et al., 1964; Newberne, 1965), led Newberne et al. (1968) to speculate that a marginal lipotrope diet may enhance the renal toxicity of AFB_1. Consequently, they evaluated the influence of "superimposing AFB_1 on a diet which induces renal lesions."

Of particular relevance to this section was a preliminary experiment in which rats reared on a basal marginal lipotrope diet (i.e., 0.1% methionine and 0.1% choline chloride) with the addition of either supplemental choline chloride (0.6%) or methionine (0.6%) or vitamin B_{12} (50 μg/kg of diet) were compared with groups fed either the unsupplemented low-lipotrope diet (basal) or the normal (i.e., adequately supplied) lipotrope diet. Their findings revealed that both vitamin B_{12} and methionine supplementation reduced the severity of marginal lipotrope-induced renal lesions, while choline supplementation was without effect. Furthermore, the effect of methionine was considerably more beneficial than that of vitamin B_{12}. However, when AFB_1 was given to rats reared on a low-lipotrope diet, it did not enhance the occurrence of renal lesions compared to unexposed controls. Thus the original hypothesis of Newberne et al. (1968) that a low-lipotrope diet (including inadequate methionine) predisposes rats to the development of AFB_1-induced renal damage was not supported.

b. Cysteine

Research concerning the mechanism by which AFB_1 causes toxicity and/or carcinogenicity has suggested that it must become transformed to an epoxide intermediate, which then initiates a biochemical lesion within either nucleic acids or proteins (Schoental, 1970). More specifically, evidence exists that suggests that the parent compound (i.e., aflatoxin B_1) is converted to aflatoxin B_1-2,3 oxide, which may bind in a covalent fashion to the nucleophilic sites on DNA, RNA, and other macromolecules (Swenson et al., 1974; Garner et al., 1971).

According to Mgbodile et al. (1975), aflatoxin B_1-2,3-epoxide, the proposed active intermediate presumably responsible for the adverse effects of AFB_1, exhibits comparable electrophilic characteristics to the epoxide of bromobenzene. Since bromobenzene is detoxified to a large extent via conjugation to glutathione (GSH), they hypothesized that aflatoxin epoxide may also be similarly detoxified. If this were true, then it would be expected that the administration of GSH or its amino acid precursors such as cysteine would enhance the detoxification of aflatoxin epoxide. In studies to evaluate this hypothesis, a 200 mg/kg dose of cysteine was given before the administration of AFB_1. As predicted, the cysteine supplementation resulted in a diminished degree of liver necrosis as well as partially reversing the decrease in the activity of liver microsomal-enzyme activity as measured by cytochrome P-450 content. Consistent with these findings were observations that diethyl maleate, an agent that depletes liver GSH, enhanced aflatoxin-induced liver toxicity.

These authors concluded that glutathione may have an important role in the detoxification of AFB_1 within the liver. It would be of further interest to evaluate whether these findings also extend to protecting against aflatoxin-induced carcinogenicity. Finally, Ferreyra et al. (1979) reported that cystamine and cysteine were unable to protect against AFB_1-induced hepatotoxic effects in rats when given as a single therapeutic dose 12 hours after treatment.

c. *Addendum*

Many of the investigations concerning the role of dietary lipotropes on the toxicity and carcinogenicity of chemical agents consider the total amount of lipotropes in the diet. The comparison is made between animals reared on a low- vs. high-lipotropic diet. For example, Newberne et al. (1968) identified their marginal lipotrope diet as having 1/6 the levels of DL-methionine and choline chloride given the control group, while vitamin B_{12} was not given in the marginal diet but was added to a level of 5.0 μg/100 g of diet for the controls. Other marginal lipotrope diets manipulate just choline, or choline and vitamin B_{12} levels, or numerous other possible arrangements. Since more than one lipotropic agent may frequently differ between treatment and control groups, it is not possible to conclude definitively what the specific function of each lipotrope may be. This is especially true of the series of investigations by Newberne and Rogers of MIT concerning the role of marginal lipotrope diets on the carcinogenicity of AFB_1, several nitrosamines, and dimethylhydrazine. In contrast to modification of the levels of several lipotropes simultaneously to establish a marginal lipotrope diet are the recent papers of Shinozuka et al. (1978, 1978a), which evaluated the influence of a single lipotropic agent, choline, on DL-ethionine carcinogenicity. This is not intended to be critical of the research of Newberne and Rogers since their work is (1) pioneering in the area, as well as (2) an attempt to create a realistic situation by providing diets marginal in lipotropes rather than totally deficient. Consequently, when the role of a low-lipotropic diet on the toxicity and/or carcinogenicity of agents is discussed, the reader will find additional information in Volume 1, Chapter 2, "The B-Vitamins", in connection with choline and/or vitamin B_{12}.

References

Ferreyra de, E.C.; Fenos de, O.M.; Bernacchi, A.S.; Castro de, C.R., and Castro, J.A. (1979). Therapeutic effectiveness of cystamine and cysteine to reduce liver cell necrosis induced by several hepatotoxins. *Toxicol. Appl. Pharm.* **48**:221–228.

Garner, R.C.; Miller, E.C.; Miller, J.A.; Garner, J.V.; and Hanson, R.S. (1971). Formation of a factor lethal for *S. typhimurium* TA 1530 and TA 1531 on incubation of aflatoxin B_1 with rat liver microsomes. *Biochem. Biophys. Res. Commun.* **45**:774–780.

Mgbodile, M.U.K.; Holscher, M.; and Neal, R.A. (1975). A possible protective role for reduced glutathione in aflatoxin B_1 toxicity: effect of pretreatment of rats with phenobarbital and 3-methylcholanthrene on aflatoxin toxicity. *Toxicol. Appl. Pharmacol.* **34**:128–142.

Newberne, P.M. (1965). Carcinogenicity of aflatoxin-contaminated peanut meal. In: *Mycotoxins in Foodstuffs*, p. 187. Edited by G.N. Wogan. MIT Press, Cambridge, MA.

Newberne, P.M.; Carlton, W.W.; and Wogan, G.N. (1964). Hepatomas in rats and hepatorenal injury in ducklings fed peanut meal or *Aspergillus flavus* extract. *Pathol. Vet.* **1**:105.

Newberne, P.M.; Rogers, A.E.; and Wogan, G.N. (1968). Hepatorenal lesions in rats fed a a low lipotrope diet and exposed to aflatoxin. *J. Nutr.* **94**:331–336.

Newberne, P.M. and Young, V.R. (1966). Effect of diets marginal in methionine and choline with and without vitamin B_{12} on rat liver and kidney. *J. Nutr.* **89**:69.

Rogers, A.E. and Newberne, P.M. (1969). Aflatoxin B_1 carcinogenesis in lipotrope-deficient rats. *Cancer Res.* **29**:1965–1972.

Schoental, R. (1970). Hepatotoxic activity of retrosine, senkirkine and hydroxysenkirkine in new-born rats, and the role of epoxides in carcinogenesis by pyrrolizidine alkaloids and aflatoxins. *Nature* **221**:401–402.

Shinozuka, H.; Lombardi, B.; Sell, S.; and Iammarino, R.M. (1978). Enhancement of DL-ethionine-induced liver carcinogenesis in rats fed a choline-devoid diet. *J. Natl. Cancer Instit.* **61**(3):813–817.

Shinozuka, H.; Lombardi, B.; Sell, S.; and Iammarino, R.M. (1978a). Early histological and functional alterations of ethionine liver carcinogenesis in rats fed a choline-deficient diet. *Cancer Res.* **38**:1092–1098.

Suit, J.L.; Rogers, A.E.; Jetten, M.E.R.; and Luria, S.E. (1977). Effects of diet on conversion of aflatoxin B_1 to bacterial mutagen(s) by rats *in vivo* and by rat hepatic microsomes *in vitro. Mutation Res.* **46**:313–323.

Swenson, D.H.; Miller, E.C.; and Miller, J.A. (1974). Aflatoxin B_1-2,3 oxide: evidence for its formation in rat liver *in vivo* and by human liver microsomes *in vitro. Biochem. Biophys. Res. Commun.* **60**:1036–1043.

3. Azo Dyes

a. Methionine

That dietary factors may influence the toxicity and/or carcinogenicity of the azo dye p-dimethylaminoazobenzene (DAB) (butter yellow) has been amply demonstrated for various nutrients, and especially for the B-vitamins (see volume 1). In addition to these vitamin interactions with carcinogenic hydrocarbons, considerable interest developed concerning the role of sulfur-containing amino acids in the detoxification of these carcinogenic agents as well. In fact, the primary reason for studying the influence of dietary methionine on DAB-induced toxicity and/or carcinogenicity was derived from a series of investigations that revealed that diets *low* in sulfur-containing amino acids enhanced the toxicity of several hydrocarbons (e.g., bromobenzene [White and White, 1938], naphthalene [Osborne and Mendel, 1919], and anthracene [Toennies and Lavine, 1936], while diets supplemented with these amino acids prevented the growth-depressing effects of benzpyrene, methylcholanthrene, and pyrene (White and White, 1939).

The first published study concerning a cystine and/or methionine-DAB interaction revealed that supplementation of either amino acid was able to offset the inhibitory effects of DAB on growth in contrast to taurine, cysteic acid, or sodium sulfate. These findings led White (1941) to conclude "that sulfur in the form of cystine, methionine, or substances giving rise to cystine or methionine are capable of functioning as detoxifying agents. It is suggested that butter yellow probably produces a specific demand for a sulfur-containing amino acid, cystine or methionine, which is needed for detoxification. As a result, the synthesis of new tissue protein becomes limited."

With respect to carcinogenicity, several studies revealed that methionine supplementation (0.5–0.72%) had no demonstrable influence on the incidence of p and m DAB-induced (0.06%) hepatic tumors in rats (White and Edwards, 1942; Clayton and Baumann,

1949), while a similar level of methionine (0.3–0.7%) was found to diminish the incidence of rat-liver tumors induced by O′ methyl p-dimethylaminoazobenzene (O′ Me DAB) (0.096%). Consistent with the protective features of methionine was the observation that methionine enhances the retention of riboflavin in the liver (also see Riesen et al., 1946; Sarett and Perlzweig, 1943). This is of some significance since riboflavin is thought to enhance the detoxification of DAB (see Volume 1, Chapter 2—"The B-Vitamins"). These findings suggest that studies designed to evaluate the influence of methionine on the carcinogenicity of azo dyes should consider the dietary status of other interacting nutrients such as riboflavin (Miller et al., 1948; Clayton and Baumann, 1949; Griffin et al., 1949). In light of the banning of butter yellow as a food additive, research on this compound has virtually stopped for many years. However, these and other nutritional interactions with azo dyes do illustrate the potential importance of diet on the occurrence of chemical carcinogenesis.

b. Cystine

While several investigations clearly demonstrated that dietary cystine supplementation could prevent or reduce the occurrence of butter yellow-induced carcinogenicity (White, 1941; Gyorgy et al., 1942), the influence of dietary cystine on the development of spontaneous and chemically induced cancer is quite complex. Dietary cystine has been found to enhance different types of tumors initiated by a variety of chemical agents. In fact, it appears that sufficient cystine may facilitate the development of chemically induced tumors (*Nutr. Rev.*, 1944; Baumann, 1948). In contrast, several studies have shown that cystine supplementation alone as well as with choline may retard the occurrence of DAB-induced cancers of the liver (Gyorgy et al., 1941; Miller et al., 1948; Harris et al., 1946, 1947). Finally, several studies have revealed that when rats are reared on a high-fat, low-casein diet and exposed to polycyclic hydrocarbon or azo-dye carcinogens that the cystine supplementation apparently acts to diminish the toxic effects of the agents (White and Mider, 1941; White and Edwards, 1942, 1942a).

Conclusions. While limited studies do suggest that both cystine and methionine prevent some of the toxic effects of a variety of polycyclic hydrocarbon and azo-dye carcinogens, the data are not well defined concerning the role of these nutrients on the course of chemically induced cancers. Studies with either nutrient have at one time or another demonstrated either a preventive or a procarcinogenic influence, especially with regard to cystine. It appeared that increasing the level of cystine in the diet markedly increased the incidence of the tumors (Baumann, 1948). However, a close look at these studies reveals that the rats reared on the high-cystine diets also consumed by far the most calories. Consequently, this confounding variable of caloric intake questions the conclusion that cystine is a procarcinogenic agent. Unfortunately, pair-feeding techniques were not employed. Despite the apparently strong research interest in the role of both cystine and methionine on the carcinogenicity of azo-compounds in the 1930s and 1940s, research in this area waned without adequate resolution of the issue.

References

Baumann, C.A. (1948). Diet and tumor development. *J. Amer. Dietetic Assoc.* **24**:573–581.

Clayton, C.C. and Baumann, C.A. (1949). Diet and azo dye tumors: effect of diet during a period when the dye is not fed. *Cancer Res.* **9**:575–582.

Griffin, A.C.; Clayton, C.C.; and Baumann, C.A. (1949). The effects of casein and methionine on the retention of hepatic riboflavin and on the development of liver tumors in rats fed certain azo dyes. *Cancer Res.* **9**:82–87.

Gyorgy, P.; Poling, E.C.; and Goldblatt, H. (1941). Necrosis, cirrhosis, and cancer of the liver in rats fed a diet containing dimethylaminoazobenzene. *Proc. Soc. Exper. Biol. Med.* **47**:41.

Gyorgy, P.; Tomarelli, R.; Ostergard, R.P.; and Brown, J.B. (1942). Unsaturated fatty acids in the dietary destruction of N,N-dimethylaminoazobenzene (butter yellow) and in the production of anemia in rats. *J. Exp. Med.* **76**:413–420.

Harris, P.N.; Krahl, M.E.; and Clowes, G.H.A. (1946). The effect of liver extract, egg albumen, cystine, and cysteine upon p-dimethylaminoazobenzene carcinogenesis in rats. *Cancer Res.* **6**:487.

Harris, P.N.; Krahl, M.E.; and Clowes, G.H.A. (1947). P-dimethylaminoazobenzene carcinogenesis with purified diets varying in content of cysteine, cystine, liver extract, protein, riboflavin, and other factors. *Cancer Res.* **7**:162–175.

Miller, E.C.; Miller, J.A.; Kline, B.E.; and Rusch, H.P. (1948). Correlation of the level of hepatic riboflavin with the appearance of liver tumors in rats fed aminoazo dyes. *J. Exp. Med.* **88**:89–98.

Nutrition Reviews (1944). Cystine and tumor formation. *Nutr. Rev.* **2**:79–81.

Nutrition Reviews (1944a). Dietary factors that influence carcinogenesis. *Nutr. Rev.* **2**:338–339.

Osborne, T.B. and Mendel, L.B. (1919). The nutritive value of the wheat kernel and its milling products. *J. Biol. Chem.* **37**:557–601.

Riesen, W.H.; Schweigert, B.S.; and Elvehjem, C.A. (1946). The effect of the level of casein, cystine, and methionine intake on riboflavin retention and protein utilization by the rat. *Arch. Biochem.* **10**:387–395.

Sarett, H.P. and Perlzweig, W.A. (1943). The effect of protein and B vitamin levels of the diet upon the tissue content and balance of riboflavin and nicotinic acid in rats. *J. Nutr.* **25**:173–183.

Toennies, G. and Lavine, T.F. (1936). The oxidation of cystine in non-aqueous media. V. Isolation of a disulfoxide of l-cystine. *J. Biol. Chem.* **113**:571–582.

White, A. (1935–1936). The production of a deficiency involving cystine and methionine by the administration of cholic acid. *J. Biol. Chem.* **112**:503–509.

White, F.R. and White, J. (1944). Effect of diethylstilbestrol on mammary tumor formation in strain C₃H mice fed a low cystine diet. *J. Natl. Cancer Instit.* **4**:413.

White, F.R. and White, J. (1946). Effect of cystine per se on the formation of hepatomas in rats following the ingestion of p-dimethylaminoazobenzene. *J. Natl. Cancer Instit.* **6**:99.

White, J. (1941). Retardation of growth of the rat ingesting p-dimethylaminoazobenzene (butter yellow). I. The effect of various dietary supplements. *J. Natl. Cancer Instit.* **1**:337–341.

White, J. and Andervont, H.B. (1943). Effect of a diet relatively low in cystine on the production of spontaneous mammary gland tumors in strain C₃H female mice. *J. Natl. Cancer Instit.* **3**:449.

White, J. and Edwards, J.E. (1942). Effect of dietary cystine on the development of hepatic tumors in rats fed p-dimethylaminozobenzene (butter yellow). *J. Natl. Cancer Instit.* **2**:535.

White, J. and Edwards, J.E. (1942a). Effect of supplementary methionine or choline plus cystine on the incidence of p-dimethylaminoazobenzene induced hepatic tumors in the rat. *J. Natl. Cancer Instit.* **3**:43–59.

White, J. and Mider, G.B. (1941). The effect of dietary cystine on the reaction of dilute brown mice to methylcholanthrene (preliminary report). *J. Natl. Cancer Instit.* **2**:95.

White, J.; Mider, G.B.; and Heston, W.E. (1944). Effect of amino acids on the induction of leukemia in mice. *J. Natl. Cancer Instit.* **4**:409.

White, J. and White, A. (1938). Inhibition of growth of rat by oral administration of methylcholanthrene. Effects of dietary cystine and methionine supplements. *Proc. Soc. Exp. Biol. Med.* **39**:527–529.

White, J. and White, A. (1939). Inhibition of growth of the rat by oral administration of methylcholanthrene, benzpyrene, or pyrene, and the effects of various dietary supplements. *J. Biol. Chem.* **131**:149–161.

White, J.; White, F.R.; and Mider, G.B. (1947). Effect of diets deficient in certain amino acids on the induction of leukemia in dba mice. *J. Natl. Cancer Instit.* **7**:199.

4. Benzene

In the chapter on the influence of protein status on pollutant toxicity, it was shown that dietary protein level is of considerable significance in affecting the degree of susceptibility of several animal species (i.e., the rat and dog) to benzene (Li and Freeman, 1945; Li et al., 1945). Of particular concern was the occurrence of a markedly greater incidence of leukopenia among the benzene-exposed animals that were reared on the low-protein diet as compared to their appropriate controls. Since benzene is excreted in part by sulfate conjugation (Li et al., 1945; Yant et al., 1936), and since protein is the major source of dietary sulfur, animals reared on low-protein diets may have a decreased capacity to resist benzene intoxication. Thus, Li and Freeman (1947) evaluated the influence of methionine on the toxicity of benzene in growing rats given a 9%-casein or low protein diet. Methionine was to be provided in amounts that exceeded growth requirements, thereby addressing the theoretical assumption that the excess sulfur would be used to detoxify the benzene.

After rearing four groups of albino rats on a common diet apparently adequate in all respects for 2 weeks, the investigators placed the respective groups on new diets that were all low in protein (9%), with two of the groups given methionine supplementation that would approximate the sulfur content of a 30%-casein diet. A supplemented and unsupplemented group were then exposed to an atmosphere with 600 ppm benzene for 40 hours per week for 12 weeks. Two other dietary groups, one supplemented, the other not, employed as controls, were kept in similar chambers and were exposed to circulating air that did not include benzene. Food and water were provided ad libitum, but consumption was carefully recorded.

Their results indicated that the methionine treatment (1) enhanced growth regardless of exposure to benzene, and (2) reduced the degree of benzene-induced leukopenia. This protection from the development of leukopenia was only partially successful in that the nonsupplemented group exposed to benzene exhibited a 50% drop in leukocytes during the last week of the study, while the methionine-supplemented group displayed a 23% decrease during the same time period.

Even though the methionine supplementation did not completely prevent the occurrence of benzene-induced leukopenia, the fact that it reduced the magnitude of this condition should be appreciated. Unfortunately, investigators have not continued to advance the line of research initiated by Li and Freeman. Without question, these data indicate that dietary levels of methionine do influence the extent of benzene toxicity. They also suggest that other dietary factors may also be operational. It would seem that further evaluation of the influence of sulfur-containing amino acids, including both methionine and cystine on benzene toxicity, may offer an exciting and socially relevant area of research.

References

Li, T.W. and Freeman, S. (1945). The effect of protein and fat content of the diet upon the toxicity of benzene for rats. *Amer. J. Physiol.* **145**:158–165.

Li, T.W. and Freeman, S. (1947). The effect of methionine on protein-deficient rats exposed to benzene. *Amer. J. Physiol.* **148**:358–364.

Li, T.W.; Freeman, S.; Hough, V.H.; and Gunn, F.D. (1945). The increased susceptibility of protein-deficient dogs to benzene poisoning. *Amer. J. Physiol.* **148**:166.

Yant, W.P.; Schrenk, H.H.; Sayers, R.R.; Horvatt, A.A.; and Reinhart, W.H. (1936). Urine sulfate determinations as measure of benzene exposure. *J. Indust. Hyg. Toxicol.* **18**:69–88.

5. Bromobenzene

The addition of bromobenzene to the diet retards the growth of rats. However, supplementation of the toxic diet by L-cystine results in a resumption of growth, presumably through an enhanced detoxification of the bromobenzene (Stekol, 1937; White and Jackson, 1935). According to White and Lewis (1932), bromobenzene is detoxified by two paths: (1) when the cystine level is low, the bromobenzene is detoxified via conjugation with sulfuric acid; and (2) when the cystine level is sufficiently high, the bromobenzene is excreted in the form of a p-bromophenylmercapturic acid. Figure 8-3 clearly illustrates the essential role of sulfur-containing amino acids in the formation of mercapturic acid derivatives.[3] The protective influence of L-cystine and other sulfur–containing amino acids suggests that these substances have a sparing effect in the presence of limited quantities of cysteine. More recently, Ferreyra et al. (1979) have reported that cystamine as well as cysteine was able to reduce bromobenzene-induced liver damage in rats when given within 12 hours after treatment.

References

Ariens, E.J.; Simonis, A.M.; and Offermeier, J. (1976). *Introduction to Toxicology.* Academic Press, p. 60.

Ferreyra de, E.C.; Fenos de, O.M.; Bernacchi, A.S.; Castro de, C.R.; and Castro, J.A. (1979). Therapeutic effectiveness of cystamine and cysteine to reduce liver cell necrosis induced by several hepatotoxins. *Toxicol. Appl. Pharm.* **48**:221–228.

Haley, F.L. and Samuelsen, G.S. (1937). Cystine metabolism. II. Detoxification of monobromobenzene. *J. Biol. Chem.* **119**:383–387.

Stekol, J.A. (1937). Studies on the mercapturic acid synthesis in animals. VII. Bromobenzene and l-cystine in relation to growth of rats on a navy bean meal diet. *J. Biol. Chem.* **122**:55–57.

White, A. and Jackson, R.W. (1935). The effect of bromobenzene on the utilization of cystine and methionine by the growing rat. *J. Biol. Chem.* **111**:507–513.

[3]Mercapturic acid may be defined as a condensation product of cysteine with compounds like bromobenzene.

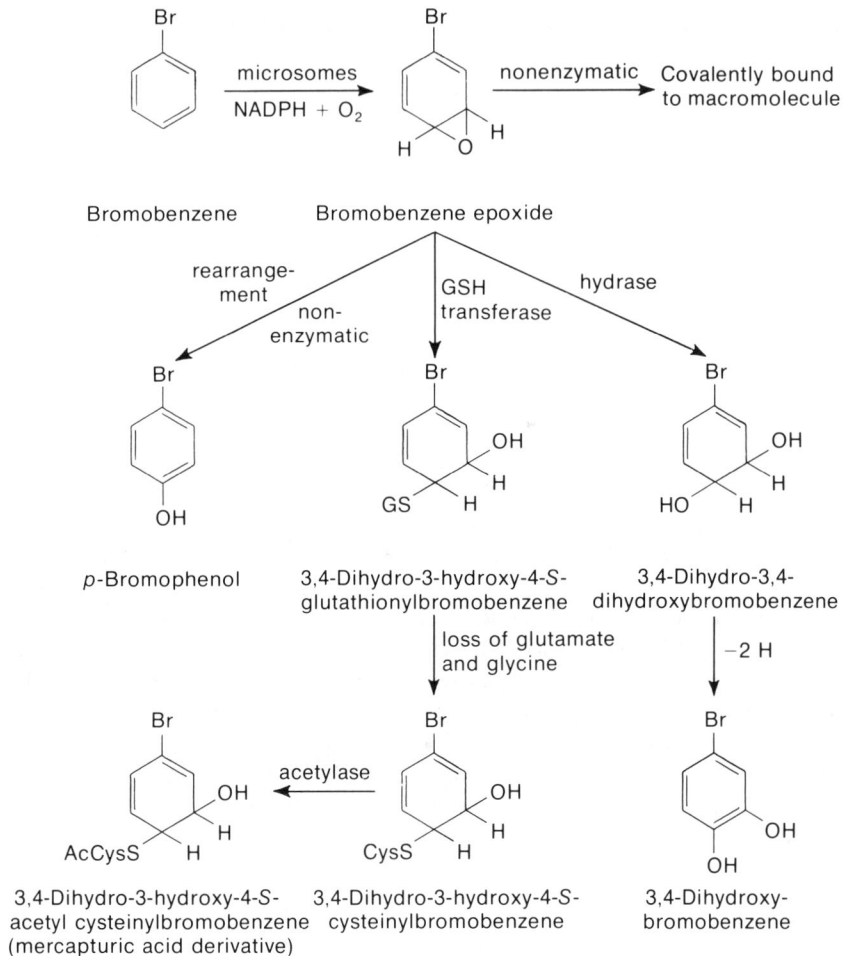

Figure 8-3. Detoxification of bromobenzene. The formation of an epoxide (biological alkylating agent) from bromobenzene followed by conjugation of the toxic intermediate by glutathione, which eventually leads to the excretion of bromobenzene as a water-soluble mercapturic acid derivative. *Source.* Ariens, E.J.; Simonis, A.M.; and Offermeier, J. (1976). *Introduction to Toxicology.* Academic Press, New York, p. 60.

White, A. and Lewis, H.B. (1932). The metabolism of sulfur. XIX. The distribution of urinary sulfur in the dog after the oral administration of monobromobenzene as influenced by the character of the dietary protein and by the feeding of 1-cystine and dl-methionine. *J. Biol. Chem.* **98**:607–624.

6. Carbon Tetrachloride

a. Methionine

That methionine administration could affect the occurrence of carbon tetrachloride (CCl_4) toxicity was first suggested by Beattie et al. in 1944. They reported one case of CCl_4-induced hepatitis that was treated successfully with methionine. This quickly led Eddy (1945) to utilize methionine in the treatment of CCl_4-induced hepatitis, also with highly successful results.

These initial clinical findings clearly suggested that methionine administration may be successfully used to diminish liver damage caused by CCl_4. Furthermore, since some of the patients treated by Eddy (1945) were consuming diets with presumably low levels of protein, it seemed that low levels of dietary methionine might also be a predisposing factor in CCl_4 toxicity. While these clinical findings were of great interest and provided the impetus to initiate further research in this area, they were not experimental studies in which adequate control groups were employed, thereby diminishing the strength of any conclusions.

Experimental studies with rats (Shaffer et al., 1946) and dogs (Shaffer et al., 1946; Sellers et al., 1950; Drill and Loomis, 1946, 1947), however, were not able to confirm the findings of Beattie et al. (1944) and Eddy (1945). Of particular significance is that these investigators evaluated the influence of methionine as well as cystine supplementation on diets that had low, average, and above average levels of protein (as casein), as well as over a wide range of CCl_4 levels. In addition, a number of CCl_4-induced effects were compared, including both functional and pathological changes in the liver as well as survival. The only supportive findings were published by Gyorgy et al. (1946)[4] who noted that methionine supplementation of low-protein diets enhanced survival of rats during chronic CCl_4 inhalation (300 ppm) 7 hours/day/5 days a week for 5 months, as well as reducing the occurrence of renal (but apparently not liver) damage.

In commenting on their findings, Gyorgy et al. (1946) stated: "In

---

[4]Hove and Hardin (1951) reported that cystine prevented the acute toxicity of CCl_4.

applying the findings of the present experiments to the condition of CCl₄ poisoning in men, supplements of methionine and of methionine-containing protein appear to be the most suitable dietary directions, especially with regard to the renal changes. Nephrosis is often the leading symptom in acute or more protracted exposure to CCl₄ in man (Smetana, 1939). Its possible management by dietary means is worthy of consideration."

This conclusion of Gyorgy et al. (1946), while not in disagreement with the findings of others, should be contrasted with the following critical assessment provided by Drill (1952) in his classic review:

"Supplements of methionine have not been shown to decrease the liver injury produced by CCl₄ in animals fed a normal diet or a moderately low protein diet, although renal injury occurring on the low protein diet may be prevented. Thus there is no experimental support for the use of methionine to combat liver injury induced by CCl₄ in patients and certainly, despite claims to the contrary, there is no good clinical evidence for such an effect. This does not deny a possible effect of methionine on other organs, or its possible value in liver lesions in the face of very severe protein depletion, which has not yet been studied. When early cirrhosis is induced in rats by CCl₄, repair of the liver occurs when a normal diet is fed, but there are no indications for supplemental methionine."

Unfortunately, research has not continued on the interactions of dietary methionine[5] with CCl₄-induced toxicity of the liver and especially the kidney. In light of the fact that workers exposed to CCl₄ are recommended to undergo periodic health examinations that include liver- and kidney-function tests (Tabershaw et al., 1977), it would seem that a strong effort should be made to further evaluate whether methionine levels in the diet do affect kidney susceptibility to CCl₄ and at what levels of exposure. It is clear that more quantitative relationships need to be derived from animal studies, as well as the initiation of prospective epidemiologic studies.

b. Cysteine

Research on the prophylactic potential of cysteine with respect to CCl₄-induced toxicity was initiated in 1974 by DeFerreyra et al. who were attempting to find a compound that would act like cystamine in

---

[5]In a recent report by Hafeman and Hoekstra (1977), dietary methionine supplementation (0.4%) markedly reduced the occurrence of CCl₄-induced lipid peroxidation in rats as measured by ethane evolution.

preventing CCl_4 toxicity, but one that would also be much less toxic. Their search was, for the most part, rewarded since these investigators found that cysteine administration (1.9 g/kg po) prevented the occurrence of CCl_4-induced necrosis and fatty liver in rats regardless of whether the cysteine was given 30 minutes before or 1 hour after CCl_4 exposure. However, cysteine treatment could not stop the irreversible binding of labeled carbon from CCl_4 to microsomal lipids; it diminished, to a certain extent, the binding to microsomal proteins at 6 hours after $^{14}CCl_4$ treatment. Additionally, cysteine could not prevent CCl_4-induced lipid peroxidation of cytochrome-P-450. These findings led the authors to conclude that cysteine acts to protect against CCl_4 toxicity at some point leading to necrosis, but not at the site of activation. They further concluded that cysteine administration may have great usefulness in the treatment of CCl_4-induced toxicity "because of its apparent effectiveness and low toxicity and because its effectiveness may be further increased by its combination with other antidotes acting more specifically (e.g., those acting on CCl_4 activation or lipid peroxidation)."

References

Beattie, J.; Herbert, P.H.; Wechtel, C.; and Steele, C.W. (1944). Studies on hepatic dysfunction. Carbon tetrachloride poisoning treated with casein digest and methionine. *Brit. Med. J.* 1:209.

Brunschwig, A.; Johnson, C.; and Nichols, S. (1945). Carbon tetrachloride injury of the liver. The protective action of certain compounds. *Proc. Soc. Exper. Biol. Med.* 60:388–391.

DeFerreyra, E.C.; Castro, J.A.; Diaz Gomez, M.I.; D'Acosta, N.; DeCastro, C.R.; and DeFenos, O.M. (1974). Prevention and treatment of carbon tetrachloride hepatotoxicity by cysteine: studies about its mechanism. *Toxicol. Appl. Pharmacol.* 27:558–568.

Drill, V.A. (1952). Hepatotoxic agents: mechanism of action and dietary interrelation. *Pharmacol. Rev.* 4:1–41.

Drill, V.A. and Loomis, T.A. (1946). Effect of methionine supplements on hepatic injury produced by carbon tetrachloride. *Science* 103:199–201.

Drill, V.A. and Loomis, T.A. (1947). Methionine therapy in experimental liver injury produced by carbon tetrachloride. *J. Pharmacol. Exp. Therap.* 90:138–149.

Eddy, J.H. (1945). Carbon tetrachloride poisoning: a preliminary report on the use of methionine in hepatitis. *JAMA* 128:994–996.

Editorial (1944). Successful treatment of carbon tetrachloride poisoning. *JAMA* 124:925–926.

Gyorgy, P.; Seifter, J.; Tomarelli, R.M.; and Goldblatl, H. (1946). Influence of dietary factors and sex on the toxicity of carbon tetrachloride in rats. *J. Exper. Med.* 83:449–462.

Hafeman, D.G. and Hoekstra, W.G. (1977). Protection against carbon tetrachloride-induced lipid peroxidation in the rat by dietary vitamin E, selenium, and methionine as measured by ethane evolution. *J. Nutr.* **107**:656–665.

Hove, E.L. and Hardin, J.O. (1951). Effect of vitamins E, B_{12} and folacin on CCl_4 toxicity and protein utilization in rats. *Proc. Soc. Exp. Biol. Med.* **77**:502–505.

Lehnher, E.R. (1935). Acute carbon tetrachloride poisoning. *Arch. Int. Med.* **56**:98–104.

Report of the Council (1947). The status of methionine in the prevention and treatment of liver injury. *JAMA* **133**:107.

Sellers, E.A.; Rosemary, W.Y.; and Lucas, C.C. (1950). Lipotropic agents in liver damage produced by selenium or carbon tetrachloride. *Proc. Soc. Exper. Biol. Med.* **75**:118–120.

Shaffer, C.B.; Carpenter, C.P.; and Moses, C. (1946). An experimental evaluation of methionine in the therapy of liver injury from carbon tetrachloride. *J. Indust. Hyg. Toxicol.* **28**:87–93.

Smetana, H. (1939). Nephrosis due to carbon tetrachloride. *Arch. Int. Med.* **63**:760–777.

Tabershaw, I.R.; Utidjian, H.M.D.; and Kawahara, B. (1977). Chemical hazards. In: *Occupational Diseases: A Guide to Their Recognition.* Edited by M.M. Key et al. U.S. DHEW, PHS, CDS, NIOSH, Washington, D.C.

7. Chloroform

Concern with chloroform toxicity was generally widespread during the 1930s and 1940s, in large measure due to its common use as an anesthetizing agent. While chloroform is no longer employed in this fashion, humans are still exposed to it in certain occupations because of its use as a solvent in the lacquer industry, in the production of certain pharmaceuticals, and in the manufacture of a variety of products including artificial silks, plastics, polishes, and fluorocarbons (Tabershaw et al., 1977). As has been pointed out elsewhere, the chlorination of drinking water with high organic content also results in the formation of chloroform at levels up to somewhat greater than 200 ppb in the more extreme instances.

While a primary concern of exposure to chloroform today is the carcinogenic risk, it has long been recognized as a potent renal and hepatotoxic agent. According to Drill (1952), chloroform was the first hepatotoxic agent for which interactions with dietary factors were carried out. Much of the early evaluations from 1914 to the 1930s involved a comparison of the influence of proteins, fats, and carbohydrates on chloroform toxicity, with the initial findings revealing that meat protein provided less protection than did a high-carbohydrate diet. After 1924 when standard diets were introduced into laboratory experimentation, it was discovered that a high-protein diet in the form of casein provided good protection as compared to the performance offered by the meat-protein diet (Drill, 1952).

Other investigations not only considered the levels of dietary protein as affecting the toxicity of chloroform but also fasting and starvation, which markedly enhanced its toxicity (Davis and Whipple, 1919; Moise and Smith, 1924). In addition, rearing dogs on a diet totally devoid of protein also markedly enhanced chloroform toxicity (Miller and Whipple, 1940). Since part of the biochemical alterations induced by acute chloroform exposure was the increased excretion of nitrogen and sulfur (Howland and Richards, 1909; Daft et al., 1936) and since dietary casein (and beef muscle) contain high quantities of these elements, especially in the form of the sulfur-containing amino acids, it was decided to evaluate whether methionine and cystine could prevent chloroform-induced liver injury.

In their test of this hypothesis, Miller et al. (1940) demonstrated that methionine given 24 to 5 hours prior to chloroform anesthesia provided nearly total protection to protein-depleted dogs. In their experiment, dogs were reared on a diet with nearly zero-protein levels from 4 to 10 weeks and then were fasted for 24 hours prior to anesthesia. Other studies of a similar nature revealed that methionine and to a more limited degree cystine, protected against chloroform intoxication when given 3 to 4 but not 4 to 6 hours after anesthesia (Miller and Whipple, 1942). In partial contrast, Drill (1952) revealed that methionine supplementation was not able to correct or reverse a chloroform-induced decrease in weight gain of rats exposed via inhalation for 70 days and reared on diets with either 8 or 20% casein. Drill (1952) concluded by stating that "the response to chloroform and the effect of methionine will vary tremendously with the degree of protein restriction and perhaps also with the chronicity of the study."

In a related study, Brunschwig et al. (1945) presented suggestive evidence that methionine and sodium thioglycollate protect against chloroform-induced liver disease (as measured by the bromsulfatein liver-function test) in dogs reared on a normal-stock diet. However, because of considerable variation with respect to the responses of this liver-function test, it cannot be confidently concluded that the methionine treatment provided a positive influence. Based on these findings, it is necessary to conclude, in agreement with Drill (1952), that methionine is protective against chloroform toxicity in dogs when the level of protein in the diet is exceptionally (i.e., unrealistically?) low for a prolonged time. Beneficial effects in animals on more normal diets remain to be established. Finally, in light of the widespread exposure to chloroform in many drinking-water supplies throughout the United States, further research on the effects of dietary levels of methionine on chronic low-level chloroform exposure is quite relevant.

References

ACGIH (1976). Documentation of TLVs. American Conference of Governmental Industrial Hygienists. Cincinnati, OH.

Brunschwig, A.; Nichols, S.; Bigelow, R.R.; and Miles, J. (1945). Sulfhydryl protection of the liver. *Arch. Path.* **40**:81–83.

Daft, F.S.; Robscheif-Robbins, F.S.; and Whipple, G.H. (1936). Liver injury by chloroform, nitrogen metabolism, and conservation. Liver function and hemoglobin production in anemia. *J. Biol. Chem.* **113**:391–404.

Davis, N.C. and Whipple, G.H. (1919). The influence of fasting and various diets on the liver injury effected by chloroform anesthesia. *Arch. Int. Med.* **23**:612–635.

Drill, V.A. (1952). Hepatotoxic agents: mechanism of action and dietary interrelationship. *Pharm. Rev.* **4**:1–42.

Drill, V.A. and Bonnycastle, D.C. Relation of methionine and protein intake to chloroform induced injury in the rat. (manuscript) (Cited in Drill, 1952).

Howland, J. and Richards, A.N. (1909). An experimental study of the metabolism and pathology of delayed chloroform poisoning. *J. Exp. Med.* **11**:344–372.

Miller, L.L.; Ross, J.F.; and Whipple, G.H. (1940). Methionine and cystine specific protein factors preventing chloroform liver injury in protein-depleted dogs. *Am. J. Med. Sci.* **200**:739–756.

Miller, L.L. and Whipple, G.H. (1940). Chloroform liver injury increases as protein stores decrease. *Am. J. Med. Sci.* **199**:204–216.

Miller, L.L. and Whipple, G.H. (1942). Liver injury, liver protection, and sulfur metabolism. Methionine protects against chloroform liver injury even when given after anesthesia. *J. Exp. Med.* **76**:421–435.

Moise, T.S. and Smith, A.H. (1924). Diet and tissue growth. I. The regeneration of liver tissue on various adequate diets. *J. Exp. Med.* **40**:13–23.

Tabershaw, I.R.; Utidjian, B.M.D.; and Kawahara, B. (1977). Chemical hazards. In: *Occupational Diseases: A Guide to Their Recognition.* Edited by M.M. Key et al. U.S. DHEW, PHS, CDC, NIOSH, Washington, D.C.

8. 1,2-Dichloroethane (Ethylene Dichloride)

In the early 1940s Heppel and his associates at the Industrial Hygiene Research Laboratory of the U.S. National Institute of Health initiated a series of toxicological investigations on the effects of 1,2-dichloroethane on rats. They were concerned with this compound because of its widespread use within certain industries as a solvent and as an intermediate in the manufacture of synthetic rubber. As part of their toxicological appraisal of this compound, they provided an assessment of a variety of dietary factors, including methionine as potential mitigating agents in 1,2-dichloroethane toxicity (Heppel et al., 1945, 1945a, 1947).

In their initial investigation, Heppel et al. (1945) utilized weanling rats that were reared on semisynthetic diets in which the level of protein and fat varied markedly depending on the treatment. Following a 3-week period of dietary acclimation, the rats were given a 4-hour inhalation exposure to 1,2-dichloroethane at 1000 ppm. It was found that rats given diets low in protein (4% casein) were much more susceptible to the 1,2-dichloroethane than controls, with respect to mortality incidence and average liver-fat levels. Increasing of the fat content of the diet also markedly enhanced these toxicologic effects. However, dietary supplementation of the low-protein, high-fat diets with both choline (0.7%) and methionine (0.7%) strikingly reduced the mortality percentage from 100% in the nonsupplemented group to only 10% in the choline-and-methionine-supplemented animals. Supplementation also markedly reduced the extent of liver fat as well. Interestingly, in another experiment in which only choline was used as a supplement, the mortality incidence was 55%, thereby implying that methionine contributes in a substantial manner to preventing the toxicity.

Subsequent studies by Heppel et al. (1947) substantiated the importance of methionine in reducing the susceptibility of rats reared on a low-casein diet to 1,2-dichloroethane. In experiments quite similar to those described above, it was found that methionine supplementation consistently reduced mortality rates that were 65 to 100% in the unsupplemented controls to 0 to 20%. Comparable experiments also revealed that dietary supplementation with L-cystine or an oral dose given 1 hour before exposure offered marked protection from the acute toxicity of 1,2-dichloroethane as well as its influence on the development of fatty liver tissue. Other studies showed that nine sulfur-free amino acids did not offer protection from 1,2-dichloroethane-induced toxicity, while limited research with L-cysteine hydrochloride revealed a protective response.

Unfortunately, these striking findings, which clearly indicate the protective effects of sulfur-containing amino acid supplementation against 1,2-dichloroethane toxicity in rats reared on low-protein diets, have not been extended.[6] This topic clearly represents an area in which

---

[6]A recent Soviet study (Mizyukova and Kokarovtseva, 1978) has revealed that acetyl-cysteine treatment was able to provide a marked therapeutic effect on 1,2-dichloro-

important advancements in our understanding of diet-pollutant interactions can be made, as well as potentially contributing to industrial hygiene practice.

References

Heppel, L.A.; Neal, P.A.; Daft, F.S.; Endicott, K.M.; Orr, M.L.; and Porterfield, V.T. (1945). Toxicology of 1,2-dichloroethane (ethylene dichloride). II. Influence of dietary factors on the toxicity of dichloroethane. *J. Ind. Hyg. Tox.* 27:15–21.

Heppel, L.A.; Neal, P.A.; Perrin, T.L.; Endicott, K.M.; and Porterfield, V.T. (1945a). The toxicology of 1,2-dichloroethane. III. Its acute toxicity and the effect of protective agents. *J. Pharmacol. Exp. Therap.* 84:53–63.

Heppel, L.A.; Porterfield, V.T.; and Sharpless, N.E. (1947). Toxicology of 1,2-dichloroethane (ethylene dichloride). IV. Its detoxication by L-cysteine, DL-methionine and certain other sulfur containing compounds. *J. Pharmacol. Exp. Therap.* 91:385–394.

Mizyukova, I.G. and Kokarovtseva, M.G. (1978). Therapeutic effect of acetylcysteine in acute ethylene dichloride poisoning. *Farmakologiia I. Toksikologiia* 41(3):350–354.

9. 1,2-Dichloropropane (Propylene Dichloride)

That dietary factors may affect the toxicity of 1,2-dichloropropane was suggested by Heppel et al. (1946) in studies with dietary protein, fat, and several amino acids including cystine and methionine. These investigators exposed weanling rats reared on a low-casein diet (with or without a methionine supplement or a combined supplement of l-cystine (0.7%) and choline (0.7%) to 1000 ppm of 1,2-dichloropropane for 7 hours per day for up to 10 days. In these experiments in which the rats were fed ad libitum, it was found that the low-casein group exposed to the 1,2-dichloropropane exhibited appreciable mortality by the fourth day of exposure, with 8 of 15 animals dying while only 1 of 15 unexposed controls reared on the low-casein diets died during the course of the study. In remarkably similar fashion to the unexposed controls, exposed animals reared on the low-casein diets but supplemented with 1% methionine exhibited only one death out of 15 animals during the study. The cystine-plus-choline supplement, while not as effective as the methionine treatment, had only 3 of 15 1,2-

---

ethane toxicity (disruption of hemopoiesis, blood coagulation, and lesions of kidneys and liver) in mice, rats, and rabbits. The acetylcysteine treatment presumably reduces the toxicity of a metabolite of 1,2-dichloroethane, chloroethane, since acetylcysteine is able to prevent toxicity from both compounds.

dichloropropane-exposed animals die during the entire course of the 10-day study.

Other experiments of a similar nature revealed a striking protective effect of methionine when the rats were reared on a low-casein, high-fat diet. In this case, the nonsupplemented group experienced 90% mortality by the fourth day of treatment, while the methionine-supplemented group exhibited 90% survivorship by the end of the same 4-day period. The methionine supplementation was also considerably more effective than supplementation with 0.7% choline.

Pair-feeding studies also supported the original findings, with the methionine supplementation providing considerable protection against 1,2-dichloropropane-induced mortality for rats reared on a low-casein, high-fat diet as well as for those supplemented with 0.7% choline. However, the methionine supplementation did not appear to offer any noticeable improvement over a combined 0.7% cystine and 0.7% choline supplementation.

Despite these impressive findings of Heppel et al. (1946), no further studies have extended this rather striking revelation that dietary methionine and cystine offer protection from 1,2-dichloropropane. Future studies should involve an evaluation of variable levels of dietary methionine and/or cystine, as well as a consideration of methionine in combination with choline and cystine on low-level, chronic exposure.

Reference

Heppel, L.A.; Highman, B.; and Porterfield, V.T. (1946). Toxicology of 1,2-dichloropropane (propylene dichloride). II. Influence of dietary factors on the toxicity of dichloropropane. *J. Pharmacol. Exp. Therap.* **87**:11–17.

10. Ethionine

In 1938, Dyer demonstrated that ethionine (S-ethylhomocysteine) caused a marked weight loss and subsequent death when given to young rats reared on a 5%-casein diet. These rather striking adverse effects of ethionine could be prevented for the most part by supplementation with methionine. Since ethionine is a methionine analogue, differing only in the presence of an S-ethyl group in place of an S-methyl group, and because methionine prevents ethionine-induced toxicity (Dyer, 1938; Harris and Kohn, 1941), it was suggested that ethionine is an antimetabolite of methionine (Stekol and Weiss, 1949).

Subsequent studies have attempted to elucidate the precise manner by which ethionine may disrupt methionine metabolism. Since methionine and its derivatives are metabolized along several metabolic pathways, it is not unexpected that the mode of ethionine's toxicological activity may be quite complex. Research in this domain has revealed that ethionine may inhibit the conversion of methionine to cystine in rodents, thereby implying that ethionine prevents the demethylation of methionine (Simpson et al., 1950). Similarly, Siekevitz and Greenberg (1950) reported that ethionine prevented the formation of formate from methionine both in vitro and in vivo. In addition, ethionine administration may result in the formation of fatty livers in female rats (Farber et al., 1950), as well as diffuse and hemorrhagic pancreatitis (Lombardi, 1976; Lombardi and Kalipatnapu-Rao, 1975; Farber and Popper, 1950). Interestingly, these adverse effects of ethionine can be reversed by methionine supplementation, but not by other amino acids such as cystine, valine, lysine, alanine, and homocysteine, as well as the B-vitamin choline. These findings were quite interesting, especially the lack of a sparing action for choline (see Farber et al., 1950; Lombardi, 1976; Lombardi and Kalipatnapu-Rao, 1975), since it has been thought that the primary lipotropic function of methionine was its capacity to provide methyl groups for the synthesis of choline. Thus if ethionine caused the occurrence of fatty liver by preventing the demethylation of methionine, it would be logically predicted that choline supplementation would relieve the symptoms of ethionine intoxication. While these findings certainly illustrate the lack of present knowledge to adequately explain the manner by which ethionine causes its adverse effects as well as the protective action of methionine, it should not lead one to conclude that the presence of choline in the diet does not markedly affect some of the adverse effects of ethionine (see Shinozuka et al., 1978, 1978a).

While the previously cited studies clearly demonstrated that ethionine is a highly toxic agent, it was not until 1956 that Farber reported that ethionine caused liver cancer in rats. In light of the research that has revealed that (1) methionine administration prevents ethionine toxicity; (2) consumption of methionine-choline-deficient diets predisposes rats (Copeland and Salmon, 1946; Salmon and Copeland, 1955), mice (Wilson, 1951; Buckley and Hartroft, 1955), and chickens (Salmon and Copeland, 1954; Salmon et al., 1955) to develop liver cancer; and (3) ethionine treatment reduces the availability of methyl groups from methionine for choline synthesis (Farber, 1949; Simmonds et al., 1950), Farber and Ichinose (1958) decided to evaluate whether methionine could also prevent ethionine-induced carcinogenicity.

In their study, male and female white Wistar rats were exposed to a basal diet containing 0.25% of DL-ethionine along with various levels of methionine (0.3 to 0.8%), choline chloride (0.3 to 0.6%), and betaine chloride (0.8%) for the specific treatment conditions. The results indicated that the diets with either 0.6 or 0.8% methionine fed for either 4.5 or 8 months completely prevented the occurrence of ethionine-induced liver cancer while unsupplemented controls exhibited 90% cancer incidence. When the level of dietary methionine was 0.3%, an intermediate level of protection was found. Thus, four of 10 rats on this diet developed tumors after 8 months. From a pathological perspective, it is important to note that animals reared on the 0.6 to 0.8% methionine-supplemented diets and exposed to ethionine had a normally appearing liver under gross and microscopic evaluations. In contrast, however, the pancreas of animals at the 0.6% level of methionine supplementation exhibited minimal to moderate levels of atrophy and a moderate degree of tubular-cell atrophy of the testis. Animals reared on the 0.8% methionine diet had normal pancreas and testicular tissue. Finally, from a comparative viewpoint methionine supplementation was considerably more effective in preventing the occurrence of ethionine-induced cancer than both butaine chloride and choline chloride, with the choline chloride being the least effective.

Biochemical explanations for how methionine supplementation prevents the occurrence of ethionine-induced cancer remain to be developed. Farber and Ichinose (1958) hypothesized that the carcinogenicity of ethionine is most likely associated with the interference of methionine cellular metabolism; however, they were unable to provide any specific mechanistic explanations. Other researchers have suggested that the presence of methionine enhances the capacity of the organism to acetylate ethionine sulfoxide, thereby preventing the synthesis of S-adenosylethionine, a step thought to be necessary for ethionine carcinogenesis (Brada et al., 1976).

The relevance of these findings for environmental/occupational health is difficult to assess, primarily because ethionine is used only for experimental purposes. Consequently, it poses no widespread concern to the general public or to industrial workers other than laboratory technicians, by whom extreme caution must be exercised. Despite the limited exposure to ethionine, these experiments have provided valuable information concerning the role of methionine in cellular and liver physiology, as well as its relationship to other nutrients including choline.

References

Brada, Z.; Bulba, S.; and Altman, N.H. (1976). The influence of DL-methionine on the metabolism of S-adenosylethionine in rats chronically treated with DL-ethionine. *Cancer Res.* **36**:1573–1579.

Buckley, G.F. and Hartroft, W.S. (1955). Pathology of choline deficiency in the mouse. *Arch. Pathol.* **59**:185–197.

Caboche, M. (1976). Methionine metabolism in BHK cells: selection and characterization of ethionine resistant clones. *J. Cell. Physiol.* **87**:321–336.

Copeland, D.H. and Salmon, W.D. (1946). The occurrence of neoplasms in the liver, lungs, and other tissue of rats as a result of prolonged choline deficiency. *Am. J. Path.* **22**:1057–1079.

Dyer, H.M. (1938). Evidence of the methylthiol group: the synthesis of S-ethyl-homocysteine (ethionine) and a study of its availability for growth. *J. Biol. Chem.* **124**:519–524.

Farber, E. (1949). The effect of amino acid analogues on the metabolism of normal and tumor tissue. Thesis, Univ. of California.

Farber, E. (1956). Carcinoma of the liver in rats fed ethionine. *Arch. Path.* **62**:445–453.

Farber, E. and Ichinose, H. (1958). The prevention of ethionine-induced carcinoma of the liver in rats by methionine. *Cancer Res.* **18**:1209–1213.

Farber, E. and Popper, H. (1950). Production of acute pancreatitis with ethionine and its prevention by methionine. *Proc. Soc. Exp. Bio. Med.* **74**:838–840.

Farber, E.; Simpson, M.V.; and Tarver, H. (1950). Studies on ethionine. II. The interference with lipid metabolism. *J. Biol. Chem.* **182**:91–99.

Harris, J.S. and Kohn, H.I. (1941). On the mode of action of the sulfonamides. II. The specific antagonism between methionine and the sulfonamides in *Escherichia coli. J. Pharmacol. Exp. Therap.* **73**:383–400.

Lombardi, B. (1976). Influence of dietary factors on the pancreatic toxicity of ethionine. *Amer. J. Path.* **84**:633–648.

Lombardi, B. and Kalipatnapu-Rao, N. (1975). Acute hemorrhagic pancreatic necrosis in mice. *Amer. J. Path.* **81**:87–99.

Rogers, A.E. (1975). Variable effects of a lipotrope-deficient high-fat diet on chemical carcinogenesis in rats. *Cancer Res.* **35**:2469–2474.

Salmon, W.D. and Copeland, D.H. (1954). Liver carcinoma and related lesions in chronic choline deficiency. *Ann. N.Y. Acad. Sci.* **57**:664–677.

Salmon, W.D.; Copeland, D.H.; and Burns, M.J. (1955). Hepatomas in choline deficiency. *J. Natl. Cancer Instit.* (Suppl.) **15**:1549–1565.

Shinozuka, H.; Lombardi, B.; Sell, S.; and Iammarino, R.M. (1978). Early histological and functional alterations of ethionine liver carcinogenesis in rats fed a choline-deficient diet. *Cancer Res.* **38**:1092–1098.

Shinozuka, H.; Lombardi, B.; Sell, S.; and Iammarino, R.M. (1978a). Enhancement of DL-ethionine-induced liver carcinogenesis in rats fed a choline-devoid diet. *J. Natl. Cancer Instit.* **61**:813–817.

Sidransky, H. and Farber, E. (1956). The effects of ethionine upon protein metabolism in the pancreas of rats. *J. Biol. Chem.* **219**:231–243.

Siekevitz, P. and Greenberg, D.M. (1950). The biological formation of formate from methyl compounds in liver slices. *J. Biol. Chem.* **186**:275–286.

Simmonds, S.; Keller, E.B.; Chandler, J.P.; and DuVigneaud, V. (1950). The effect of ethionine on transmethylation from methionine to choline and creatine *in vivo*. *J. Biol. Chem.* **182**:191–195.

Simpson, M.V.; Farber, E.; and Tarver, H. (1950). Studies of ethionine. I. Inhibition of protein synthesis in intact animals. *J. Biol. Chem.* **182**:81–89.

Stekol, J.A. and Weiss, K. (1949). A study on growth inhibition by D-, L-, and DL-ethionine in the rat and its alleviation by the sulfur-containing amino acids and choline. *J. Biol. Chem.* **179**:1049–1056.

Wilson, J.W. (1951). Hepatomas in mice fed a synthetic diet low in protein and deficient in choline. *Cancer Res.* **11**:290.

Yamada, M. and Takahashi, J. (1977). Reversal of ethionine intoxication in the domestic fowl with methionine and adenine sulphate. *Br. Poult. Sci.* **18**:567–571.

11. Marijuana and Tobacco Smoke

A recent report by Leuchtenberger and Leuchtenberger (1977) has investigated whether L-cysteine and vitamin C could protect hamster lung cultures from developing carcinogenic effects of fresh smoke from tobacco and marijuana cigarettes. The rationale for such a study was derived from a number of earlier investigations, which demonstrated that:

1. Inhalation by mice of cigarette smoke and exposure of hamster and human lung-tissue cultures to tobacco and marijuana smoke resulted in abnormal cellular and chromosomal content of DNA, irregular cell division along with abnormal proliferations, and increased inclination toward malignant cell transformation (Leuchtenberger and Leuchtenberger, 1970; Leuchtenberger et al., 1963, 1973, 1973a, 1976, 1976a, 1976b).

2. The degree of sulfhydryl reactivity and NO levels of the smoke were directly related to the ability of the smoke to cause abnormal growth and malignant transformation of hamster lung cultures (Leuchtenberger et al., 1974, 1976; Davies et al., 1975).

3. There is a direct association between elevated sulfhydryl reactivity of the smoke and a decrease in lysosomes and the later development of malignant transformation (Davies et al., 1975; Leuchtenberger and Leuchtenberger, 1976a).

4. Cigarette smoke inhibits sulfhydryl-dependent enzyme systems (Lange, 1961; Powell and Green, 1972).

5. Lysosomal damage has been implicated in carcinogenesis (Allison and Paton, 1965; Allison, 1969).

Based on these data, Leuchtenberger and Leuchtenberger (1977a) decided to evaluate whether lung cell cultures could be protected from the sulfhydryl reactivity of smoke by the thiol, L-cysteine, since it had been previously reported to react with cigarette smoke (Fenner and Braven, 1968; Leuchtenberger et al., 1976a) and could protect the enzyme glyceraldehyde-3-phosphate dehydrogenase from the inhibitory influence of the vapor phase of cigarette smoke (Powell and Green, 1972). In addition, they investigated whether vitamin C would also have a protective influence because: (1) Pelletier (1975) had found lower levels of vitamin C in smokers than in nonsmokers, (2) Mirvish (1975) reported that vitamin C could block the effects of NO compounds, and (3) vitamin C has a stimulatory influence on lysosomal activity (Leuchtenberger and Leuchtenberger, 1977).

To test this hypothesis, hamster lung-tissue cultures were grown in either a normal media (NM), or NM plus L-cysteine (0.1–0.3 g per liter) or NM plus vitamin C (8 mg or 20 mg per liter). The cultures were exposed three times each week to puffs (25 ml puff volume) of smoke from tobacco, and six puffs from fresh smoke or the gas-vapor phase of marijuana cigarettes for up to 3 to 6 months.

With respect to the L-cysteine, its treatment led to an enhancement of lysosomes and protection against abnormal growth and malignant transformation from both types of smoke. In addition, subsequent studies revealed that vitamin C treatment could also partially reverse the malignant transformation caused by smoke from tobacco and/or marijuana as revealed by a gradual reversal from disorganized fibroblastic growth to epitheloid and epithelial growth. In their discussion it was noted that "L-cysteine in media evoked in hamster lung cultures not only a change in morphology and growth rate of cells but also altered their response to repeated exposure to fresh smoke from either tobacco or marijuana cigarettes, when compared with hamster lung cultures grown in NM only." These striking findings should encourage continued research in this area.

References

Allison, A.C. (1969). Lysosomes and cancer. In: *Lysosomes in Biology and Pathology.* Edited by J.T. Dingle and H.B. Fell. Amsterdam, London, North Holland Publishing Co., p. 178.

Allison, A.C. and Paton, G.R. (1965). Chromosome damage in human diploid cells following activation of lysosomal enzymes. *Nature* **207**:1170.

Davies, P.; Kistler, G.S.; Leuchtenberger, C.; and Leuchtenberger, R. (1975). Ultrastructural studies on cells of hamster lung cultures after chronic exposure to whole smoke or the gas vapor phase of cigarettes. *Beitr. Path. Bd.* **155**:168.

Fenner, M.L. and Braven, J. (1968). The mechanism of carcinogenesis by tobacco smoke. *Brit. J. Cancer* **22**:474.

Lange, R. (1961). Inhibiting effect of tobacco smoke on some crystalline enzymes. *Science* **134**:52.

Leuchtenberger, C. and Leuchtenberger, R. (1970). Effects of chronic inhalation of whole fresh cigarette smoke and of its gas phase on pulmonary tumorigenesis in Snell's mice. In: *Morphology of Experimental Respiratory Carcinogenesis,* p. 329. U.S. Atomic Energy Commission, 21st AEL Symposium Series.

Leuchtenberger, C. and Leuchtenberger, R. (1976). Cytological and cytochemical studies of the effects of fresh marijuana cigarette smoke on growth and DNA metabolism of animal and human lung cultures. In: *The Pharmacology of Marihuana,* p. 595. Edited by M.C. Braude and S. Szara. Raven Press, N.Y.

Leuchtenberger, C. and Leuchtenberger, R. (1976a). Protection of hamster lung cultures by L-cysteine against carcinogenic effects of fresh smoke from tobacco or marihuana cigarettes. Abst. of paper presented at the 1st International Congress of Cell Biology. September 5–10, 1976. *J. Cell. Biol.* **70**:44a.

Leuchtenberger, C. and Leuchtenberger, R. (1977). L-cysteine or vitamin C influence cellular growth and prolong survival of normal adult human lung tissue in culture. *Cell. Biol. Intern. Repts.* **1**:317.

Leuchtenberger, C. and Leuchtenberger, R. (1977a). Protection of hamster lung cultures by L-cysteine or vitamin C against carcinogenic effects of fresh smoke from tobacco or marihuana cigarettes. *Brit. J. Exper. Pathol.* **58**(6):625–634.

Leuchtenberger, C.; Leuchtenberger, R.; Ritter, V.; and Invi, N. (1973a). Effects of marijuana and tobacco smoke on DNA and chromosomal complement in human lung explants. *Nature* **242**:403.

Leuchtenberger, C.; Leuchtenberger, R.; Ruch, F.; Tanaka, K.; and Tanaka, T. (1963). Cytological and cytochemical alterations in the respiratory tract of mice after exposure to cigarette smoke, influenza virus, and both. *Cancer Res.* **23**:555.

Leuchtenberger, C.; Leuchtenberger, R.; and Schneider, A. (1973). Effects of marijuana and tobacco smoke on human lung physiology. *Nature* **241**:137.

Leuchtenberger, C.; Leuchtenberger, R.; and Zbinden, I. (1974). Gas vapor phase constituents and SH reactivity of cigarette smoke influence lung cultures. *Nature* **247**:565.

Leuchtenberger, C.; Leuchtenberger, R.; Zbinden, I.; and Schleh, E. (1976). SH reactivity of cigarette smoke and its correlation with carcinogenic effects on hamster lung cultures. *Sozialund Praventivmed.* **21**:47.

Leuchtenberger, C.; Leuchtenberger, R.; Zbinden, I.; and Schleh, E. (1976a). Cytological and cytochemical effects of whole smoke and of the gas vapor phase from marihuana cigarettes on growth and DNA metabolism of cultured mammalian cells. In: *Marihuana: Chemistry, Biochemistry, and Cellular Effects,* p. 243. Edited by G.G. Nahas. Springer Verlag, N.Y.

Leuchtenberger, C.; Leuchtenberger, R.; Zbinden, I.; and Schleh, E. (1976b). *Significance of oxides of nitrogen (NO) and SH Reactive Components in Pulmonary Carcinogenesis.* In SERM Symposium Series. **52**:73.

Mirvish, S.S. (1975). Blocking the formation of nitroso compounds with ascorbic acid *in vitro* and *in vivo*. *Ann. N.Y. Acad. Sci.* **258**:175.

Pelletier, O. (1975). Vitamin C and cigarette smokers. In: Second Conference on Vitamin C. New York Acad. of Science, *Ann. N.Y. Acad. Sci.* **258**:156.

Powell, G.M. and Green, G.M. (1972). Cigarette smoke—a proposed metabolic lesion in alveolar macrophages. *Biochem. Pharmacol.* **21**:1785.

12. Methyl Chloride

Methyl chloride (CH_3Cl) has been widely employed as a methylating and chlorinating agent in organic chemistry laboratories. It is also employed as an extractant for greases, oils, and resins in the refining of petroleum (Tabershaw et al., 1977). These authors go on to note that methyl chloride is also a solvent in the synthetic rubber industry, as a refrigerant and as a propellant in polystyrene-foam production.

Toxicological investigations of the effects of methyl chloride have revealed that it is a neurotoxic agent in both experimental animals (Sayers et al., 1929) and humans (Patty, 1963; McNally, 1946; Hansen et al., 1953; Mackie, 1961). Symptoms of methyl chloride toxicity includes ataxia, staggering gait, weakness, tremors, vertigo, difficulty in speech, and blurred vision (see ACGIH, 1976). In addition to its neurotoxic effects, methyl chloride may also cause renal and liver damage as well as depression of bone marrow activity (Tabershaw et al., 1977). The results of industrial hygiene surveys, which demonstrated that a range of average exposures of from 195 to 475 ppm was associated with the above mentioned neurological symptoms while levels less than 195 ppm were not associated with illness, led to the derivation of the present federal standard of 100 ppm (210 mg/m^3) as an 8-hour TWA (ACGIH, 1976; Tabershaw et al., 1977).

Very limited research has been carried out concerning the potential interaction of sulfur-containing amino acids (i.e., cystine and methionine) with methyl chloride. One such study in 1946 by Smith revealed that dietary supplementation with cystine and methionine markedly prolonged the survival of methyl chloride-induced mortality and neurological symptoms in rats exposed to 2000 ppm of this compound for 6 hours/day, 6 days/week until death.

References

ACGIH (1976). Documentation of TLVs. American Conference of Governmental Industrial Hygienists. Cincinnati, OH.

Hansen, H.; Weaver, N.K.; and Venable, F.S. (1953). Methyl chloride intoxication. Report of fifteen cases. *Arch. Ind. Hyg. Occup. Med.* **8**:328.

Mackie, I.J. (1961). Methyl chloride intoxication. *Med. J. Aust.* **1**:203.

McNally, W.D. (1946). Eight cases of methyl chloride poisoning with three deaths. *J. Ind. Hyg. Toxicol.* **28**:94–97.

Patty, F.A. (1963). *Industrial Hygiene and Toxicology.* Vol. II, 2nd ed., p. 1248. Interscience, N.Y.

Sayers, R.R.; Yant, W.P.; Thomas, G.H.; and Berger, L.B. (1929). Physiological response attending to exposure to vapors of methyl bromide, methyl chloride, ethyl bromide and ethyl chloride. *Pub. Health Bull.* **185**:56

Smith, W.W. (1946). The protective action of cystine and methionine in rats exposed to methyl chloride. *Fed. Proc.* **5**:97–98.

Tabershaw, I.R.; Utidjian, H.M.B.; and Kawahara, B. (1977). Chemical hazards. In: *Occupational Diseases: A Guide to Their Recognition.* Edited by M.M. Key et al. U.S. DHEW, PHS, CDC, NIOSH, Washington, D.C.

13. Naphthalene

Naphthalene ($C_{10}H_8$) is a widespread industrial irritant causing erythema and dermatitis. In addition to causing local effects, naphthalene may also cause intravascular hemolysis, renal tubular blockade, ocular neuritis, and a number of gastrointestinal and related disorders such as nausea, vomiting, profuse sweating, etc. The present federal standard for exposure to naphthalene is 10 ppm and is designed to prevent ocular effects. However, according to the ACGIH (1976), it is not known whether this standard sufficiently protects against naphthalene-induced hemolysis in G-6-PD-deficient individuals.

Exposure to naphthalene may occur in a variety of industrial environments since it is employed as a chemical intermediate for the synthesis of phthalic, anthranilic, hydroxyl (naphthol), amino (naphthylamines), and sulfuric compounds that are employed in the production of dyes (Tabershaw et al., 1977). These authors also noted that naphthalene may also be used to produce hydronaphthalenes, synthetic resins, lampblack, smokeless powder, and celluloid, as well as being commonly used as a moth repellent.

While it is widely recognized that individuals with a G-6-PD deficiency are at increased risk to the hemolytic activities of naphthalene, little attention has been directed toward the identification of other factors that may enhance susceptibility to this compound. However, one study has been published that does suggest that sulfur-containing amino acids may affect the toxicity of naphthalene (Stekol, 1937).

The rationale that dietary sulfur-containing amino acids may affect the toxicity of naphthalene was derived from a study by White and Jackson (1935), which indicated that when bromobenzene was given to growing rats reared on a diet low in organic sulfur but sufficient for moderate growth, the growth ceased, but was resumed again when the diet was supplemented with the sulfur-containing amino acids l-cystine or methionine. Since studies with a variety of species (i.e., dogs, swine, and rabbits) (Stekol, 1935, 1936; Bourne and Young, 1934) revealed that naphthalene and halogenated benzenes (Stekol, 1937; White and Lewis, 1932) act in a similar manner, Stekol (1937) hypothesized that sulfur-containing amino acids in the diet may also serve to modify the toxicity of naphthalene. The results of the Stekol (1937a) study did in fact support the above stated hypothesis in that the addition of dl-methionine and l-cystine, when added to the naphthalene-containing diet, enhanced the growth and increased the food consumption of rats.

Unfortunately, this study has not been followed up. Thus, the relevance of the potential interaction of methionine and L-cystine with naphthalene is not well defined. Needless to say, further study in this area is required.

References

ACGIH (1976). Documentation of TLVs. American Conference of Governmental Industrial Hygienists, Cincinnati, OH.

Bourne, M.C. and Young, L. (1934). The metabolism of naphthalene in rabbits. *Biochem. J.* **28**:803–808.

Stekol, J.A. (1935). Metabolism of naphthalene in adult and growing dogs. *J. Biol. Chem.* **110**:463–469.

Stekol, J.A. (1936). Comparative studies in the sulfur metabolism of the dog and pig. *J. Biol. Chem.* **113**:675–682.

Stekol, J.A. (1937). Studies on the mercapturic acid synthesis in animals. I. The extent of the synthesis of p-bromophenyl mercapturic acid in dogs as affected by diets of varying sulfur content. *J. Biol. Chem.* **117**:147–157.

Stekol, J.A. (1937a). Studies on the mercapturic acid synthesis in animals. V. The effect of naphthalene on the growth of rats as related to diets of varying sulfur content. *J. Biol. Chem.* **121**:87–91.

Tabershaw, I.R.; Utidjian, H.M.B.; and Kawahara, B. (1977). Chemical hazards. In: *Occupational Diseases: A Guide to Their Recognition*. Edited by M.M. Key et al. U.S. DHEW, PHS, CDC, NIOSH, Washington, D.C.

White, A. and Jackson, R.W. (1935). The effect of bromobenzene on the utilization of cystine and methionine by the growing rat. *J. Biol. Chem.* **111**:507–513.

White, A. and Lewis, H.B. (1932). The metabolism of sulfur. XIX. The distribution of urinary sulfur in the dog after the oral administration of monobromobenzene as influenced by the character of the dietary protein and by the feeding of l-cystine and dl-methionine. *J. Biol. Chem.* **98**:607–624.

14. N-nitroso Compounds

The toxicity and carcinogenicity of N-nitroso compounds is now widely recognized. It has been speculated that the mechanism by which N-nitroso compounds cause these adverse effects is via "the decomposition to short-lived highly reactive electrophiles which react with nucleophilic sites on DNA bases leading to altered bases" (Gutenplan, 1977). Based on this speculation of N-nitroso initiation of carcinogenesis, Gutenplan (1977) theorized that it may be possible to prevent N-nitroso-induced carcinogenesis by finding a relatively innocuous compound that may be able to interfere with the electrophilic attack of the DNA. The ideal situation was thought to be a naturally occurring, relatively nontoxic nucleophilic compound that could outcompete the DNA for the electrophilic mutagen. Of course it would help if this compound were more nucleophilic than the DNA, and present near DNA in sufficient quantities. Among the potentially eligible compounds meeting these fundamental criteria to varying degrees were ascorbic acid, creatine-H_2O, cysteine-HCl, serine, tyrosine, tryptophan, and methionine.

In testing the potential effectiveness of these nucleophilic compounds to prevent N-nitroso mutagenesis, Gutenplan (1977) utilized the microbial test organism *Salmonella typhimurium* TA 1500 in direct and in liver-assisted assays, while testing the mutagenicity of N-methyl-N-nitrosoguanidine (MNNG). While ascorbic acid proved to be highly effective (99% reduction) in preventing the mutagenicity of MNNG, methionine was only marginally preventive (17% reduction). Serine, tyrosine, tryptophan, creatine-H_2O, and cysteine-H_2O were reasonably effective, showing approximately 50–80% reductions. According to Gutenplan (1977), the levels of all the compounds tested except ascorbate were considerably higher than levels normally found in the urine. As for ascorbic acid, it would not be unexpected to find even higher levels in the urine. Consequently, at least with respect to preventive activity in the urinary bladder, ascorbic acid would seem to be highly superior to the other compounds tested. Thus the role of methionine relative to other naturally occurring nucleophiles in potentially preventing the mutagenicity of MNNG seems quite modest. Whether this type of experiment accurately predicts the potentially protective action of nucleophiles against N-nitroso compounds in animal models and humans is clearly an important area of research that should be vigorously pursued.

Reference

Gutenplan, J.B. (1977). Inhibition by L-ascorbate of bacterial mutagenesis induced by two N-nitroso compounds. *Nature* **268**:368–370.

15. Pesticides

Several studies have offered preliminary evidence that dietary exposure to chlorinated hydrocarbon insecticides such as DDT (Phillips, 1963) and dieldrin (Lee et al., 1964) diminish liver stores of vitamin A. For instance, Phillips (1963) reported that DDT markedly decreased liver vitamin-A storage when rats were fed a semipurified diet, while Lee et al. (1964) also demonstrated that dieldrin reduced liver vitamin-A levels in rats. However, it has also been recognized that dietary status can markedly influence the effect of chlorinated hydrocarbons on vitamin-A liver storage. Tinsley (1969) noted that the DDT-induced reduction of liver vitamin-A stores was inversely related to the level of dietary methionine. Other studies revealed that high-protein diets (25%) provided some protection to rats from the adverse effects of dieldrin (Lee et al., 1964), while others revealed that when weanling albino rats were maintained on a diet with one-third of the normal quantity of protein, they became slightly more susceptible to the DDT toxicity via an oral dose (Boyd and DeCastro, 1968). Subsequent research by Young et al. (1973) supported the earlier studies of Lee et al. (1964) and Boyd and DeCastro (1968), in that the degree of DDT-induced decreases in liver vitamin-A stores depends, in large part, on both the quality (soybean vs. casein) and quantity (10% vs. 20%) of dietary protein as well as on the presence or absence of methionine.

The results of the Young et al. (1973) study suggest that the quantity of protein affects the amount of DDT and its metabolites stored in the liver. This suggestion is consistent with the findings of Stoewsand and Bourkes (1968) who reported that rats given high quantities of protein (25 and 50%) have an increased urinary and fecal excretion of DDT metabolites and lower dieldrin levels in various tissues including the liver, brain, and epididymal adipose. However, Tinsley and Claeys (1970) and Young et al. (1973) have found that methionine increases residues of DDT, DDD, and DDE in the liver of the rat when fed on a soybean-protein diet. Young et al. (1973) also found this to be true for a casein diet at 10%, but when the percentage was increased to 20% no effect was noted. The findings, which indicate that dietary supplementation with methionine increases the liver residues of DDT and some of its metabolites, are especially interesting in light of the apparent capability of methionine to prevent a DDT-induced depletion of liver vitamin-A stores.

Tinsley and Claeys (1970) have attempted to explain how methionine supplementation causes an increase in the liver residues of DDT. They suggest that this increased residue of DDT may be related to the influence of methionine on lipid transport. They inferred that reducing the amount of methionine limits the formation of chylomicrons, thereby diminishing the degree of lipid transport (see Hyams et al., 1966; Sabesin and Isselbacher, 1965). As a corollary, since DDT is most likely associated with chylomicrons in the chyle, its transport may be similarly affected. It follows that when levels of dietary methionine are increased, fat transport would also be increased and thus more DDT would be absorbed and transported to the liver. Tinsley and Claeys (1970) concluded "that feeding proteins low in methionine would not accentuate the chronic response to DDT. Low levels of methionine result in lower levels of DDT and its metabolites assimilating in the tissue."

In terms of using diet to reduce the potential toxic effects of pollutants, it appears that one is faced with an ambivalent situation with respect to the DDT and methionine. On the positive side, sulfur-containing amino acids, especially methionine (Koyanagi and Odagiri, 1961; Tinsley, 1966), can prevent DDT-induced depletion of liver vitamin-A stores. However, on the negative side, dietary methionine supplementation causes greater retention of DDT in the liver. It would be interesting to investigate the influence of other sulfur-containing amino acids (e.g., cystine) on DDT-induced liver vitamin-A depletion as well as on DDT retention.

References

Boyd, E.M. and DeCastro, E.S. (1968). Protein-deficient diet and DDT toxicity. *Bull. WHO* 38:141.

Hyams, D.E.; Sabesin, S.M.; Greenberger, N.J.; and Isselbacher, K.J. (1966). Inhibition of intestinal protein synthesis and lipid transport by ethionine. *Biochim. Biophys. Acta.* 125:166.

Koyanagi, T. and Odagiri, S. (1961). Effects of the sulfur amino acids on the vitamin A content in liver of rats. *Nature* 192:168.

Lee, M.; Harris, K.; and Trowbridge, H. (1964). Effect of the level of dietary fat on the toxicity of dieldrin for the laboratory rat. *J. Nutr.* **84**:136–144.

Phillips, W.E.J. (1963). DDT and the metabolism of vitamin A and carotene in the rat. *Can. J. Biochem. Physiol.* **41**:1793–1803.

Sabesin, S.M. and Isselbacher, K.J. (1965). Protein synthesis inhibition: mechanism for the production of impaired fat absorption. *Science* **147**:1149.

Stoewsand, G.S. and Bourkes, J.B. (1968). The influence of dietary protein on the resistance to dieldrin toxicity in the rat. *Indus. Med. Surg.* **37**:526.

Tinsley, I.J. (1966). Nutritional interactions in dieldrin toxicity. *J. Agr. Food Chem.* **14**:563–565.

Tinsley, I.J. (1969). DDT effect on rats raised on alpha-protein rations: growth and storage of liver vitamin A. *J. Nutr.* **98**:319.

Tinsley, I.J. and Claeys, R.R. (1970). Influence of dietary methionine on metabolism of DDT in the rat. *J. Agr. Food Chem.* **18**:107.

Young, M.L.; Mitchell, G.V.; and Seward, C.R. (1973). Effect of protein and methionine on vitamin A liver storage in rats fed DDT. *J. Nutr.* **103**:218–229.

16. Pyridine

That pyridine toxicity may be influenced by modifications in the diet is well known for several nutrients including vitamin E (Hove, 1953), protein levels in general, and sulfur-containing amino acids such as cystine and methionine (Drill, 1952; Baxter, 1947). The hypothesis that dietary methionine levels may affect pyridine toxicity was first offered by Baxter (1947). He felt that since pyridine is metabolized in part via the process of methylation, that substances capable of donating methyl groups (such as methionine) to this process may be markedly diminished over the course of a prolonged exposure. Consequently, it was thought that (1) pyridine exposure may enhance the occurrence of a methionine deficiency, and (2) low levels of dietary methionine enhance pyridine toxicity by retarding the detoxification process.

In his study, Baxter (1947) reported that the addition of pyridine (0.1 to 0.2%) to a diet low in protein (10% casein) adversely affects growth and causes death with liver and kidney injury. Increasing either the amount of casein to 20% or the addition of 0.15% methionine permitted the rats to grow, but according to the authors, this level of supplementation did not significantly increase the rate of survival. However, when the level of methionine was increased to 0.5%, it markedly enhanced survival so that 30 to 90% of the rats survived, depending on the experiment, in contrast to 0% of previous studies. Furthermore, dietary methionine supplementation of up to 1.0% markedly enhanced survival in rats given pyridine citrate in the diet at a level of 1.0%.

Subsequent studies by Coulson and Brazda (1948) and Baxter (1949) also revealed that dietary supplementation with methionine and cystine as well as cystine plus choline (but not choline alone), when added to diets containing 10 to 25% casein, enhanced the survival of pyridine-treated rats.

The significance of these findings is difficult to interpret since the level of exposure is quite high and the route of exposure is oral. Human exposure to pyridine is within the occupational setting, with the present federal standard being 5 ppm (15 mg/m³). While the ACGIH (1976) noted that "the TLV of 5 ppm should be low enough to prevent systemic effects (i.e., damage to the liver, kidneys and bone marrow), provided skin absorption is not permitted . . .," no consideration was given to the role of dietary factors, including methionine, in the derivation of the industrial limit.

While this lack of consideration is probably legitimate in light of the limited data base, the results of these investigations should raise concern that certain segments of the working population may be at increased risk to pyridine toxicity. Further research should be devoted toward clarifying the interaction of methionine and pyridine, especially in experimental conditions that more closely simulate human exposures.

References

ACGIH (1976). Documentation of TLVs. American Conference of Governmental Industrial Hygienists, Cincinnati, OH.

Baxter, J.H. (1947). Studies of the mechanisms of liver and kidney injury. III. Methionine protects against damage produced in rat by diets containing pyridine. *J. Pharmacol. Exp. Therap.* **91**:345–349.

Baxter, J.H. (1949). Pyridine liver and kidney injury in rats; the influence of diet, with particular attention to methionine, cystine and choline. *Bull. Johns Hopkins Hosp.* **85**:138–167.

Coulson, R.A. and Brazda, F.G. (1948). The influence of choline, cystine, and methionine on toxic effects of pyridine and certain related compounds. *Proc. Soc. Exp. Biol. Med.* **69**:480–487.

Drill, V.A. (1952). Hepatotoxic agents: mechanism of action and dietary interrelationship. *Pharm. Rev.* **4**:1–41.

Hove, E.L. (1953). The relation of pyridine toxicity in rats to dietary vitamin E. *J. Nutr.* **50**:361–372.

Tabershaw, I.R.; Utidjian, H.M.B.; and Kawahara, B. (1977). Chemical hazards. In: *Occupational Diseases: A Guide to Their Recognition.* Edited by M.M. Key et al. U.S. DHEW, PHS, CDC, NIOSH, Washington, D.C.

17. TNT

That dietary status may affect the toxicity of TNT has been hypothesized since the First World War when toxicity symptoms seemed to be related to the adequacy of the diet. The dietary factors evaluated included protein, fat, and carbohydrate levels, as well as ascorbic acid and the sulfur-containing amino acids cystine and methionine.

With respect to methionine, very little research has been published concerning whether it may affect the occurrence of TNT-induced toxicity. Despite its extremely limited data base, what information is available is impressive. In the one study that addressed this issue, Smith et al. (1943) compared the response of white rats of the Wistar strain on different diets to dietary TNT (0.3%). The seven dietary treatments included (1) 5% casein, (2) 5% casein + 2% ascorbic acid, (3) 5% casein + 0.1% cystine, (4) 5% casein + 0.5% cystine, (5) 5% casein + 1% methionine, (6) 37% casein, and (7) 18% casein, with the food being provided ad libitum.

Their results indicated that cystine (but especially methionine) supplementation provided protection from the effects of TNT toxicity as well as from the adverse effects of a low-protein diet. For instance, while every other dietary group (including cystine supplementation) experienced some degree of abnormal liver function[7] ranging from as "low" as 20% in the 18%-casein animals to 100% of those on the 5%-casein and 5%-casein + 2%-ascorbic-acid diets, no abnormal functioning was found in the methionine-treated group. Similarly, all dietary treatments except the methionine-supplemented one exhibited some degree of fatty livers, with the percentage ranging from 20 (in the case of the 18%-casein group) to 70 (in the case of the 5%-casein group).

These findings are so striking that it is disappointing that this potentially very significant finding has not been pursued. One possible reason for this period of benign neglect may stem from the total lack of emphasis provided by Smith et al. (1943) in their reporting of the data; that is, their major intention was to provide an evaluation of the influence of ascorbic acid on TNT poisoning in a variety of species (rats, guinea pigs, rabbits, cats), because of its potential role in the process of conjugate glucuronidation. That methionine was considered in their research protocol seems almost an afterthought, with no rationale provided to support why it was evaluated. Thus it appears that this finding may have been buried along with the other findings of this

[7]As measured by the Rose Bengal retention test.

article, which were not particularly exciting except for the influence of protein levels in the diet. In any case, the findings of Smith et al. (1943) suggest further research should be directed toward a more comprehensive assessment of the role of dietary methionine on TNT-induced hepatotoxicity.

References

Shils, M.E. and Goldwater, L.J. (1949). Nutritional factors affecting the toxicity of some aromatic hydrocarbons with special reference to benzene and nitrobenzene compounds: a review. *J. Ind. Hyg. Tox.* **31**(4):175.

Smith, M.I.; Westfall, B.B.; and Stohlman, E.F. (1943). Experimental trinitrotoluene poisoning with attempts at detoxification. *J. Ind. Hyg. Tox.* **25**(9):391.

C. AMINO ACIDS—POLLUTANT INTERACTIONS— A PERSPECTIVE

It has been shown that the administration of a variety of sulfur-containing amino acids including methionine, cystine, and cysteine may affect the toxicity and/or carcinogenicity of over 40 compounds (see Table 2). In the overwhelming number of cases, these amino acids clearly reduce both the incidence and severity of the particular adverse condition. The exceptions to this generalization include the interactions of methionine with aflatoxin, lead, and chlorinated hydrocarbon insecticides. In these exceptions the administration of methionine has not conclusively been shown to enhance their toxicity or carcinogenicity. In fact, for aflatoxin-induced renal disease, methionine does not have an obvious influence, while for both lead and the DDT-like pesticides it has been demonstrated that methionine may either enhance their absorption from the gastrointestinal tract and/or enhance tissue retention, presumably enhancing toxicity, although the later presumption remains to be demonstrated.

In addition to the overall impression that these amino acids reduce the toxicity of a large number of quite unrelated compounds, one is struck by the general inconclusiveness of most of the studies. For example, many of the interactions of cystine, cysteine, or methionine with individual pollutants have fewer than five articles published about them and in a number of instances only one reference has been found. Thus, striking findings reported for the protective influence of methionine against the toxicity of benzene, 1,2-dichloroethane, 1,2-dichloropropane, pyridine, and other compounds are highly suggestive but certainly not conclusive. Perhaps the most conclusive interaction

Table 2. Summary—The Influence of Amino Acids on Pollutant Toxicity and Carcinogenicity

A. Inorganic Substances		
Antimony	Cysteine administration has been found to detoxify this compound	Launoy, 1934
Arsenic	Limited animal and human studies have revealed that methionine or cystine administration prevent arsenical-induced liver injury and enhance liver recovery from arsenical damage	Goodell et al., 1944 Peters et al., 1944, 1945
	Cystine and especially cysteine were effective in reducing the acute toxicity of arsphenamine, while glycine was not effective. While these results may appear to be in partial contrast to Versari (1937), who reported that glycine decreased the toxicity of arsphenamine, their experiment protocols differed slightly, possibly accounting for the contradictory findings. However, cysteine enhanced the toxicity of pentavalent arsenic by reducing it to its trivalent form. Both glycine and calcium glucuronate did not affect the toxicity, while ascorbic acid reduced the toxicity	Martin and Thompson, 1943 Versari, 1937 Lambert, 1937
Bismuth	Cystine administration reduced the acute toxicity of bismuth by about 20% while treatment with glycine, calcium glycuronate, and ascorbic acid was not effective	Martin and Thompson, 1943

Cadmium	Cysteine prevented cadmium-induced testicular damage in rats; however, the minimum dose of cysteine required to prevent damage was 500 times greater than cadmium dose. In contrast to its protective activity, cysteine was not effective in preventing cadmium lethality and in fact enhanced it by facilitating cadmium-induced renal damage	Gunn et al., 1966, 1968, 1968a Bordas et al., 1976
Cobalt	Limited animal research indicates that cobalt toxicity is diminished by methionine and/or cystine; relevance to the human situation is questionable due to the low probability of excessive exposure	Griffith et al., 1942
Copper	Low levels of methionine or cystine are known to enhance the toxicity of copper in several farm animals including poultry, cattle, and sheep. Relevance to the human situation remains to be evaluated	Jensen and Maurice, 1979
Cyanide	Strong biochemical evidence to support an important role for sulfur-containing amino acids in the detoxification of cyanide; limited epidemiological investigations are consistent with the biochemical theory	Anonymous, 1969 Wilson 1965 Wood and Cooley, 1956
Fluoride	Administration of cysteine did not prevent the enhancing influence of supplemental fat on the development of fluorosis in the rat	Miller and Phillips, 1955

Table 2. (Continued)

Gold	Cystine, cysteine, and methionine administration reduced the acute toxicity in mice of a medicinal gold compound. Glycine administration did not affect gold-induced acute toxicity	Martin and Thompson, 1943
Lead	Recent experiments suggest that methionine enhances the gastrointestinal absorption of lead. Earlier investigations suggested that methionine prevented lead toxicity; further research is needed to resolve these apparently contradictory findings	Baernstein and Grand, 1942 Conrad and Barton, 1978
Mercury	Cystine (0.4% in diet) was found to reduce several indications of mercury toxicity in rats; it was suggested that cystine may offer sulfur-binding sites in proteins that complex with mercury or change methylmercury to a less toxic form	Stillings et al., 1974
	Cystine, cysteine, glycine, ascorbic acid, and calcium glucuronate did not affect the acute toxicity of mercuric acetate in mice	Martin and Thompson, 1943
Molybdenum	Supplementation with methionine markedly prevented the toxicity of excessive dietary molybdenum in rats; methionine was more effective than copper; cystine and methionine reduced alteration of enzymatic processes in rats	Gray and Daniel, 1954
Radiation	The administration of multiple radioprotective agents including cysteine (along with glutathione, bromide hydrobromide, serotonin, and others) reduced the acute toxicity of irradiation in mice	Maisin and Mattelin, 1967 Straube et al., 1950

Selenium	Methionine supplementation to the diet will reduce the toxicity of selenium, especially in the presence of sufficient α-tocopherol, which is thought to facilitate the donation of methyl groups from methionine molecules for the ultimate detoxication of selenium	Levander and Morris, 1970
	Cystine supplementation was unable to prevent selenium-induced toxicity	Schneider, 1936 Smith and Stohlman, 1940
Strontium	The amino acids lysine and arginine have been found to markedly enhance the gastrointestinal uptake of calcium and strontium, especially the latter. Eighteen other amino acids, including those essential for the rat, were found to have little or no influence	Wasserman et al., 1956
Thallium	Methionine supplementation partially prevents toxic manifestations of thallium exposure; cystine, another amino acid, however, is markedly protective; theoretical biochemical explanation is provided within the text	Gross et al., 1948
B. Organic Substances		
Acetaldehyde/ ethanol	Administration of several amino acids (cysteine, lysine, glycine, arginine, ornithine) reduces the toxicity of these compounds	Breglia et al., 1973 Sprince et al., 1975
Acetyl amino fluorine (AAF)	Male rats given 0.006% AAF in an adequate diet, to which a large quantity of methionine, (2%) cystine, or casein was added, exhibited a decreased incidence of liver tumors	Miller and Miller, 1972

Table 2. (Continued)

Aflatoxin B$_1$	Administration of cysteine reduced the degree of aflatoxin B$_1$-induced hepatotoxicity by presumably enhancing its conjugation to glutathione; in contrast, later findings indicated that cystamine and cysteine could not prevent liver necrosis in rats when given 12 hours after AFB$_1$ treatment	Mgbodile et al., 1975 Ferreyra et al., 1979
	Methionine supplementation to a deficient diet did not affect the occurrence of aflatoxin-induced renal lesions	Newberne et al., 1968
Allyl alcohol	Cystine was highly effective in reducing the toxicity of this compound in rats; more recent investigations using rats revealed that cystamine and cysteine were unable to reduce the portal necrosis caused by allyl alcohol	Eger, 1956 Ferreyra et al., 1979
Azo dyes	Limited animal experimentation reveals that methionine may reduce DAB intoxification; however, studies concerning the role of methionine in affecting DAB-induced carcinogenicity are equivocal	Griffin et al., 1949 Clayton and Baumann, 1949
Benzene	Methionine supplementation was found to reduce the extent of benzene-induced leukopenia in rats	Li and Freeman, 1947
Bromobenzene	Methionine supplementation enhances the excretion of this compound in the rat	White and Lewis, 1932 White and Jackson, 1935 Drill, 1952 Dessi, 1965

Carbon tetrachloride	Cystamine and/or cysteine administration to rats 3 to 12 hours after bromobenzene treatment were protected from developing liver necrosis	Ferreyra et al, 1979
	While empirical clinical studies suggest that methionine supplementation reduces CCl_4-induced liver damage, experimental studies with animal models do not; however, experimental studies do indicate that methionine may prevent CCl_4-induced renal damage	Drill, 1952 Gyorgy et al., 1946
	Cysteine administration prevented CCl_4-induced hepatotoxicity in rats	DeFerreyra et al., 1974
Chloroform	Methionine dietary supplements have been found to prevent chloroform-induced toxicity, especially to the liver of dogs previously reared on a low-protein diet; studies on chronic low-level exposure to chloroform as may occur in drinking water remain to be carried out	Drill, 1952 Miller et al., 1940 Miller and Whipple, 1942
Dimethylnitrosamine	Cysteine administration of 0.3 g/day s.c. significantly decreased the toxicity of DMN but not N-nitroso diethylamine	Mizrahi and Emmelot, 1962, 1963
	Treatment with cystamine and/or cysteine offered protection from DMN-induced liver necrosis in rats when given 3 and 6 hours after DMN treatment, respectively	Ferreyra et al, 1979
1,2-dichloroethane	Supplementation of low-protein diets with methionine or cystine markedly reduces mortality and liver-fat levels in rats	Heppel et al., 1945, 1945a, 1947

Table 2. (Continued)

1,2-dichloropropane	Methionine and/or cystine supplementation to a low-protein diet markedly reduces the toxicity of this agent	Heppel, 1946
Ethanol	Pretreatment of rodents with L-lysine resulted in a significant increase in survival, increased LD_{50} of ethanol, a decrease in ethanol-enhanced sleeping time, and decrease in ethanol levels in blood	Ward et al., 1972 Dorato et al., 1977 Jamall et al., 1979
	Methionine supplements reduce the occurrence of alcohol-induced fatty infiltration of the liver in rats	Klatskin et al., 1954
Ethionine	Methionine and/or cystine administration prevents the occurrence of ethionine-induced toxicity and carcinogenicity in a dose-dependent fashion	Farber and Ichinose, 1958
Marijuana	Cysteine protects against premalignant tissue changes caused by marijuana smoke in hamster lung culture	Leuchtenberger and Leuchtenberger, 1977
Methyl chloride	Neurological symptoms of methyl chloride toxicity were reduced in rats given diets supplemented with methionine and cystine	Smith, 1946
Methylcholanthrene (MCA)	Mice reared on a diet deficient in phenylalanine-tyrosine showed an enhanced susceptibility to MCA-induced tumorigenesis, while dietary deficiencies of leucine and isoleucine did not predispose mice toward developing MCA-induced cancer	Worthington et al., 1978

Naphthalene	Preliminary findings suggest that sulfur-containing amino acids including methionine and cystine reduce the toxicity of this compound in rats as determined by growth rates and food consumption	Stekol, 1937
Nicotine	Dietary supplements of cystine and ascorbic acid gave rats protection against chronic nicotine poisoning. "Exogenous and possibly dietary factors may account, in part, for the difference in individual susceptibility to nicotine in man and animals"	Hueper, 1943
N-nitroso compounds	Methionine was not very effective as a nucleophilic agent in protecting bacterial DNA from electrophilic attack by MNNG, an N-nitroso carcinogen	Gutenplan, 1977
Pesticides	Methionine supplementation has been found to enhance the transport of fat-soluble chlorinated hydrocarbon pesticides (i.e., DDT) and their retention in the liver	Tinsley, 1966
Phenolic/biphenolic compounds	Low levels of methionine and cystine in the diets of rats markedly reduces their capacity to detoxify compounds of a phenolic or biphenolic nature via sulfoconjugation	Magdalov et al., 1979
Pyridine	Pyridine-induced lethality was markedly reduced by cystine or methionine supplementation in rats	Baxter, 1947 Coulson and Brazda, 1948

Table 2. (Continued)

Sulfanilamide	Supplementation of a 7%-protein diet with cystine to simulate the amount of cystine in a 30%-protein diet did not affect sulfanilamide toxicity, but a joint supplementation of cystine and methionine did reduce the mortality rate but not the sulfanilamide-induced anemia	Smith et al., 1941
Thioacetamide	Treatment with cystamine and/or cysteine reduced the occurrence of thioacetamide induced liver damage in rats when given 12 hours after exposure to the hepatotoxin.	Ferreyra et al., 1979
TNT	Limited but striking findings suggested that methionine supplementation may markedly reduce TNT-induced hepatotoxicity	Smith et al., 1943
Tri-o-cresyl phosphate (TOCP)	Dietary supplementation with 1% cystine was able to substantially improve the growth of TOCP-treated rats as compared to those reared on the basal or control diet. In contrast, supplementation with methionine (1%) depressed growth relative to the controls. The authors hypothesized that the enhanced growth by cystine treatment may have resulted from being contaminated with selenium, or the TOCP may prevent the conversion of methionine to cystine	Shull and Cheeke, 1973
Tyrosine	Supplementation with methionine reduced the toxicity to rats of diets with excessive levels of tyrosine	Yamamoto et al., 1976

Urethane	Methionine administration to the diet of rats reduced the incidence of urethane-induced tumors after 4 and 6 months, respectively, as well as enhancing a retention of liver riboflavin. More recent studies have not supported this finding	Miller et al., 1948 French, 1978
Mutagenicity of: N-methyl-N'-nitro-N- nitrosoguanidine N-acetoxy-2- acetylaminofluorine N-hydroxy-2- acetylaminofluorine 4-nitroguinoline-1-oxide methylmethanesulfo- nate 5-nitro-2-furaldehyde semicarbazone 2-(2 furyl)-3- (5-nitro-2-furyl) acrylamide aflatoxin B$_1$ nitrosation production of methylurea and methylguanidine	At nontoxic levels, cysteine markedly decreased the frequency of mutations in bacterial testing system. Mechanism of cysteine protection is highly speculative, but may involve competing for nucleophilic sites on DNA by the electrophilic mutagen	Rosin and Stich, 1978

of methionine with a toxic substance is with ethionine, which is now recognized as having many characteristics of a methionine anti-metabolite. The relevance of these data to the ambient and industrial environments is quite limited.

Without question, the strongest aspect of this information is the suggestion that further research concerning the interrelationships of methionine and a wide range of toxic substances is a potentially fruit-ful area. For example, the notion that methionine supplementation may reduce the occurrence of benzene-induced leukopenia is a highly important finding to investigate further. So, too, is the synergistic interaction of methionine and ascorbic acid in reducing methemoglo-bin to hemoglobin or its use in detoxifying cyanide and thallium (see the specific sections on these pollutants).

Research concerning the influence of methionine and cystine on pollutant toxicity was quite active during the 1940s, especially with respect to hepatotoxic agents such as chloroform, CCl_4, and azo dyes. However, with the phase out of the use of carcinogenic azo dyes in foods as well as the replacement of chloroform in anesthesia, it seems as if research interest in the interactions of these amino acids with hepatotoxic agents also diminished. Of course, there are exceptions to these casual observations such as the research with selenium, ethionine, and several others that continued to have considerable interest shown in them during the 1950s. However, more recently there seems to have been a revival of interest with respect to the potential interactions of the sulfhydryl compounds of the sulfur-containing amino acids and toxic substances, especially with regard to N-nitroso compounds (Rosin and Stich, 1978; Gutenplan, 1977), afla-toxin (Rogers, 1975), and cigarette and marijuana smoke (Leuchten-berger and Leuchtenberger, 1977), as well as the role of lipotropic amino acids like methionine in chemoprevention.

In some of the most important research to date with experimental animal models on the role of diet affecting the occurrence of chemically induced cancers, Rogers and Newberne (1969) have repeatedly em-ployed low-lipotrope diets that have included marginal levels of choline, vitamin B_{12}, and methionine. Thus, while it is not possible to distinguish the influence of methionine in these studies, it is critical not to overlook its potential role in affecting the occurrence and sever-ity of chemical carcinogenesis. In fact, it is in the occurrence of multi-ple interactions as seen in the Rogers and Newberne (1969) research, that more realistic conditions are achieved.

How amino acid nutritional status affects the occurrence of adverse health effects resulting from pollutant exposure is an area of outstanding research potential that will hopefully yield many improvements in the public's health. For not only do these sulfur-containing amino acids have the capacity to serve as potent reducing agents and thereby directly diminish the potential toxicity of many environmental oxidant stressor agents, they may also participate in the formation of conjugation products (as in the case of the detoxification of bromobenzene and related compounds), as well as possibly forming complexes with toxic molecules such as acetaldehyde. This diversity of biochemical reactivity provides the physiological foundations for the capacity of these amino acids to reduce the toxicity of such a broad and seemingly unrelated grouping of toxic substances.

While it is true that the vast majority of the effects of dietary supplementation of amino acids helps to alleviate the toxicity of certain pollutants, it must be emphasized that amino acids, when given in excess, may also cause severe intoxication (Harper et al., 1970). For example, additions of 0.3 to 0.9% of L-cystine to diets with 16% casein have caused acute kidney damage (Cox et al., 1929; Griffith and Wade, 1940). Other studies with excess cystine supplementation have demonstrated that cystine is a hepatotoxic agent as well (Harper et al., 1970; Lillie, 1932). Similar precautions must be directed toward the other amino acids discussed herein, especially with respect to methionine (i.e., also a renal and liver toxicant), the amino acid generally considered the most toxic. Not only is excessive methionine toxic, it may also result in an enhanced requirement for other nutrients including the B-vitamin pyridoxine. For example, only a small addition of methionine (0.45%) to a low-protein (15% casein) pyridoxine-deficient diet markedly diminished survival time of rats (Cerecedo and DeRenzo, 1950). These precautionary words are not intended to dampen the enthusiasm of researchers investigating the potential use of amino acids as prophylactic and therapeutic agents against pollutant toxicity and/or carcinogenicity, but to make people realize the limitations of dietary manipulation of amino acids.

References

Anonymous. (1969). Chronic cyanide neurotoxicity. *Lancet* **2**:942–943.

Baernstein, H.D. and Grand, J.A. (1942). The relation of protein intake to lead poisoning in rats. *J. Pharm. Exp. Therap.* **74**:18–24.

Baxter, J.H. (1947). Studies of the mechanisms of liver and kidney. III. Methionine protects against damage produced in rat by diets containing pyridine. *J. Pharmacol. Exp. Therap.* **91**:345–349.

Bordas, E.; Gabor, S.; and Papilian, V.V. (1976). The role of cysteine in cadmium induced experimental testicular damage. *Arch. Toxicol.* **36**:163–168.

Breglia, R.J.; Ward, C.O.; and Jarowski, C.I. (1973). Effect of selected amino acids on ethanol toxicity in rats. *J. Pharm. Sci.* **62**(1):49–55.

Cerecedo, L.R. and DeRenzo, E.C. (1950). Protein intake and vitamin B_6 deficiency in the rat. III. The effect of supplementing a low-protein, vitamin B_6 deficient diet with tryptophan and with other sulfur-free amino acids. *Arch. Biochem.* **29**:273–280.

Clayson, C.C. and Baumann, C.A. (1949). Diet and azo dye tumors: effect of diet during a period when the dye is not fed. *Cancer Res.* **9**(10):575–582.

Conrad, M.E. and Barton, J.C. (1978). Factors affecting the absorption and excretion of lead in the rat. *Gastroenterology* **74**:731–740.

Coulson, R.A. and Brazda, F.G. (1948). The influence of choline, cystine, and methionine on toxic effects of pyridine and certain related compounds. *Proc. Soc. Exp. Biol. Med.* **69**:480–487.

Cox, G.J.; Smythe, C.V.; and Fishback, C.F. (1929). The nephropathogenic action of cystine. *J. Biol. Chem.* **82**:95–103.

DeFerreyra, E.C.; Castro, J.A.; Diaz Gomez, M.I.; D'Acosta, N.; DeCastro, C.R.; and DeFenos, D.M. (1974). Prevention and treatment of carbon tetrachloride hepatotoxicity by cysteine; studies about its mechanism. *Toxicol. Appl. Pharmacol.* **27**: 558–568.

Dessi, P. (1965). Azioni di omologhi superiori della metionina nell'intossicazione da bromobenzene. *Societa Italiana di Biologia Specimentale* **41**:973–976.

Diplock, A.T.; Green, J.; Bunyan, J.; McHale, D.; and Muthy, I.R. (1967). Vitamin E and stress. 3. The metabolism of D-L-tocopherol in the rat under dietary stress with silver. *Brit. J. Nutr.* **21**:115–125.

Dorato, M.A.; Lynch, V.D.; and Ward, C.O. (1977). Effect of lysine and diethanolamine-rutin on blood levels, withdrawal reaction and acute toxicity of ethanol in mice. *J. Pharmacol. Sci.* **66**:35–39.

Drill, V.A. (1952). Hepatotoxic agents: mechanism of action and dietary interrelationship. *Pharmacol. Rev.* **4**:1–41.

Eger, (1956). *Virchows Arch. Path. Anat. Physiol.* **328**:536. (Cited in Diplock et al. [1967]). *Brit. J. Nutr.* **21**:124.

Farber, E. and Ichinose, H. (1958). The prevention of ethionine-induced carcinoma of the liver in rats by methionine. *Cancer Res.* **18**:1209–1213.

Ferreyra de, E.C.; Fenos de, O.M.; Bernacchi, A.S.; Castro de, C.R.; and Castro, J.A. (1979). Therapeutic effectiveness of cystamine and cysteine to reduce liver cell necrosis induced by several hepatotoxins. *Toxicol. Appl. Pharm.* **48**:221–228.

French, F.A. (1978). The influence of nutritional factors on pulmonary adenomas in mice. In: *Inorganic and Nutritional Aspects of Cancer*, pp. 281–292. Edited by G.N. Schrauzer. Plenum Press, N.Y.

Goodell, J.P.B.; Hanson, P.C.; and Hawkins, W.B. (1944). Methionine protects against mapharsen liver injury in protein-depleted dogs. *J. Exp. Med.* **79**:625–632.

Gray, L.F. and Daniel, L.J. (1954). Some effects of excess molybdenum on the nutrition of the rat. *J. Nutr.* **53**:43–51.

Griffin, A.C.; Clayton, C.C.; and Baumann, C.A. (1949). The effects of casein and methionine on the retention of hepatic riboflavin and on the development of liver tumors in rats fed certain azo doses. *Cancer Res.* **9**:82–87.

Griffith, W.H.; Paucek, P.L.; and Mulford, D.J. (1942). The relation of the sulphur amino acids to the toxicity of cobalt and nickel in the rat. *J. Nutr.* **23**:603–612.

Griffith, W.H. and Wade, N.J. (1940). Choline metabolism. II. The interrelationship of choline, cystine, and methionine in the occurrence and prevention of hemorrhage degeneration in young rats. *J. Biol. Chem.* **132**:627–637.

Gross, P.; Runne, E.; and Wilson, J.W. (1948). Studies on the effect of thallium poisoning of the rat. *J. Invest. Dermatol.* **10**:119–134.

Gunn, S.A.; Gould, T.C.; and Anderson, W.A.D. (1966). Protective effect of thiol compounds against cadmium-induced damage to testis. *Proc. Soc. Exp. Biol. Med.* **122**:1036.

Gunn, S.A.; Gould, T.C.; and Anderson, W.A.D. (1968). Specificity in protection against lethality and testicular toxicity from cadmium. *Proc. Soc. Exp. Biol. Med.* **128**:591–595.

Gunn, S.A.; Gould, T.C.; and Anderson, W.A.D. (1968a). Mechanisms of zinc, cysteine and selenium protection against cadmium-induced vascular injury to mouse testis. *J. Reprod. Fert.* **15**:65–70.

Gutenplan, J.B. (1977). Inhibition by L-ascorbate of bacterial mutagenesis induced by two N-nitroso compounds. *Nature* **268**:368–370.

Gyorgy, P.; Seifter, J.; Tomarelli, R.M.; and Goldblatt, H. (1946). Influence of dietary factors and sex on the toxicity of carbon tetrachloride in rats. *J. Exper. Med.* **83**:449–462.

Harper, A.E.; Benevenga, N.J.; and Wohlhueter, R.M. (1970). Effects of ingestion of disproportionate amounts of amino acids. *Physiol. Rev.* **50**(3):428–558.

Heppel, L.A.; Highman, B.; and Porterfield, V.T. (1946). Toxicology of 1,2-dichloropropane (propylene dichloride). II. Influence of dietary factors on the toxicity of dichloropropane. *J. Pharmacol. Exp. Therap.* **87**:11–17.

Heppel, L.A.; Neal, P.A.; Daft, F.S.; Endicott, K.M.; Orr, M.L.; and Porterfield, V.T. (1945). Toxicology of 1,2-dichloroethane (ethylene dichloride). II. Influence of dietary factors on the toxicity of dichloroethane. *J. Indust. Hyg. Toxicol.* **27**:15–21.

Heppel, L.A.; Neal, P.A.; Perrin, T.L.; Endicott, K.M.; and Porterfield, V.T. (1945a). The toxicology of 1,2-dichloroethane. III. Its acute toxicity and the effect of protective agents. *J. Pharm. Exp. Therap.* **84**:53–63.

Heppel, L.A.; Porterfield, V.T.; and Sharpless, N.F. (1947). Toxicology of 1,2-dichloroethane (ethylene dichloride). IV. Its detoxication by L-cysteine, DL-methionine and certain other sulfur containing compounds. *J. Pharmacol. Exp. Therap.* **91**:385–394.

Hueper, W.C. (1943). Experimental studies in cardiovascular pathology. VIII. Chronic nicotine poisoning in rats and in dogs. *Arch. Path.* **35**:846–856.

Jamall, I.S.; Mignano, J.E.; Lynch, V.D.; Bidanset, J.H.; Lau-Cam, C.; and Greening, M. (1979). Protective effects of zinc sulfate and L-lysine on acute ethanol toxicity in mice. *Environ. Res.* **19**:112–120.

Jensen, L.S. and Maurice, D.V. (1979). Influence of sulfur amino acids on copper toxicity in chicks. *J. Nutrit.* **109**:91–97.

Klatskin, G.; Krehl, W.A.; and Conn, H.O. (1954). The effect of alcohol on the choline requirement. I. Changes in the rats' liver following prolonged ingestion of alcohol. *J. Exp. Med.* **100**:605–614.

Lambert, L. (1937). De l'emploi d'une solution de glycocolle comme solvant des arseno benzenes dans le traitement de la syphilis chez les indigenes du Senegal. *Bull. Soc. Path. Exot.* **30**:131–134.

Launoy, L. (1934). Action de la cysteine sur la toxicite de l'antimoine. *Compt. Rend.* **199**:646.

Leklem, J.E.; Linkswiler, H.M.; Brown, R.R.; Rose, D.P.; and Anand, C.R. (1977). Metabolism of methionine in oral contraceptive users and control women receiving controlled intake of vitamin B_6. *Amer. J. Clin. Nutr.* **30**:1122–1128.

Leuchtenberger, C. and Leuchtenberger, R. (1976). Protection of hamster lung cultures by L-cysteine against carcinogenic effects of fresh smoke from tobacco or marihuana cigarettes. *J. Cell. Biol.* **70**:44a.

Leuchtenberger, C. and Leuchtenberger, R. (1977). Protection of hamster lung cultures by L-cysteine or vitamin C against carcinogenic effects of fresh smoke or marihuana cigarettes. *Brit. J. Exper. Pathol.* **58**(6):625–634.

Levander, O.A. and Morris, V.C. (1970). Interactions of methionine, vitamin E, antioxidants in selenium toxicity in the rat. *J. Nutr.* **100**:1111–1118.

Li, T.W. and Freeman, S. (1947). The effect of methionine on protein-deficient rats exposed to benzene. *Amer. J. Physiol.* **148**:358–364.

Lillie, R.D. (1932). Histopathologic changes produced in rats by the addition to the diet of various amino acids. *U.S. Pub. Health Repts.* **47**:83–93.

Magdalov, J.; Steimetz, D.; Batt, A.M.; Poullain, B.; Siest, G.; and Debry, G. (1979). The effect of dietary sulfur-containing amino acids on the activity of drug-metabolizing enzymes in rat-liver microsomes. *J. Nutr.* **109**:864–871.

Maisin, J.R. and Mattelin, G. (1967). Reduction in radiation lethality by mixtures of chemical protectors. *Nature* **214**:207–208.

Martin, G.J. and Thompson, M.R. (1943). Therapeutic and prophylactic detoxication. Chemotherapeutic metallic compounds. *Exp. Med. Surg.* **1**:38–50.

Mgbodile, M.V.K.; Holscher, M.; and Neal, R.A. (1975). A possible protective role for reduced glutathione in aflatoxin B_1 toxicity: effect of pretreatment of rats with phenobarbital and 3-methyl-cholanthrene on aflatoxin toxicity. *Toxicol. Appl. Pharmacol.* **34**:128–142.

Miller, E.C. and Miller, J.A. (1972). Approaches to the mechanism and control of chemical carcinogenesis. Bertner Foundation Award Lecture. In: *Environment and Cancer*, pp. 5–39. 24th Annual Symposium, M.D. Anderson Hospital, Baltimore. William & Wilkins.

Miller, E.C.; Miller, J.A.; Kline, B.E.; and Rusch, H.P. (1948). Correlation of the level of hepatic riboflavin with the appearance of liver tumors in rats fed aminoazo dyes. *J. Exp. Med.* **88**:89–98.

Miller, L.; Dow, M.J.; and Kokkeler, S.C. (1978). Methionine metabolism and vitamin B_6 status in women using oral contraceptives. *Am. J. Clin. Nutr.* **31**:619–625.

Miller, L.L.; Ross, J.F.; and Whipple, G.H. (1940). Methionine and cystine specific protein factors preventing chloroform liver injury in protein-depleted dogs. *Amer. J. Med. Sci.* **200**:739–756.

Miller, L.L. and Whipple, G.H. (1942). Liver injury, liver protection, and sulfur metabolism. Methionine protects against chloroform liver injury even when given after anesthesia. *J. Exp. Med.* **76**:421–435.

Miller, R.F. and Phillips, P.H. (1955). The enhancement of the toxicity of sodium fluoride in the rat by high dietary fat. *J. Nutr.* **56**:447–454.

Mizrahi, I.J. and Emmelot, P. (1962). The effect of cysteine on the metabolic changes produced by 2 carcinogenic N-nitroso-dialkylamines in the rat liver. *Cancer Res.* **22**:339–351.

Mizrahi, I.J. and Emmelot, P. (1963). Counteraction by sulphhydryl compounds of the enzymic conversion of and the metabolic lesions produced by two carcinogenic N-nitroso-dialkylamines in rat liver. *Biochem. Pharmacol.* **12**:55–63.

Newberne, P.M.; Rogers, A.E.; and Wogan, G.N. (1968). Hepatorenal lesions in rats fed a low lipotrope diet and exposed to aflatoxin. *J. Nutrition* **94**:331–336.

Peters, R.A.; Thompson, R.H.S.; King, A.J.; Williams, D.L.; and Nicol, C.S. (1944). Sulphur-containing amino acids and jaundice. *Nature* **153**:773.

Peters, R.A.; Thompson, R.H.S.; King, A.J.; Williams, D.L.; and Nicol, C.S. (1945). The treatment of postarsphenamine jaundice with sulphur-containing amino acids. *Quart. J. Med.* **14**:35–56.

Rogers, A.E. (1975). Variable effects of a lipotrope-deficient high-fat diet on chemical carcinogenesis in rats. *Cancer Res.* **35**:2469–2474.

Rogers, A.E. and Newberne, P.M. (1969). Aflatoxin B₁ carcinogenesis in lipotrope-deficient rats. *Cancer Res.* **29**:1965.

Rosin, M.P. and Stich, H.F. (1978). The inhibitory effect of cysteine on the mutagenic activities of several carcinogens. *Mutation Res.* **54**:73–81.

Schneider, H.A. (1936). Selenium in nutrition. *Science* **83**:22.

Shull, L.R. and Cheeke, P.R. (1973). Antiselenium activity of tri-o-cresyl phosphate in rats and Japanese quail. *J. Nutr.* **103**:560–568.

Smith, M.I.; Lillie, R.D.; and Stohlman, E.F. (1941). The influence of dietary protein on the toxicity of sulfanilamide. *U.S. Pub. Health Rept.* **56**:24.

Smith, M.I. and Stohlman, E.F. (1940). Further observations on the influence of dietary protein on the toxicity of selenium. *J. Pharmacol. Exp. Therap.* **70**:270–278.

Smith, M.I.; Westfall, B.B.; and Stohlman, E.F. (1943). Experimental trinitrotoluene poisoning with attempts at detoxification. *J. Ind. Hyg. Tox.* **25**(9):391.

Smith, W.W. (1946). The protective action of cystine and methionine in rats exposed to methyl chloride. *Fed. Proc.* **5**:97–98.

Sprince, H.; Parker, C.M.; Smith, G.G.; and Gonzales, L.J. (1975). Protective action of ascorbic acid and sulfur compounds against acetaldehyde toxicity: Implications in alcoholism and smoking. *Agents and Actions* **5**(2):164–173.

Stekol, J.A. (1937). Studies on the mercapturic acid synthesis in animals. I. The extent of the synthesis of p-bromophenyl mercapturic acid in dogs as affected by diets of varying sulfur contents. *J. Biol. Chem.* **117**:147–157.

Stillings, B.R.; Lagally, H.; Bauersfield, P.; and Soares, J. (1974). Effect of cystine, selenium, and fish protein on the toxicity and metabolism of methylmercury in rats. *Toxicol. Appl. Pharmacol.* **30**:243–254.

Straube, R.L.; Patt, H.M.; Smith, D.E.; and Tyree, E.B. (1950). Influence of cysteine on the radiosensitivity of Walker rat carcinomas. *Cancer Res.* **10**:243–244.

Tinsley, I.J. (1966). Nutritional interactions in dieldrin toxicity. *J. Agr. Food. Chem.* **14**:563–565.

Van Reen, R. and Williams, M.A. (1956). Studies on the influence of sulfur compounds on molybdenum toxicity in rats. *Arch. Biochem. Biophys.* **63**:1–8.

Versari, A. (1937). Ricerche sperimentali sulla azione svelenatrice della glicacolla per gli arsenobenzoli. *Riforma Med.* **53**:1443–1445.

Ward, C.O.; Lau-Cam, C.A.; Tang, A.S.M.; Bregalia, R.J.; and Jarowski, C.I. (1972). Effect of lysine on toxicity and depressant effects of ethanol in rats. *Toxicol. Appl. Pharmacol.* **22**:422.

Wasserman, R.H.; Comar, C.L.; and Nold, M.M. (1956). The influence of amino acid and other organic compounds on the gastrointestinal absorption of calcium[45] and strontium[89] in the rat. *J. Nutr.* **59**:371.

White, A. and Jackson, R.W. (1935). The effect of bromobenzene on the utilization of cystine and methionine by the growing rat. *J. Biol. Chem.* **11**:507–511.

White, A. and Lewis, H.B. (1932). The metabolism of sulfur. XIX. The distribution of urinary sulfur in the dog after the oral administration of monobromobenzene as influenced by the character of the dietary protein and by the feeding of l-cystine and dl-methionine. *J. Biol. Chem.* **98**:607–624.

Wilson, J. (1965). Leber's hereditary optic atrophy: A possible defect of cyanide metabolism. *Clin. Sci.* **29**:505–515.

Wood, J.L. and Cooley, S.L. (1956). Detoxication of cyanide by cystine. *J. Biol. Chem.* **218**:449–457.

Worthington, B.S.; Syrotuck, J.A.; and Ahmed, S.I. (1978). Effects of essential amino acid deficiencies on syngenic tumor immunity and carcinogenicity in mice. *J. Nutr.* **108**:1402–1411.

Yamamoto, Y.; Katayama, H.; and Muramatsu, K. (1976). Beneficial effect of methionine and theonine supplements on tyrosine toxicity in rats. *J. Nutr. Sci. Vitaminol.* **22**:467–475.

Fofats

A. INORGANIC SUBSTANCES

1. Fluoride

Many dietary factors have been found to influence the toxicity of fluoride. While considerable attention has been directed to the interactions of calcium and ascorbic acid with fluoride, more limited discussion has been directed toward elucidating the relationship of dietary fat ingestion to fluoride toxicity. However, evidence that elevated levels of dietary fat may enhance the toxicity and/or body burden of fluoride has been gradually emerging within recent years and will be critically assessed in the subsequent narrative.

The initial investigation concerning whether elevated levels of dietary fat could affect the toxicity of fluoride was published in 1935 by Phillips and Hart. They really were not concerned so much with elevated levels of dietary fat but with the combination of low-carbohydrate and high-fat diet. This was because fluoride was generally accepted as an inhibitor of carbohydrate metabolism (i.e., glycolysis). It was reasoned that the body could "out-maneuver" the fluoride if it (i.e., the body) was provided only a small amount of carbohydrate and a high-fat diet. In this case, the dietary energy source (i.e., fat) would not be wasted, as it would if the normal high-carbohydrate diet was provided. Subsequent experimentation with rats revealed that a high-fat, low-carbohydrate diet did not diminish the chronic toxic effects of fluoride. This hypothesis was not examined again for two decades.

From 1955 to 1976 there were a number of studies that attempted to further evaluate the role of dietary fat on fluoride toxicity. These studies were in fundamental agreement in that they revealed that a high-fat diet enhanced the toxicity (Miller and Phillips, 1955) and/or increased the body burden[1] of fluoride in a variety of tissues, including the carcass, femur, liver, kidney, and plasma of rats (Miller and Phillips, 1955; Buttner and Muhler, 1957, 1958; McGown and Suttie, 1974; McGown et al., 1976) and chicks (Bixler and Muhler, 1960). For instance, Miller and Phillips (1955) reported that increasing the dietary fat from 5 to 15% markedly increased the growth-retarding effects of fluoride at 0.1% in the diet during pair-feeding experiments.

The major question emerging from an experimental perspective was discovering how the high-fat diets were influencing an enhancement of fluoride toxicity as well as an increased body burden of fluoride. Sievert and Phillips (1959) had reported that the reduced growth of fluorotic rats given a high-fat diet may have resulted from an enhanced excretion of nitrogen, fat, and total dry matter in the feces, with the increased excretion of fecal fat being of greatest concern. Follow-up studies by Suttie and Phillips (1960) revealed that fluoride treatment caused a decreased lipase activity in the intestine of rats orally (but not intraperitoneally) administered fluoride, thereby partially explaining the elevated level of fecal lipid in fluorotic animals.

While the findings of Suttie and Phillips (1960) are of interest in trying to elucidate the nature of the fat-fluoride interaction, a major breakthrough occurred in 1974 by McGown and Suttie and was confirmed in 1976 by McGown et al. They revealed that the presence of elevated levels of fat and fluoride in the diet result in a delayed gastric emptying. This most likely provides the means by which more fluoride can be absorbed into the blood, thereby ultimately increasing the body burden of fluoride. McGown et al. (1976) concluded by stating that dietary fat does not increase the metabolic toxicity of fluoride, but merely increases the percentage absorbed from the gastrointestinal tract, and therefore increases the percentage of the fluoride to which the tissues are exposed.

[1]In contrast, Ericsson (1968) noted no differences in femur accumulation of ^{18}F 4 hours after administration of 4 ppm F with 28% olive oil (Tween emulsion), compared to controls that were given only ^{18}F and water.

While these recent findings by McGown and associates begin to delineate more clearly the influence of dietary fat on the body burden and potential toxicity of fluoride in an experimental setting, their relevance for the human condition is far from certain. The primary problem is that these investigations used fluoride levels of 400 ppm in the diet, a value greatly exceeding that occurring in the human experience. Thus, whether the combination of a high-fat diet and fluoride exposure at normally encountered levels would behave in a similar fashion remains to be determined. (See Table 1 for a listing of the studies evaluating a dietary fat-fluoride interaction.)

References

Bixler, D. and Muhler, J.C. (1960). Retention of fluoride in soft tissue of chickens receiving different fat diets. *J. Nutr.* **70**:26–30.

Buttner, W. and Muhler, J.C. (1957). The effect of fluoride administration on fluoride deposition in tissue and on serum cholesterol in the rat. *J. Nutr.* **63**:263.

Buttner, W. and Muhler, J.C. (1958). The retention of fluoride by the skeleton, liver, heart, and kidney as a function of dietary fat intake in the rat. *J. Nutr.* **65**:259–266.

Ericsson, Y. (1968). Influence of NaCl and other food components on fluoride absorption in the rat. *J. Nutr.* **96**:60–68.

Johnson, R.B. and Lardy, H.A. (1950). Orthophosphate uptake during the oxidation of fatty acids. *J. Biol. Chem.* **184**:235.

McGown, E.L.; Kolstad, D.C.; and Suttie, J.W. (1976). Effect of dietary fat on fluoride absorption and tissue fluoride retention in rats. *J. Nutr.* **106**:575–579.

McGown, E.L. and Suttie, J.W. (1974). Influence of fat and fluoride on gastric emptying of rats. *J. Nutr.* **104**:909–915.

Miller, R.F. and Phillips, P.H. (1955). The enhancement of the toxicity of sodium fluoride in the rat by high dietary fat. *J. Nutr.* **56**:447–454.

Phillips, P.H. and Hart, E.B. (1935). The effect of organic dietary constituents upon chronic fluorine toxicosis in the rat. *J. Biol. Chem.* **109**:657–663.

Sievert, A.H. and Phillips, P.H. (1959). Metabolic studies on the sodium fluoride fed rat. *J. Nutr.* **68**:109–120.

Suttie, J.W. and Phillips, P.H. (1960). Fat utilization in the fluoride fed rat. *J. Nutr.* **72**:429–434.

2. Lead

That dietary fat may affect the toxicity of lead has been a topic of interest for well over 100 years when Tanquerel des Planches (1848) recommended the use of foods high in fat to prevent lead intoxication. Despite this early interest in a fat-lead interaction, it was not until 1933 that further research interest was shown. In apparent contrast

Table 1. Listing of the Studies Evaluating a Dietary Fat-Fluoride Interaction

Authors	Animal Model	Comment
Phillips and Hart, 1935	Rats	A high-fat, low-carbohydrate diet did not lessen the chronic toxic effects of fluoride.
Miller and Phillips, 1955	Rats	(a) Increasing level of fat in diet from 5 to 15% augmented the growth-retarding effects of a diet with 0.1% sodium fluoride. (b) Different fats were equally effective in enhancing toxicity (i.e., butter fat and cottonseed oil).
Buttner and Muhler, 1957	Rats	Dietary fat seems to enhance the retention of fluoride in a variety of soft tissues.
Buttner and Muhler, 1958	Rats	Increasing the level of fat in the diet from 5 to 20% resulted in an increased fluoride body burden in the whole carcass, femur, and soft tissue (liver and kidney).
Bixler and Muhler, 1960	Chickens	Increased dietary fat enhances the retention of fluoride in a variety of soft tissues of chickens.
Suttie and Phillips, 1960	Rats	High level of fecal fat excreted by fluorotic animals; found to be related to a fluoride-induced inhibition of lipase activity in the intestine.
Ericsson, 1968	Rats	No differences were demonstrated in femur accumulation of ^{18}F 4 hours after the administration of 4 ppm F with 28% olive oil (Tween emulsion), compared to controls that were given only ^{18}F and water.

Table 1. (Continued)

Authors	Animal Model	Comment
McGown and Suttie, 1974	Rats	Fluoride found to cause a delayed emptying of stomach contents, thus allowing a greater chance for fluoride absorption.
McGown et al., 1976	Rats	High levels of dietary fat increase the body burden of fluoride in plasma, liver, and femur due to increased absorption. Supporting this interpretation were data indicating that the rats given the high-fat diets also exhibited increased urinary excretion of fluoride and decreased fecal excretion of fluoride.

to the earlier suggestion of Tanquerel des Planches concerning the prophylactic action of dietary fat with respect to lead toxicity, Weyrauch and Necke (1933) reported that high levels of fat (i.e., oil and margarine) in the diet actually enhanced the absorption of lead in rabbits by greater than a factor of 10. Stephens and Waldron (1975) were quite critical of this conclusion, since the authors did not indicate the level of dietary calcium. Recent studies by Barltrop and Khoo (1975) and Barltrop (1976) have also revealed that lead retention is greatly influenced by the quantity of fat in the diet. For instance, when the level of corn oil in the diet of male albino rats was increased from 5 to 40%, a marked increase in the lead retention of various tissues occurred. However, decreasing the level of dietary fat from 5 to 0% had no effect on lead absorption (Table 2). These findings are consistent with the recommendation of several researchers who have suggested the use of a low-fat diet for lead workers (Boyadzhiev, 1960; Buckup et al., 1956; Zielhuis, 1960; Sand, 1965). For example, Sand (1965) advocated the use of skimmed milk in place of whole milk for lead workers because fat was believed to solubilize ingested lead (see Weyrauch and Necke, 1933).

With respect to the quality of dietary fats, Barltrop (1976) reported that butterfat caused the largest increase in lead absorption, while fats high in polyunsaturated fatty acids (rapeseed and sunflower oils) demonstrated only a minor influence. In light of his findings, Barltrop (1976) concluded by stating that "although the enhanced absorption associated with butterfat would seem to be of particular relevance to the normal human diet, further studies are required for a more detailed evaluation of the effects of individual fatty acids."

In other research on the influence of the type (or quality) of dietary fat on lead absorption, Quarterman et al. (1977) (see Levander, 1979 for a review) demonstrated that lecithin, mixed bile salts, and choline enhanced the uptake of lead. They hypothesized that the enhancing effect of dietary fat on the uptake of lead was related to the presence of the phospholipids and to the occurrence of bile flow, which would provide phospholipids and bile salts to the lumen contents. Supporting this contention was the observation that rats with cannulated and exteriorized bile ducts did not absorb a significant quantity of an oral dose of labeled lead.

While the above studies supported the notion that both the quantity and quality of dietary fats affect the absorption and/or retention of lead, Tompsett (1939) reported that dietary fat (i.e., olive oil) did not seem to noticeably affect the absorption of lead from the gut in mice. Finally, Stephens and Waldron (1975) reported that Kello and Kostial (1973) "did not find a clear correlation between fat and gastrointestinal absorption," thereby not supporting the hypothesis that dietary fat affects the absorption and/or retention of lead. On closer inspection, however, Kello and Kostial (1973) reported that "the body retention of the orally applied lead-203 was much higher in animals on a milk diet than in controls." All the animal groups given milk con-

Table 2. Effects of Dietary Fat on Lead Absorption (ratio of mean retention experimental: control)

Diet (% fat)	Blood	Kidneys	Femur	Liver	Carcass
0	1	1	1	1	1
2.5	1	1	1	1	1
5 (control)	1	1	1	1	1
10	1.9	2	1.5	1.5	1.8
15	9.6	7.5	4.8	4.2	5.2
20	7.9	5.5	4.6	4.4	4.2
40	13.6	14.2	10.8	7.1	8.9

Source. Barltrop, D. and Khoo, H.E. (1975). The influence of nutritional factors on lead absorption. *Postgrad. Med. J.* **51**:795–800.

sumed considerably more fat than the nonmilk-fed controls. Those on the various milk diets consumed in a range of 1.7 to 3.0 grams of fat each day while the controls ingested only 0.6 gm/day. While there are numerous confounding variables with respect to differential consumption of other potentially influential nutrients (e.g., protein, carbohydrates, vitamin D, calcium, phosphorus, and iron) that make any definite conclusion on the relationship of dietary fat and lead impossible, it is accurate to say that those animals given the milk diets retained more lead than the controls. The major inconsistency is that a group consuming 2.4 g of fat/day retained more lead than a group consuming 3.0 gm of fat/day. However, both of these milk-fed groups retained more lead than the controls (as mentioned previously) as well as a milk-fed group given 1.7 g/day.

While considerable research remains to be conducted on the nature of the relationship between dietary fats and oral-lead exposure, the studies with animal models, primarily rodents, have revealed that diets high in fat, especially those with a high degree of saturation, markedly enhance the absorption and/or retention of orally administered lead. At this time, it would seem important to evaluate the mechanism by which the dietary fat affects lead retention; that is, could it be affecting both absorption and excretion. Epidemiological research should also be performed to evaluate whether the animal-model studies can be validated with human populations.

References

Barltrop, D. (1976). The influence of nutritional factors on the absorption of lead. Final Report to U.S. Dept. Health, Education, and Welfare, Center for Disease Control, Atlanta, GA.

Barltrop, D. and Khoo, H.E. (1975). The influence of nutritional factors on lead absorption. *Postgrad. Med. J.* **51**:795–800.

Boyadzhiev, V. (1960). Vlizanie na kraveto mlyako i maslo vuskhu vuznikraneto i proichaneto na slovonoto otravyane mezhdu akumulatomi rabotnitsi. *Nauchni trud. vissh. Med. Inst.* Vulko Chervenkov **39**:143.

Buckup, H.; Böhm, M.; Zimmermann, H.; Remy, R.; Portheine, F.U.; and Voss, C. (1956). Nahrungskomponenten und ihre Bedeutung fur die Prophylaxie beruflicher Bleivergiftung (Experimentelle Untersuchungen am Kaninchen). *Zentbl. ArbMed. ArbSchutz* **6**:29.

Kello, D. and Kostial, K.C. (1973). The effect of milk diet on lead metabolism in rats. *Environ. Res.* **6**:355–360.

Levander, O. (1979). Lead toxicity and nutritional deficiencies. *Environ. Health Perspect.* **29**:115.

Quarterman, J.; Morrison, J.N.; and Humphries, W.R. (1977). The role of phospholipids and bile in lead absorption. *Proc. Nutr. Soc.* **36**:104A.

Sand, T. (1965). Milchgabe an Bleiarbeiter. Eine Literatursichtung. *Zentbl. Arb. ArbSchutz* **15**:190.

Stephens, R. and Waldron, H.A. (1975). The influence of milk and related dietary constituents on lead metabolism. *Food Cosmet. Toxicol.* **13**:555–563.

Tanquerel des Planches, L. (1848). *Lead Diseases: A Treatise.* With notes and additions on the use of lead pipe and its substitutes. Translated by S.L. Dana, p. 333. Bixby & Co., Lowell, MA.

Tompsett, S.L. (1939). The influence of certain constituents of the diet upon the absorption of lead from the alimentary tract. *Biochem. J.* **33**:1237.

Weyrauch, F.U. and Necke, A. (1933). Zur Frage der MilchSchleimsuppenund Feltprophylaxe bei der Bleivergiftung. *Z. Hyg. Infekt.-Krankh.* **114**:629.

Zielhuis, R.L. (1960). De Betekenis van de voeding voor het onstaan en het verloop van de industriële lookintoxicatie. *Voeding* **21**:399.

B. ORGANIC SUBSTANCES

1. Aflatoxin

While a major public health concern is the reduction of aflatoxin B_1 exposure to humans to the greatest extent possible due to its hepatotoxic and carcinogenic activities, aflatoxicosis is of great concern to those who rear broilers as well. Aflatoxicosis in broilers may be frequently characterized by poor growth rates and inefficient feed utilization (Smith et al., 1971; Gardiner and Oldroyd, 1965; Carnaghan et al., 1966). In attempting to prevent the adverse effects of aflatoxicosis in chicks, one may attempt to decrease the level of aflatoxin exposure and/or increase the adaptive capacity of the chicken to ward off the adverse effects of this stressor agent. Since these two approaches are not mutually exclusive and because it is extremely difficult to avoid using feed with some level of contamination with preformed aflatoxin, Smith et al. (1971) decided to evaluate dietary factors that may enhance the resistance to aflatoxin.

In support of their proposed endeavor, Smith et al. (1971) cited the work of several groups of researchers who had previously demonstrated that dietary factors, including protein, various vitamins, and lipotropic compounds, could modify the expression of aflatoxin toxicity under defined experimental conditions (Newberne et al., 1968; Todd et al., 1968; Madhavan and Gopalan, 1965; Marcos and Lebshtein, 1963; McLean and McLean, 1967). For instance, Newberne et al. (1968) reported that a diet low in lipotropes enhanced the hepatotoxic effects of aflatoxin in rats, while Madhavan and Gopalan (1965) demonstrated that low levels of dietary protein (4% casein) resulted in rats being considerably more susceptible to aflatoxin-induced liver damage than controls reared on a 20%-casein diet.

In a well-designed study using isocaloric diets and a completely randomized selection of chicks, Smith et al. (1971) revealed that aflatoxicosis was markedly influenced by dietary factors. Increasing the protein level from 10% to 30% prevented, for the most part, the occurrence of reduced growth and hypoproteinemia caused by dietary aflatoxin (5 ppm) (see Brown and Abrams, 1965). (See protein section of this volume.) In addition, they reported that a high-lipid diet offered protection from the lethal effects of 10 ppm aflatoxin, presumably by reducing the amount of aflatoxin absorbed via the gastrointestinal tract. In addition, high levels of several lipids (i.e., safflower oil and olive oil) were also found to enhance growth, "but the growth increase with olive oil was not commensurate with the decrease in mortality if nonabsorption is the only answer." Thus, Smith et al. (1971) concluded that "increased dietary lipids apparently have two different effects on aflatoxicosis in broiler chickens. Lipids appear to have a mortality sparing effect which does not depend on the degree of unsaturation and which does not appear to be the result of decreased absorption of aflatoxin from the intestinal tract. The other effect is a promotion of growth rate which is correlated with the degree of unsaturation of the dietary lipid, since a high level of coconut oil or animal fat which is low in unsaturated fatty acids did not promote growth, while a high level olive oil or safflower oil which are high in unsaturates promoted growth." Further support for the hypothesis that increased levels of dietary fat offer protection to poultry from the adverse effects of afla-toxin exposure was offered by Hamilton et al. (1972), who reported that increasing the level of fat in the diet from 6 to 18% resulted in a marked decrease in mortality from 27.5 to 5%. However, the increase in fat content of the diet did not seem to offset the adverse effects of aflatoxin treatment (1 ppm) on growth rate.

While these research findings have direct implications for those in the poultry-rearing business, they may also be of relevance to the human condition. First, the response of chickens was similar to that of rats with respect to the influence of dietary protein in preventing the adverse effects of aflatoxin. Such comparability implies a greater generalizability of these data than just to poultry alone. Furthermore, that dietary lipids may prevent the absorption of aflatoxin is worthy of further investigation. Finally, Wilson (1978) has attempted to develop a risk assessment for aflatoxin-induced liver cancer in humans who consume peanut butter on a regular basis (according to levels of aflatoxin in U.S. peanut butter in 1973 and on a downward extrapolation of rat studies). However, since peanut butter has an appreciable amount of oil along with the aflatoxin contamination, it may be possible that the oil in the peanut butter may serve to reduce the amount of aflatoxin absorbed and thereby diminish the risk of developing a liver cancer. While all this is speculation, it does suggest that further research concerning the influence of dietary fats on aflatoxin absorption is an area in which important new contributions may be made.

References

Brown, J.M.M. and Abrams, L. (1965). Biochemical studies on aflatoxicosis. *Ondersteport. J. Vet. Res.* **32**:119–146.

Carnaghan, R.B.A.; Lewis, G.; Patterson, D.S.P.; and Allcroft, R. (1966). Biochemical and pathological aspects of ground nut poisoning in chickens. *Path. Vet.* 3:601–615.

Gardiner, M.R. and Oldroyd, B. (1965). Avian aflatoxicosis. *Australian Vet. J.* 41:272–276.

Hamilton, P.B.; Tung, H.T.; Harris, J.R.; Gainer, J.H.; and Donaldson, W.E. (1972). The effect of dietary fat on aflatoxicosis in turkeys. *Poult. Sci.* **51**:165–170.

Madhavan, T.V. and Gopalan, C. (1965). Effect of dietary protein on aflatoxin liver injury in weanling rats. *Arch. Path.* **80**:123–126.

Marcos, S.R. and Lebshtein, A.K. (1963). Proteins and toxicity: the effect of different dietary levels of protein on the changes produced by the "groundnut toxin" in chicks. *Arab. Vet. Med. Assoc. J.* **23**:375–380.

McLean, A.E.M. and McLean, E.K. (1967). Protein depletion and toxic liver injury due to carbon tetrachloride and aflatoxin. *Proc. Nutr. Soc.* **26**:13.

Newberne, P.M.; Rogers, A.E.; and Wogan, G.N. (1968). Hepatorenal lesions in rats fed a low lipotrope diet and exposed to aflatoxin. *J. Nutr.* **94**:331–343.

Smith, J.W.; Hill, C.H.; and Hamilton, P.B. (1971). The effect of dietary modifications on aflatoxicosis in the broiler chicken. *Poult. Sci.* **50**:768–774.

Todd, G.C.; Shalkop, W.T.; Dooley, K.L.; and Wiseman, H.G. (1968). Effects of ration modifications on aflatoxicosis in the rat. *Am. J. Vet. Res.* **29**:1855–1861.

Wilson, R. (1978). Risks caused by low levels of pollution. *Yale J. Biol. Med.* **51**:37–41.

2. Benzene

Very little research has evaluated the influence of dietary fat intake on the toxicity and carcinogenicity of benzene. However, from the research that has been published, evidence does exist that high levels of dietary fat may enhance the toxicity of benzene (Li and Freeman, 1945; Li et al., 1945). In their studies, Li and associates were concerned with evaluating how both dietary protein and fat may affect benzene toxicity (see protein chapter). While these researchers offered no specific rationale for why dietary fat may influence the expression and extent of benzene-induced adverse effects, there was a fairly sizable literature already available that implicated dietary factors as agents that could modify benzene toxicity (see Shils and Goldwater, 1949 for a review of the earlier literature).

In their experiments Li, Freeman, and their associates utilized both dogs and rats and exposed them to 600 ppm benzene for 42 hours each week for 12 weeks (in the case of rats), or until they died, or up to a year (in the case of dogs). As indicated previously, the influence of four different diets was assessed: (1) high protein (21%)-low fat (15%); (2) high protein (25%)-high fat (33%); (3) low protein (8.5%)-high fat (33%); and (4) low protein (10%)-high fat (33%). While varying the fat level of the dogs' diet did not result in any noticeable influence on benzene toxicity in general, the average survival time was least for the high-fat, low protein group. With respect to the rat model, the benzene treatment resulted in a greater incidence of leukopenia in those rats reared on the high-fat diets regardless of the level of protein in the diet.

The results with the rat model are particularly alarming in the light of present concern about benzene being a possible cause of leukemia. Unfortunately, these very interesting findings were not followed up. As a result of the continued widespread use of benzene, further study along this line is clearly warranted.

References

Li, T.W. and Freeman, S. (1945). The effect of protein and fat content of the diet upon the toxicity of benzene for rats. *Amer. J. Physiol.* **145**:158–165.

Li, T.W.; Freeman, S.; Hough, V.H.; and Gunn, F.D. (1945). The increased susceptibility of protein-deficient dogs to benzene poisoning. *Amer. J. Physiol.* **145**:166–176.

Shils, M.E. and Goldwater, L.J. (1949). Nutritional factors affecting the toxicity of some aromatic hydrocarbons with special reference to benzene and nitrobenzene compounds: a review. *J. Ind. Hyg. Tox.* **31**:175.

3. Diethylstilbestrol

Of great concern has been the recognition that exposure to diethylstilbestrol (DES) is a cause of cervical cancer in an apparently very small percentage ($\leq 0.4\%$) of female children born to women who had been treated with DES to prevent miscarriages (McLachlan and Dixon, 1976; Lanier et al., 1973). The magnitude of this problem is of considerable public concern, since between 500,000 to 2 million pregnant women were treated with DES in the United States from about 1950 to 1970 (Noller and Fish, 1974). The main question of concern with regard to this book is why some individuals developed a DES-induced cancer while most did not. It is certainly expected that differential exposure to DES may be an important factor affecting the occurrence of the cancer. However, there may be other factors, including nutritional status and developmental processes that influence susceptibility to DES-induced cancer.

While it is well established that age and sex are important factors affecting susceptibility to DES-induced carcinogenicity, limited research has also suggested that diet may be implicated as well. In carefully controlled studies, Dunning et al. (1949) compared the incidence of DES[2]-induced mammary cancer in paired rats (12 pairs in this experiment) given isocaloric high- and low-fat diets. From their study, which lasted nearly two years, it was shown that the rats given the high-fat diets developed considerably more tumors as identified at autopsy (i.e., 167 tumors vs. 78) and had a shorter latency period for those tumors that did develop than appropriate controls.

While the biomedical significance of this information is uncertain, it suggests that diet may influence the occurrence of DES-induced tumors; that is, some individuals may be at greater risk than others because of diet. It is unfortunate that this initial study of Dunning et al. (1949) was not followed up, especially in light of subsequent revelations concerning the established link between DES and vaginal cancer in humans. Of further interest and of great continuing concern is whether dietary factors such as high-fat diets can sufficiently enhance the susceptibility to DES-induced cancer so that trace levels that have been found in certain foods may be identified as a serious public health hazard.

References

Dunning, W.F.; Curtis, M.R.; and Maun, M.E. (1949). The effect of dietary fat and carbohydrate on diethylstilbestrol-induced mammary cancer in rats. *Cancer Res.* **9**:354–361.

Lanier, A.P.; Noller, K.L.; Decker, D.G.; Elveback, L.R.; and Kurland, L.T. (1973). Cancer and stilbestrol: a follow-up of 1,719 persons exposed to estrogens in utero and born 1943-1959. *Mayo Clinic Proc.* **48**:793–799.

McLachlan, J.A. and Dixon, R.L. (1976). Transplacental toxicity of diethylstilbestrol: a special problem in safety evaluation. In: *New Concepts in Safety Evaluation*, pp. 423–442. Edited by M.M. Mehlman, R.E. Shapiro and H. Blumenthal. Hemisphere Publishing Corp.

Noller, K.L. and Fish, C.R. (1974). Diethylstilbestrol usage: its interesting past, important presence, and questionable future. *Med. Clin. North Am.* **58**:793–810.

[2]Cholesterol pellets with 4 to 6 mg of DES were implanted SC into the scapular region.

4. DNT

Since numerous investigators had demonstrated that various dietary factors could markedly affect the toxicity and carcinogenicity of the azo dye dimethylaminoazobenzene (Nakahara et al., 1939; Kensler et al., 1941; Gyorgy et al., 1941; DuVigneaud et al., 1942; Antopolis and Unna, 1942; Smith et al., 1943; Miner et al., 1943; Miller et al., 1944), Clayton and Baumann (1944) suggested that other N-containing compounds such as dinitrotoluene (DNT) may also have their toxicity affected by dietary factors. These researchers chose DNT for evaluation because of its industrial importance and because after reduction of the NO_2 groups in the body (Lipschitz, 1920; Lipschitz and Osterroth, 1924; Perkin, 1919; Schwartz, 1939), it may yield compounds similar to the cleavage products of various carcinogenic azo dyes. In their study, mice were found to be more resistant to DNT fed in a diet with 30% fat (partially hydrogenated vegetable oil) as compared to a low-fat diet. The mice fed the high-fat diets grew considerably better than their counterparts on the low-fat diet and their survival was noticeably greater.

Despite the obvious protective effect of the high-fat diets with respect to DNT toxicity, it was not possible to separate the influence of the dietary fat on DNT toxicity from the protective influence of enhanced caloric intake in those rats on the high-fat diet. Thus it was not possible to make an unequivocal judgment on the influence of dietary fat on DNT toxicity. Consequently, Clayton and Baumann (1948) addressed this issue by determining the relative influence of fat and caloric intake on DNT toxicity. Their findings revealed that even when caloric intakes were equalized between experimental groups, the original findings (Clayton and Baumann, 1944) were supported; that is, the mice reared on the high-fat diet were protected from the adverse effects of DNT relative to those maintained on a low-fat diet. Of further interest is that a wide variety of fats were found to reduce the toxicity of DNT in mice. These included cottonseed oil, corn oil, peanut oil, partially hydrogenated cottonseed oil (Crisco), hydrogenated coconut oil, lard, and butterfat. In marked contrast, rancid hydrogenated cottonseed oil enhanced the toxic effects of the DNT.

Unfortunately, these interesting findings have not been followed up in terms of their applicability to the human situation. DNT is an agent commonly used in the production of certain dyes and explosives and has a TLV of 1.5 mg/m^3 (Tabershaw et al., 1977). Whether persons consuming low-fat diets would be at increased risk to experiencing some of the adverse health effects associated with prolonged exposure to DNT is unknown. There are certainly animal research studies as reviewed here that suggest that possibility. Yet unless more data are forthcoming, it is not possible to make policy initiatives with such a limited data base. Once again, it is necessary to suggest that epidemiologists make use of these highly suggestive animal studies to initiate prospective industrial studies that would help to provide the basis on which quantifiable risk assessment may ultimately be derived.

References

Antopolis, W. and Unna, K. (1942). The effect of riboflavin on the liver changes produced in rats by p-dimethylaminoazobenzene. *Cancer Res.* **2**:694–696.

Clayton, C.C. and Baumann, C.A. (1944). Some effects of diet on the resistance of mice toward 2,4-dinitrotoluene. *Arch. Biochem. Biophys.* **5**:115–120.

Clayton, C.C. and Baumann, C.A. (1948). Effect of fat and calories on the resistance of mice to 2,4-dinitrotoluene. *Arch. Biochem. Biophys.* **16**:415–422.

DuVigneaud, V.; Spangler, J.M.; Burk, D.; Kensler, C.J.; Sugiura, K.; and Rhoads, C.J. (1942). The procarcinogenic effect of biotin in butter yellow tumor formation. *Science* **95**:174–176.

Gyorgy, P.; Poling, E.C.; and Goldblatt, H. (1941). Necrosis, cirrhosis and cancer of liver in rats fed a diet containing dimethylaminoazobenzene. *Proc. Soc. Exp. Biol. Med.* **47**:41–44.

Kensler, C.J.; Sugiora, K.; Halter, N.F.; and Rhoads, C.P. (1941). Partial protection of rats by riboflavin with casein against liver cancer caused by dimethylaminoazobenzene. *Science* **93**:308–310.

Lipschitz, W. (1920). *Z. Physiol. Chem.* **109**:189. (Cited in Clayton and Baumann, 1944.)

Lipschitz, W. and Osterroth, J. (1924). *Arch. Ges. Physiol.* **205**:354. (Cited in Clayton and Baumann, 1944.)

Miller, J.A.; Kline, B.E.; Rusch, H.P.; and Baumann, C.A. (1944). The carcinogenicity of p-dimethylaminoazobenzene in diets containing hydrogenated coconut oil. *Cancer Res.* **4**:153–158.

Miner, D.L.; Miller, J.A.; Baumann, C.A.; and Rusch, H.P. (1943). The effect of pyridoxine and other B vitamins on the production of liver cancer with p-dimethylaminoazobenzene. *Cancer Res.* **3**:296–302.

Nakahara, W.; Mori, K.; and Fujiwara, T. (1939). Inhibition of experimental production of liver cancer by liver feeding; study in nutrition. *Gann.* **33**:406–427.

Perkin, R.G. (1919). *U.S. Pub. Health Repts.* **34**:2335. (Cited in Clayton and Baumann, 1944.)

Schwartz, L. (1939). *Pub. Health Bull.* 249. (Cited in Clayton and Baumann, 1944.)

Smith, M.I.; Lillie, R.D.; and Stohlman, E.F. (1943). The toxicity and histopathology of some azo compounds as influenced by dietary protein. *U.S. Pub. Health Repts.* **58**:304.

Tabershaw, I.R.; Utidjian, H.M.D.; and Kawahara, B.C. (1977). Chemical hazards. In: *Occupational Diseases: A Guide to Their Recognition.* Edited by M.M. Key et al. U.S. DHEW, PHS, CDC, NIOSH, Washington, D.C.

5. Pesticides

While there is a substantial literature concerning the interactions of dietary protein and pesticides, there is only a meager amount of research published concerning how dietary fat may affect the toxicity of pesticides. The only research found on this topic was published in the 1930s and 1940s and concerned the toxicity of the well-known insecticide rotenone. Rotenone is a plant extract with insecticidal activity. The OSHA standard for rotenone, which is 5 mg/m^3, is based on a very limited data base (ACGIH, 1976), although Tabershaw et al. (1977) are of the opinion that, as normally used, rotenone does not present any serious health concern to insecticide workers. That the toxicity of rotenone may be affected by dietary fat was first suggested by Lightbody and Mathews (1936), who reported that when rotenone is dissolved in olive oil and given gastrically to rats and guinea pigs, its toxicity is enhanced relative to when water is used as the carrier. Similar observations were made by Ambrose and Haag (1936) with respect to the insecticide derris in rats and rabbits.

In light of these data, Ambrose et al. (1943) advanced the hypothesis that individuals consuming a high-fat diet may have their susceptibility to such insecticides modified. In an effort to evaluate this hypothesis, these researchers exposed male albino rats to either derris or rotenone for 140 days, according to dietary schemes that offered variable amounts of fat as Crisco. Their findings, in marked contrast to the earlier studies reported above, revealed that a high-fat diet did not enhance the toxicity of either derris or rotenone. Of course, the previous study used olive oil as a "fat source" in contrast to Crisco, and they also were concerned with acute in contrast to chronic toxicity. In light of the limited scope of these investigations as well as a total lack of follow-up studies, it is not possible to draw definite conclusions with respect to fat-pesticide (e.g., rotenone) interactions.

References

ACGIH (1976). Documentation of TLVs. American Conference of Governmental Industrial Hygienists. Cincinnati, OH.

Ambrose, A.M.; DeEds, F.; and Cox, A.J., Jr. (1943). The effect of high fat diet on chronic toxicity of derris and rotenone. *J. Pharmacol. Exp. Therap.* **78**:90–92.

Ambrose, A.M.; DeEds, F.; and McNaught, J.B. (1942). *Ind. Eng. Chem.* **34**:684 (cited in Ambrose, A.M., et al. (1943). *J. Pharmacol. Exper. Therap.* **78**:90–92).

Ambrose, A.M.; and Haag, H.B. (1936). *Ind. Eng. Chem.* **28**:815 (cited in Ambrose, A.M., et al. (1943). *J. Pharmacol. Exper. Therap.* **78**:90–92).

Lightbody, H.D. and Mathews, J.A. (1936). *Ind. Eng. Chem.* **28**:809 (cited in Ambrose, A.M., et al. (1943). *J. Pharmacol. Exp. Therap.* **78**:90–92).

Tabershaw, I.R.; Utidjian, H.M.D.; and Kawahara, B. (1977). Chemical hazards. In: *Occupational Diseases: A Guide to Their Recognition.* Edited by M.M. Key et al. U.S. DHEW, PHS, CDC, NIOSH, Washington, D.C.

6. Polycyclic Aromatic Hydrocarbons (e.g., Dimethylbenzanthracene)

Introduction. That dietary fat may play an important role in the etiology of chemically induced cancer has been the subject of considerable research for the past 50 years. In 1930, Watson and Mellanby clearly demonstrated that dietary fat can affect the incidence of skin tumors induced in mice by repeated application of coal tar. These authors reported that the presence of 12.5 to 25% butter in a basal diet of bread and oats resulted in a considerable increase in the incidence of the coal tar-induced tumors. This section will trace the progress of subsequent research on the role of dietary fats on chemical carcinogenesis with respect to both animal model and human epidemiological investigations. Included within this assessment will be a consideration of not only the amount of fat in the diet but also the type or quality of fats. The latter point may be of considerable importance, since more recent investigations have suggested that the presence of unsaturated fats may enhance chemical carcinogenesis in animal models while saturated fats have been widely implicated in the genesis of cardiovascular disease.

Skin Cancer. The original striking findings of Watson and Mellanby (1930) that dietary fat enhanced the carcinogenicity of coal tars were confirmed and extended in a series of studies by Baumann and associates, which revealed that elevated levels of dietary fat not only enhanced the incidence of hydrocarbon-induced tumors but also those caused by ultraviolet light (Baumann and Rusch, 1939; Baumann et al., 1939; Jacobi and Baumann, 1940; Lavik and Baumann, 1941). Other research published several years later also suggested a promotional role for dietary fat in chemical carcinogenesis. Carroll and Khor (1975) have provided a summary of these early investigations (Table 3). These initial reports clearly indicated that a variety of fats including coconut oil, wheat-germ oil, Crisco, butter, and lard promoted the occurrence of chemically (3,4-benzpyrene, methylcholanthrene, and 1,2,5,6-dibenzanthracene) induced cancer as determined by the time needed for 50% of the mice to develop tumors after treatment.

From these consistent research findings, several questions emerged.

Table 3. Effects of Dietary Fat on Incidence of Skin Tumors in Mice

Strain[a] and Sex	Carcinogenic Agent	Frequency of Treatment	Type of Fat	Level in Diet (%)	Length of Experiment	Tumor Incidence[b] (%)		References[g]
						Low Fat[c]	High Fat	
	coal-tar	twice weekly for 120 days for 90 days	butter	12.5–25 19–25	330 days 240 days	(34)[d] (59)[d]	(57)[d] (82)[d]	Watson and Mellanby [125]
A♂	UV light	1 h daily	Primex[f]	30	7.5 months	(55)[e]	(75)[e]	Baumann and Rusch [6]
C	UV light benzpyrene (0.3–0.5% sol. in benzene)	1 h daily twice weekly	Crisco[f] Crisco	25 25	4.5 months 5.5 months	5/16 (33) 12/18 (67)	12/14 (87) 15/16 (94)	Baumann et al. [5]
	methylchol-anthrene (0.2–0.3% sol. in dioxane)	twice weekly for 2 months	coconut oil Primex	15 15	4 months 6 months	1/15 (6) 3/17 (17)	10/12 (83) 18/21 (86)	Lavik and Baumann [77]
Jax Swiss♀	benzpyrene (0.3% sol. in benzene)	32 application over 20 weeks	Kremit[f]	28	42 weeks	22/43 (51)	28/42 (67)	Tannenbaum [114]
C57BL♂		twice weekly for 13 weeks	Kremit	31	49 weeks	13/49 (27)	17/50 (35)	
DBA♂		twice weekly for 10 weeks	Kremit	31	56 weeks	34/50 (68)	39/50 (78)	

[a]Strain and sex were not specified in some cases.

[b]Tumor incidence is expressed in most cases as the percentage of animals with tumors out of the total number alive when the first tumor appeared. The original papers frequently give tumor incidence at various times after the start of treatment with carcinogenic agent.

[c]Various natural diets containing not more than 2–3% fat were used. Cod-liver oil was given in some cases.

[d]Percentage of surviving mice with tumors estimated from charts. 70 mice per group used in the first experiment and 90 per group in the second experiment.

[e]From 28 to 37 out of 50 mice were alive at the end of these experiments.

[f]Partially hydrogenated cottonseed oil.

[g]Numbers refer to the references in the source of the table.

Source. Carroll, K.K. and Khor, H.T. (1975). Dietary fat in relation to tumorigenesis. *Progr. Biochem. Pharmacol.* **10**:311.

What other chemically induced tumorous growths, in addition to skin cancer, can be enhanced by dietary fats? Are there any quantifiable differences in the capacity to promote chemical carcinogenesis by moderate vs. high levels of fat in the diet (i.e., the development of a dose-response relationship)? What components within the fat itself may be responsible for this promotional activity? If the fat is actually serving as a promoter in the classical sense, then shouldn't fat be most effective if given after carcinogen treatment and, if so, how long after treatment?

Cancer at Other Sites. Considerable research has also revealed that the incidence of chemically induced mammary tumors and hepatomas in mice and rats are enhanced by high levels of dietary fat (Carroll and Khor, 1975), while limited evidence also exists that dietary fat may affect tumorigenesis of the eye (Engel and Copeland, 1951; Copeland and Engel, 1950; Engel, 1950), and hypophyseal tissue (Silberberg and Silberberg, 1953). In contrast, hydrocarbon-induced sarcomas have not been found to be affected by dietary fat in mice and rats (Tannenbaum, 1942; Lavik and Baumann, 1943; Baumann et al., 1939). In addition, chemically induced cancer of the lung (benzo[a]pyrene) (Tannenbaum, 1942), ear duct (2-acetylamino fluorene) (Engel and Copeland, 1951), submaxillary gland (methylcholanthrene) (Lavik and Baumann, 1943), and leukemia (methylcholanthrene) (Lawrason and Kirschbaum, 1944) were not found to be enhanced by dietary fat.

Quantity of Fat—Role in Carcinogenesis—Dose-Promoting Response. With regard to evaluation of the dose-promotion response of fat in chemical carcinogenesis, Silverstone and Tannenbaum (1950) reported that the tumor incidence increased as the levels of fat in the diet increased, but that any quantitative relationships are far from clear. For example, there was a proportionate increase in tumor incidence as the level of dietary fat increased from 2 to 6–8%. However, the rate of tumor increase as the level of dietary fat increased from 6–8% to 24–26% was not as dramatic as the rate when the level of fat increased from 2 to 6–8%. Carroll and Khor (1975) cautioned against trying to establish a clearly defined, direct linear relationship according to intermediate levels of dietary fat. Yet comparisons between the low- and high-fat groups do yield the expected differential tumor incidence.

Quality of Fat—Role in Carcinogenesis. While a number of studies have supported the conclusion that the increase in tumorigenicity is more a function of the amount than the type of fat in the diet (Haven and Bloor, 1956; Jacobi and Baumann, 1940), there is evidence to suggest that the quality of diet may be a contributing factor as well (Gammal et al., 1967, 1968; Carroll and Khor, 1970, 1971, 1975; King et al., 1979).

As was the case in the genesis of skin cancer, a number of different fats (i.e., partially hydrogenated cottonseed oil, egg lipids, lard, olive oil, corn oil) were found to enhance the incidence of mammary tumors from a variety of chemical agents including stilbestrol (Dunning et al., 1949), 2-AAF (Engel and Copeland, 1951), as well as DMBA (Carroll and Khor, 1970, 1971; Farber, 1972) (Table 4). Other studies by Gammal et al. (1967) revealed that corn oil was considerably more effective than coconut oil in enhancing the occurrence of DMBA-induced mammary cancer in rats with respect to the tumor incidence, number of tumors per animal, and reducing the latent period. More systematic experimentation on an expanded number of edible fats and oils revealed that with the sole exception of rapeseed oil, rats reared on diets with unsaturated fats developed more adenocarcinomas following DMBA exposure than similarly exposed rats reared on diets with saturated fats. More specifically, the differential tumor incidence was primarily due to differences in the number of tumors per rat and in the percentage of animals developing tumors (Figure 9-1).

In attempting to extrapolate their animal studies to the human conditions, Carroll and Khor (1971) noted that "the high fat diets used in [their] studies contain about the same level of fat (20% by weight=approximately 40% of total calories) as typical American diets, whereas a low-fat diet [control groups] which was effective in decreasing the incidence of mammary tumors in rats is comparable in fat content (5% by weight=approximately 10% by calories) to diets in countries such as Japan where the death rate from breast cancer is much lower than in America. The fact that unsaturated fats appeared to enhance the yield of mammary tumors to a greater extent than saturated fats in experiments with rats also suggests that caution should be exercised in recommending a large-scale shift to more highly unsaturated fats in human diets. [See King et al. (1979) for more recent support for this position.]

Liver Cancer. As indicated earlier, dietary fat may affect the occurrence of azo dye-induced cancers (Opie, 1944; Miller et al., 1944, 1944a; Miller and Miller, 1953). In studies by Miller et al. (1944, 1944a), it was shown that rats reared on a diet with 0.06% DAB developed a high incidence of hepatomas (53 to 73%) when the diet con-

Table 4. Effects of Dietary Fat on Incidence of Mammary Tumors in Female Mice and Rats

Species and Strain	Carcinogenic Agent	Type of Fat	Level in diet (%)	Length of Experiment	Tumor Incidence[a] (%)		References[f]
					Low Fat[b]	High Fat	
Mouse DBA	none	Kremit[c]	12	38 weeks to death	14/44 (32)	24/44 (55)	Tannenbaum [114]
			12	24 weeks to 2 years	16/50 (32)	32/50 (64)	
Rat	none	Primex[c]	30	30 months	3/33 (9)	2/32 (6)	Lavik and Baumann [78]
Rat A × C line 9935	Stilbestrol (4–6 mg implanted s.c. in cholesterol pellets)	Crisco[c]	46	av. survival 383–392 days	9/12 (75)	12/12 (100)[d] 11/12 (92)	Dunning et al. [33]
Rat AES strain	2-acetylamino-fluorene (0.03% in diet)	lard	15	av. survival 28–29 weeks	0/8 (0)	46/62 (74)	Engel and Copeland [38]
			26	31 weeks	1/6 (17)	6/6 (100)	
Rat Sprague-Dawley	none	olive oil	20	10 months	3/25 (12)[c]	5/13 (39)[e]	Benson et al. [7]
Rat Sprague-Dawley	7,12-dimethyl-benz(α)anthra-cene (DMBA) (10mg orally)	corn oil	20	4 months	15/21 (71)	21/22 (96)	Gammal et al. [46]
		coconut oil	20			16/21 (76)	

[a] Results expressed as in table 3.

[b] Various neutral and purified diets were used. The level of fat in the basal diet varied from 0.5 to 3%, except for the experiments of Dunning et al. where the level was 6.5%.

[c] Partially hydrogenated cottonseed oil.

[d] The first group was pair-fed with the low-fat controls and the second group was fed ad libitum.

[e] Only animals over 18 months of age were included in the evaluation because no tumors developed in younger animals.

[f] Numbers refer to references in the source of the table.

Source. Carroll, K.K. and Khor, H.T. (1975). Dietary fat in relation to tumorigenesis. *Progr. Biochem. Pharmacol.* **10:**315.

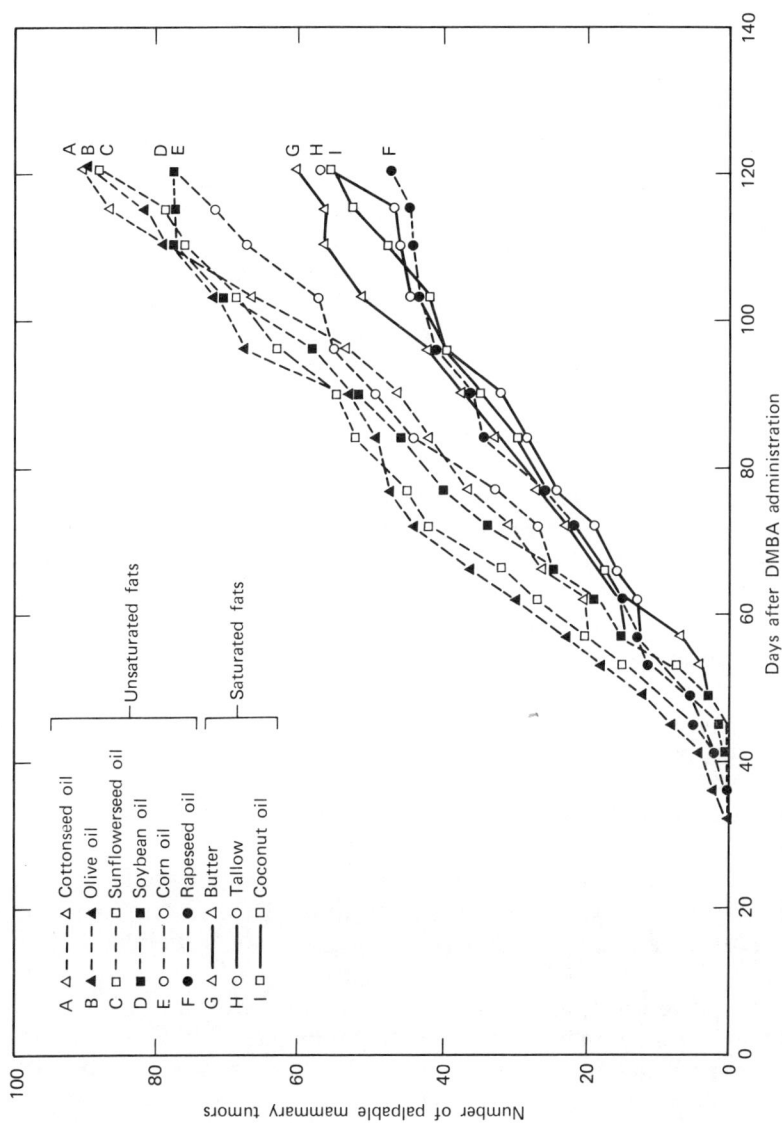

Figure 9-1. Effect of different dietary fats and oils fed as 20% by weight of the diet on cumulative number of palpable mammary tumors in female Sprague-Dawley rats given a single oral dose of 5 mg of DMBA at 50 days of age. 30 rats per group. [*Source.* Carroll, K.K. and Khor, H.T. (1975). Dietary fat in relation to tumorigenesis. *Progr. Biochem. Pharmacol.* **10**:316.]

tained 5% corn oil, while in controls given similar diets but with 5% hydrogenated coconut oil instead of corn oil, the tumor incidence was only between 0 to 8%, depending on the study.

Mechanism of Action. Perhaps the most likely hypothesis to explain the role of dietary fats in chemical carcinogenesis is that of its action as a cocarcinogen, or promoter. The most striking evidence to support this role for dietary fats is seen in rat studies when a high-fat diet caused an enhancement of chemically induced cancer only when the fat is given after exposure to the carcinogenic agent; that is, after initiation (Lavik and Baumann, 1941). However, precisely how fat may promote carcinogenesis is not especially well defined.

Early investigators suggested that dietary fat may promote carcinogenesis by enhancing the absorption of the carcinogenic agent (Watson and Mellanby, 1930). However, subsequent studies by Lavik and Baumann (1943) suggested that this could not entirely explain the influence of dietary fat on chemically induced skin cancer. Others have hypothesized that dietary fat may influence the occurrence of DMBA-induced mammary cancer by causing a change in the distribution of the carcinogenic agent (Gammal et al., 1967). However, subsequent studies by these investigators could not support their original contention (Gammal et al., 1968; Carroll and Khor, 1975). In their review, Hopkins and West (1976) speculated that dietary fats may enhance carcinogenesis by facilitating alterations in a number of biological systems including (1) enzymatic detoxification-intoxication processes, (2) the structure and function of membranes, (3) immunocompetence, (4) DNA repair potential, and (5) endocrine function.

Recent Animal Studies—Colon Cancer. While the earlier discussed studies have focused primarily on skin, mammary, and liver cancer, more recent investigations stimulated by epidemiological research (Wynder et al., 1969; Stemmermann, 1970; Armstrong and Doll, 1975) have considered the role of high levels of dietary protein and fat on colon cancer (Gross and Newberne, 1976). From a conceptual perspective, the working hypothesis is that "bile acids and cholesterol metabolites of the lumen of the large bowel help to modify large bowel carcinogenesis and that these compounds, whether directly or indirectly, are derived from dietary factors and subsequently are modified by the gut bacteria" (Reddy et al., 1976).

Using this concept as their framework, Reddy et al. (1976) conducted experiments with a known colon carcinogen (dimethylhydrazine [DMH]) with rats reared on diets with different levels of protein and fats (Reddy et al., 1976, 1976a). Their studies revealed that diets with high levels of fat (i.e., 20% corn oil or 20% lard) and/or diets high in both fat (i.e., 20% corn oil) and protein (i.e., 22% casein) exhibited a significantly greater incidence of colon tumors than rats reared on low-fat diets (5% corn oil or lard).

While the precise explanation of how fat enhances DMH-induced colon cancer remains to be determined, Reddy et al. (1974) speculated the fat may enhance the conversion of the DMH to its ultimate carcinogenic form by facilitating its enzymatic conversion and/or by altering of intestinal microflora which, in turn, may affect the required transformation. While exposure to DMH does not tend to occur among the general public, the findings of Reddy et al. (1974, 1976, 1976a) are of potential significance with respect to their speculation that fats may alter the biochemical transformation of precarcinogens to their ultimate carcinogenic state.

Epidemiological Studies. There have been extensive epidemiologic investigations concerning the association of dietary fat consumption and the incidence of death by different types of cancer among various countries. Highly positive correlations between per capita consumption of dietary fats for many countries and age-adjusted mortality from cancers of various sites including the female breast (+ 0.935 correlation coefficient), male (+ 0.928) and female (+ 0.911) intestine, prostate (+ 0.892), male (+ 0.857) and female (+ 0.838) leukemia and aleukemia, male (+ 0.834) and female (+ 0.786) rectum, ovary, fallopian tube and broad ligament (+ 0.726), male lung, bronchus and trachea (+ 0.710), male pancreas (+ 0.666), male (+ 0.634) and female (+ 0.550) skin, and others (Carroll and Khor, 1975).

While these statistical associations strongly support a role for dietary fat in a variety of human cancers, high levels of fat consumption are also highly associated with other factors (i.e., calorie and protein intake) that may also affect carcinogenesis. Thus the highly positive association of dietary fat consumption and cancer incidence must be cautiously evaluated when discussing its role as a potential causative agent.

The animal studies reviewed here clearly illustrate that elevated levels of dietary fat consumption enhance the carcinogenicity of a variety of substances. The epidemiologic studies to date have focused on associations of fat consumption and cancer mortality. What is missing is information on whether dietary fat consumption in humans may enhance the carcinogenicity of environmental agents. For instance, while the occurrence of skin cancer mortality is moderately correlated with fat consumption, does this imply that high levels of dietary fat consumption enhance the carcinogenicity of UV-induced skin cancer? This is certainly a hypothesis worth investigating, since animal model studies have previously demonstrated such an occurrence (Baumann and Rusch, 1939). However, the complexity of the relationships involved in trying to understand nutrient-cancer interactions must be recognized so that the limitations and strengths of the epidemiological perspective may be appreciated. For example, in order to evaluate the potential role of dietary fat on the incidence of skin cancer, it is necessary to take into account exposure to sunlight and coal tar products, as well as the latitude of the countries or areas where the subjects live, and the natural pigmentation of the inhabitants. To the extent that these confounding variables are not accounted for, the strength of any conclusions will be diminished. In addition, since latency periods within humans tend often to be greater than 15 years, it is necessary to try to consider the dietary consumption and exposure levels at a much earlier time. This is clearly a factor that has discouraged epidemiological research in this area.

One of the most interesting hypotheses developed from the animal model studies has been that consumption of diets high in unsaturated fats may enhance the carcinogenicity of certain hydrocarbons such as DMBA. In this regard, Pearce and Dayton (1971) evaluated the incidence of cancers between groups of individuals participating in a dietary trial that was originally set up to test the ability of polyunsaturated fats to reduce coronary heart disease. In this 8-year controlled clinical trial, these researchers reported more deaths due to cancer in the polyunsaturated-diet group than those on a normal diet. Other studies with long-term dietary trials have not supported this hypothesis (West and Redgrave, 1974; Ederer et al., 1971). However, Hopkins and West (1976) have pointed out that these trials were not designed to test the hypothesis that dietary fat may enhance the incidence of death from causes other than coronary heart disease such as cancer. These authors further state that "it would be difficult to carry out a worthwhile trial to examine the role of dietary fats in carcinogenesis especially [since] fat almost certainly does not act as a carcinogen but as a co-carcinogenic agent."

Conclusions.   Research over the past 50 years with animal models has clearly established that diets with elevated levels of fats markedly predispose the animals to experience chemically induced cancer. Skin, mammary glands, and the liver are sites that are particularly sensitive to the promoting activity of dietary fats, while other sites such as muscle are not. From the initial study in 1930 that indicated that dietary fats enhance the carcinogenicity of coal-tars, subsequent research has considerably expanded the number of agents to include, among others, BAP, DMBA, methylcholanthrene, DMH, stilbestrol, and ultraviolet radiation. Studies from a variety of investigators indicate that the promotional activity of fats is directly related to its level in the diet. While the amount of fat in the diet, therefore, is of critical importance with respect to susceptibility to chemical carcinogenesis, so too is the quality of fat. Of interest in this regard is the hypothesis that diets high in unsaturated fats may enhance carcinogenesis of chemical agents. Since diets high in unsaturated fats may be consumed by persons trying to reduce their risk to coronary heart disease, this hypothesis should be given more than casual reflection.

In light of the knowledge that dietary fats enhance the occurrence of tumors in a number of tissues by a variety of agents, considerable efforts should be made to initiate research on occupationally exposed workers who may be at enhanced risk to develop a job-related cancer. For if it is true that workers who consume diets high in fats have their risk to a job-related cancer enhanced, then educational programs can be instituted to encourage workers to adopt and maintain appropriate life-styles.

References

Anonymous (1944). Dietary factors that influence carcinogenesis. *Nutr. Rev.* November, pp. 338–339.

Armstrong, B. and Doll, R. (1975). Environmental factors and the incidence and mortality from cancer in different countries with special reference to dietary practices. *Int. J. Cancer* 15:617–631.

Baumann, C.A. (1948). Diet and tumor development. *J. Amer. Dietet. Assoc.* 24:573–581.

Baumann, C.A.; Jacobi, H.P.; and Rusch, H.P. (1939). The effect of diet on experimental tumor production. *Amer. J. Hyg.* Sect. A. 30:1–6.

Baumann, C.A. and Rusch, H.P. (1939). Effect of diet on tumors induced by ultraviolet light. *Amer. J. Cancer* 35:213–221.

Carroll, K.K. and Khor, H.T. (1970). Effects of dietary fat and dose level of 7,12-dimethylbenz[a]anthracene on mammary tumor incidence in rats. *Cancer Res.* 30:2260–2264.

Carroll, K.K. and Khor, H.T. (1971). Effects of level and type of dietary fat on incidence of mammary tumors induced in female Sprague-Dawley rats by 7,12-dimethylbenz(α)anthracene. *Lipids* 6(6):415–420.

Carroll, K.K. and Khor, H.T. (1975). Dietary fat in relation to tumorigenesis. *Progr. Biochem. Pharmacol.* 10:308–353.

Caster, W.O.; Wade, A.E.; Greene, F.E.; and Meadows, J.S. (1970). Effect of different levels of corn oil in the diet upon the rate of hexobarbital, heptachlor and aniline metabolism in the liver of the male white rat. *Life Sci.* **9**:181–190.

Chan, P. and Cohen, L.A. (1974). Effect of dietary fat, anti-estrogen, and antiprolactin on the development of mammary tumors in rats. *J. Natl. Cancer Instit.* **52**:25–30.

Copeland, D.H. and Engel, R.W. (1950). Eye tumors in female rats produced by feeding 2-acetylaminofluorene. *Cancer Res.* **10**:211–215.

Doll, R. (1969). The geographic distribution of cancer. *Brit. J. Cancer* **23**:1–8.

Dunning, W.F.; Curtis, M.R.; and Maun, M.E. (1949). The effect of dietary fat and carbohydrate on diethylstilbestrol-induced mammary cancer in rats. *Cancer Res.* **9**:354–361.

Ederer, F.; Leven, P.; Turpeinen, O.; and Frantz, I.D., Jr. (1971). Cancer among men on cholesterol-lowering diets. Experience from five clinical trials. *Lancet* **ii**:203–206.

Engel, R.W. (1950). Dietary factors in influencing the carcinogenicity of 2-acetyl-aminofluorene. *Cancer Res.* **10**:215.

Engel, R.W. and Copeland, D.H. (1951). Influence of diet on the relative incidence of eye, mammary, ear-duct and liver tumors in rats fed 2-acetylaminofluorene. *Cancer Res.* **11**:180–183.

Enig, M.G.; Munn, R.J.; and Koeney, M. (1978). Dietary fat and cancer trends—a critique. *Fed. Proc.* **37**:2215–2220.

Farber, E.C. (1972). Chemical carcinogenesis. In: Anfinsen, Polter and Schechter, *Current Research in Oncology*, pp. 95–123. Academic Press, N.Y.

Gammal, E.B.; Carroll, K.K.; and Plunkett, E.R. (1967). Effects of dietary fat on mammary carcinogenesis by 7,12-dimethylbenz(a)anthracene in rats. *Cancer Res.* **27**:1737–1742.

Gammal, E.B.; Carroll, K.K.; and Plunkett, E.R. (1968). Effects of dietary fat on the uptake and clearance of 7,12-dimethylbenz(a)anthracene by rat mammary tissue. *Cancer Res.* **28**:384–385.

Giese, J.E.; Clayton, C.C.; Miller, E.C.; and Baumann, C.A. (1946). The effect of certain diets on hepatic tumor formation due to m-methyl-p-dimethylaminoazobenzene and O'-methyl-p-dimethylaminoazobenzene. *Cancer Res.* **6**:679–684.

Gross, R.L. and Newberne, P.M. (1976). Nutrients modifying chemical carcinogenesis. In: *Advances in Exp. Med. and Biol.* **73**, pt A:434–440.

Gyorgy, P.; Tomarelli, R.; Ostergard, R.P.; and Brown, J.B. (1942). Unsaturated fatty acids in the dietary destruction of N,N-dimethylaminoazobenzene (butter yellow) and in the production of anemia in rats. *J. Exp. Med.* **76**:413–420.

Haven, F.L. and Bloor, W.R. (1956). Lipids in cancer. *Adv. Cancer Res.* **4**:237–314.

Hopkins, G.J. and West, C.E. (1976). Possible roles of dietary fats in carcinogenesis. *Life Sci.* **19**:1103–1116.

Jacobi, H.P. and Baumann, C.A. (1940). The effect of fat on tumor formation. *Amer. J. Cancer* **39**:338–342.

Kensler, C.J.; Sugiura, K.; Young, N.F.; Halter, C.R.; and Rhoads, C.P. (1941). Partial protection of rats by riboflavin with casein against liver cancer caused by dimethylaminoazobenzene. *Science* **93**:308–310.

King, M.M.; Balley, D.M.; Gibson, D.D.; Pitna, J.V.; and McCoy, P.B. (1979). Incidence and growth of mammary tumors induced by 7,12-dimethylbenz[a]anthracene as related to the dietary content of fat and antioxidant. *J. Natl. Cancer Inst.* **63**(3):657–663.

Lavik, P.S. and Baumann, C.A. (1941). Dietary fat and tumor formation. *Cancer Res.* **1**:181–187.

Lavik, P.S. and Baumann, C.A. (1943). Further studies on the tumor promoting action of fat. *Cancer Res.* **3**:749–756.

Lawrason, F.D. and Kirschbaum, A. (1944). Dietary fat with reference to the spontaneous appearance and induction of leukemia in mice. *Proc. Soc. Exp. Biol. Med.* **56**:6–7.

Lu, A.Y.H. (1976). Liver microsomal drug-metabolizing enzyme system fractional components and their properties. *Fed. Proc.* **35**:2460–2463.

Marshall, W.J. and McLean, A.E.M. (1971). A requirement of dietary lipids for induction of cytochrome P-450 by phenobarbitone in rat liver microsomal fraction. *Biochem. J.* **122**:569–573.

Miller, J.A. (1947). Studies on the mechanism of the effects of fats and other dietary factors on carcinogenesis by the azo dyes. *Ann. N.Y. Acad. Sci.* **49**:19–28.

Miller, J.A.; Kline, B.E.; Rusch, H.P.; and Baumann, C.A. (1944). The carcinogenicity of p-dimethylaminoazobenzene in diets containing hydrogenated oil. *Cancer Res.* **4**:153–158.

Miller, J.A.; Kline, B.E.; Rusch, H.P.; and Baumann, C.A. (1944a). The effect of certain lipids on the carcinogenicity of p-dimethylaminoazobenzene. *Cancer Res.* **4**:756–761.

Miller, J.A. and Miller, E.C. (1953). The carcinogenic amino azo dyes. *Adv. Cancer Res.* **1**:339–396.

Miller, J.A.; Miner, D.L.; Rusch, H.P.; and Baumann, C.A. (1941). Diet and hepatic tumor formation. *Cancer Res.* **1**:699–708.

Narisawa, T.; Magadia, N.; Weisburger, J.H.; and Wynder, E.L. (1974). Promoting effect of bile acids on colon carcinogenesis after intrarectal instillation of N-methyl-N'-nitro-N-nitrosoguanidine in rats. *J. Natl. Cancer Instit.* **53**:1093–1097.

Narkahara, W.; Mori, K.; and Fujiwara, T. (1939). Inhibition of experimental production of liver cancer by liver feeding. A study in nutrition. *Gann.* **33**:406–428.

Norred, W.P. and Wade, A.E. (1972). Dietary fatty acid-induced alterations of hepatic microsomal drug metabolism. *Biochem. Pharmacol.* **21**:2887–2897.

Opie, E.L. (1944). The influence of diet on the production of tumors of the liver by butter yellow. *J. Exp. Med.* **80**:219–236.

Pearce, M.L. and Dayton, S. (1971). Incidence of cancer in men on a diet high in polyunsaturated fat. *Lancet* **1**:464–467.

Ray, S.C. and Morin, R.J. (1965). Interaction of 4-dimethylaminoazobenzene and dietary fat in the regulation of hepatic microsomal ascorbic acid synthesis. *Nature* **207**:1294–1295.

Reddy, B.S.; Narisawa, T.; Vukusich, D.; Weisburger, J.H.; and Wynder, E.L. (1976). Effect of quality and quantity of dietary fat and dimethylhydrazine in colon carcinogenesis in rats. *Proc. Soc. Exp. Biol. Med.* **151**:237–239.

Reddy, B.S.; Narisawa, T.; and Weisburger, J.H. (1976a). Effect of a diet with high levels of protein and fat on colon carcinogenesis in F344 rats treated with 1,2-dimethylhydrazine. *J. Natl. Cancer Instit.* **57**:567–569.

Reddy, B.S.; Weisburger, J.H.; and Wynder, E.L. (1974). Effects of dietary fat level and dimethylhydrazine on fecal acid and neutral sterol excretion and colon carcinogenesis in rats. *J. Natl. Cancer Instit.* **52**:507–511.

Reddy, B.S. and Wynder, E.L. (1973). Large-bowel carcinogenesis: fecal constituents of populations with diverse incidence rates of colon cancer. *J. Natl. Cancer Instit.* **50**:1437–1442.

Rogers, A.E. (1975). Variable effects of a lipotrope-deficient, high-fat diet on chemical carcinogenesis in rats. *Cancer Res.* **35**:2469–2474.

Rusch, H.P.; Kline, B.E.; and Baumann, C.A. (1945). The influence of caloric restriction of dietary fat on tumor formation with ultraviolet radiation. *Cancer Res.* **5**:431–435.

Silberberg, R. and Silberberg, M. (1953). Hypophyseal tumors produced by radioactive iodine (I^{131}) in mice of various strains fed a high fat diet. *Proc. Amer. Assoc. Cancer Res.* **i**:52–53.

Silverstone, H. and Tannenbaum, A. (1950). The effect of the proportion of dietary fat on the rate of formation of mammary carcinoma in mice. *Cancer Res.* **10**:448–453.

Stemmermann, G.N. (1970). Patterns of disease among Japanese living in Hawaii. *Arch. Environ. Health* **20**:266–273.

Sugiura, K. (1941). Effect of feeding wheat germ oil on production of liver cancer by butter yellow. *Proc. Soc. Exp. Biol. Med.* **47**:17–19.

Sugiura, K. and Rhoads, C.P. (1941). Experimental liver cancer in rats and its inhibition by rice-bran extract, yeast and yeast extract. *Cancer Res.* **1**:3–16.

Tannenbaum, A. (1942). The genesis and growth of tumors. III. Effects of a high fat diet. *Cancer Res.* **2**:468–475.

Tannenbaum, A. (1959). Nutrition and cancer. In: *The Physiopathology of Cancer*, pp. 517–562. Edited by F. Homburger. Huebber-Harper, N.Y.

Wade, A.E. and Norred, W.P. (1976). Effect of dietary lipid on drug-metabolizing enzymes. *Fed. Proc.* **35**:2475–2479.

Watson, H.F. and Mellanby, E. (1930). Tar cancer in mice. II. The condition of the skin when modified by external treatment on diet, as a factor in influencing the cancerous reaction. *Brit. J. Exper. Path.* **11**:311–322.

West, C.E. and Redgrave, T.G. (1974). *Search* **5**:90–94 [cited in Hopkins, G.J. and West, C.E. (1976). *Life Sciences* **19**:1103–1116].

Wynder, E.L.; Kajiteni, T.; Ishikawa, S.; et al. (1969). Environmental factors of cancer of the colon and rectum. II. Japanese epidemiological data. *Cancer* **23**:1210–1220.

Wynder, E.L. and Klein, V.E. (1965). The possible role of riboflavin deficiency in epithelial endoplasia. 1. Epithelial changes of mice in simple deficiency. *Cancer* **18**:167–180.

7. TNT

That dietary fat may affect the toxicity of TNT was first experimentally tested more than 50 years ago by Voegtlin et al. (1920, 1921). Based on occupational exposure to TNT during World War I, which implicated dietary factors in TNT toxicity, these researchers decided to compare how dogs reared on three fundamentally different diets (i.e., high carbohydrate, protein, and mixed [white bread, milk, and medium-fat beef]) would be affected by TNT. While the studies were quite crude according to today's standards, they did suggest that mixed and meat diets with their higher protein levels were more protective (i.e., less severe anemia, longer survival). However, since these diets differed in fat, protein, and carbohydrate levels as well as vitamins and minerals, it was not possible to delineate the specific nutrient(s) that may have affected the toxicity of TNT.

According to Shils and Goldwater (1949), the next effort to evaluate this diet-TNT interaction was in 1942 by Himsworth and Glynn, using the rat model and three different diets (i.e., diets high in either protein, fat, or carbohydrate). Their findings indicated that rats reared on the high-fat diet (bacon fat) were highly susceptible to TNT toxicity, while those on the high-protein diet were seemingly unaffected, and those on the high-carbohydrate diet were only slightly affected. While it appeared that the obvious conclusion was that high-fat diets enhance the toxicity of TNT, Shils and Goldwater (1949) pointed out that the high-fat diet was also low in protein (while the high-carbohydrate diet contained more than twice as much protein on a per-100-calories-of-diet basis). Thus, were the rats fed on a high-fat diet very susceptible to TNT because of the high-fat diet, or the absence of sufficient protein in their diet, or a combination of both?

In a test of this hypothesis, Shils and Goldwater (1950) compared the influence of diets either high or low in fat but with a constant amount of protein (moderate or low depending on the experiment) on the toxicity of TNT. Their findings revealed "that TNT may be somewhat more toxic in a high fat diet than on a low fat diet when the relative growth of the control groups is taken as a criterion. However, it is quite clear that the level of fat in the diet is not a serious factor affecting TNT toxicity under the conditions of [their] experiments." Not only did Shils and Goldwater (1950) consider the quantity of fat in the diet but also the quality as well. They compared the influence of corn oil, hydrogenated cottonseed oil, and lard and also found no differential response of the animals.

The findings of Shils and Goldwater (1950) are in striking contrast to those of Himsworth and Glynn (1942). For not only did Shils and Goldwater (1950) not find any influence of fat on the toxicity of TNT but protein level of the diet was also not an important factor. Why these two studies did not agree is unclear. Among the possible reasons for different findings is that the diets used in both studies differed to a considerable extent. For example, in contrast to the Shils and Goldwater (1950) report, Himsworth and Glynn (1942) included yeast and wheat in the diet. Thus the findings of either study seem to lack the generalizability that most researchers desire and should be considered valid only for their specific experimental protocol, pending more extensive study (Anonymous, 1952).

Unfortunately, there has been little interest concerning the influence of dietary fats on TNT toxicity over the past 30 years. Whether dietary fat affects the toxicity of TNT is still an open question despite the negative findings of Shils and Goldwater (1950). A reevaluation of this issue with both animal models and epidemiological protocol is warranted.

References

Anonymous (March, 1952). Diet and poisons. *Nutr. Rev.* pp. 72–73.

Goldwater, L.J. and Shils, M.E. (1949). Some relationships of nutrition to detoxification. *Amer. Ind. Hyg. Assoc. J.* **10**:17–20.

Himsworth, H.P. and Glynn, L.E. (1942). Experimental trinitrotoluene poisoning; the effect of diet. *Clin. Sci.* **4**:421.

Shils, M.E. and Goldwater, L.J. (1949). Influence of dietary protein and fat on the toxicities of trinitrotoluene (TNT) and 2,4-dinitrotoluene (DNT) for the rat. *Fed. Proc.* **8**:397.

Shils, M.E. and Goldwater, L.J. (1950). The effect of diet on the susceptibility of rats to poisoning by 2,4,6-trinitrotoluene (TNT). *J. Nutr.* **41**:293–309.

Voegtlin, C.; Hooper, C.W.; and Johnson, J.M. (1920). Trinitrotoluene poisoning. Hygienic Lab. Bull. No. 126. U.S. Govt. Printing Off., Washington, D.C.

Voegtlin, C.; Hooper, C.W.; and Johnson, J.M. (1921). Trinitrotoluene poisoning—its nature, diagnosis and prevention. *J. Indust. Hyg.* **3**:229.

C. OTHER

1. Microsomal Enzymes and Lipids

Biochemical evidence exists that may support the studies of Carroll and Khor (1971) that unsaturated fats enhance the carcinogenicity of hydrocarbon carcinogens as compared to saturated fats. More specifically, several investigators have compared the influence of saturated vs. unsaturated fats on the metabolism of various xenobiotic compounds by the liver microsomal enzymes. Since metabolism by these enzymes may result in either detoxification or biointoxication including metabolic conversion to the ultimate carcinogenic state, any differential influence on the metabolism of xenobiotics by saturated vs. unsaturated fats may be of potential clinical significance. Specific examples of this differential response include the following: (1) Century (1969, 1973) demonstrated that rats fed 7% beef fat (i.e., saturated fats) metabolized hexobarbital and aminopyrine more slowly than rats reared on a diet with unsaturated fatty acids (i.e., 7% corn oil, 7% linseed oil, or 7% menhaden oil); (2) Marshall and McLean (1971) found that the level of cytochrome P-450 reached after induction with phenobarbital is principally determined by the quality of the dietary fat, with the highest degree of induction occurring in rats fed on diets with higher levels of unsaturated fat; (3) Norred and Wade (1973) revealed that the presence of 3% coconut oil (a saturated fat) was not nearly as effective in supporting phenobarbital induction of hexobarbital oxidase or aniline hydroxylase as a diet with corn oil.

Not only does the quality of fat in the diet affect the capacity of microsomal enzymes to metabolize xenobiotic compounds, so too does the *quantity* of dietary fat. For instance, dietary polyunsaturated or essential fatty acids induced greater mixed-function oxidase activity than a fat-free diet (Caster et al., 1968; Norred and Wade, 1973; Wade et al., 1969). In a typical study, rats reared on diets with 3 or 10% corn oil for 21 days exhibited considerably more liver microsomal enzyme activity than controls reared on a fat free diet. For example, aniline hydroxylation, hexobarbital oxidation, and heptachlor epoxidation were increased by an average of 31%, 80%, and 160%, respectively, in male rats reared on a 3%-corn oil diet compared to those reared on a fat free diet (Wade and Norred, 1976). A comparison of the 3% vs. 10% corn oil diets in male rats revealed that a 3%-corn oil diet may provide maximal metabolism of aniline and ethylmorphine, while up to or more than 10% corn oil is needed for maximal metabolism of hexobarbital (Wade and Norred, 1976).

While these findings demonstrate convincingly that the quantity and quality of dietary fat may markedly affect the capacity of microsomal enzymes to metabolize a wide range of xenobiotic compounds, Wade and Norred (1976) have emphasized that "*in vitro* metabolic changes induced by dietary lipid have not been always correlated with changes in *in vivo* activity." Despite a lack of apparent coordination between some in vitro and in vivo studies, these biochemical investigations on the influence of dietary fats on the metabolism of naturally occurring and foreign compounds provide an approach to developing a more accurate explanation of mechanisms in the promotional role of dietary fats. Future studies that will be evaluating the role of fats in chemically induced cancer should include a biochemical assessment of the relationship of changes in microsomal enzyme induction with pathogenesis.

Finally, for those interested in acquiring some background information concerning the role of lipids in microsomal enzyme function, an outstanding review by Wade and Norred (1976) should be consulted, from which the following quotation encapsulating such evidence is taken:

Drug-metabolizing enzymes are associated with the lipoprotein membranes of endoplasmic reticulum. About 30–40% of the dry weight of hepatic endoplasmic reticulum is lipid, most of which is phospholipid (Glaumann and Dallner, 1968; Siekevitz, 1963). Several lines of evidence indicate that lipids are essential for proper function of enzymes bound to these membranes: 1) Treatment of microsomes with detergents or phospholipases or subjecting them to enhanced peroxidation diminishes enzyme activity (Kamataki and Kitagawa, 1973; Lu et al., 1969; Wills, 1971). 2) Hydrolysis of phospholipids to the corresponding α, β-diglycerides or phosphatidic acid with phospholipase C or D, or extraction with isooctane or l-butanol and acetone, alters substrate binding to cytochrome P-450 and inhibits Type I substrate metabolism (Chaplin and Mannering, 1970; Eling and DiAugustine, 1971; Vore et al., 1974; Young et al., 1971). 3) Phosphatidylcholine restores metabolic activity to a solubilized cytochrome P-450-NADPH cytochrome P-450 reductase system and also restores activity to microsomes treated with phospholipases or extracted with isooctane or l-butanol and acetone (Coon et al., 1971; Lu et al., 1969; Strobel et al., 1970; Vore et al., 1974). 4) Phospholipid cholesterol, and triglyceride concentrations of microsomes increase as proteins increase during enzyme induction with phenobarbital (Cooper and Feuer, 1972; Glaumann and Dallner, 1968; Infante et al., 1971; Orrenius et al., 1965, 1969; Young et al., 1971). 5) Phenobarbital or 3-methylcholanthrene induction increases the incorporation of linoleate into phospholipid at almost the exact time that the concentrations of other components of the drug hydroxylation system increase (Davison and Wills, 1974). 6) The sex difference in phospholipid content of rat hepatic microsomes may be related to their sex differences in drug metabolizing activity, since the elevated phospholipid functions seen in males are the same ones that increase during induction of drug metabolizing enzymes (Belina et al., 1975). 7) Phospholipid appears to be essential for the NADPH-dependent reduction of cytochrome P-450 since electron transfer from NADPH to cytochrome P-450 occurs at a rate sufficient to support substrate hydroxylation only when phosphatidylcholine is present.

References

Belina, H.; Cooper, S.D.; Farkas, R.; and Feuer, G. (1975). Sex difference in the phospholipid composition of rat liver microsomes. *Biochem. Pharmacol.* **24**:301–303.

Bull, A.W.; Soullier, B.K.; Wilson, P.S.; Hayden, M.T.; and Nigro, N.D. (1979). Promotion of azoxymethane-induced intestinal cancer by high-fat diet in rats. *Cancer Res.* **39**:4956–4959.

Carroll, K.K. and Khor, H.T. (1971). Effects of level and type of dietary fat on incidence of mammary tumors induced in female Sprague-Dawley rats by 7,12 DMBA. *Lipids* **6**(6):415–420.

Caster, W.O.; Wade, A.E.; Greene, F.E.; and Meadows, J.S. (1968). Effect of small changes in dietary thiamine or essential fatty acid in altering the rate of drug detoxication in the liver of the rat. *Fed. Proc.* **27**:549.

Century, B. (1969). *Drugs Affecting Lipid Metabolism.* Edited by W.H. Holmes. p. 629. Plenum, N.Y.

Century, B. (1973). A role of the dietary lipid in the ability of phenobarbital to stimulate drug detoxification. *J. Pharmacol. Exp. Therap.* **185**:185–194.

Chaplin, M.D. and Mannering, G.J. (1970). Role of phospholipids in the hepatic microsomal drug-metabolizing system. *Mol. Pharmacol.* **6**:631–640.

Coon, M.J.; Strobel, H.W.; Autor, A.P.; Heidema, J.; and Duppel, W. (1971). Functional components of the liver microsomal enzyme system catalysing fatty acid, hydrocarbon and drug hydroxylation. *Biochem. J.* **125**(2):2p.

Cooper, S.D. and Feuer, G. (1972). Relation between drug-metabolizing activity and phospholipids in hepatic microsomes. I. Effects of phenobarbital, carbon tetrachloride, and actinomycin D. *Canad. J. Physiol. Pharmacol.* **50**:568–575.

Davison, S.C. and Wills, E.D. (1974). Studies on the lipid composition of the rat liver endoplasmic reticulum after induction with phenobarbitone and 20-methylcholanthrene. *Biochem. J.* **140**:461–468.

Eling, T.E. and DiAugustine, R.P. (1971). A role for phospholipids in the binding and metabolism of drugs by hepatic microsomes. *Biochem. J.* **123**:539–544.

Forbes, J.C.; Leach, B.E.; and Outhouse, E.L. (1941). Studies on fat metabolism and susceptibility to carbon tetrachloride. *J. Pharm. Exper. Therap.* **72**:202–210.

Glaumann, H. and Dallner, G. (1968). Lipid composition and turnover of rough and smooth microsomal membranes in rat liver. *J. Lipid Res.* **9**:720–729.

Hammer, C.T. and Wills, E.D. (1979). The effect of dietary fats on the composition of the liver endoplasmic reticulum and oxidative drug metabolism. *Brit. J. Nutrit.* **41**:465.

Infante, R.; Petit, D.; Polononski, J. and Caroli, J. (1971). Microsomal phospholipid biosynthesis after phenobarbital administration. *Experientia* **27**:640–642.

Kamataki, T. and Kitagawa, H. (1973). Effects of lipid peroxidation on activities of drug-metabolizing enzymes in liver microsomes of rats. *Biochem. Pharmacol.* **22**:3199–3207.

Lu, A.Y.H.; Junk, K.W.; and Coon, M.J. (1969). Resolution of the cytochrome P-450-containing ω-hydroxylation system of liver microsomes into three components. *J. Biol. Chem.* **244**:3714–3721.

Marshall, W.J. and McLean, A.E.M. (1971). A requirement for dietary lipids for induction of cytochrome P-450 by phenobarbitone in rat liver microsomal fraction. *Biochem. J.* **122**:569–573.

Norred, W.P. and Wade, A.E. (1972). Dietary fatty acid-induced alterations of hepatic microsomal drug metabolism. *Biochem. Pharmacol.* **21**:2887–2897.

Norred, W.P. and Wade, A.E. (1973). Effect of dietary lipid ingestion on the induction of drug-metabolizing enzymes by phenobarbital. *Biochem. Pharmacol.* **22**:432–436.

Orrenius, S.; Das, M.; and Gnosspelius, Y. (1969). In: *Microsomes and Drug Oxidations.* Edited by J.R. Gillette, A.H. Connery, G.J. Cosmides, R.W. Estabrook, J.R. Fouts, and G.J. Mannering. p. 251. Academic, N.Y.

Orrenius, S.; Ericsson, J.L.E.; and Ernster, L. (1965). Phenobarbital-induced synthesis of the microsomal drug-metabolizing enzyme system and its relationship to the proliferation of endoplasmic membranes. *J. Cell. Biol.* **25**(1):627–639.

Siekevitz, P. (1963). Protoplasm: Endoplasmic reticulum and microsomes and their properties. *Ann. Rev. Physiol.* **25**:15–40.

Strobel, H.W.; Lu, A.Y.H.; Heidema, J.; and Coon, M.J. (1970). Phosphatidylcholine requirement in the enzymatic reduction of hemoprotein P-450 and in fatty acid, hydrocarbon and drug hydroxylation. *J. Biol. Chem.* **245**:4851–4854.

Vore, M.; Hamilton, J.G.; and Lu, A.Y.H. (1974). Organic solvent extraction of liver microsomal lipid. I. The requirement of lipid for 3,4-benzpyrene hydroxylase. *Biochem. Biophys. Res. Commun.* **56**:1038–1044.

Wade, A.E.; Caster, W.O.; Greene, F.E.; and Meadows, J.S. (1969). *Arch. Int. Pharmacodyn. Ther.* **181**:466.

Wade, A.E. and Norred, W.P (1976). Effect of dietary lipid on drug-metabolizing enzymes. *Fed. Proc.* **35**:2475–2479.

Wills, E.D. (1971). Effects of lipid peroxidation on membrane-bound enzymes of the endoplasmic reticulum. *Biochem. J.* **123**:983–991.

Young, D.L.; Powell, G.; and McMillan, W.O. (1971). Phenobarbital-induced alterations in phosphatidylcholine and triglyceride synthesis in hepatic endoplasmic reticulum. *J. Lipid Res.* **12**:1–8.

2. Ultraviolet Radiation

In the late 1930s, it was reported that an increase in the fat content of the diet from 5% to 25–30% enhanced the occurrence of ultraviolet-induced tumors in male albino mice (Baumann and Rusch, 1939). An examination of their research methodology reveals that the mice were allowed to consume food and water ad libitum. Since isocaloric diets were not given to both the exposed and controls, these investigators introduced a possible confounding variable (i.e., possible differential consumption of calories between the two experimental groups). This is of significance since experimental evidence has revealed that diets with high fat or caloric intake enhance the occurrence of a variety of tumors in the mouse (Baumann et al., 1939; Baumann and Rusch, 1939; Rusch et al., 1939; Jacobi and Baumann, 1940; Tannenbaum, 1942), while a restricted caloric intake reduces the occurrence of the cancer and/or extends the latency period of experimentally induced and spontaneously occurring tumors in the mouse (Tannenbaum, 1940, 1942; Visscher et al., 1942). Since mice given the diets with high-fat levels voluntarily consume more calories than animals on the control diets (Lavik and Baumann, 1943), Rusch et al. (1945) decided to reevaluate the hypothesis that a high-fat diet enhanced the expression of UV-induced tumors under closely controlled experimental procedures in which confounding of differential caloric consumption was eliminated. These findings, in marked contrast to the Baumann and Rusch (1939) study, revealed that most (but not all) of the accelerating action of fat on UV-induced tumor formation can be explained on the basis of an increased caloric intake. It appears that when the total caloric intake is particularly restricted that higher levels of fat in the diet can enhance the occurrence of UV-induced tumors. Yet at higher levels of permitted caloric intake, the phenomenon was reversed with the higher level of fat being protective.

The primary importance of this section is not that dietary factors may influence the occurrence of UV-induced tumors, but the need to eliminate confounding variables so that legitimate conclusions can be drawn from experiments. This is a problem that continuously reoccurs and must be carefully guarded against in the development of research protocol, as well as in the interpretation of the published literature. Finally, these data do suggest that dietary levels of fat may affect the expression of UV-induced cancer. In light of the high incidence of skin cancer (90 to 140/100,000 Caucasians), especially in areas where the latitude is low (i.e., Honolulu, Dallas) relative to other areas (i.e., Philadelphia, Minneapolis) (30 to 50/100,000 Caucasians), it is important to investigate the role that diet may have in affecting this environmental hazard, realizing that protective clothing is probably the most important preventive measure that could be easily implemented.

References

Baumann, C.A.; Jacobi, H.P.; and Rusch, H.P. (1939). The effect of diet on experimental tumor production. *Amer. J. Hyg.* **30**:1–6.

Baumann, C.A. and Rusch, H.P. (1939). Effect of diet on tumors induced by ultraviolet light. *Amer. J. Cancer* **35**:213–221.

Jacobi, H.P. and Baumann, C.A. (1940). Effect of fat on tumor formation. *Amer. J. Cancer* **39**:338–342.

Lavik, P.S. and Baumann, C.A. (1943). Further studies on the tumor-promoting action of fat. *Cancer Res.* **3**:749–756.

Rusch, H.P.; Baumann, C.A.; and Kline, B.E. (1939). Effect of local applications on development of ultraviolet tumors. *Proc. Soc. Exp. Med. Biol.* **42**:508–512.

Rusch, H.P.; Kline, B.E.; and Baumann, C.A. (1945). The influence of caloric restriction and of dietary fat on tumor formation with ultraviolet radiation. *Cancer Res.* **5**:431–435.

Tannenbaum, A. (1940). The initiation and growth of tumors. I. Effects of underfeeding. *Amer. J. Cancer* **38**:335–350.

Tannenbaum, A. (1942). The genesis and growth of tumors. II. Effects of caloric restriction per se. *Cancer Res.* **2**:460–465.

Visscher, M.B.; Ball, Z.B.; Barnes, R.H.; and Silvertsen, I. (1942). The influence of calorie restriction upon the incidence of spontaneous mammary carcinoma in mice. *Surgery* **11**:48–55.

D. FATS—POLLUTANT INTERACTIONS—A PERSPECTIVE

Since the turn of the century and even further back in some instances, researchers have been interested in the influence of dietary fat on pollutant toxicity and/or carcinogenicity. Over thirty toxic agents have had their adverse effects either enhanced or diminished to a certain extent by dietary fat (Table 5). However, despite the long history of interest in fat-pollutant interactions and the sizable listing of substances whose toxicity may be affected, the role of dietary fats in modifying pollutant toxicity is only reasonably well defined for just a few specific compounds such as fluoride, lead, and hydrocarbon carcinogens. Even with these "reasonably well defined" dietary fat-pollutant interactions, a reading of each of these sections reveals that our understanding of the biochemical mechanisms for such interactions are, for the most part, speculation. Many other dietary fat-pollutant interactions are often based on fewer than three studies, all over 30 years old (e.g., 1,2-dichloroethane, 1,2-dichloropropane, arsenic, phenol, uranium nitrate, potassium chromate, and others). Thus, while some of these studies are highly suggestive that dietary fat may markedly affect pollutant toxicity, the data base is so limited as to not permit any firm generalizations. However, despite all the above-stated limitations, it seems reasonably safe to say that with only a few exceptions (i.e., the toxic effects of aflatoxin and DNT, and possibly some carcinogenic responses), elevated levels of fat in the diet in the animal models tested (usually rodents and dogs) enhance the adverse effects of the pollutants considered.

The two most important areas of fat-pollutant interactions are with lead and chemical carcinogens. The importance stems from (1) the severity of the adverse effects caused by these agents, (2) that elevated levels of fat are hypothesized to enhance the adverse effects, and (3) the data base is sufficiently robust as to provide theorists at least some basis on which to formulate conceptual frameworks for further study. It is interesting to note that both the quantity and quality of dietary fats have been found to influence the adverse effects of lead and several chemical carcinogens. Recognition of this finding is important if one is to appreciate the complexity of the experimental protocols in this area and the frequent difficulty of comparing one study to another. Thus it is important to know not just how much fat was used in the diet but what type of fats, what proportion of saturated vs. unsaturated fats, and so on.

Since lead poisoning in children remains a problem of considerable proportions in the United States today primarily because of the

Table 5. Summary—Studies from Substances with Limited Data Concerning a Fat-Pollutant Interaction

Substance	Animal	Effect	Reference
Aflatoxin	Chickens Turkeys	Increased levels of dietary fat reduce some of the adverse effects of aflatoxin, including mortality incidence	Smith et al., 1971 Hamilton et al., 1972
Arsenic	Dogs	High-fat diet enhances the toxicity of arsphenamine in dogs. (Contrary findings were reported by Craven [1931] with arsphenamine and Packman et al. [1961] with arsenic trioxide.)	Messinger and Hawkins, 1940
Atabrine	Rats	Rats reared on a high-protein, low-fat diet were less susceptible to atabrine-induced hepatotoxic effects than rats reared on a low-protein or high-protein, high-fat diet	Scudi and Hamlin, 1944
Carbon tetrachloride	Rats	Oral administration of fat several hours prior to the time of poisoning enhances the toxicity of CCl_4	Forbes et al., 1941 Gyorgy et al., 1946
Chloroform	Rats	Diet high in fat enhances the toxicity of chloroform relative to those animals given substantial quantities of meat	Opie and Alford, 1914, 1914a Goldschmidt et al., 1939
Cyanide	Rats	Mortality incidence of rats on high-fat diets was less than those on high-protein and carbohydrate diets	Rothe Meyer, 1939
1,2-dichloro-ethane (ethylene di-chloride)	Rats	A high-fat diet in combination with either low or normal casein dietary levels markedly enhanced toxicity (i.e., death; pathological changes in liver). Combination of low-protein and high-fat diet seems to result in a synergistic response. Supplementation with choline and methionine markedly reduced toxicity, but not completely. (See protein chapter for more detailed discussion of research protocol of this study.)	Heppel et al., 1945

Table 5. (Continued)

1,2-dichloro-propane (propylene dichloride)	Rats	The combination of a low-protein, high-fat diet markedly enhanced the toxicity of this compound via inhalation exposure. Supplementation of both choline and methionine markedly diminished toxicity (i.e., death; liver pathology), but not totally. (See protein chapter for more detailed discussion of research protocol.)	Heppel et al., 1946
Phenol	Rats	No obvious differences between groups receiving differential levels of fat and carbohydrate with respect to mortality. Rats on high-fat diets had somewhat greater mortality than those on high-protein diet	Rothe Meyer, 1939
Phosphorus	Rats	Toxicity of phosphorus is greater in rats given a diet of meat as compared to one higher in either carbohydrates or fat	Opie and Alford, 1914a, 1915, 1915a
Polychlorinated biphenyls	Hybrid Broiler Cockerels	No consistent differences between controls and those fed on either low-protein or high-fat diets	Hansen et al., 1976
Potassium chromate	Rats	Diets with meat were more toxic than those of fat	Opie and Alford, 1914a, 1915a
Radiation	Mice	Erythrocytes of mice reared on diets with either high levels of saturated (coconut oil) or unsaturated (safflower oil) fatty acids were evaluated for susceptibility to radiation damage (in-vitro studies). Cells from mice on the unsaturated diet were more resistant	Prince and Little, 1973

Selenium	Rats	A diet low in protein and high in fat gave better protection to rats from selenium (10 ppm in diet) toxicity than a diet low in protein and high in carbohydrates. However, a high-protein, low-carbohydrate diet was the most protective diet employed. It was assumed "that the protective action of the high fat diet may be due to its protein sparing action."	Smith, 1939
Sulfanilamide	Rats	High-fat diet (40.8% Crisco) offered slight protection from sulfanilamide-induced lethality relative to controls fed a diet with 22.8% Crisco	Kapnick et al., 1942
Uranium nitrate	Rats	A high fat diet enhances the toxicity of uranium nitrate relative to one of meat. However, a carbohydrate diet is more protective than a fat diet	Opie and Alford, 1914a, 1915a

ingestion of leaded paints, it is important to provide parents and their children with all the help they can get to avoid lead intoxication. If experimentation indicates that consumption of skimmed milk significantly reduced the absorption and/or retention of ingested lead as compared to buttered or whole milk, then serious consideration should be given within state Public Health Departments to develop educational programs that will reach parents of high-risk children. While it is clearly better to remove the lead, what does one do in the meantime, especially when parental supervision of the child is often less than adequate? Nutritional prophylaxis is not THE ANSWER to preventing lead intoxication, but it may be part of a strategy to deal with reducing the risk. Unfortunately, the data on how fat affects lead absorption and retention are somewhat equivocal. However, since several studies have demonstrated highly significant interactions with lead absorption, a strong effort should be made by the federal government to resolve this issue.

As for dietary fat and chemical carcinogenesis, this is an area where great strides have been made, especially within recent years. However, the nature of carcinogen interactions is quite complex. For here we are dealing with problems of latency, tissue sensitivity, and a wide range of chemicals, as well as the quantity and quality of the dietary fat. Obtaining answers for the dietary fat-lead interaction hypothesis, while difficult and time-consuming, is relatively simple compared to developing a coherent and consistent model that explains how dietary fats affect the incidence and extent of chemically induced cancers. Perhaps the most frustrating aspect is that prospective epidemiological studies that may be used to test theories derived from animal model investigations are quite expensive and difficult to successfully carry out, especially because of the latency variables as well as other competing causes of death and the adequacy of one's sample size.

Even though investigators are faced with innumerable difficulties in obtaining reliable data in this area and there are many gaps in our present understanding, sufficient information has emerged that has established that dietary fat does play a role in the development of chemically induced cancers in animals. This has been demonstrated time and again. Even the quality of the fat is important in this regard. Numerous epidemiologic investigations have also associated differential fat consumption with cancer mortality. At this point, though, it is not known whether elevated levels of dietary fat enhance chemically induced cancer in humans. However, it would be surprising if this phenomenon, which is so striking in the animal models, does not occur in humans. Research to evaluate this hypothesis should be given a high priority.

References

Craven, E.B. (1931). Importance of diet in preventing acute yellow atrophy during arsphenamine treatment. *Johns Hopkins Hosp. Bull.* **48**:131–142.

Forbes, J.C.; Leach, B.E.; and Outhouse, E.L. (1941). Studies of fat metabolism and susceptibility to carbon tetrachloride. *J. Pharmacol. Exp. Therap.* **72**:202–210.

Goldschmidt, S.; Vars, H.M.; and Ravdin, I.S. (1939). The influence of the foodstuffs upon the susceptibility of the liver to injury by chloroform, and the probable mechanism of their action. *J. Clin. Invest.* **18**:277–289.

Gyorgy, P.; Seifter, J.; Tomarelli, R.M.; and Goldblatt, H. (1946). Influence of dietary factors and sex on the toxicity of carbon tetrachloride in rats. *J. Exp. Med.* **83**:449–462.

Hamilton, P.B.; Tung, H.T.; Harris, J.R.; Gaines, H.H.; and Donaldson, W.E. (1972). The effect of dietary fat on aflatoxicosis in turkeys. *Poult. Sci.* **51**:165–170.

Hansen, L.G.; Beamer, P.D.; Wilson, D.W.; and Metcalf, R.L. (1976). Effects of feeding polychlorinated biphenyls to broiler cockerels in three dietary regimes. *Poult Sci.* **5**:1084–1088.

Heppel, L.A.; Highman, B.; and Porterfield, V.T. (1946). Toxicology of 1,2-dichloropropane (propylene dichloride). II. Influence of dietary factors on the toxicity of dichloropropane. *J. Pharmacol. Exp. Therap.* **87**:11–17.

Heppel, L.A.; Neal, P.A.; Daft, F.S.; Endicott, K.M.; Orr, M.L.; and Porterfield, V.T. (1945). Toxicology of 1,2-dichloroethane (ethylene dichloride). II. Influence of dietary factors on the toxicity of dichloroethane. *J. Ind. Hyg. Tox.* **27**:15–21.

Kapnick, I.; Lyons, C.; and Stewart, J.D. (1942). Influence of diet on sulfanilamide toxicity. *J. Pharmacol. Exp. Therap.* **74**:284–289.

Messinger, W.I. and Hawkins, W.B. (1940). Arsphenamine liver injury modified by diet. Protein and carbohydrate protective, but fat injurious. *Amer. J. Med. Sci.* **199**:216–225.

Opie, E.L. and Alford, L.B. (1914). The influence of diet on hepatic necrosis and toxicity of chloroform. *JAMA* **62**(12):895–896.

Opie, E.L. and Alford, L.B. (1914a). Influence of diet on the toxicity of substances which produce lesions of the liver or the kidney. *JAMA* **63**:136–137.

Opie, E.L. and Alford, L.B. (1915). The influence of diet upon necrosis caused by hepatic and renal poisons. Part I. Diet and the hepatic lesions of chloroform, phosphorus, or alcohol. *J. Exp. Med.* **21**:1–20.

Opie, E.L. and Alford, L.B. (1915a). Influence of diet upon necrosis caused by hepatic and renal poisons. Part II. Diet and the nephritis caused by potassium chromate, uranium nitrate, or chloroform. *J. Exp. Med.* **21**:21–37.

Packman, E.W.; Abbott, D.D.; and Harrison, J.W.E. (1961). The acute oral toxicity in rats of several diet-arsenic trioxide mixtures. *Agric. Food Chem.* **9**(4):271–279.

Prince, E.W. and Little, J.B. (1973). The effect of dietary fatty acids and tocopherol on the radiosensitivity of mammalian erythrocytes. *Rad. Res.* **53**:49–64.

Rothe Meyer, A. (1939). Influence of diet on intoxication with phenol and cyanide. *Proc. Soc. Exp. Biol. Med.* **41**:402–403.

Scudi, J.V. and Hamlin, M.T. (1944). Biochemical aspects of the toxicity of atabrine. II. The influence of the diet upon the effects produced by repeated doses of the drug. *J. Pharmacol. Exp. Therap.* **8**:150–159.

Smith, J.W.; Hill, C.H.; and Hamilton, P.B. (1971). The effect of dietary modifications on aflatoxicosis in the broiler chicken. *Poult. Sci.* **50**:768–774.

Smith, M.I. (1939). The influence of diet on the chronic toxicity of selenium. *Pub. Health Repts.* **54**:1441.

10

Carbohydrates and Related Compounds

1. Interactions with Dietary Protein

In the majority of studies in which the influence of dietary protein on the toxicity and/or carcinogenicity of various agents were evaluated, the level of carbohydrates was altered inversely with respect to the protein. In other words, if one were comparing the influence of a low-protein diet on the toxicity of lead, the control diet might have 25% of casein and 55% carbohydrates, while the low-protein diet might have only 5% protein but 75% carbohydrates. At least two variables were introduced: the level of protein and of carbohydrate. However, in almost all the studies of this type, the authors conclude that a low-protein diet is responsible for the effect rather than the combination of a low-protein, high-carbohydrate diet. A notable exception to the trend of imprecise scientific reporting is a study by Swann and McLean (1971) concerning dimethylnitrosamine. Persons interested in the influence of carbohydrate-protein interactions on pollutant toxicity should refer to the protein section.

Reference

Swann, P.F. and McLean, A.E.M. (1971). Cellular injury and carcinogenesis: the effect of a protein-free high-carbohydrate diet on the metabolism of dimethylnitrosamine in the rat. *Biochem. J.* **124**:283–288.

2. Citric Acid

Considerable research on the influence of citric acid on the toxicity of lead has been conducted, especially in the early 1950s. The findings associated with these studies have been reviewed by Stephens and Waldron (1975). In general, it has been found that large doses of sodium citrate have been reported to prevent the occurrence of lead intoxication in a number of animal models and humans (Hsu and Yao, 1958; Kety and Letonoff, 1941; Moeschlin and Schechterman, 1952; Mokranjac et al., 1958; Rossi et al., 1954; Shibata, 1957; Shiels et al., 1950; Suntych, 1953; Hardy et al., 1951). In contrast, Masuda (1959) reported that potassium sodium citrate displayed only a minor therapeutic influence on rabbits orally intoxicated with lead.

Other studies have revealed that inhalation of calcium sodium citrate and zirconium citrate had no prophylactic influence on individuals exposed to lead (Niemoller, 1957). These findings were supported by Sano (1953), who demonstrated that sodium citrate given orally to guinea pigs did not modify the urinary excretion of lead that was either inhaled or ingested. According to Stephens and Waldron (1975), this lack of protection results because citrate is quickly metabolized within the Krebs cycle. They cited further support for this notion from the research of Schubert and Lindenbaum (1960), who injected small amounts of monofluoroacetic acid into lead-poisoned rats so that citric acid accumulated as a result of the inhibition of enzymes in the Krebs cycle. Injection of modest doses of sodium citrate then provided the animals with protection against lead poisoning.

In a more recent study by Garber and Wei (1974) it was reported that both sodium citrate (5%) (0.1 ml/mouse) and orange juice (0.1 ml/mouse) significantly enhanced the gastrointestinal absorption[1] of lead in mice by factors of approximately 3 and 2, respectively. In light of the apparent discrepancy between the findings of Garber and Wei (1974) and the numerous earlier studies reviewed by Stephens and Waldron

[1]Values concerning lead absorption do not include possible resecretion of the absorbed lead back to the intestine or the excretion of lead via the urine or feces.

(1975) with respect to the influence of citric acid on the absorption and toxicity of lead (as well as the fact that sodium citrate and citric acid are common food additives), further research should be directed toward assessing in a quantitative fashion the influence of citric acid on the uptake, retention, tissue distribution, and toxicity of lead.

References

Garber, B.T. and Wei, E. (1974). Influence of dietary factors on the gastrointestinal absorption of lead. *Toxicol. Appl. Pharmacol.* **27**:685–691.

Hardy, H.L.; Bishop, R.C.; and Maloof, C.C. (1951). Treatment of lead poisoning with sodium citrate. Report of four cases. *Arch. Ind. Hyg. Occ. Med.* **3**:267.

Hsu, J.H. and Yao, K.P. (1958). Sodium citrate in the prevention and treatment of lead poisoning. *Chin. J. Int. Med.* **6**:97, 836.

Kety, S.S. (1942). The lead citrate complex ion and its role in the physiology and therapy of lead poisoning. *J. Biol. Chem.* **142**:181.

Kety, S.S. and Letonoff, T.V. (1941). Treatment of lead poisoning with sodium citrate. *Proc. Soc. Exper. Biol. Med.* **46**:476.

Masuda, Y. (1959). The effects of potassium sodium citrate on lead intoxication. *Nichida: Igaka Zasshi* **18**:2983.

Moeschlin, S. and Schechterman, L. (1952). Comparative study of therapeutic effect of 2, 3-dimercaptopropanol (BAL) or sodium citrate on experimental lead poisoning. *Schweiz. Med. Wschn.* **82**:1164.

Mokranjac, M.S.; Radmic, S.; and Soldatovic, D. (1958). Action of certain drugs on guinea pigs intoxicated with lethal doses of lead. *Acta Pharm. Jugosl.* **8**:197.

Niemoller, H.K. (1957). Zur Prophyllaxie der Bleivergiftung. Inhalationsversuche mit verchiedenen Chemikalien. *Dt. Med. Wschr.* **82**:738.

Rossi, L.; Vitacca, L.; and Pagano, R. (1954). Azione del citrato di sodio nell'intossicazione da piombo. Contributo clinico e sperimentale. *Folia Med.* **37**:967.

Sano, S. (1953). Milchgabe an Bleiarbeiter. Eine Literatursichtung. *Zentbl. ArbMed. ArbSchutz* **15**:190.

Schubert, J. and Lindenbaum, A. (1960). The mechanism of action of chelating agents on metallic elements in the intact animal. In: *Metal Binding in Medicine,* p. 68. Edited by J.J. Sevenand and L.A. Johnson. Lippincott, Philadelphia.

Schubert, J. and White, M.R. (1952). Effect of sodium and zirconium citrates on distribution and excretion of injected radiolead. *J. Lab. Clin. Med.* **39**:260.

Shibata, S. (1957). Pharmacological studies on the antidotal action of chelating agents. *Nippon Yukurigaki Zasshi* **53**:602.

Shiels, D.O.; Thomas, W.C.; and Palmer, G.R. (1950). The effects of sodium citrate in lead poisoning and lead absorption. *Med. J. Aust.* **2**:886.

Stephens, R. and Waldron, H.A. (1975). The influence of milk and related dietary constituents on lead metabolism. *Fd. Cosmet. Toxicol.* **13**:555–563.

Suntych, F. (1953). Nase zkusenosti s techov outravy olovem citranem sodvym. *Pracovni Lek.* **5**:320.

3. Lactose

Stephens and Waldron (1975) have suggested that lactose may play an important, though indirect, role in the absorption of lead via the gastrointestinal tract. This notion is based on the observations in many species, including rats (Bergeim, 1926), dairy calves (Robinson et al., 1929), dogs (Greenwald and Gross, 1929), chicks (Kline et al., 1932), and humans (Mills et al., 1940) that lactose enhances the absorption of calcium. Lactose is also known to enhance markedly the gastrointestinal absorption of strontium in the rat (Wasserman and Comar, 1959). In light of the abundance of lactose in milk, Stephens and Waldron (1975) suggested that further research on the influence of lactose on lead uptake is of potential significance.

References

Bergeim, O. (1926). Intestinal chemistry. V. Carbohydrates and calcium and phosphorus absorption. *J. Biol. Chem.* **70**:35.

Greenwald, I. and Gross, J. (1929). The prevention of the tetany of parathyroidectomized dogs. II. Lactose-containing diets. *J. Biol. Chem.* **82**:531.

Kline, O.L.; Keenan, J.A.; Elvehjem, C.A.; and Hart, E.B. (1932). Lactose in nutrition. *J. Biol. Chem.* **98**:121.

Mills, R.; Breiter, H.; Kempster, E.; McCay, B.; Pickens, M.; and Outhouse, J. (1940). The influence of lactose in calcium retention in children. *J. Nutr.* **20**:467.

Robinson, C.S.; Huffman, C.F.; and Mason, M.F. (1929). The results of the ingestion of certain calcium salts and lactose. *J. Biol. Chem.* **84**:257.

Stephens, R. and Waldron, H.A. (1975). Influence of milk and related dietary constituents on lead metabolism. *Fd. Cosmet. Toxicol.* **13**:555–563.

Wasserman, R.H. and Comar, C.L. (1959). Carbohydrates and gastrointestinal absorption of radiostrontium and radiocalcium in the rat. *Proc. Soc. Exp. Biol. Med.* **101**:314.

Dietary Fiber

11

A. INTRODUCTION

Every year in the United States there are approximately 100,000 newly diagnosed cases of colorectal cancer, with nearly 50,000 cases per year resulting in death (Spiller et al., 1978). The occurrence of colorectal cancer has been found to be associated with Western dietary patterns, which include a high intake of fats as well as a low intake of fiber. For instance, 40% of the caloric intake in the United States is from dietary fat while in Japan where the incidence of colonic cancer is quite low, only 12% of the caloric intake is from fats. As for dietary fiber, Burkitt et al. (1972) reported a correlation between the amount of fiber in the diet and the incidence of large-bowel cancer. They noted that groups of people who consume a high-fiber diet have a low incidence of this disease, while the reverse is true. Presumably, the presence of high levels of dietary fiber reduces the intestinal transit time, thereby diminishing exposure of the mucosa to carcinogens and promoting agents. This chapter will critically review the biomedical literature concerning the influence of dietary fiber on the development of chemically induced cancer as well as other adverse effects resulting from exposure to toxic environmental agents.

425

In order to facilitate a greater understanding of the strengths and limitations of subsequent studies concerned with the capacity of dietary fiber to modify the toxicity and/or carcinogenicity of chemical agents, it is necessary to discuss briefly what is meant by the term "dietary fiber." Among those on the leading edge of dietary fiber research there is considerable debate over what should be included within the definitional framework of fiber. There is also much debate over whether the term "fiber" should be replaced by a more accurate phrase (Spiller et al., 1978). For the sake of this review, dietary fiber is defined as "plant material that is not digested by enzymes of the human gastrointestinal tract" (Kritchevsky, 1979). Table 1 identifies the types of dietary fiber naturally present in foods, including several of their distinguishing chemical characteristics (Dwyer et al., 1978). It is important to note that it was not until quite recently that researchers have been able to make more quantitative assessments of the composition of fiber. Previously, fiber determinations involved treatments that destroyed all components except cellulose and lignin. This residual fraction was called crude fiber. Thus the amount of crude fiber often grossly underestimated the total amount of fiber originally present. For example, the total dietary fiber content in grams per 100 grams of broccoli and cocoa powder is 4.1 and 43.3, respectively, while their crude fiber level is 1.5 and 4.3. This is an important consideration, since the early research concerning fiber and carcinogenicity from 2-acetylaminofluorene (AAF) (Wilson and DeEds, 1950; Engel and Copeland, 1952) lacked the more quantitative determinations.

As can be seen from Table 1, many substances are included within the umbrella of what is commonly referred to as dietary fiber. Unless researchers carefully characterize the type of fiber constituents employed in their studies, attempts at replication may not infrequently prove futile.

The first indications that dietary fiber may help prevent chemically induced cancer were published approximately 30 years ago. Wilson and DeEds (1950) gave rats diets with 3.0% (diet A) or 6.0% (diet B) crude fiber. However, these diets also differed somewhat in their protein, fat, ash, and nitrogen-free extract levels. When the diet contained 0.062% AAF, rats on diet B displayed considerably fewer carcinogenic responses than their diet A comparison animals. Similar findings were observed by Engel and Copeland (1952), who noted that rats reared on a stock diet developed fewer AAF-induced tumors than those given semi-purified and modified stock diets. These early reports suggested that low levels of crude dietary fiber may enhance the carcinogenicity

Table 1. Characteristics of Dietary Fiber

Form in which Fiber Appears	Name	Chemistry	Absorb Water or Water-soluble	Degraded by Intestinal Bacteria	Other Characteristics Relevant to Clinical Medicine
Dietary fiber naturally present in foods	Components of plant cell walls:				
	Pectin	Complex polymer of the sugar uronic acid and its derivatives	Yes	Yes	Form gels and thus alter water-holding capacity of residues. React with metal ions such as calcium to form insoluble pectates; this may influence nutrient absorption
	Hemicelluloses A and B	Structural polysaccharides composed of glucose units	Yes	Yes	When attacked by intestinal bacteria, produce volatile short-chain fatty acids (acetic, butyric, propionic). In addition to organic acid production, metabolism of hemicellulose by gut flora leads to increased stool-water loss, increased fecal fat, and nitrogen excretion

427

Table 1. (Continued)

Form in which Fiber Appears	Name	Chemistry	Absorb Water or Water-soluble	Degraded by Intestinal Bacteria	Other Characteristics Relevant to Clinical Medicine
	Cellulose	Structural polysaccharides composed of glucose units	No	Yes	
	Lignins	Heterogeneous, amorphous, random polymers of phenylpropane units making up the skeleton of the plant	No	No	Absorb bile acids, particularly secondary bile acids such as deoxycholic acid. Degree of polymerization (lignification) depends on age, type of plant, etc., so lignins differ considerably even if from the same source. These differences in lignification affect the digestibility of the celluloses present in food
Components found elsewhere in plants:	Waxes, cutins, etc.	Unavailable lipid substances forming part of skin or rind of plant	No	No	

Food fractions particularly high in fiber	Materials found associated with dietary fiber	—	—	
Brans, husks, germs of various cereals	Unavailable nitrogen, trace elements, enzymes, minerals, salts, etc., present in vegetable cell walls			
Naturally occurring gums	Unavailable polysaccharides, colloids	Yes	?	Dissolve or disperse in water to make a viscous mucilaginous solution or suspension
Carageenan (Irish moss extract)	Unavailable polysaccharides, colloids	Yes	?	Water extract of certain red algae seaweeds. Seaweeds themselves are used in the Orient
Aginic acid, algen	Unavailable polysaccharides, colloids	Yes	?	Extract from brown algae
Agar	Unavailable polysaccharides, colloids	Yes		Seaweed derivative often used for making sweetened, flavored gels
Furacellan	Unavailable polysaccharides, colloids	Yes		A seaweed extract

Table 1. (Continued)

Form in which Fiber Appears	Name	Chemistry	Absorb Water or Water-soluble	Degraded by Intestinal Bacteria	Other Characteristics Relevant to Clinical Medicine
Additives providing fiber sometimes present in processed foods	Naturally occurring gums (see above)				
	Synthetic gums	Unavailable polysaccharides existing in a colloidal form	Yes	?	These substances have been approved by the FDA for use in foods, but if they are used as dietary supplements the amounts used may surpass approved levels. Therefore, they are not presently recommended for supplement use
	Avicel	Microcrystalline cellulose			
	CMC	Carboxymethyl cellulose			
	Methylcellulose	Cellulose derivative			

Bulk-producing hydrophilic colloids	Hydroxymethyl-cellulose	Cellulose derivative		
	PVP	Polyvinyl pyrolidine		
	Carbopal	Polyvinyl polymer		
	Polyox Gantrezan	Polyethylene oxide		
	Psyllium hydro-philic colloid (Metamucil)		Yes	?

Source. Dwyer et al. (1978). *Am. J. Hosp. Pharm.* **35:**279–280.

of AAF in rats. However, the influence of other confounding dietary variables do not permit any general conclusions.

While other research was conducted from the 1950s to the present indicating that dietary fiber may alter the toxicity of a wide range of agents including "oestrogens (Ershoff, 1964), glucoascorbic acid (Ershoff, 1954 and 1957), Tween 60 (Ershoff and Hernandez, 1959; Ershoff and Marshall, 1975), chlorazanil hydrochloride (Ershoff, 1959), the red dye, amaranth (Ershoff and Thurston, 1974), sodium cyclamate (Ershoff, 1972), PCBs (Kiriyama et al., 1973), DDT (Kiriyama et al., 1973), heavy metals (Arkhipova and Zorina, 1965), and X-rays (Ershoff et al., 1967, 1969)" (Chadwick et al., 1978), it was not until the 1970s with the previously cited study of Burkitt et al. (1972) that interest was renewed about the possibility that fiber could play a critical role affecting one's susceptibility to developing colon cancer.

B. SPECIFIC POLLUTANTS

1. Chemical Carcinogens

In order to study the influence of dietary fiber on the colonic cancer incidence in animal models, one approach is to see whether low levels of fiber enhance or high levels of fiber retard the development of tumors induced by an agent that is known to cause such colon cancers. The most widely used procedure for testing this hypothesis is to expose rodents (mice and rats) to dimethylhydrazine (DMH). Dimethylhydrazine must undergo metabolic activation to become an alkylating agent responsible for initiating carcinogenesis (Figure 11-1). LaMont and O'Gorman (1978) noted that "because of their chemical stability, high yield of colon cancers, and short latency period, DMH and its derivative azoxymethane (AOM) have become the most widely used colonic carcinogens." In addition, these authors have reported that the clinical and pathological characteristics of DMH-induced colon tumors are quite similar to human colonic tumors. As for rodents, they make excellent animal models since they rarely develop spontaneous colorectal cancer.

As of this writing, 11 studies have been published since the Burkitt et al. (1972) paper concerning the hypothesis that dietary fiber affects the incidence of chemically induced colon cancer. Of these 11 studies, two (Cruse et al., 1978; Watanabe et al., 1978a) did not find that fiber protected against at least one form of intestinal cancer. Of the partially supportive studies, Wilson et al. (1977) reported that a high-fiber

1,2-Dimethylhydrazine $CH_3-NH-NH-CH_3$

$\downarrow$

Azomethane $CH_3-N{=}N-CH_3$

$\downarrow$

Azoxymethane $CH_3-N{=}N-CH_3$
                         $|$
                         O $\downarrow$

Methylazoxymethanol $CH_3-N{=}N-CH_2OH \longleftarrow CH_3-N{=}N-CH_2-O-glucose$
                              $|$ $|$
                              O $\downarrow$ O

Methyldiazonium $CH_3-N\,^{\cdot}{\equiv}N$ Cycasin

$\downarrow$

Carbonium $H_3C^{\cdot} + N_2$

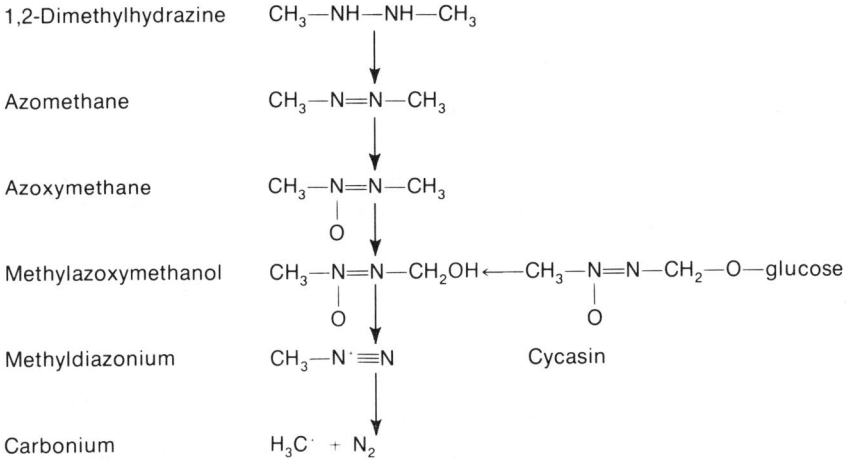

Figure 11-1. Metabolic activation of dimethylhydrazine. 1,2-Dimethylhydrazine, azoxymethane, methylazoxymethanol, and cycasin are colonic carcinogens and are converted to the alkylating agent, methyldiazonium. This compound decomposes spontaneously to generate a highly reactive carbonium ion. *Source.* LaMont and O'Gorman (1978). *Gastroenterology* **75**:1158.

(wheat bran) diet prevented DMH-induced benign but not malignant tumors, while Ward et al. (1973) reported that cellulose (20 or 40%) did not reduce AOM-induced colon cancer but did diminish the frequency of small intestine tumors. With these exceptions, the remaining seven studies found that high levels of dietary fiber were able to reduce the incidence of histopathological changes and/or tumor formation within the colon (Nigro et al., 1979; Chen et al., 1978; Freeman et al., 1978; Fleiszer et al., 1978; Barbolt and Abraham, 1978; Clinton et al., 1978; Watanabe et al., 1978). These studies have utilized a wide range of experimental protocols including: (1) exposures via subcutaneous injection or by gastrointubation; (2) a variety of rat models, including male and female rats of various strains and ages; (3) a variety of fiber types such as cellulose, wheat bran, and alfalfa. However, several of these supportive studies may be questioned (although not totally disregarded), either because of other confounding dietary factors (Fleiszer et al., 1978) or the occurrence of more than 50% of the DMH-exposed animals dying before 15 weeks because of toxicity and not cancer (Chen et al., 1978), and because the bran-DMH group exhibited significantly lower growth rates than controls, thereby causing a decreased growth of tumors probably related to caloric intake (Barbolt and Abraham, 1978).

Despite the limitations of the above reports, there are several studies (Nigro et al., 1979; Freeman et al., 1978; Watanabe et al., 1978) that clearly support the notion that high levels of dietary fiber reduce DMH- or AOM-induced colon cancer. Of particular interest was the recent report of Nigro et al. (1979), which revealed that a 10%-fiber supplement to a diet with 35% fat did not prevent AOM-induced colonic tumor. However, when 20 or 30% fiber was added to a low-fat (6%) diet, AOM-induced tumors were markedly reduced. Such findings clearly suggest that fiber and fat may interact in affecting the incidence of chemically induced colon cancer.

While some of the supportive studies deserve a certain amount of criticism so too does the Cruse et al. (1978) report; for while their research protocol was appropriate and they did not find any protective influence of fiber, it must be recognized that the level of DMH employed caused cancer in all experimental animals whether given fiber supplements or not. Clearly, the possibility exists that these researchers gave such a large dose that it may have totally eliminated any protective influence of the fiber. Thus, it cannot be concluded that their study offered a legitimate test of the hypothesis.

On balance, the findings to date suggest that high levels of dietary fiber reduce the incidence of DMH- and AOM-induced colonic cancers in rodents. However, the occurrence of numerous inconsistencies among the supportive studies and the occurrence of nonsupportive experiments as well indicate that more research is needed in this important area before firm conclusions can be drawn.

One of the major problems in trying to replicate the work of previous authors is the indefinite fiber composition. For example, Barbolt and Abraham (1978) used a wheat-bran supplement, realizing that "wheat bran contains 14% protein, 3% fat, and numerous vitamins and minerals as well as 11% crude fiber." Thus if one were to replicate their work, it would be necessary to utilize an exact replica of their wheat bran, which is probably an impossible task. One can only praise the recent effort of Freeman et al. (1978), which used only highly purified microcrystalline cellulose and no other fiber components. This approach at least offers the chance to provide direct comparisons with other work.

Of further significance is that various fiber differentially prevent the absorption of divalent heavy metals such as zinc. Dietary levels of zinc are known to affect the occurrence of chemical carcinogenesis at least for nitrosamines. How fiber may be indirectly affecting the process of chemical carcinogenesis via modifying the absorption of other nutrients is worth considering.

The level of dietary fiber used in the above reported studies grossly exceeds that consumed by humans. While the average U.S. daily consumption values for total fiber vary between 10–20 g (i.e., less than 5%) (Dwyer et al., 1978), it is not uncommon to find 20–40% of the diets of the experimental animals composed of fiber. Thus efforts should be made to utilize more realistic levels of dietary fiber in the experimentation.

2. Radiation

It has been reported that the level of fiber in the diet markedly affects the susceptibility of rodents to radiation-induced periodontal lesions (Ershoff et al., 1967) and tumor formation (Ershoff et al., 1969). However, the first report noting such a relationship between fiber and radiation exposure was published in 1961 by Greulich and Ershoff, who noted that 100% of mice reared on a highly purified diet and given multiple sublethal doses of total body X-irradiation (six weekly exposures of 200 R each) developed severe periodontal lesions four months after the initial X-ray exposure. In contrast, a comparison group of mice exposed to the identical radiation treatment but reared on a natural food stock diet was much less susceptible to the radiation-induced lesions.

These findings and the confirmative report of Ershoff et al. (1967) are of particular interest in light of the fact that Reichborn-Kjennerud (1963) has demonstrated that gingival inflammation and destruction of periodontal bone may occur in humans following treatment of jaw tumors with radiation.

Not only does the purified diet enhance the development of radiation-induced periodontal lesions, it also enhances the occurrence of radiation- (six weekly exposures of 200 R each) induced tumors (adenocarcinoma of the uterus, lung adenoma, mandibular lymphosarcoma, thymus lymphosarcoma) in mice as compared with controls reared on a stock diet. In their study, the influence of six somewhat different semipurified diets were compared with the stock diet treatment. With respect to the ratio of tumors per mouse, the incidence of tumors ranged from 0.70 to 2.33 for the semipurified diets, while it was only 0.36 on the stock diet (Kritchevsky, 1977).

These findings are quite striking and are clearly in need of further research. How the stock diet provided greater protection from the carcinogenic effects of radiation than a semipurified diet is not known. Generally, the protective effects of fiber with respect to other toxic agents is thought to be via interactions in the gastrointestinal tract. However, this clearly does not appear to be the case with the radiation. Ershoff et al. (1969) speculated that the stock diet may contain higher levels of dietary antioxidants, which may help reduce the adverse effects of the radiation. However, since no measurements of vitamin E and other antioxidants in tissues and blood were made, no correlations could be developed.

3. Bacterial Challenge

While all the previous sections have indicated that dietary fiber exhibits either a neutral or protective influence with respect to pollutant toxicity, this is certainly not the case for susceptibility to bacterial challenge. Several studies have shown that the resistance of mice to Type 1 pneumococcus was increased if reared on a purified diet as compared to a stock diet (Hutchings and Falco, 1946, 1946a). Why this is so was not assessed. However, it was speculated that "some factor essential to the rapid multiplication of the pneumococcus . . . would be absent from, or in low concentration in, the synthetic diet." Regardless of the viability of the theoretical means of protection, it must be realized that this apparent interaction of diet with bacteria is known for only one bacterial strain and may or may not be applicable to others.

4. Fiber—Interactions with Other Toxic Substances

Long before the present intense interest in the role of dietary fiber on the occurrence of colorectal cancer, several groups of researchers systematically evaluated the interaction of fiber with selected toxic substances. The leader in this area concerning dietary fiber-toxic substance interactions has been Dr. Benjamin H. Ershoff whose publications on this topic have spanned over 20 years, and a variety of types of fiber and pollutants.

Stimulating the research program of Dr. Ershoff were several suggestive findings in the 1940s and early 1950s. For instance, azo dyes were found to be more carcinogenic in rats reared on a rice diet compared to controls fed diets with wheat, rye, or millet (Rusch, 1944). Other reports, as previously mentioned, had also indicated that rodents reared on a purified diet were more susceptible than controls administered a high fiber stock diet to the carcinogenic effects of AAF

(Wilson and DeEds, 1950; Engel and Copeland, 1952; Miller et al., 1949) and 4-acetyl-aminobiphenyl (Tuba et al., 1953). However, the first study that Ershoff followed up on was a report by Wooley and Krampitz (1943) concerning the influence of dietary factors on the toxicity of glucoascorbic acid.

a. Glucoascorbic Acid

In their investigations, Wooley and Krampitz (1943) noted that immature mice reared on a purified diet with 5–10% glucoascorbic acid exhibited a failure of growth, developed diarrhea, subcutaneous hemorrhages, alopecia, and premature death. However, these adverse effects did not develop in mice given identical doses of glucoascorbic acid and fed either with a natural food stock ration or with a purified diet supplemented with dry grass. Subsequent studies by Ershoff (1954, 1957) revealed that supplementation of a purified diet with alfalfa meal (10% in diet) was also able to prevent the adverse effects of this toxic agent in both mice and rats. Further experimentation revealed that the alfalfa residue fraction and not the dried alfalfa juice was the component responsible for the protective effect. In addition, other fibrous grasses including dehydrated rye grass, orchard grass, wheat grass, fescue grass, and oat grass were also effective in preventing the toxicity of glucoascorbic acid. Of interest was that supplemental cellulose was also protective, but not to the extent of the aforementioned grasses.

b. Chlorazanil Hydrochloride

Not only could a diet high in fiber diminish the toxicity of glucoascorbic acid, subsequent reports by Ershoff in the late 1950s and early 1960s revealed that such diets could also reduce adverse effects resulting from excessive exposure to chlorazanil hydrochloride (Ershoff, 1959) and several nonionic surface-active agents (Chow et al., 1953; Ershoff and Hernandez, 1959; Ershoff, 1960).

According to Ershoff (1959, 1974), chlorazanil hydrochloride is "a potent, orally active, nonmercurial diuretic which has been effectively employed in Europe and the United States in patients with edema due to congestive heart failure, toxemia of pregnancy, peripheral vascular disease, hepatic cirrhosis, renal disease and other conditions. It is particularly suitable for long-term therapy since with continued administration of the recommended therapeutic dosage, disturbances in the concentrations of plasma electrolytes are not induced and the incidence of side effects is low. In some patients, however, an increase in blood nitrogen occurs, particularly at the higher dosage levels." Of potential significance is that dietary supplementation of a purified diet with alfalfa (20%) partially offset several adverse effects (i.e., growth retardation, increase in serum nonprotein N, urea N, and creatinine) of elevated levels of this drug, which occurred in a comparison group reared on a purified diet.

c. Nonionic Surface-Active Agents

Chow et al. (1953) became interested in the toxicity of nonionic surface-active agents since they had been broadly employed in the processing of common foods. They found that exposure to Tween 60 at 5% or greater in a purified diet with low fiber resulted in a variety of toxic effects in weanling rats, and that these effects could be prevented by the presence of bulk-forming substances in the diet. Later experiments by Ershoff and Hernandez (1959) and Ershoff (1960) revealed that a wide range of fibrous materials (i.e., alfalfa meal, dehydrated rye grass, and orchard grass) were effective in preventing toxicity from this and several other nonionic agents.

d. Amaranth (trisodium salt of 1-(4-sulfo-1-naphthylazo) 2 naphthol-3,6-disulfonic acid); FD and C Red No. 2

Ershoff and Thurston (1974) have reported that the toxicity of the red dye amaranth may be markedly enhanced by feeding rats a purified diet, in contrast to a similar diet supplemented with 10% cellulose, 10% alfalfa meal, or several other fiber-containing substances. While the level of amaranth used in this study was greater than 1000 times the 1972 FDA maximum tolerance for this agent (FDA, 1972), these findings underscore the need to identify conditions that may enhance the toxicity of xenobiotic substances.

e. Sodium Cyclamate

With so much public debate about the safety of continued use of saccharin as an artificial sweetener, there has been discussion that the merits of sodium cyclamate may also be publicly reviewed, since its use as an artificial sweetener may be again petitioned to the FDA. Regardless of what the future holds in store for sodium cyclamate, Ershoff (1972) observed that cyclamate toxicity was markedly affected by diet, with rats (Sprague-Dawley) reared on a semipurified diet being markedly more sensitive than those given a stock diet. In fact, after as early as 3 days on 2.5% cyclamate treatment, the experimental rats experienced diarrhea, alopecia, and growth retardation, while only at the 10% level was there some growth retardation in the stock diet fed rats. Other experiments by Ershoff (1972) revealed that supplementation of the semipurified diet with 20% alfalfa completely eliminated cyclamate-induced toxicity.

Ershoff (1972) contended that "the amount of cyclamate that caused growth retardation in rats fed a purified diet was similar when expressed as percent of the diet to that which has been ingested in the past by many human subjects. For example, 3 bottles of a soft drink, (when cyclamates were permitted as an additive to beverages in the U.S.) could contain a total of 4 g cyclamate. These amounts consumed daily with a normal food intake (400 g dry weight, 2400 calories) would result in a diet containing 1 percent cyclamate. . . . Many persons would habitually consume 8 bottles of soft drink per day, which together with other sources of cyclamate would result in a diet containing in excess of 2.5 percent cyclamate, a level that was toxic to rats fed a purified diet. No data are available as to whether man when fed certain diets would react in the same manner to cyclamate feeding as the rat. However, in view of the wide diversity of diets consumed by human subjects and in view of the fact that the general population is composed not only of normal individuals but also of metabolically defective and sick individuals who may possess varying susceptibilities to toxic agents, the possibility exists that cyclamate when ingested in amounts comparable to that ingested in the past may constitute a hazard in many persons."

f. DBH (2,5-di-t-butylhydroquinone)

Ershoff (1963) extended the list of substances (e.g., DBH) whose toxicity in rats was enhanced in the presence of a semipurified diet as compared to consumption of a stock diet. Such consistent findings led Ershoff (1963) to conclude that "in view of the wide variety of diets that may be ingested by a potential consumer of the test substance, there would appear to be some question as to the validity of assessing the toxicity or nontoxicity of a test compound on findings based on the use of a single diet."

g. Heavy Metals—Cadmium and Lead

Two papers have been published that considered the influence of fiber on cadmium toxicity. The first was by Wilson and DeEds (1950) who reported that rats given a diet with 6% crude fiber were protected from the harmful effects (low weight gain, bleaching of teeth, and anemia) of cadmium at 125 ppm $CdCl_2$ in diets, while rats given only 3% crude fiber in diet were quite susceptible to these Cd induced effects. However, since these two diets differed in other factors, it is not possible to attribute the enhanced susceptibility to the lower amount of fiber. The second study was published in 1977 by Muto and Omori and revealed that the absence of fiber in the diet was associated with enhanced cadmium toxicity. However, since these authors were studying the influence of multiple dietary variables (i.e., protein, calcium, phosphorus, and fiber), it again was not possible to assess the extent, if any, of the contribution of fiber to the occurrence of enhanced cadmium toxicity. As for lead, in the one study published on this topic, Barltrop and Khoo (1975) found that the presence of fiber in the form of cellulose at 3% had no influence on the blood lead levels (as % of ingested dose) as compared to those controls reared on a diet without fiber. However, the presence of only 3% fiber in the diet may not have been enough to have obtained the protective effect. A follow up study with a 10% fiber differential between treatment and controls may be worthwhile.

h. Pesticides—Lindane, an Organochlorine Insecticide

Chadwick et al. (1978) evaluated the influence of several dietary fibers on the metabolism of lindane in Sprague-Dawley weanling female rats. The animals were reared for 28 days on their respective treatments, which included a low-residue diet (LR), LR + 10% pectin, LR + 10% agar, LR + 10% cellulose, or Purina Cat chow, and orally exposed to 2.87 mg of lindane and then sacrificed 24 hours later. The study revealed that the LR group excreted less of the labeled insecticide and that selected tissue samples of the LR group also had low levels of the lindane. Follow up studies with pectin and Purina chow revealed that these two diets affected marked changes in the metabolism of lindane relative to the LR diet. These changes included, among others, an enhanced excretion of radiolabeled products, more conjugated chlorophenols and polar metabolites, and a significant change in the proportions of the excreted chlorophenols. These striking findings of Chadwick et al. (1978) provided clear evidence that at least some fiber types can markedly alter the metabolism of lindane within an animal model. Future studies are needed to extend these findings to other insecticides.

i. Synthetic and Natural Estrogens

Ershoff (1964) reported that stock diets prevented an enlargement of the pituitary gland with several estrogens, including ethinyl estradiol and DES. Furthermore, those rats on the stock diets were more resistant to ethinyl estradiol-induced tumors of the uterus and ovaries.

References

Arkhipova, O.G. and Zorina, L.A. (1965). The use of pectin for the prophylaxis of poisoning by metals: clinical experimental studies. In: *Occupational Diseases in the Chemical Industry,* p. 210. Meditsina, Moscow.

Barbolt, T.A. and Abraham, R. (1978). The effect of bran on dimethylhydrazine-induced colon carcinogenesis in the rat. *Proc. Soc. Exp. Biol. Med.* **157**:656–659.

Barltrop, D. and Khoo, H.E. (1975). The influence of nutritional factors on lead absorption. *Postgrad. Med. J.* **51**:795–800.

Brown, S.M. and Falk, H.L. (1978). Dietary fiber and chemically induced bowel tumours. *Lancet* **2**:1252.

Burkitt, D.P.; Walker, A.R.; and Painter, N.S. (1972). Effect of dietary fiber on stools and transit times, and its role in the causation of disease. *Lancet* **2**:1408–1412.

Chadwick, R.W.; Copeland, M.F.; and Chadwick, C.J. (1978). Enhanced pesticide metabolism, a previously unreported effect of dietary fibre in mammals. *Fd. Cosmet. Toxicol.* **16**:217–225.

Chen, W.F.; Patchefsky, A.S.; and Goldsmith, A.S. (1978). Colonic protection from dimethylhydrazine by a high fiber diet. *Surgery, Gynecology and Obstetrics* **147**:503–506.

Chow, B.F.; Burnett, J.M.; Ling, C.T.; and Barrows, L. (1953). Effects of basal diets on the response of rats to certain dietary non-ionic surface-active agents. *J. Nutr.* **49**:563–577.

Clinton, S.K.; Truex, C.R.; and Visek, W.J. (1978). A model system for evaluating the role of dietary fiber in chemical carcinogenesis. *Biochem. Pharmacol.* **27**:1393–1396.

Crofts, T.J. (1979). Bran and experimental colon cancer. *Lancet* **1**:108.

Cruse, J.P.; Lewin, M.R.; and Clark, C.G. (1978). Failure of bran to protect against experimental colon cancer in rats. *Lancet* **2**:1278–1280.

Cummings, J.H. (1978). Dietary factors in the aetiology of gastrointestinal cancer. *J. Human Nutr.* **32**:455–465.

Dwyer, J.T.; Goldin, B.; Gorbach, S.; and Patterson, J. (1978). Drug therapy reviews: dietary fiber and fiber supplements in the therapy of gastrointestinal disorders. *Amer. J. Hosp. Pharm.* **35**:278–287.

Engel, R.W. and Copeland, D.H. (1952). Protective action of stock diets against the cancer-inducing action of 2-acetylaminofluorene in rats. *Cancer Res.* **12**:211–215.

Ershoff, B.H. (1954). Protective effects of alfalfa in immature mice fed toxic doses of glucoascorbic acid. *Proc. Soc. Exp. Biol. Med.* **87**:134–136.

Ershoff, B.H. (1957). Beneficial effects of alfalfa and other succulent plants on glucoascorbic acid toxicity in the rat. *Proc. Soc. Exp. Biol. Med.* **95**:656–659.

Ershoff, B.H. (1959). Beneficial effects of alfalfa meal on chlorazanil hydrochloride toxicity in the rat. *Exp. Med. Surg.* **17**:204–209.

Ershoff, B.H. (1960). Beneficial effects of alfalfa meal and other bulk-containing or bulk-forming materials on the toxicity of nonionic surface active agents in the rat. *J. Nutr.* **70**:484–490.

Ershoff, B.H. (1963). Comparative effects of a purified and stock diet on DBH (2,5-di-tertbutylhydroquinone) toxicity in the rat. *Proc. Soc. Exp. Biol. Med.* **112**:362–365.

Ershoff, B.H. (1964). Effects of diet on pituitary tumor induction by estrogens. *Expl. Med. Surg.* **22**:28–32.

Ershoff, B.H. (1972). Comparative effects of a purified diet and stock ration on sodium cyclamate toxicity in rats. *Proc. Soc. Exp. Biol. Med.* **141**:857–862.

Ershoff, B.H. (1974). Antitoxic effects of plant fiber. *Am. J. Clin. Nutr.* **27**:1395.

Ershoff, B.H.; Bajwa, G.S.; Field, J.B.; and Bavetta, L.A. (1969). Comparative effects of purified diets and a natural food stock ration on the tumor incidence of mice exposed to multiple sublethal doses of total body X-irradiation. *Cancer Res.* **29**:780–788.

Ershoff, B.H.; Bajwa, G.S.; Shapiro, M.; and Bernick, S. (1967). Comparative effect of a purified diet and natural food stock rations on the periodontium of mice exposed to multiple sublethal doses of total body X-irradiation. *J. Dent. Res.* **46**:1051–1057.

Ershoff, B.H. and Hernandez, H.J. (1959). Beneficial effects of alfalfa meal and other bulk containing or bulk-forming material on symptoms of Tween 60 toxicity in the immature mouse. *J. Nutr.* **69**:172–178.

Ershoff, B.H. and Marshall, W.E. (1975). Protective effects of dietary fiber in rats fed toxic doses of sodium cyclamate and polyoxyethylene sorbitan monostearate (Tween 60). *J. Fd. Sci.* **40**:357.

Ershoff, B.H. and Thurston, E.W. (1974). Effects of diet on amaranth (FD & C Red No. 2) toxicity in the rat. *J. Nutr.* **104**:937–942.

Fleiszer, D.; Murray, D.; MacFarlane, J.; and Brown, R.A. (1978). Protective effect of dietary fibre against chemically induced bowel tumours in rats. *Lancet* **2**:552–553.

Food and Drug Administration, Dept. of HEW (1972). Color additive FD and C Red No. 2. Proposed limit on ingestion. *Fed. Reg.* No. 129, pp. 13181–13182.

Freeman, H.J.; Spiller, G.A.; and Kim, Y.S. (1978). A double-blind study on the effect of purified cellulose dietary fiber on 1,2-dimethylhydrazine induced rat colonic neoplasia. *Cancer Res.* **38**:2912–2917.

Greulich, R.C. and Ershoff, B.H. (1961). Delayed effects of multiple sublethal doses of total body X-irradiation on the periodontium and teeth of mice. *J. Dent. Res.* **40**:1211–1224.

Hill, M.J. (1978). Some leads to the etiology of cancer of the large bowel. *Surgery Annual* **10**:135–149.

Hutchings, G.H. and Falco, E.A. (1946). Effect of nutrition on susceptibility of mice to pneumococcal infection. *Proc. Soc. Exp. Biol. Med.* **61**:54–57.

Hutchings, G.H. and Falco, E.A. (1946a). Effects of whole-wheat and white bread diets on susceptibility of mice to pneumococcal infection. *Science* **104**:568–569.

Kiriyama, S.; Inoue, S.; Machinaka, T.; and Yoshida, A. (1973). Effect of addition of nonnutritive polysaccharides on toxicity of dietary polychlorinated biphenyls (PCB) and 1,1,1-trichloro-2,2-bis (p-chlorophenyl) ethane (p,p'-DDT). *J. Jap. Soc. Fd. Nutr.* **26**:15.

Kritchevsky, D. (1977). Modification by fiber of toxic dietary effects. *Fed. Proc.* **36**(5):1692–1695.

Kritchevsky, D. (1979). Metabolic effects of dietary fiber. *Western J. Med.* **130**(2):123–127.

LaMont, J.H. and O'Gorman, T.A. (1978). Experimental colon cancer. *Gastroenterology* **75**:1157–1169.

Lowenfels, A.B. (1979). Bran and experimental colon cancer. *Lancet* **1**:108.

Matzkies, F. and Berg, G. (1978). Dietary fiber syndrome as the cause of disease in civilized societies. *Acta Hepato-Gastroenterol.* **25**:402–407.

Miller, E.C.; Miller, J.A.; Sandin, R.B.; and Brown, R.K. (1949). The carcinogenic activities of certain analogues of 2-acetylaminofluorene in the rat. *Cancer Res.* **9**:504–509.

Modan, B. (1977). Role of diet in cancer etiology. *Cancer* **40**:1887–1891.

Muto, Y. and Omori, M. (1977). Nutritional influence on the onset of renal damage due to long-term administration of cadmium in young and adult rats. *J. Nutr. Sci. Vitaminol.* **23**:349–360.

Newcombe, R.G. (1979). Bran and experimental colon cancer. *Lancet* **1**:108.

Nigro, N.D.; Bull, A.W.; Klopfer, B.A.; Pak, M.S.; and Campbell, R.L. (1979). Effect of dietary fiber on azoxymethane-induced intestinal carcinogenesis in rats. *J. Natl. Cancer Inst.* **62**:1097–1102.

Reddy, B.S. (1976). Dietary factors and cancer of the large bowel. *Seminars in Oncology* **3**(4):351–359.

Reichborn-Kjennerud, I. (1963). Dento-alveolar resorption in periodontal disorders. In: *Mechanisms of Hard Tissue Destruction,* Sognnaes, R.E., editor, pp. 297–319. Washington, D.C., AAAS.

Rusch, H.P. (1944). Extrinsic factors that influence carcinogenesis. *Physiol. Rev.* **24**:177–204.

Spiller, G.A. and Arnen, R.J. (1975). Dietary fiber in human nutrition. *CRC Crit. Rev. Food Sci. Nutr.* **7**:39.

Spiller, G.A. and Shipley, E.A. (1977). Perspectives in dietary fiber in human nutrition. *Wld. Rev. Nutr. Diet* **27**:105–131.

Spiller, G.A.; Shipley, E.A.; and Blake, J.A. (1978). Recent progress in dietary fiber (Plantix) in human nutrition. *CRC Crit. Rev. Food Sci. Nutr.* **10**:31–90.

Thorne, M.C. (1979). Bran and experimental colon cancer. *Lancet* **1**:10.

Tuba, J.; Rawlinson, H.S.; Fraser, M.S.; and Jeske, I. (1953). Hyperplastic nodules in rat mammary glands following feeding of 4-acetylamino biphenyl. *Canad. J. Res.* **31**:95–98.

Ward, J.M.; Yamamoto, R.S.; and Weisburger, J.H. (1973). Cellulose dietary bulk and azoxymethane-induced intestinal cancer. *J. Natl. Cancer Inst.* **51**:713–715.

Watanabe, K.; Reddy, B.S.; and Kritchevsky, D. (1978). Effect of various dietary fibers and food additives on azoxymethane or methylnitrosourea-induced colon carcinogenesis in rats. *Federat. Proc.* **37**:262.

Watanabe, K.; Reddy, B.S.; Wong, C.O.; and Weisburger, J.H. (1978a). Effect of dietary undergraded carrageen on colon carcinogenesis in F344 rats treated with azoxymethane or methylnitrosourea. *Cancer Res.* **38**:4427–4430.

Wilson, R. and DeEds, F. (1950). Importance of diet in studies of chronic toxicity. *Arch. Ind. Hyg. Occup. Med.* **1**:73–80.

Wilson, R.; Hutcheson, D.P.; and Wideman, L. (1977). Dimethylhydrazine-induced colon tumors in rats fed diets containing beef fat or corn oil with and without wheat bran. *Amer. J. Clin. Nutr.* **30**:176–181.

Wooley, D.W. and Krampitz, L.O. (1943). Production of a scurvy-like condition by feeding a compound structurally related to ascorbic acid. *J. Exptl. Med.* **78**:333.

C. EVALUATION OF SPECIFIC FIBROUS MATERIAL

1. Alginate and Pectate

a. *Strontium*

The exposure of humans to radioactive strontium from atmospheric testing of nuclear weapons and the prospective danger of an inadvertent release of radioactive substances from nuclear power plants is an important public health concern. Since radioactive strontium is a well-known carcinogen that is rapidly deposited in bone, efforts have been made to assess the efficacy of removing strontium from the bone as well as preventing its absorption from the gastrointestinal tract. While attempts to remove strontium from bone have not proven to be very successful (see Chapter 1 of this volume), very promising results have been obtained through dietary manipulation via the use of sodium alginate, a derivative of kelp. This acts to selectively inhibit the gastrointestinal absorption of strontium, thereby reducing the potential retention of strontium by the body. The intention of this section is to review the development of the use of sodium alginate in preventing the uptake of strontium in animal models and humans and to assess its efficacy as a prophylactic treatment.

Considerable research during the early to mid-1960s was directed toward the discovery of substances (i.e., naturally occurring macromolecular compounds with ion-exchange properties [Kahn et al., 1963; Paul et al., 1964; Skoryna et al., 1964]) that could possibly serve to diminish the intestinal absorption of strontium. After preliminary testing, a polymer of mannuronic and guluronic acid called alginic acid emerged as the most effective agent (Figure 11-2).

Initial testing of this compound by Skoryna et al. (1964a) revealed that the administration of sodium alginate into ligated intestinal segments of rats markedly diminished the intestinal absorption, blood level, and bone uptake of simultaneously administered strontium[90]. Of further importance was the concomitant observation that sodium alginate administration exhibited a negligible effect on the absorption and uptake of calcium[45]. Subsequent studies by Skoryna and his associates revealed that sodium alginate reduced the absorption of strontium in rats when introduced directly into the stomach by intubation (Paul et al., 1964), as well as when given orally in food or in drinking water (Waldron-Edward et al., 1964; Skoryna et al., 1965). In the Waldron-Edward et al. (1964) study, the amount of strontium absorbed was inversely related to the amount of dietary alginate. In fact, when the diet consisted of 24% alginate, strontium[89] uptake was reduced by

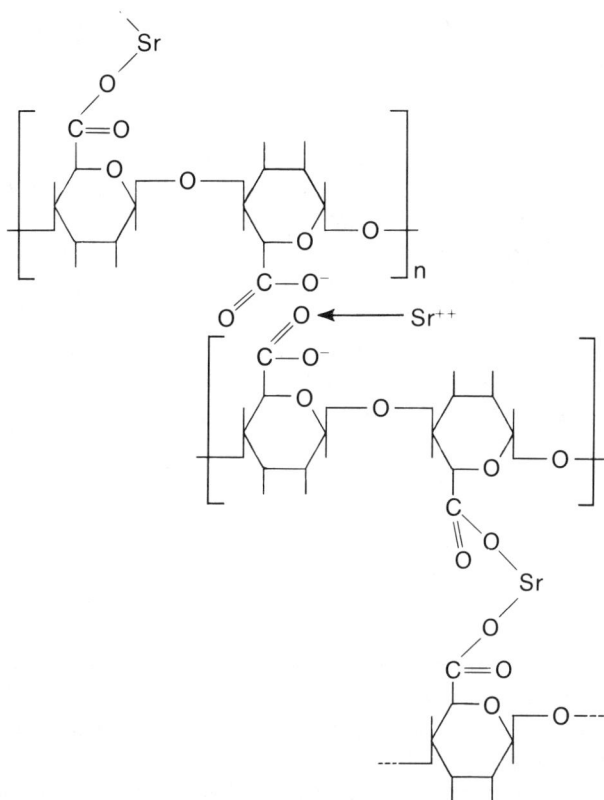

Figure 11-2. Proposed structure of strontium salt of polymannuronic acid. *Source.* Skoryna et al., 1964.

83%. At low levels of alginate (i.e., 3%), no influence on calcium uptake was observed. However, as the concentration increased to 24%, a 47% decrease in calcium[45] uptake occurred. According to the authors, these findings were of potential significance for human studies since the form in which sodium alginate was applied (i.e., in jelly form) proved to be palatable and did not cause disruptions of digestive tract function, including a lack of constipation and no alteration in the electrolyte balance. In addition, the alginate does not bind to alkali metals and while at low concentrations, does not disrupt calcium metabolism.

Several other research groups have also verified the initial finding that sodium alginate reduces the gastrointestinal absorption of strontium in rats (Moore and Elder, 1965; Waldron-Edward et al., 1965; Harrison et al., 1966; Light et al., 1970).

Some of these investigations considered the potential usefulness of nontoxic and nonabsorbable polyelectrolytes other than sodium alginate that have been employed in food preparation. In this regard Waldron-Edward et al. (1965) reported that polygalacturonic acid, carboresin, Rexyn 101, and pectic acid were effective in reducing the uptake of strontium in rats. While several substances were found that could discriminate against strontium absorption, further research indicated some chemical factors that may contribute to the differential capabilities of certain polyelectrolytes to prevent strontium absorption. For example, Harrison et al. (1966) have shown that alginate that contained higher proportions of guluronic acid relative to mannuronic acid exhibits enhanced ability to discriminate against strontium.

Several studies have also indicated that strontium uptake in humans is markedly reduced by the concomitant ingestion of sodium alginate (Hesp and Ramsbottom, 1965; Harrison et al., 1966; Hodgkinson et al., 1967; Sutton, 1967; Sutton et al., 1971). In a study in which only 1.5 gm of alginate was administered on a single occasion, a twofold reduction in strontium uptake was observed (Harrison et al., 1966). Higher doses of alginate of up to 10 grams resulted in further reductions (up to a factor of 9) in the amount of strontium absorbed (Hesp and Ramsbottom, 1965). As in the case with animal model studies, humans were also found to have greater strontium discrimination when the alginate contained a greater guluronic/mannuronic acid ratio (Hodgkinson et al., 1967).

The theory behind how the alginate discriminates against the uptake of strontium is, as implied above, by an ion-exchange mechanism. Since this is an ion-exchange process, it is expected that the alginate would also be effective against other ions (Hodgkinson et al., 1967):

"Thus, the binding of one molecule of strontium, calcium, or magnesium was accompanied by the release of two molecules of sodium into solution while one molecule of ferric iron displaced three sodium (atoms). Secondly, binding was dependent upon pH. Finally, the affinity of sodium alginate for ferric iron, strontium, calcium, and magnesium appeared to decrease in the following order: Fe > Sr > Ca > Mg. The binding process might therefore be depicted as follows":

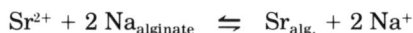

$$Sr^{2+} + 2\,Na_{alginate} \rightleftharpoons Sr_{alg.} + 2\,Na^+$$

In light of these ion-exchange properties, the prolonged ingestion of sodium alginate might be predicted to reduce the absorption of iron and other essential metals; in fact, this was observed by Hodgkinson et al. (1967) with human subjects. However, this observation was not confirmed by Harrison (1967), who reported no reduction in the absorption of Na, K, Ca, Mg, or Zn or in the body retention of P in rats fed a diet with 10% sodium alginate for over a year.

Conclusions. It has been shown that the absorption of strontium in rats and humans can be markedly diminished by the concomitant ingestion of sodium alginate, an extract of brown algae. Since sodium alginate preparations have been made that are palatable to humans, the possibility of their use by humans is quite apparent. However, adoption of the widespread use of sodium alginate as a strategy for reducing one's strontium body burden is hopefully one that it will not be necessary to consider. Within the past several years there has been potential concern over the strontium-90 contamination of cow's milk due to the atmospheric testing of nuclear weapons by the People's Republic of China. Usually in these situations the U.S. government orders dairy farmers to put their cows in barns and feed them uncontaminated food. Whether sodium alginate could be used by farmers for their milking cows may be of some interest. In general, if there was a high enough level of strontium-90 contamination to suggest the use of alginate, then the level of contamination would probably be high enough to call for an evacuation.

b. Lead

Several investigators have evaluated the influence of alginate on the absorption of lead in rats (Carr et al., 1969) and humans (Harrison et al., 1969). According to Harrison et al. (1969), "the expected stability constants of other metal alginates indicate that such dietary supplements may suppress the absorption of certain heavy metals, many of which are regarded as toxic. In particular, the ionotropic series quoted by Haug (1964) shows that lead is much more strongly bound to alginate than is strontium. If the absorption of lead could be diminished by alginate supplementation, this would be of interest, especially because of the continued occurrence of lead intoxication in children primarily via the consumption of leaded paint chips. However, despite the theoretical predictions that alginate may reduce lead absorption, it was found to be without apparent effect in the limited human studies of Harrison et al. (1969) and actually stimulated absorption (i.e., 3.7 vs. 9.1%) in rats.

Besides alginate and an alginate-like polyuronate produced by certain bacteria (Carlson and Matthews, 1966; Linker and Jones, 1966), Paskins-Hurlburt et al. (1977) have reported that the only other naturally occurring polyuronate is pectate. Because of its similarity to alginate in its chemical interactions, Paskins-Hurlburt et al. (1977) decided to test its capacity to affect the uptake of lead in rats, using the ligated intestinal-segment technique and duodenal-section procedures. The pectate treatment resulted in up to an 87% reduction in the amount of lead absorbed, resulting in a marked diminution in the amount of lead in the blood (Figure 11-3), kidneys, and liver. Based on these findings, the authors concluded that the biological effectiveness of pectate [in preventing lead absorption] is significant, for it may well explain the difference in the blood-lead levels of people of various backgrounds. Pectates are present in citrus fruits and other plants and the varying levels of dietary intake of these foodstuffs may be reflected in the wide range of concentrations of lead found in the blood. Not only does pectate bind with lead but also with a number of other cations,

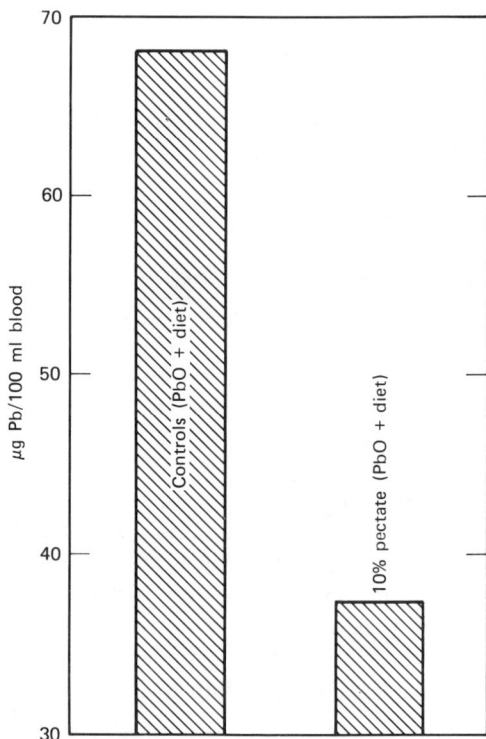

Figure 11-3. Effect of pectate on the blood-lead levels of weanling rats. [*Source.* Paskins-Hurlburt, A.J.; Tanaka, Y.; Skoryna, S.C.; Moore, W., Jr.; and Stara, J.F. (1977). The binding of lead by a pectic polyelectrolyte. *Environ. Res.* **14:**128–140.

including the highly toxic heavy metals strontium, nickel, and cadmium.

Recent industrial studies have supported the hypothesis that consumption of pectin reduces the occurrence of lead toxicity. Stantschev et al. (1979) reported that consumption of 48% esterified apple pectin in 100 g of yogurt for 28 days markedly reduced lead-induced hematological changes (e.g., increased punctured erythrocytes and reticulocytes) as well as enhancing the excretion of lead in the urine in 28 lead-exposed workers. Twenty-five industrially exposed individuals serving as controls not only did not show improved values but showed a further deterioration of such values. Based on these findings, these researchers recommended "the administration of about 50% esterified apple pectin as an antidote and prophylactic agent to those exposed to lead."

References

Carlson, M.C. and Matthews, L.W. (1966). Polyuronic acids produced by *Pseudomonas aeruginosa*. *Studies Polyuronic Acids* **5**:9.

Carr, T.E.F.; Harrison, G.E.; Humphreys, E.R.; and Sutton, A. (1968). Reduction in the absorption and retention of dietary strontium in man by alginate. *Int. J. Radiat. Biol.* **14**:225–233.

Carr, T.E.F.; Nolan, J. and Durakovic, A. (1969). Effect of alginate on the absorption and excretion of ^{203}Pb in rats fed milk and normal diets. *Nature* **224**:1115.

Comar, E.L. (1965). *Ann. Rev. Nucl. Sci.* **15**:175.

Feldman, H.S.; Urbach, K.; Naegele, C.F.; Regan, F.D.; and Doerner, A.A. (1952). Cation absorption by alginic acid in humans. *Proc. Soc. Exp. Biol. Med.* **79**:439–441.

Fischer, F.G. and Dorfel, H. (1962). *Z. Physiol. Chem.* **302**:186.

Harrison, G.E. (1967). *Symposium on Diagnosis and Treatment of Deposited Radionuclides.* Richland, WA.

Harrison, G.E.; Carr, T.E.F.; Sutton, A.; Humphreys, E.R.; and Rundo, J. (1969). Effect of alginate on the absorption of lead in man. *Nature* **224**:1115–1116.

Harrison, G.E.; Humphreys, E.R.; Sutton, A.; and Shepherd, H. (1966). Strontium uptake in rats on alginate-supplemented diet. *Science* **152**:655–666.

Harrison, J.; McNeill, K.G.; and Janiga, A. (1966). The effect of sodium alginate on the absorption of strontium and calcium in human subjects. *Canad. Med. Assoc. J.* **95**:532–534.

Haug, A. (1964). Report No. 30. Composition and properties of alginates. Norwegian Inst. of Seaweed Research, Trondheim, 74. (Cited in Harrison et al., 1969).

Haug, A. and Larsen, B. (1962). Quantitative determination of the uronic composition of alginates. *Acta Chem. Scand.* **16**:1908–1918.

Hava, A. (1959). Ion exchange properties of alginate fractions. *Acta Chem. Scand.* **13**:1250–1251.

Hesp, R. and Ramsbottom, B. (1965). Effect of sodium alginate in inhibiting uptake of radiostrontium by the human body. *Nature* **208**:1341–1342.

Hodgkinson, A.; Nordin, B.E.C.; Hambleton, J.; and Oxby, C.B. (1967). Radiostrontium absorption in man: suppression by calcium and by sodium alginate. *Canad. Med. Assoc. J.* **97**:1139–1143.

Kahn, D.S.; Makhani, J.S.; and Skoryna, S.C. (1963). Studies of the late effects of internal irradiation by radioactive strontium in the rat. *Laval Med.* **34**:169–183.

Light, J.M.; Stookey, G.K.; and Muhler, J.C. (1970). The effects of sodium alginate and other untested polymers on radiostrontium retention in the rat. *Proc. Soc. Exp. Biol. Med.* **133**:1259–1264.

Linker, A. and Jones, R.S. (1966). Á new polysaccharide resembling alginic acid isolated from Pseudomonads. *J. Biol. Chem.* **241**:3845–3851.

McDowell, R.H. (1958). *Chemistry and Industry.* 1401.

Millis, J. and Reed, F.B. (1947). The effect of sodium alginate on the absorption of calcium. *Biochem. J.* **41**:273–275.

Moore, W. and Elder, R.L. (1965). Effect of alginic acid on the movement of strontium-85 and calcium-45 across surviving ileal segments. *Nature* **206**:841–842.

Paskins-Hurlburt, A.J.; Tanaka, Y.; Skoryna, S.C.; Moore, W., Jr.; and Stara, J.F. (1977). The binding of lead by a pectic polyelectrolyte. *Environ. Res.* **14**:128–140.

Patrick, G.; Carr, T.E.F.; and Humphreys, E.R. (1967). Inhibition by alginates of strontium absorption studied *in vitro* and *in vivo*. *Intern. J. Rad. Biol.* **12**:427–434.

Paul, T.M.; Edward, D.W.; and Skoryna, S.C. (1964). Studies on inhibition of intestinal absorption of radioactive strontium. II. Effects of administration of sodium alginate by orogastric intubation and feeding. *Canad. Med. Assoc. J.* **91**:553–557.

Paul, T.M.; Waldron–Edward, C.; and Skoryna, S.C. (1964a). *Proc. Canad. Fed. Biol. Soc.* **1**:40.

Rosenthal, M.W. (1960). Radioisotope absorption and methods of elimination: factors influencing elimination from the body. In: A symposium on radioisotopes in the biospheres. Edited by R.S. Caldecott and L.A. Snyder. University of Minnesota, Minneapolis, October 19–23, 1959. Univ. of Minn. Press, p. 541.

Skoryna, S.C.; Paul, T.M.; and Waldron-Edward, D. (1964). Studies on inhibition of intestinal absorption of radioactive strontium. I. Prevention of absorption from ligated intestinal segments. *Canad. Med. Assoc. J.* **91**:285–288.

Skoryna, S.C.; Paul, T.M.; and Waldron-Edward, D. (1964a). Rapp. Teme Comg. Int. de Gastroenterologue. **3**:291.

Skoryna, S.C.; Paul, T.M.; and Waldron-Edward, D. (1965). Studies on inhibition of intestinal absorption of radioactive strontium. IV. Estimation of the suppression effect of sodium alginate. *Canad. Med. Assoc. J.* **93**:404–407.

Stantschev, von St.; Kratschanov, Chr.; Popova, M.; Kirtschev, N.; and Martschev, M.C. (1979). Administration of granulated pectin to workers exposed to lead. *Zeit. Ges. Hygiene Grenzgebiete* **25**:585–87.

Stara, J. and Waldron-Edward, D. (1968). *Symposium on Diagnosis and Treatment of Deposited Radionuclides.* Edited by H.A. Kornberg and N.D. Norwood. p. 340. Richland, WA.

Sutton, A. (1967). Reduction of strontium absorption in man by the addition of alginate to the diet. *Nature* **216**:1005–1007.

Sutton, A.; Harrison, G.E.; Carr, T.E.F.; and Barltrop, D. (1971). Reduction in the absorption of dietary strontium in children by an alginate derivative. *Int. J. Radiat. Biol.* **19**:79–85.

Van der Borght, O.; Colard, J.; van Puymbroeck, S.; and Kirshman, R. (1966). Radioecological concentration processes. *Proc. Intern. Sym.*, Stockholm, p. 589.

Waldron-Edward, D.; Paul, T.M.; and Skoryna, S.C. (1964). Studies on the inhibition of intestinal absorption of radioactive strontium. *Canad. Med. Assoc. J.* **91**:1006–1010.

Waldron-Edward, D.; Paul, T.M.; and Skoryna, S.C. (1965). Suppression of intestinal absorption of radioactive strontium by naturally occurring non-absorbable polyelectrolytes. *Nature* **205**:1117–1118.

D. DIETARY FIBER—POLLUTANT INTERACTIONS— A PERSPECTIVE

There is a rapidly growing interest in the health implications of dietary fiber. How much fiber should be consumed for optimal health? What kind of fiber? What are the negative features of too much or too little dietary fiber? While biomedical researchers are actively pursuing answers to such questions, there is sufficient evidence to indicate that the amount and type of fiber in the diet does affect susceptibility of animal models to a wide range of toxic and carcinogenic substances.

Most of the early investigations employed the use of stock versus purified or semipurified diets. While it is evident that a major difference between such diets is the level and type of fiber, there are numerous other potential dietary differences that may have contributed to the impressive findings of these earlier studies. Nevertheless, attempts to specifically locate the "source of protection" by the addition of specific fibrous agents to semipurified diets unquestionably supported the protective role of such substances as alfalfa, cellulose, and others. In general, the mechanism by which fiber may prevent pollutant toxicity is unknown. However, fiber is thought to (1) dilute the concentration of the toxic agent, and (2) reduce its contact with the intestinal mucosa by speeding up fecal elimination. These two factors should assist in minimizing the potential for colo–rectal carcinogens to initiate carcinogenesis. How fiber reduces the toxicity of substances such as Tween 60, sodium cyclamate, DMB, and others remains to be seen. Perhaps there is considerable binding of the toxic substances to the fiber (as is the case for alginate and pectate), thereby preventing its absorption and thus eliminating the agent(s) from reaching the site of action. Experimentation along these lines is certainly feasible and worthwhile.

As is usually the case, the level of fiber studied often exceeded a level well above that normally consumed in human populations. Generally about 2.5–5.0% of the U.S. diet is composed of fiber. However, for vegetarians the percentage of fiber in the diet may be between 5 and 10%. Yet many studies cited here utilized a 20% value, with some studies going as high as 40%. Clearly, future studies should use a fiber level that is within a normal range of consumption.

Another area of great concern is the capacity of fiber to preferentially bind with various dietary components, especially divalent cations such as calcium and zinc. Since this book has shown that changes in the nutritional status of these other elements may markedly affect pollutant toxicity, it is important for future fiber-pollutant research to consider the metal-binding capacity of fiber.

12

Synthetic Antioxidants

IT HAS BEEN DEMONSTRATED that antioxidants such as α-tocopherol and selenium may help reduce or prevent the occurrence of cancers in mice induced by certain polycyclic hydrocarbons and promoted by croton oil (Shamberger, 1970). If naturally occurring antioxidants may provide some degree of protection from environmental cancer, it may be hypothesized that synthetic antioxidants such as butylated hydroxyanisole (BHA) and butylated hydroxytoluene (BHT) may also act via a similar chemopreventive fashion. The potential significance of this suggestion becomes quite apparent when it is realized that these phenolic antioxidants are widely employed as preservatives in foods consumed by human populations. In fact, it has been estimated that the amount of phenolic antioxidants ingested per capita is about 2 mg/day in the United States (Collings and Sharratt, 1970).

In 1972, Wattenberg published the first evaluation of this hypothesis. He reported that the antioxidants BHA, BHT, and ethoxyquin were very effective in preventing several types of cancer (i.e., mammary and forestomach cancer) caused by benzo[a]pyrene (BP) and 7,12-dimethylbenz[a]anthracene (DMBA) in rodents. In addition, BHA

453

decreased dietary DMBA-induced lethality in mice while all three antioxidants prevented DMBA-induced adrenal necrosis in female rats.

Subsequent reports by Wattenberg (1972a, 1973, 1974) confirmed and considerably extended his earlier findings. Experiments with BHA revealed that intraperitoneal administration of this antioxidant resulted in a reduced number of diethylnitrosamine (DEN) and 4-nitroquinoline-N-oxide induced pulmonary adenomas (Wattenberg, 1972a), while dietary BHA protected against pulmonary neoplasia from a wide variety of carcinogens including BP, DMBA, urethan, and uracil mustard.

These original and striking findings of Wattenberg, as could be expected, generated considerable interest within the scientific community. Consequently, there has been a growing number of research papers published in this area since 1972. In general, most investigators have confirmed the original finding that BHA and BHT may protect against previously known and several previously untested chemical carcinogens (e.g., N-2-fluorenylacetamide, N-hydroxy-N-2-fluorenylacetamide) (Ulland et al., 1973; Slaga and Bracken, 1977; Clapp et al., 1974, 1976; Clapp, 1978; Cumming and Walton, 1973; King et al., 1977), and acute toxicity from several nitrosamines, X-irradiation (Clapp, 1978), and UV light-induced erythema (DeRios et al., 1978) and viral infection (Brugh, 1977). In addition, Shamberger et al. (1973) reported that BHT affected a 63.8% reduction in the occurrence of chromosomal breaks in human leukocyte cultures treated with DMBA. Other studies utilizing a combination of antioxidants including ascorbic acid, α-tocopherol, BHT, and others have indicated that such a treatment reduces the occurrence of UV-induced tumors in mice (Black and Chan, 1975; Black, 1974).

As a result of these studies, which consistently indicated that BHT and BHA prevent the occurrence of tumors from a range of chemical carcinogens, several questions emerge. What are the mechanisms by which these compounds prevent toxicity and carcinogenicity? Could other synthetic antioxidants be developed that are even more effective in preventing carcinogenicity, especially once the mechanism of action is determined? Since all animal studies have been with rodents, how accurate are these models in predicting the response in humans? Could the ingestion of these synthetic antioxidants in the human diet be a protection against the adverse effects of low-level exposure to ubiquitous carcinogenic agents such as BP, nitrosamines, and others?

Some progress has been made in elucidating the mechanism(s) by which these agents may prevent carcinogenesis. Wattenberg (1975) has stated that these agents may (1) have some form of direct interaction with the reactive species of carcinogens, or they (2) may act more indirectly, such as the modification of enzyme activity.

It is widely known that phenolic antioxidants modify the microsomal mixed-function oxidase (MFO) system. For example, they alter the activities of aminopyrine demethylase, hexobarbitone oxidase, and nitroanisole demethylase (Creaven et al., 1966; Gilbert et al., 1969; Martin and Gilbert, 1968). Since the MFO system can both detoxify chemical carcinogens and/or bioactivate them to proximate or ultimate carcinogenic forms, a clarification of how phenolic antioxidants affect this system may help explain their anticarcinogenic activities.

An interesting observation by Speier and Wattenberg (1975) revealed that incubation of BP and DNA with microsomes from BHA-fed mice caused a marked reduction (i.e., by 50%) in the binding of BP metabolites to DNA as compared to controls (Table 1). Presumably, this reduction in binding capacity to DNA may diminish the opportunity for initiation.

Table 1. Microsomal AHH Activity and Binding of BP Metabolites to DNA in Livers of Mice Fed BHA and Corresponding Controls

Experiment Number	AHH Activity in		Binding of BP Metabolites to DNA[a]			
	BHA-Fed Mice (U/mg wet wt)[b]	Controls (U/mg wet wt)[b]	μCi/80 μg BP Added to Reaction Mixture	BHA-Fed Mice (dpm/ mg DNA)	Controls (dpm/ mg DNA)	Ratio of BHA/ Control
1	4.2	4.8	0.25	162	279	0.58
2	9.8	9.1	0.25	288	683	0.42
3	8.5	9.0	0.25	221	564	0.39
4	8.0	7.9	0.25	306	701	0.44
5	5.7	5.2	0.45	499	847	0.59
6	8.6	8.4	0.45	437	894	0.49
7	8.6	8.2	1.80	2,735	5,512	0.50

[a]Binding of BP metabolites to calf thymus DNA in a reaction mixture also containing ^{14}C-BP, liver microsomes, and NADPH.
[b]1 U = fluorescence equivalent to 0.1 ng 3-hydroxybenzo[α]pyrene/minute.

Source. Speier, J.L. and Wattenberg, L.W. (1975). Alterations in microsomal metabolism of benzo[a]pyrene in mice fed butylated hydroxyanisole. *J. Natl. Cancer Inst.* **55**(2):470.

Another report (Grantham et al., 1973) has revealed that BHT administration enhances the excretion of carcinogens (N-2-fluorenylacetamide and N-hydroxy-N-2-fluorenylacetamide) via conjugation with glucuronic acid. In addition, the BHT also reduced the binding of the carcinogen to DNA 48 hours after injection of the carcinogen in agreement with Speier and Wattenberg (1975). As consistent as these findings may be with respect to elucidating the chemopreventive mechanism of BHT and BHA, it must be remembered that these compounds are also free-radical scavengers and may affect their protective function in a manner involving this characteristic as well.

Wattenberg (1972) has tried to develop an extrapolation of his findings to the human condition for the purpose of risk assessment. First, one must accept the usual assumptions that mice and humans respond identically to the BHA and BP and that the BP acts according to a nonthreshold process. He then goes on to state that "5 mg BHA/g of diet exerted an inhibitory effect against 1 mg BP/g of diet [Table 2]. This was [the] most favorable experiment in terms of obtaining inhibition with a low ratio of antioxidant to carcinogen. . . . A dietary intake of 2 mg antioxidant [e.g., the average daily human exposure] could protect against 0.5 mg carcinogen. This amount [of hydrocarbon carcinogen] probably exceeds the ordinary human consumption." It may therefore be suggested that the present exposure to these antioxidants may in fact be providing a significant amount of protection to the human population. While this extrapolation is useful for establishing a practical perspective, its degree of accuracy is totally unknown. In light of the consistency of the animal data summarized here, and the obvious importance of the topic for the public health, a strong epidemiologic effort should be initiated to validate the animal studies and begin to establish the role, if any, of the synthetic antioxidants in affecting human responses to chemical and physical carcinogens.

Before concluding this section it should be pointed out that several researchers have reported that BHT may also promote the occurrence of chemically induced cancers in controlled animals studies (Peraino et al., 1977; Weisburger et al., 1977; Witschi et al., 1977). For example, Witschi et al. (1977) have recently indicated that intraperitoneal injections of BHT after exposure to the carcinogen urethan enhanced tumorigenesis in mouse lung tissue. High doses of BHT stimulate a proliferation of type II alveolar cells and these cells are also the target tissue of urethan carcinogenesis. The doses needed to produce such cell growth in the mouse lung exceed the quantity consumed by humans by a factor of 1000 to 10,000. Incidentally, treatment with BHT alone at all concentrations employed was not carcinogenic. While these findings

Table 2. Effect of Antioxidants on BP-Induced Neoplasia of Forestomach of A/HeJ Mice

Experimental Diet		Num- ber of Mice	Diet Intake[a] (g/mouse/ day)	Body Weight (g)		Tumors of Forestomach		
Carcinogen (per g diet)	Antioxidant (per g diet)			At 9 Weeks[b]	At 21 Weeks[c]	Number of Mice with Tumors	Percentage of Mice with Tumors	Number of Tumors/Mouse[d]
BP, 1.0 mg	None	12	4.8	21	29	12	100	2.3 ± 0.25
BP, 1.0 mg	BHA, 5 mg	12	4.7	20	26	2	17[e]	0.2 ± 0.11[e]
BP, 1.0 mg	BHT, 5 mg	9	4.3	20	25	2	22[e]	0.3 ± 0.24[e]
None	None	12	4.8	20	29	0	0	0
None	BHA, 5 mg	12	4.8	21	28	0	0	0
None	BHT, 5 mg	10	4.1	20	28	0	0	0

[a]Diet intake during 2-week period of feeding experimental diets.

[b]Age of mice at start of experimental diets.

[c]Age of mice when killed.

[d]Mean ± SE.

[e]$P < 0.001$.

Source. Wattenberg, L.W. (1972). Inhibition of carcinogenic and toxic effects of polycyclic hydrocarbons by phenolic antioxidants and ethoxyquin. *J. Natl. Cancer Inst.* **48**:1428.

do not contradict nor should they diminish the potential significance of previously cited studies, they do infer the vast complexity of such interrelationships and our limited data base.

Addendum. King et al. (1977) have recently reported that BHT was effective in reducing the occurrence of DMBA induced mammary tumors in rats reared on high-fat diets. However, the degree of BHT protection was considerably greater for those rats reared on highly saturated as compared to highly polyunsaturated diets.

References

Black, H.S. (1974). Effects of dietary antioxidants on actinic tumor induction. *Res. Commun. Chem. Pathol. Pharmacol.* **7**(4):783–786.

Black, H.S. and Chan, J.T. (1975). Suppression of ultraviolet light-induced tumor formation by dietary antioxidants. *J. Invest. Dermatol.* **65**:412–414.

Brugh, M. (1977). Butylated hydroxytoluene protects chickens exposed to Newcastle disease virus. *Science* **197**:1291–1292.

Clapp, N.K. (1978). Interactions of ionizing radiation, nitrosamines, sulfononyalkanes and antioxidants as they affect carcinogenesis and survival in mice. *Amer. Ind. Hyg. Assoc. J.* **39**:448–453.

Clapp, N.K.; Klima, W.C.; and Satterfield, L.C. (1976). Dependent protection against diethylnitrosamine-induced squamous cell carcinomas of forestomach by concomitant administration of food additive, butylated hydroxytoluene. *Proc. Amer. Assoc. Cancer Res.* **17**:168.

Clapp, N.K.; Tyndall, R.L.; Cumming, R.B.; and Otten, J.A. (1974). Effects of butylated hydroxytoluene alone or with diethylnitrosamine in mice. *Food Cosmet. Toxicol.* **12**:367–371.

Collings, A.J. and Sharratt, M. (1970). The BHT content of human adipose tissue. *Fd. Cosmet. Toxicol.* **8**:409–412.

Creaven, P.J.; Davies, W.H.; and Williams, R.T. (1966). The effect of butylated hydroxytoluene, butylated hydroxyanisole and acetyl galate upon liver weight and biphenyl-4-hydroxylase activity in the rat. *J. Pharm. Pharmacol.* **18**:485–489.

Cumming, R.B. and Walton, M.F. (1973). Modification of the acute toxicity of mutagenic and carcinogenic chemicals in the mouse by prefeeding with antioxidants. *Food Cosmet. Toxicol.* **11**:547–553.

DeRios, G.; Chan, J.T.; Black, H.S.; Rudolph, A.H.; and Knox, J.M. (1978). Systemic protection by antioxidants against UVL-induced erythema. *J. Invest. Dermatol.* **70**:123–125.

Frankfurt, O.S.; Lipchina, L.P.; Bunto, T.V. et al. (1967). The influence of 4-methyl-2, 6-terbutylphenol (Ionol) on the development of hepatic tumors in rats. *Bull. Exp. Biol. Med.* **8**:86–88.

Gilbert, D.; Martin, A.D.; Gargolli, S.D.; Abraham, R.; and Goldberg, L. (1969). The effect of substituted phenols on liver weights and liver enzymes in the rat: structure-activity relationships. *Food Cosmet. Toxicol.* **7**:603–619.

Grantham, P.H.; Weisburger, J.H.; and Weisburger, E.K. (1973). Effect of the antioxidant butylated hydroxytoluene (BHT) on the metabolism of the carcinogens N-2-fluorenylacetamide and N-hydroxy-N-2-fluorenylacetamide. *Fd. Cosmet. Toxicol.* **11**:209–217.

Kahl, R. and Wulff, V. (1979). Induction of rat hepatic epoxide hydratase by dietary antioxidants. *Toxicol. Appl. Pharm.* **47**:217–227.

King, M.M.; Bailey, D.M.; Gibson, D.D.; Pitha, J.V.; and McCay, P.B. (1977). Effect of antioxidant in diets containing different types and amounts of fat on mammary tumor incidence induced by a single dose of 7,12-dimethylbenzanthracene. *Fed. Proc.* **36**:1148. Abst. No. 4635.

Martin, A.D. and Gilbert, D. (1968). Enzyme changes accompanying liver enlargement in rats treated with 3-tert-butyl-4-hydroxyanisole. *Biochem. J.* **106**:22.

Peraino, C.; Fry, R.J.M.; Staffeldt, E.; and Christopher, J.P. (1977). Enhancing effects of phenobarbital and butylated hydroxytoluene on 2-acetylaminofluorene-induced hepatic tumorigenesis in the rat. *Food Cosmet. Toxicol.* **15**:93–96.

Shamberger, R.J. (1970). Relationship of selenium to cancer. I. Inhibitory effect of selenium on carcinogenesis. *J. Natl. Cancer Inst.* **44**:931–936.

Shamberger, R.J.; Baughman, F.F.; Calchert, S.L.; Willis, C.E.; and Hoffman, G.E. (1973). Carcinogen-induced chromosomal breakage decreased by antioxidants. *Proc. Nat. Acad. Sci. USA* **70**(5):1401–1403.

Slaga, T.J. and Bracken, W.M. (1977). The effects of antioxidants on skin tumor initiation and aryl hydrocarbon hydroxylase. *Cancer Res.* **37**:1631–1635.

Speier, J.L. and Wattenberg, L.W. (1975). Alterations in microsomal metabolism of benzo[a]pyrene in mice fed butylated hydroxyanisole. *J. Natl. Cancer Inst.* **55**(2):469–472.

Ulland, B.M.; Weisburger, J.H.; Yamamoto, R.S.; and Weisburger, E.K. (1973). Antioxidants and carcinogenesis: butylated hydroxytoluene, but not diphenyl-p-phenylenediamine, inhibits cancer induction by N-2-fluorenylacetamide and by N-hydroxy-N-2-fluorenylacetamide in rats. *Fd. Cosmet. Toxicol.* **11**:199–207.

Wattenberg, L.W. (1966). Chemoprophylaxis of carcinogenesis: a review. *Cancer Res.* **26**:1520–1526.

Wattenberg, L.W. (1972). Inhibition of carcinogenic and toxic effects of polycyclic hydrocarbons by phenolic antioxidants and ethoxyquin. *J. Natl. Cancer Inst.* **48**:1425–1430.

Wattenberg, L.W. (1972a). Inhibition of carcinogenic effects of diethylnitrosamine and 4-nitroquinoline-N-oxide by antioxidants. *Fed. Proc.* **31**:633.

Wattenberg, L.W. (1973). Inhibition of chemical carcinogen-induced pulmonary neoplasia by butylated hydroxyanisole. *J. Natl. Cancer Inst.* **50**:1541–1544.

Wattenberg, L.W. (1974). Inhibition of carcinogenic and toxic effects of polycyclic hydrocarbons by several sulfur-containing compounds. *J. Natl. Cancer Inst.* **52**:1583–1587.

Wattenberg, L.W. (1975). Effects of dietary constituents on the metabolism of chemical carcinogens. *Cancer Res.* **35**:3326–3331.

Wattenberg, L.W. (1976). Inhibition of chemical carcinogenesis by antioxidants and some additional compounds. In: *Fundamentals of Cancer Prevention.* Edited by S. Takayama and T. Sugimura. Proc. 6th Intern. Symp. of the Princess Takamatsu Cancer Research Fund. Univ. Park, Baltimore.

Wattenberg, L.W. and Leong, J.L. (1965). Effect of phenothiazines on protective systems against polycyclic hydrocarbons. *Cancer Res.* **25**:365.

Weisburger, E.K.; Evarts, R.P.; and Wenk, M.L. (1977). Inhibitory effect of butylated hydroxytoluene (BHT) on intestinal carcinogenesis in rats by azoxymethane. *Food Cosmet. Toxicol.* **15**:139–141.

Witschi, H.; Williamson, D.; and Lock, S. (1977). Enlargement of urethan tumorigenesis in mouse lung by butylated hydroxytoluene. *J. Natl. Cancer Inst.* **58**:301–305.

Index

THE MEASUREMENT OF AIRBORNE PARTICLES
Richard D. Cadle

ANALYSIS OF AIR POLLUTANTS
Peter O. Warner

ENVIRONMENTAL INDICES
Herbert Inhaber

URBAN COSTS OF CLIMATE MODIFICATION
Terry A. Ferrar, Editor

CHEMICAL CONTROL OF INSECT BEHAVIOR: THEORY AND APPLICATION
H. H. Shorey and John J. McKelvey, Jr., Editors

MERCURY CONTAMINATION: A HUMAN TRAGEDY
Patricia A. D'Itri and Frank M. D'Itri

POLLUTANTS AND HIGH RISK GROUPS
Edward J. Calabrese

METHODOLOGICAL APPROACHES TO DERIVING ENVIRONMENTAL AND
OCCUPATIONAL HEALTH STANDARDS
Edward J. Calabrese

NUTRITION AND ENVIRONMENTAL HEALTH—Volume I: The Vitamins
Edward J. Calabrese

NUTRITION AND ENVIRONMENTAL HEALTH—Volume II: Minerals and Macronutrients
Edward J. Calabrese

SULFUR IN THE ENVIRONMENT, Parts I and II
Jerome O. Nriagu, Editor

COPPER IN THE ENVIRONMENT, Parts I and II
Jerome O. Nriagu, Editor

ZINC IN THE ENVIRONMENT, Parts I and II
Jerome O. Nriagu, Editor